Handbook of Behavioral Group Therapy

APPLIED CLINICAL PSYCHOLOGY

Series Editors:
Alan S. Bellack, *Medical College of Pennsylvania at EPPI, Philadelphia, Pennsylvania,*
and Michel Hersen, *University of Pittsburgh, Pittsburgh, Pennsylvania*

Recent Volumes in this Series

REHABILITATION OF THE BRAIN-DAMAGED ADULT
Gerald Goldstein and Leslie Ruthven

SOCIAL SKILLS ASSESSMENT AND TRAINING WITH CHILDREN
An Empirically Based Handbook
Larry Michelson, Don P. Sugai, Randy P. Wood, and Alan E. Kazdin

BEHAVIORAL ASSESSMENT AND REHABILITATION OF THE TRAUMATICALLY BRAIN DAMAGED
Edited by Barry A. Edelstein and Eugene T. Couture

COGNITIVE BEHAVIOR THERAPY WITH CHILDREN
Edited by Andrew W. Meyers and W. Edward Craighead

TREATING CHILD-ABUSIVE FAMILIES
Intervention Based on Skills Training Principles
Jeffrey A. Kelly

ISSUES IN PSYCHOTHERAPY RESEARCH
Edited by Michel Hersen, Larry Michelson, and Alan S. Bellack

SUBSTANCE ABUSE AND PSYCHOPATHOLOGY
Edited by Arthur I. Alterman

HANDBOOK OF BEHAVIORAL GROUP THERAPY
Edited by Dennis Upper and Steven M. Ross

forthcoming

RESEARCH METHODS IN APPLIED BEHAVIOR ANALYSIS
Issues and Advances
Edited by Alan Poling, R. Wayne Fuqua, and Roger Ulrich

SEVERE BEHAVIOR DISORDERS IN THE MENTALLY RETARDED
Nondrug Approaches to Treatment
Edited by Rowland P. Barrett

Handbook of Behavioral Group Therapy

EDITED BY

DENNIS UPPER

Lahey Clinic Medical Center
Burlington, Massachusetts
and Harvard Medical School
Boston, Massachusetts

AND

STEVEN M. ROSS

Veterans Administration Medical Center
and University of Utah School of Medicine
Salt Lake City, Utah

PLENUM PRESS • NEW YORK AND LONDON

Library of Congress Cataloging in Publication Data

Main entry under title:

Handbook of behavioral group therapy.

(Applied clinical psychology)
Includes bibliographies and index.
1. Behavior therapy. 2. Group psychotherapy. I. Upper, Dennis, 1942- . II. Ross, Steven M. III. Series. [DNLM: 1. Behavior Therapy. 2. Psychotherapy, Group. WM 425 H2358]
RC489.B4H349 1985 616.89′142 85-20496

DOI 10.1007/978-1-4684-4958-7

MyCopy version of the original edition 1985
A Division of Plenum Publishing Corporation
233 Spring Street, New York, N.Y. 10013

Contributors

DAVID O. ANTONUCCIO
Veterans Administration Medical Center, Reno, Nevada

BILLY A. BARRIOS
University of Mississippi, University, Mississippi

JEFFREY R. BEDELL
University of South Florida and Florida Mental Health Institute, Tampa, Florida

PERRY L. BELFER
Newton-Wellesley Hospital, Newton Lower Falls, Massachusetts and Harvard Medical School, Boston, Massachusetts

JAMES N. BRECKENRIDGE
Veterans Administration Medical Center, Palo Alto, California

JULIA STEINMETZ BRECKENRIDGE
Veterans Administration Medical Center, Palo Alto, California

NANCY B. COHN
Veterans Administration Medical Center, Salt Lake City, Utah

GERARD J. CONNORS
University of Texas Medical School at Houston, Houston, Texas

PAUL M. G. EMMELKAMP
Academic Hospital, Groningen, Netherlands

JOHN V. FLOWERS
Chapman College, Orange, California

DOLORES E. GALLAGHER
Veterans Administration Medical Center, Palo Alto, California

BRUCE S. GOTTLIEB
Pain Management and Behavioral Medicine Center, Farmington, Connecticut

J. STEPHEN HAZEL
University of Kansas, Lawrence, Kansas

STEVEN H. JENSEN
Private practice, 1225 N. W. Murray Road, Suite 215, Portland, Oregon

LYLE E. KANTOR
Department of Behavioral Medicine and Psychiatry, Lahey Clinic Medical Center, Burlington, Massachusetts

DAVID J. KOLKO
Western Psychiatric Institute and Clinic and University of Pittsburgh School of Medicine, Pittsburgh, Pennsylvania

ANTOINETTE C. M. KUIPERS
Psychiatric Hospital "Lichten Kracht," Assen, Netherlands

RONALD J. KULICH
Lahey Clinic Medical Center, Burlington, Massachusetts

CRAIG W. LECROY
Arizona State University, Tempe, Arizona

PHILIP LEVENDUSKY
McLean Hospital, Belmont, Massachusetts and Harvard Medical School, Boston, Massachusetts

PETER M. LEWINSOHN
University of Oregon, Eugene, Oregon

STEPHEN A. MAISTO
Veterans Administration Medical Center, Providence, Rhode Island

NEAL H. MAYERSON
Behavioral Medicine Associates, Salt Lake City, Utah

KEVIN B. MCGOVERN
Private practice, 1225 N. W. Murray Road, Suite 214, Portland, Oregon

DIANN DEE MICHAEL
University of South Florida and Florida Mental Health Institute, Tampa, Florida

PETER M. MONTI
Brown University and Veterans Administration Medical Center, Providence, Rhode Island

SHELDON D. ROSE
University of Wisconsin, Madison, Wisconsin

STEVEN M. ROSS
Veterans Administration Medical Center and University of Utah School of Medicine, Salt Lake City, Utah

JEAN BRAGG SCHUMAKER
University of Kansas, Lawrence, Kansas

BERNARD SCHWARTZ
Santa Ana College, Santa Ana, California

JAN SHELDON
University of Kansas, Lawrence Kansas

JAMES A. SHERMAN
University of Kansas, Lawrence, Kansas

LINDA C. SOBELL
Addiction Research Foundation and University of Toronto, Toronto, Ontario, Canada

MARK B. SOBELL
Addiction Research Foundation and University of Toronto, Toronto, Ontario, Canada

MARTIN SUNDEL
Graduate School of Social Work, The University of Texas at Arlington, Arlington, Texas

SANDRA STONE SUNDEL
Private practice, Arlington, Texas

LINDA TERI
University of Washington, Seattle, Washington

LARRY W. THOMPSON
Veterans Administration Medical Center, Palo Alto, California

REX W. TURNER
Veterans Administration Medical Center, Salt Lake City, Utah

Preface

In 1977, the current editors contributed a review article on behavioral group therapy to a volume of Hersen, Miller, and Eisler's *Progress in Behavior Modification* series (1977). At that time we noted that, despite the advantages to both clinicians and clients of conducting behavioral treatments in groups, clinical developments and research in this area were still at a relatively rudimentary level. The majority of studies in the behavioral group therapy literature we reviewed reported the direct transfer of an individual behavior therapy procedure, such as systematic desensitization, to a group of clients with homogeneous problems, such as snake phobia or test anxiety. Groups were used in many studies merely to generate sufficient numbers of subjects to allow various types of interventions to be compared, rather than to examine group process variables *per se*. Only a limited amount of attention had been given to whether these group interaction variables (such as group discussion, sharing ideas and feelings, and mutual feedback and reinforcement) might enhance individually oriented procedures applied in a group.

The 8 years since this original chapter was written have seen a significant growth in both the breadth and depth of clinical research and work in the behavioral group therapy field. This growth was documented in part in a three-volume series on behavioral group therapy by the current editors (Upper & Ross, 1979, 1980, 1981). Although each of these books focused on some aspects of behavioral group therapy (e.g., descriptions of institutional programs, group therapy with court-adjudicated clients), none attempted to provide a state-of-the-art overview of the field, as this present handbook does.

In designing this handbook, we endeavored to present chapters that cover the most significant issues, clinical populations, and problems being addressed by behavioral group therapists and that were written by experienced and knowledgeable clinicians and researchers in this field. Chapter authors were asked to review and critique the relevant literature in the area being discussed, to describe and discuss their own behavioral group therapy work, and to speculate upon the directions of future developments. They especially were encouraged to provide detailed descriptions of intervention procedures, to make liberal use of clinical case or group examples, and to offer specific suggestions for dealing with potential problems or pitfalls.

This handbook is intended to address both theoretical issues, such as whether behavioral group approaches will allow us to better understand group psychotherapy as a lawful and predictable process, and practical ones, such as how we can better match behavioral group interventions to the clinical populations and problematic behaviors being addressed. It is intended not only to provide clinicians, researchers, and students "state-of-the-art" information about a broad variety of behavioral group approaches, but also to raise interesting questions and to identify promising areas for future research as well.

DENNIS UPPER
STEVEN M. ROSS

REFERENCES

Upper, D., & Ross, S. M. Behavioral group therapy: 1. Emotional, avoidance, and social skills problems of adults. In M. Hersen, R. M. Eisler, & P. M. Miller (Eds.), *Progress in behavior modification* (Vol. 5). New York: Academic Press, 1977.

Upper, D., & Ross, S. M. (Eds.), *Behavioral group therapy, 1979: An annual review*. Champaign, Ill.: Research Press, 1979.

Upper, D., & Ross, S. M. (Eds.), *Behavioral group therapy, 1980: An annual review*. Champaign, Ill.: Research Press, 1980.

Upper, D., & Ross, S. M. (Eds.), *Behavioral group therapy, 1981: An annual review*. Champaign, Ill.: Research Press, 1981.

Contents

I

Procedural and Process Issues

Part I is composed of six chapters that address a number of important methodological issues pertaining to the implementation and evaluation of behavioral group therapy programs in applied settings. Among these are the relationship of the intervention model used to the clinical procedures employed, the cost-effectiveness of the interventions, the training and evaluation of behavioral group therapists, and potential improvements in the delivery of therapeutic services.

In Chapter 1, Sundel and Sundel present a model for planning, conducting, and evaluating time-limited behavioral group treatment. Significant features of their model are its focus on individual goal identification and attainment, on the development of a group problem-solving framework, and on programming enhanced generalization of newly acquired skills from the group to the natural environment. The detailed discussion of how to "troubleshoot" typical problems encountered in behavioral groups (e.g., noncompletion of assignments, problem switching) should prove particularly useful to behavioral group therapists, just as the description of the specific elements of a therapist training program should be of special interest to trainers.

Monti and Kolko, in Chapter 2, review the clinical and research literature on individual and group social skills training and present a detailed model for social skills training in an outpatient psychiatric setting. A notable feature of the research reported here is the use of one consistent evaluative measure (the Social Skills Intake Interview) across a number of treatment outcome studies, which permits more detailed and enlightening cross-study comparisons. Also of note are the authors' suggestions concerning the need to lengthen follow-up intervals and the value of involving family members in social skills training programs.

In Chapter 3, Cohn and Mayerson summarize the research on procedures for preparing patients for psychotherapy and discuss the goals of pretherapy training for both individual and group therapy. The authors' advocacy of using pretraining procedures aimed at specific, measurable ingroup verbal behaviors and their specific suggestions regarding pretraining for behavioral group therapy are of special note.

In Chapter 4, Bedell and Michael discuss the theoretical bases of a psychoeducational problem-solving skills training program and describe in detail the use of such a program with chronic mental patients. Of particular interest to clinicians should be the many examples of detailed program materials and the liberal inclusion of case examples to illustrate the application of this model to treatment.

Belfer and Levendusky, in Chapter 5, propose an integrated model of long-term, process-oriented behavioral group therapy. Among the variables that are seen as being of particular importance to this integrated model are the style of group leadership, the group contract, choice and development of group norms, and the stages of group development over time.

In Chapter 6, Flowers and Schwartz present a behavioral theory and methodology for applying a varied set of behavioral techniques with a group of patients with heterogeneous problems. The authors break down behavioral group therapy into the specific processes of disclosure, assessment, narrowing or focusing, intervention, and feedback, and they provide a detailed and clinically relevant discussion of each.

1

Behavior Modification in Groups

A Time-Limited Model for Assessment, Planning, Intervention, and Evaluation

MARTIN SUNDEL AND SANDRA STONE SUNDEL

The past decade has witnessed considerable growth in the research and application of behavior modification approaches to groups (Lawrence & Sundel, 1972, 1975; Lawrence & Walter, 1978; Rose, 1972, 1977, 1980; Sundel & Lawrence, 1970, 1974, 1977; Upper & Ross, 1979, 1980, 1981). Mental health professionals have become increasingly interested in the application of behavioral principles and techniques to group settings. The high cost of delivering individual services and the increased emphasis on brief therapies (Budman, 1981) have contributed to this favorable climate, especially for group treatment offered on a short-term or time-limited basis.

The purpose of this chapter is to present a time-limited model of behavioral group treatment and describe its applications to various problems and settings. The main features of the model are reviewed, emphasizing the assessment, planning, intervention, and evaluation components. Various aspects of this model have been described elsewhere (Lawrence & Sundel, 1972; Lawrence & Walter, 1978; Sundel & Lawrence, 1970, 1974, 1977; Sundel & Sundel, 1985).

A hallmark of behavior therapy has been its brevity in contrast to traditional psychodynamic approaches. Brief behavior therapy programs of up to 25 weekly sessions are frequently reported in the literature (e.g., Miller, 1980; Wilson, 1981; Sobell & Sobell, 1978). An upper limit of 25 weekly sessions has been reported for behavioral treatment groups and training groups, with the most frequent range being between 10 and 18 sessions (Rose, 1977). More intensive treatment programs meeting more frequently during the initial weeks or days have been suggested for weight loss groups (Rose, 1977).

MARTIN SUNDEL • Graduate School of Social Work, The University of Texas at Arlington, Arlington, Texas 76019. SANDRA STONE SUNDEL • Private practice, Arlington, Texas 76011.

Overview of Model

The model of group work presented in this chapter combines behavior modification principles and small-group theory to treat client problems. A significant feature of the model is its emphasis on individual goal attainment. The objective is to change the behavior of each member outside the group where the problem occurs. The therapist establishes group-functioning goals to optimize appropriate participation of group members. Group-functioning objectives such as cohesiveness or cooperation are established to help participants achieve their goals rather than as ends in themselves. These group process objectives are secondary, although they are necessary to the pursuit of individual goals. The behaviors that constitute appropriate participation of a group member are specified at the start of the group. Group members are expected to perform certain behaviors that contribute to optimum group functioning while they work on their own goals.

This treatment approach structures group sessions in order to achieve the following client objectives and group participation conditions:

1. *Treatment norms are established within the group:*

a. Members are expected to attend every session.

Group members are told that they are expected to attend every session as a condition of treatment. Attendance at every session is crucial to fulfilling the tasks required at each stage of the problem-solving process. Members learn through didactic material as well as through personal and observational training, and each session builds on the knowledge and skills developed in the previous sessions. As part of role induction (Lennard & Bernstein, 1970), members are told that attendance demonstrates a commitment to change that is a prerequisite to goal attainment.

b. Group discussions related to clients' problems are considered confidential within the group.

Confidentiality within the group is a central ethical issue related to group treatment (Corey, 1981). The therapist instructs group members to refrain from discussing members' problems outside of the group.

c. Socializing among members outside of meetings is discouraged.

Members are told to refrain from socializing with other group members outside of meetings for the duration of the group. The purpose of this rule is to prevent personal relationships from developing among members based on their shared experiences in the group. Discussing group meetings outside the group could create cliques or alliances that detract from objective participation in the group. In some groups, however, this rule might be waived, for example, in order to allow group members to assist each other in developing social skills.

d. Discussion of members' problems focuses on current events and observable data.

The focus of behavioral treatment is on present conditions rather than interpretation of early experiences. The behavioral approach involves systematic observation and recording of target behaviors. This may involve self-monitoring as well as monitoring the behavior of others.

e. Members are required to perform assignments outside the group.

Performance of behavioral assignments structures activities between group sessions and gives clients practice in performing desired behaviors in the natural environment.

Enforcement of group norms. The previously mentioned treatment norms are provided as guidelines for optimal functioning of the group within this treatment model. Although the therapist can enforce these norms unilaterally, pressure for compliance can be exerted by group members. In addition, the therapist tries to arrange conditions in which there is a strong commitment by each member to adhere to group norms by (a) engaging members in problem-solving activities that require member interaction to achieve individual goals (e.g., role plays, discussions) and (b) providing social reinforcement, along with other group members, for performance of desired behaviors.

2. *Members prioritize their problems.* The following criteria are used to help clients prioritize their problems and select one for immediate attention:

a. The problem of immediate concern to the client and/or significant others (for example, family, friends, employer)
b. The problem that has severe aversive or negative consequences for the client, significant others, or society if not handled immediately
c. The problem that can be corrected most quickly, considering resources and obstacles
d. The problem that requires handling before other problems can be treated (Sundel & Sundel, 1982)

3. *Members help each other in the assessment of their problems and in establishing behavioral change goals.* Members apply their knowledge of behavioral concepts, learned in the group, to the analysis of each individual's problems. Vague, general statements made by a client are followed by requests for specification of target responses, antecedents and, consequences. Client data obtained outside the group are examined in terms of measures of response strength and controlling conditions. If an individual has difficulty identifying target behaviors and controlling conditions, role plays are devised by the therapist in which group members assume the roles of the client or significant others.

After the client collects and presents desired assessment data, the group helps the client establish behavioral change goals. Various desirable behaviors and supporting environmental conditions are suggested and discussed. Successful experiences of particular group members in similar circumstances can be used in formulating appropriate responses.

4. *Members contribute suggestions for change and solutions to each other's problems.* An intervention plan is developed with each client based on the goals that are established. The therapist encourages group members to offer suggestions for resolving each other's problems. This input from group members expands the range of interventions available to the clients. Clients may also be more amenable to acting on these suggestions because they are supported by other members of the group.

5. *Members participate actively in role playing and educational procedures designed to teach problem-solving skills.* After intervention plans are established for the clients, role plays are devised to provide opportunities for them to practice

desired behaviors in the group. Subgroups of 2 to 4 individuals may be formed to allow clients to practice desired behaviors in role plays while the therapist and other members provide prompting, corrective feedback, and social reinforcement. For example, a client can learn assertive behaviors by roleplaying increasingly difficult situations in which he or she is required to be assertive. A client can learn how to remain calm and relaxed in stressful situations by roleplaying difficult situations in which he or she remains relaxed.

An educational component is included in this model to help group members efficiently work on problems during the course of group treatment and to help members apply this knowledge to new problems that may arise after the group terminates. The therapist teaches assessment concepts to group members that show how a problem can be broken down into parts that are functionally related to each other. The concepts of reinforcement, extinction, and punishment are used to illustrate conditions influencing the performance of desired and undesired behaviors. A variety of examples are drawn from the group members' experiences to facilitate the learning of these concepts.

6. *Members provide social reinforcement and constructive feedback to each other.* The therapist shows group members how to provide social reinforcement in the form of praise, recognition, and encouragement for complying with group norms, actively participating in problem-solving activities, performing behavioral assignments outside the group, and reporting their data. Social reinforcement is also given for member participation in role plays and offering suggestions for appropriate behaviors. Constructive feedback is given by group members in the form of pinpointing behaviors that were performed appropriately as well as providing suggestions for improvement. This feedback is based on observations of the individual's behaviors in role plays and the consequences they produce. Members are told to refrain from negative evaluations of the individual, accusations, or verbal attacks. The therapist serves as a model for providing social reinforcement and constructive feedback to members throughout the course of the group.

Group Problem-Solving Framework

The model is based on a treatment-planning cycle that has the following components: assessment, planning, intervention, and evaluation. This logical, problem-solving framework requires systematically working through each phase of the cycle for each problem while managing the group process (Sundel, Glasser, Sarri, & Vinter, 1985). The model presented here is for an 8-week treatment program. The time limit of 8 weeks was established based on the therapist's experience of the time required to teach group participants basic problem-solving concepts for assessing and treating their problems and evaluating the outcomes. The number of sessions can be varied, however, according to the characteristics of particular groups, such as size of group, length of sessions, number of therapists, and similarity of problems.

Treatment groups have typically consisted of five to seven individuals. The groups have been composed of men and women ranging in age from 20 to 54. They have been predominantly middle- and lower-middle-income individuals seen in public and private agency settings. Client problems treated in this type of group have included job stress, marital discord, child management, depression, self-control, anxiety, and interpersonal difficulties with friends, family, work associates, and superiors. The clients had no previous psychiatric history, although many had sought help for their problems from other agencies and therapists. The groups typically were heterogeneous with regard to presenting problem, sex, and age. Once the group had been formed, no new members were accepted. The groups met for 2½ hours once a week for 8 weeks and were led by co-therapists. Other groups using this model, however, have been conducted by a single therapist.

Assessment

Intake

Prospective group members are interviewed individually by one of the therapists to identify problems that are appropriate for short-term group treatment. The time limitation necessitates careful selection of individuals who have problems amenable to resolution within an 8-week course of treatment.

Individuals are often referred for group treatment because of problems in interpersonal functioning. The advantages of working on social skills in groups include (a) the opportunity to view more than one model demonstrate appropriate behaviors; (b) the availability of corrective feedback for practicing these skills from more than one person; and (c) opportunities for reinforcement for appropriate performance from more than one person. Advantages of group over individual treatment have been discussed (e.g., Upper & Ross, 1977).

Two basic criteria used for client selection were (a) Will the client contribute to problem-solving activities in the group? and (b) Will the client interact appropriately with group members? Candidates suitable for short-term group treatment included individuals who could talk about their problems, who agreed to adhere to the proposed group norms, and who agreed to help others solve their problems as well as work on solving their own. Individuals with severe behavioral disorders, such as avoidance of social contact, or individuals who are suicidal or who exhibit extremely hostile or aggressive behaviors are less suitable candidates for this type of short-term group treatment (Corey, 1981; Lazarus, 1971, 1976). Their problems are more appropriately treated in individual sessions.

During the intake session, the therapist discussed the norms of the group, and the prospective member agreed to follow the rules governing the group's operation. Clients were told that if they followed the prescribed procedures, it was likely that they could achieve their goals within the period of group treatment. The short-term program established the expectation that behavioral change goals could be accomplished in that length of time. The limited time frame made it necessary for clients and therapists to organize their group time and to work on problem-solving activities between group sessions.

The therapist's objectives for intake were to obtain (a) a verbal agreement to follow the rules for group participation; (b) a statement from the client of his or her willingness to participate in group treatment; (c) a behaviorally specific description of the client's problem(s); and (d) a statement of the client's goals for treatment.

The following six procedures were used by the therapists to achieve the preceding objectives.

Procedure 1. Orientation to the Initial Interview. Prior to the intake interview, each prospective group member completed a problem checklist (Sundel & Lawrence, 1974, pp. 341–342). The checklist was used to identify relationship problems. The client was asked to indicate the relationship that was of most concern and to describe the problem and what was desired in the way of change. By examining the client's checklist, the therapist determined what to focus on in the interview. In addition, the form helped to structure the way in which the client presented the problem.

Procedure 2. Establishment of an Initial Treatment Contract. The initial treatment contract consisted of the therapist's statement of the requirements for group membership (treatment norms) and the client's verbal agreement to comply with these conditions. During the contract discussion, the therapist answered the client's questions and explained the rationale for the procedures that would be used during treatment. The conditions of the verbal contracts made with each client were discussed and reconfirmed during the first group meeting.

Procedure 3. Role Induction. Teaching a client who comes for group treatment how to behave as a group member and what to expect from the therapist and other group members is necessary to prepare him or her to assume a particular role in the group. Role induction in psychotherapy has been discussed as an orderly social process requiring certain complementarity of behaviors and expectations (Lennard & Bernstein, 1970).

Several expectations for the behavior of group members were established during the intake interview.

1. The problem selected for treatment was expected to improve during the course of the group.
2. The client was expected to comply with the norms stated by the therapist for group participation: members were expected to attend every session; group discussions of client problems were confidential; socializing outside the group was discouraged; focus of group discussions of client problems was on current events and observable data; and members were expected to perform assignments outside of the group.
3. The client was expected to actively participate in problem solving with regard to both his or her own problem and in assisting other group members.
4. The client was expected to acquire knowledge and skill in behavior modification concepts, recording and measurement and to apply this knowledge and skill in problem solving.

Procedure 4. Description of Problems in Behaviorally Specific Terms. Clients frequently describe their problems in vague statements (for example, "My life is all messed up"). In addition, they often make assumptions about what caused their problems (for example, "If only I were more attractive, I wouldn't be lonely"); or how they could be solved (for example, "The only way to solve our family problems is to send our son away to school"). To avoid choosing interventions on the basis of faulty assumptions, the therapist asked the client to specify the problem within the context of the person and circumstances involved. For example, "When my supervisor criticizes my work unfairly, I remain silent or apologize"; "When I say 'no' to my son, he runs into his room and slams the door."

The therapist then asked the client to give two or more recent examples of each problem. If these examples were inconsistent with the client's statement of the problem, the statement was revised to accurately depict the problem.

Procedure 5. Identification of Problems to Work on in the Group. During the initial interview, the therapist discussed each problem area with the client and encouraged him or her to bring up any others that might exist. The client and therapist then narrowed down this list of problems to a few that would be appropriate to work on in the group. Criteria for establishing problem priorities were reviewed with the client.

Procedure 6. Discussion of Treatment Goals. The discussion of goals included what the client could reasonably expect to achieve in group treatment and the client's statement of the behaviors he or she wanted to alter.

Although behavioral specificity was attempted during intake, goals could not be formulated completely until the more detailed process of behavioral assessment took place during group meetings. The following example illustrates a tentative statement of a goal:

PROBLEM: When my supervisor criticizes my work unfairly, I remain silent or apologize.
REASONABLE GOAL: When my supervisor criticizes my work unfairly, I will state my disagreement in a clear voice.

RAC-S

In order to learn effective problem-solving skills, group members are taught a method for assessing problem behaviors (Lawrence & Sundel, 1972). This method, referred to as RAC-S (Sundel & Sundel, 1982), includes the following components: (a) response; (b) antecedents; (c) consequences; and (d) strength. The specification of these four elements is required of each member during the assessment phase. Assessment objectives, therefore, require each member to provide (a) a clear definition of the problem indicating undesired responses, their antecedents, and consequences; and (b) measures of the strength of the problem behaviors, using response rate or duration data.

For example, John complained that his wife did not understand him. The therapists and group members asked him to describe a typical incident between him and his wife and indicate what each of them said and did. Based on his examples, the group helped John identify his undesired responses (R), their antecedents (A), and consequences (C).

One of John's problematic responses was that he continued to read the newspaper (R) when his wife asked him how his day had gone (A). As a result, she screamed at him (C) until he put the newspaper down. John was given an assignment to record the number and duration of such incidents during the next week (S).

Behavioral reenactment is a role-playing technique used to obtain RAC-S information regarding a client's behaviors in the problematic situation by observing the client roleplay an incident that simulates the problem (Sundel & Lawrence, 1974). This technique is effective in a group setting because it can help the group pinpoint discrepancies between a client's description of the behavior and what is actually observed in the role play. For example, a behavioral reenactment of John's problematic situation revealed that he kept his head down and eyes focused on the newspaper when his wife asked him questions about work. There was a scowl on his face, and when he finally put the paper down, he threw it on the floor. John's previous description failed to identify these behaviors. Behavioral reenactment can help the therapists and group members identify problematic behavioral chains in which a stimulus that serves as a reinforcer for one response also acts as a discriminative stimulus (S^D) for the next response. By observing individuals in the role play, the group can specify the stimuli and responses in the chain that require modification. For example, John's scowling (R) was followed by his wife's screaming, which served both as a reinforcer (C) for his scowling and an S^D for throwing the paper down.

Planning and Intervention

After RAC-S assessment data are collected, individual goals are formulated with each member. Group members contribute to the goal statements of other members based on their RAC-S data as well as on observations of an individual's interactions in the group and in behavioral reenactments. Although a goal might be stated initially in broad terms, it is delineated into specific components including desired responses (R), antecedents (A), and consequences (C).

For example, John's goal stated that when his wife asked him questions about his work (A), he would put down the newspaper, look at her, and answer her questions (R). The potential positive consequences would be avoiding arguments and having pleasant conversations (C). This scenario should occur in the evenings when John comes home from work and sits down to read the paper (A). An alternative goal might be for John to ask his wife to allow him 20 minutes to read the newspaper in silence (R) after which they would have a pleasant conversation (C).

After desired behaviors are specified in treatment goals, each group member is given instructions on how to perform them. Members practice these behaviors in the group, with feedback from the therapists and other group members. Instructions, prompting, and cueing are provided to help shape appropriate behaviors. Behavioral rehearsals allow group members to practice desired behaviors in a controlled environment until they are ready to perform them in the natural environment.

A major advantage of the group is the availability of individuals who can serve as models in performing desired behaviors. Multiple models provide diverse examples of how desired behaviors can be performed and allow the group member to imitate the model that is most acceptable. Another advantage is that group members provide reinforcement to each other for appropriate behaviors. This can be more effective than if only the therapists were providing the reinforcement. The therapists serve as role models for group members by modeling desired behaviors as well as by demonstrating how to provide instructions, cues, and positive reinforcement.

After members have demonstrated desired behaviors in the group, they are assigned to perform them in their natural environment. The behavioral assignments involve tasks to be performed by the client outside the group setting between sessions. They are used to provide continuity between the group setting and the natural environment. They also help structure the time between group sessions so that members can continue to work toward their treatment goals.

A distinctive feature of this behavioral group model is the explicit, systematic treatment-planning framework that involves specifying the objectives and tasks to be accomplished during the group meetings. In order to pursue group maintenance and treatment goals, the therapists prepare objectives prior to each meeting. A session-by-session plan specifies what is to be accomplished during meetings, including behaviors each member is expected to perform and interventions that could be used to achieve these objectives. This plan is revised on the basis of weekly evaluations of the group's progress. Session plans are sufficiently flexible to allow the therapists to respond spontaneously to unexpected events.

The 8-week group treatment model was designed to implement individual treatment programs for clients. The eight sessions were carefully designed to include the following four methods:

1. *Development of group norms.* The therapists establish rules for participation and model appropriate behavioral techniques to foster protreatment behaviors in the group.

2. *Education.* The therapists teach basic principles of behavioral assessment and modification to participants and teach them how to apply these principles to their individual problems and circumstances.

3. *Problem solving.* The therapists lead the group in systematically assessing the problems of each member, formulating relevant goals, prescribing viable solutions, monitoring progress, and evaluating outcomes of interventions.

4. *Behavioral training and practice.* The therapists teach group members how to perform desired behaviors using modeling, prompting, shaping, behavioral rehearsal, corrective feedback, and reinforcement. Clients practice these behaviors in the group before trying them out in the natural environments. Group members also participate in behavioral training by serving as models and significant others in role plays, providing corrective feedback, and suggesting alternative behaviors. The group provides a controlled environment in which to improve performance of desired behaviors. If clients cannot demonstrate mas-

tery of desired behaviors in the group, they probably will have difficulty performing these behaviors in their natural environment.

Planning for Group Meetings

In treatment groups, co-therapists have certain advantages over a single therapist. While one therapist assumes the active role, the other attends to the nonverbal behaviors of group members and manages the group process. The therapists switch roles periodically so that each one has a chance to observe and manage the group process. The leader who is observing analyzes interactions among members and instigates changes to affect the group's functioning or problem-solving activities. If the therapist who is the active leader misses an important statement or nonverbal behavior, the other therapist can pick up on it. Other benefits of co-leadership are that group members have two professional role models in addition to the other group members, another professional's perspective on their problems, and an additional source of reinforcement. Because of the intensity of the 2½-hour sessions and the detailed information covered in each session, the presence of compatible co-therapists can keep the group focused on productive activities. In describing his model of behavioral group therapy, Flowers (1979) indicated that two leaders were required.

In order for the leaders to coordinate their efforts, they plan an agenda before group meetings and analyze the results of each meeting. The planning sessions involve discussions of each member's progress both as a group member and as a problem solver. Objectives for each group meeting are established. The activities and roles of each therapist are specified, including which therapist will begin the session, the kinds of role plays the co-therapists will structure, and the behaviors or techniques they will model and reinforce. In discussing each member's progress and participation in the group, the co-therapists also plan intervention strategies for modifying member behaviors that impede inidividual or group functioning.

Co-therapists typically establish operating rules that govern their behavior in group sessions. These rules include procedures for handling differences of opinion between co-therapists during group meetings, structuring role plays and assignments, and making educational presentations.

The first two group sessions focus on problem identification and assessment of individual behaviors, establishment of problem-solving norms in the group, and presentation of basic principles of behavioral analysis. During sessions 3 and 4, behavioral assessments are completed for all members. Intervention plans are established and implemented for individuals whose assessments were completed in previous sessions. Sessions 5 through 7 focus on behavioral training, and assignments are given for members to implement desired behaviors in their natural environment. Session 8 is devoted to evaluating clients' achievements in regard to goal attainment and to scheduling follow-up meetings.

Some typical objectives for the sessions are given next.

Session 1: objectives: (a) each member states his or her problem in behavioral terms and gives examples specifying undesired behaviors; (b) each member identifies an undesired behavior to observe and count during the next week; and (c) each member participates in determining problem priorities for other members.

The procedures established to achieve these objectives include

1. *Orientation:* Members are introduced to each other, the group's purpose is explained, and a description of the treatment approach is given. The rules for group participation are discussed.

2. *Educational:* The concept of response is taught. The therapists teach group members the technique of specifying responses by demonstrating how to convert vague descriptions into observable, measurable statements. Role plays are conducted to give members an opportunity to acquire and practice this skill.

3. *Confirmation or redefinition of client problems:* Members verify or revise their problem statements.

4. *Group tasks:* The therapists and group discuss with each member the problem selected for treatment. Each member affirms his or her willingness to comply with the group norms stated by the therapists. The therapists model and reinforce appropriate participation.

5. *Assignment:* Members are assigned to observe and record the frequency of their problem behaviors on a data sheet and to report the results to the group. Table 1 is a sample data sheet filled in by a client and brought to the group.

The therapists structure the first session to establish the clients' expectations for participation in the group. Group members are shown how to assume an active role in analyzing their problems as well as in helping other individuals to solve problems.

Session 2: Objectives: (a) each member reports data from the recording assignment; (b) each member identifies target responses, their controling antecedents and consequences, and measures of response strength; and (c) each member asks questions, participates in role plays or provides social reinforcement to other group members.

The procedures established to achieve these objectives include

1. *Data gathering:* Members present measures of their target responses that

TABLE 1. Sample Data Sheet

		Response strength	
Days	Description of problematic response	Frequency	Duration
Sun.	Reading newspaper at dinner table	1	10 min.
Mon.	Reading newspaper at dinner table	1	20 min.
Tues.		0	
Wed.	Reading newspaper at dinner table	1	10 min.
Thurs.		0	
Fri.	Reading newspaper at dinner table	1	5 min.
Sat.	Reading newspaper at dinner table	1	15 min.
		TOTAL: 5 times/week; average 12 min.	

they recorded since the last meeting. The data-gathering procedures and experiences of members are discussed. If clients had difficulty in carrying out the assignment, the therapists and group analyze the difficulty and demonstrate correct procedures.

2. *Educational:* The therapists teach the RAC-S behavioral assessment framework (Sundel & Sundel, 1982), giving various examples that illustrate its application. The concept of positive reinforcement, particularly its effect in maintaining target behaviors, is also taught.

3. *Group Tasks:* The therapists and group provide social reinforcement to members for completing assignments. Members discuss difficulties encountered in identifying and specifying target behaviors and in observing and recording them. Members participate in role plays that reenact reported incidents in order to allow the group to observe typical problematic behaviors.

4. *Assignment:* Members are assigned to record target behaviors and their frequency of occurrence, describe relevant antecedents and consequences, and report the results to the group. Table 2 shows sample data from a behavioral recording chart filled in by a client and brought to the group.

Sessions 3 and 4: Objectives: (a) each member reports data from the assignments; (b) each member presents examples of target responses, their strength (frequency and duration data), and controlling conditions; (c) each member specifies a behavioral change goal and identifies examples of positive and negative reinforcement contingencies from his or her data; and (d) each member participates in prescribing intervention strategies for members who have provided sufficient assessment data.

Procedures are as follows:

TABLE 2. Sample of Behavioral Recording Chart

Response to be observed: Reading newspaper at dinner table			
Day and time	Response strength (How often? For how long?)	Antecedent (What happened just before?)	Consequences (What happened just after?)
Monday			
Morning	—	—	—
Afternoon	—	—	—
Evening	10 minutes	Seated at table with wife	Wife yelled, "Put that paper down."
Tuesday			
Morning	—	—	—
Afternoon	—	—	—
Evening	15 minutes	Seated at table with wife	Wife complained about lack of conversation.

1. *Data gathering:* Members discuss the data they recorded regarding target responses and their strength, and relevant antecedents and consequences. If members experience difficulty, additional instructions are given until they demonstrate mastery of the recording assignments.

2. *Educational:* The therapists teach members how to formulate goals based on RAC-S data. Positive and negative reinforcement contingencies are examined in relation to their effects in maintaining target behaviors.

3. *Behavioral training and practice:* In role plays, members demonstrate the behaviors they have agreed to perform in the natural environment. Appropriate behaviors are shaped in the group setting based on feedback from the therapists and group members. This feedback is used by members in refining the behaviors to be performed outside the group.

4. *Group tasks:* The therapists and group provide social reinforcement to members for completing assignments. The group examines the assessment data available for each member to determine conditions that maintain target behaviors.

> For example, Thomas rarely completed his class assignments before 2 A.M. His data indicated that he engaged in highly reinforcing behaviors early in the evening that were incompatible with studying—removing his shoes, sitting down with the newspaper and turning on the television.

After assessment is completed and a treatment goal is formulated in behaviorally specific terms, the group develops an intervention strategy to achieve the goal.

> For example, in order to increase "studying between 6 and 10 P.M.," Thomas was instructed to leave his shoes on when he came home from school in the afternoon. He was to take a snack as he sat down with his assignments. Thomas was told to study for 30-minute intervals, after which he could read the newspaper for 5-minute intervals.

5. *Assignments:* Continue recording RAC-S data; carry out behavioral assignments given by the therapists and group.

Sessions 5–7: Objectives: (a) each member reports data from the assignments; (b) each member evaluates progress towards goal attainment; (c) each member performs behavioral tasks and assignments designed to achieve his or her goals; and (d) group members participate in role plays and give each other feedback on their performances.

Procedures are as follows:

1. *Data gathering:* An evaluation form is distributed to group members who are asked to complete it. The form includes a description of problems worked on in the group and instructs members to rate the extent to which their goals were achieved. Each member presents evaluative data indicating his or her progress, including examples of modified behaviors and conditions.

2. *Behavioral training and practice:* Group members perform tasks in the group that are directed toward goal achievement, including participation in role-play techniques such as behavioral rehearsal, modeling, and role reversal. In addition, members are given assignments to perform the appropriate behaviors rehearsed in the group in their natural environment.

3. *Group tasks:* Members provide feedback to each other in role plays, offer

suggestions, serve as role models, provide reinforcement to each other for completing tasks and assignments, and evaluate each other's progress toward goal attainment. The therapists gradually fade out their role in directing all group activities, allowing the group to take over such functions as suggesting behavioral rehearsals, giving assignments, and reinforcing appropriate or improved behaviors.

4. *Assignments:* Carry out behavioral assignments given by therapists and group.

Session 8: Objectives: (a) each member evaluates his or her progress toward attainment of treatment goals; (b) each member describes a procedure for maintaining his or her treatment gains; and (c) members arrange individual follow-up interviews.

Procedures are as follows:

1. *Data gathering:* An evaluation form is distributed to group members who are asked to complete it. The form includes a description of problems worked on in the group and instructs members to rate the extent to which their goals were achieved. Each member presents evaluative data indicating his or her progress, including examples of modified behaviors and conditions.

2. *Educational:* The therapists discuss ways to maintain the changes achieved. Unless the desired behaviors are well established and reinforced in the clients' natural environment, they are unlikely to be sustained.

3. *Group tasks:* Members discuss their plans and summarize their experiences in the group. Members reinforce each other for treatment gains and encourage each other to follow through with the maintenance plans.

4. *Follow-up:* Members are scheduled to return individually for a 1-month follow-up meeting. A second follow-up meeting is arranged at that time.

Evaluation

Evaluation of treatment progress is based primarily on the extent to which the clients' goals are accomplished. This is determined by observation of treatment-related behaviors in the group and client self-evaluation forms (Sundel & Lawrence, 1974, pp. 344–346). Measures of satisfaction from clients obtained after intervention are compared with their assessment of the target behaviors prior to implementation of the behavioral change plan, to determine their perceptions of the extent of change and the benefits of group treatment.

In evaluating the efficacy of the group treatment program, the therapists consider the client's appraisal of the program's success. Measures of the client's satisfaction with the results should be consistent with his or her attainment of the treatment goals (Sundel & Sundel, 1982). The therapists discuss objective measures of progress toward goal achievement with the client and relate these measures to the client's satisfaction with behavioral change so that objective measures of goal progress and the client's perceptions of improvement can be compared. If the client's goals are achieved, but he or she is dissatisfied, this may indicate faulty assessment or failure in establishing goals that the client considered important.

On the other hand, a client who is showing minimal progress in achieving behavioral change goals may report satisfaction with the group treatment program. This individual may be deriving sufficient reinforcement from social interactions in the group to compensate for lack of goal progress. The therapist can help the client realistically evaluate progress toward attainment of treatment goals and separate this appraisal from the client's evaluation of group membership.

Follow-up interviews were held with each group member individually 1 month and 6 months after the group terminated. These sessions were designed to (a) evaluate the extent to which treatment gains had been maintained; (b) provide additional interventions if necessary for the problem worked on during group treatment; (c) determine if additional treatment was necessary for problems not dealt with in the group or that had developed after termination of group treatment; and (d) determine if the clients had applied knowledge and skills learned in the group to other problems. Maintenance of treatment gains for each client was evaluated by his or her responses to a self-evaluation form filled out at the follow-up interview (see Sundel & Lawrence, 1974). The therapists discussed the client's responses to the self-evaluation form in conducting the follow-up interviews.

Research Findings

In an exploratory study using this model with three groups, 15 of the 17 (88%) group members rated their problems "much better" or "completely solved" 6 months after treatment. In addition, 12 of the 17 (71%) reported that they had successfully applied the behavioral concepts they learned in the group to other problems (Lawrence & Sundel, 1972; Sundel & Lawrence, 1977).

Lawrence and Walter (1978) used a controlled outcome study to further test the group model with clients in a family service agency and a community mental health clinic. These clients presented interpersonal problems with family members, acquaintances, and work associates. Forty-eight subjects were randomly assigned to two conditions: the behavioral group model or a no-treatment control group. The experimental condition consisted of four groups of five or six members. Each group was led by two therapists. Subjects in the control group were placed on a waiting list until evaluation posttests were administered 9 weeks later. The behavioral group model was implemented over an 8-week period. The control group then received the same treatment.

The behavioral group model was found to be more effective than no treatment according to a problem-rating form filled out by each client ($\chi^2 = 12.60$, $df = 1$, $p < .001$). Changes from pretest to posttest were observed to be greater within the treatment group than within the control group on a number of other measures used (a behavioral problem-solving test, ratings of two judges, the Rathus [1973] Assertiveness Scale, and two social effectiveness tests). A 3-month follow-up mail survey of treated clients showed that 74% of the clients either made further improvement or maintained what they had previously achieved according to a self-rating form (Lawrence & Walter, 1978).

Problems in Group Functioning

In working with groups, therapists encounter various situations that can detract from problem solving and pursuit of individual treatment goals. These issues involve inappropriate behaviors of group members that take time from the task and maintenance functions of the group.

Problem Switching or Treatment Avoidance

In problem switching or treatment avoidance, the client presents the problem with the most immediate aversive effects to work on, which changes from session to session, thereby avoiding objective analysis of any problem. When a client switches problems, the therapists and group help him or her select one problem and carry out an assessment and treatment plan for that problem.

During the first group meeting, Linda decided that she did not want to work on the original work-related problem that she had selected during intake. She said that she was quitting her job and that her real problem was her "inability to say 'no' to requests made by her friends and relatives." She responded to the group's questions for RAC-S information with vague, nonspecific answers. To help her identify RAC-S data, she was given an assignment to describe the occasions when she agreed to do something a friend or relative requested, including relevant antecedents and consequences.

At this point, it appeared reasonable for Linda to choose the new problem to work on; however, at the next session Linda had not completed her assignment and presented a different problem to work on. The therapists and group members pointed out Linda's inappropriate problem switching and failure to adhere to the group's problem-solving procedure. The therapists and group instructed Linda to stick to one problem and reinforced her for presenting RAC-S data and developing a treatment plan for that problem.

When a client fails to complete an assignment, the therapists and group examine the conditions responsible. Some of the reasons for noncompliance and how to handle them include

1. The client lacks skills in recording the data. Additional instruction in observational and recording techniques is given.
2. The client objects to doing the assignment. The group first listens to the objections and then either attempts to persuade the client to perform the assignment or negotiates an alternative assignment that the client agrees to perform.
3. The client has been reinforced previously for substituting excuses for performance. In such situations, the therapists restate the treatment con-

tract and secure the client's commitment to cooperate before resuming treatment.

4. The assignment involves behaviors that the client has not learned sufficiently well. Role playing and rehearsal of the desired behaviors in the group until the client demonstrates satisfactory performance is indicated. If the assignment is too difficult, an approximation is given, including behaviors that the client can perform more readily. The original assignment is given when the client has demonstrated proficiency in performing the assigned behaviors.

Irrelevant or Excessive Talking

Kevin spent an excessive amount of time presenting his data to the group. He digressed frequently from discussing his data and elaborately described tangentially related events. He typically prefaced his reports with elaborate justifications of his behavior, apparently attempting to present himself favorably to the group. These digressions interfered with assessment of his problems and drew complaints from group members about his monopolizing the group's time.

In addressing this problem, the therapists explained how Kevin's self-justifying remarks interfered with analysis of his problem and gave him suggestions for decreasing such remarks. In addition, group members were instructed on how to refocus Kevin's reporting. For example, members were taught to interrupt Kevin when he rambled by asking him questions pertinent to reporting his data and by reinforcing concise answers. As Kevin learned to present his data effectively, intervention from group members decreased.

Applications of the Model to Other Populations and Settings

Since first reported (Sundel & Lawrence, 1970), this behavioral group treatment model has been applied to a wide range of populations, including prisoners, drug addicts, mental patients, alcoholics, and juvenile delinquents. The model has been applied in outpatient mental health clinics, psychiatric hospitals, and parent training seminars. Many of these groups have been conducted in practice settings without controlled experimental conditions and data collection. Unpublished and informal reports by practitioners have shown that the model, with minor variations, is applicable to many populations and diverse settings.

Two examples of how the model has been adapted will be presented. The first is a method for training graduate students, and the second is a model for short-term community education groups.

A Student Training Method

Lawrence and Sundel (1975) taught a course to social work graduate students at the University of Michigan in which the students participated in self-modification groups as part of their training in group treatment. They found this to be a viable alternative when fieldwork opportunities for learning the behavioral group treatment model were unavailable, either because of lack of trained supervisors or agency opposition to behavior modification. The students were taught this model by following the guidelines developed by Sundel and Lawrence (1970) and Lawrence and Sundel (1972).

The students were assigned to groups of five and six members who met outside of class to work on preselected problems. The professors screened these problems to ensure that they were appropriate for the time-limited groups. Problems selected by the students included poor study habits, nail biting, forgetting names, overeating, smoking, and nonparticipation in class discussions. The groups met for 2-hour sessions over a period of 6 to 7 weeks. Group members rotated weekly in the roles of group leader, observer, and recorder. The professor consulted with the student leader for each week to help plan the next meeting. Weekly class lectures and discussions focused on topics that paralleled the issues and tasks to be addressed as the groups developed.

In one class of 22 students divided into four groups, Lawrence and Sundel (1975) reported the following results: 14 members achieved their behavioral change goals; 5 made significant improvements; and 3 failed to make significant improvements according to self-reports. The authors noted that the relatively poor performance of one group—2 failures, 3 partial successes—was associated with poor attendance, disruptive behaviors, and leadership difficulties.

Four years of experience using this student-training model revealed the following to be among the most significant benefits for the students:

1. Opportunity to learn behavioral group treatment skills under the guidance of an experienced practitioner
2. Observing, experiencing, and handling a variety of group-functioning problems similar to those encountered in client groups
3. Gaining a perspective on being a client in this kind of group
4. First-hand observation of the effectiveness of the behavioral group model in obtaining desired behavior changes (Lawrence & Sundel, 1975)

Short-Term Groups in Community Education

The availability of psychological knowledge through the mass media and the growth of the self-help movement, among other factors, have created a market for short-term groups that focus on self-improvement. Community-sponsored courses such as assertiveness training, personal growth, overcoming shyness, stress management, coping with divorce, child management, weight control, and smoking cessation, proliferate in communities around the country. In this consumer-oriented environment, individuals are increasingly self-diagnosing their deficits and seeking out courses that would appear to address their concerns and interests.

Assertiveness training groups have proven to be of interest to the public (Alberti & Emmons, 1974; Jakubowski & Lange, 1978; Sundel & Sundel, 1980).

The authors have conducted assertiveness training groups for such diverse clientele as women law students, women's political caucus groups, realtors, health and human service professionals, and administrative staff in federal and state agencies.

Sandra Sundel has offered assertiveness training courses to the community through a university-based continuing education program. Participants signed up for a 5-week, 10-hour course described in the continuing education brochure. The course has attracted both men and women participants, including college students, senior citizens, blue-collar workers, artists, business executives, middle managers, and clerical workers. Problems presented by group members have included interpersonal difficulties with family, friends, work associates, superiors, and self-assessed "low self-esteem." The typical size of these groups has been 12 members, with a range of 10–24.

The behavioral group model has been adapted for use in this setting, including the assessment, planning, intervention, and evaluation format. The following is a summary of the model's adaptation for an assertiveness-training course.

Orientation and Assessment

All individuals who sign up for the course are considered as group members who will learn assertive skills through interaction with each other as well as from didactic presentations from the instructor/leader. They usually present a specific problem area to work on. At the first meeting, the group leader explains the purpose of the course and its operating procedures. To optimize the time available for problem solving, an initial group goal is to establish conditions conducive to group members discussing their personal problem of nonassertiveness. For example, the chairs are arranged in a horseshoe or circle, so that the members and group leader are facing each other. The leader assumes an active role in directing group activities during the first and second meetings. The leader models behaviors that are unfamiliar or difficult for group members to perform, such as reinforcing members for discussing their problems in the group, for asking each other relevant questions, and for giving each other constructive comments and feedback. Members are given the assignment of keeping a diary of problematic situations and their responses to them.

The leader's role for sessions 1 and 2 is to (a) help each member identify an assertiveness problem to work on in the group; and (b) teach group members how to specify target behaviors and their controlling conditions (antecedents and consequences). The members are taught a behavioral assessment format for analyzing their problems: situation (antecedents)—target behavior (response)—consequences (positive and/or negative) (Sundel & Sundel, 1980). This format is a simplified version of RAC-S geared to the general population. Nontechnical language, such as *situation* instead of *antecedents* and *target behavior* instead of *response*, is used to place the emphasis on the educational rather than therapeutic focus of the group. This simplified format appears to facilitate comprehension and application of the concepts in the brief time frame of the course.

Planning and Intervention

The major tasks of the group leader during the third and fourth sessions are to help each member (1) specify desired assertive responses; and (2) evaluate the benefits and risks of acting assertively. The group leader sets up role plays, coaches individuals during the role plays, and models assertive responses. The leader also demonstrates for group members how to model and coach each other and give feedback. Feedback is designed to acknowledge assertive behaviors the individual has performed and give suggestions for improving future role-play performances.

Group members are encouraged to become actively involved in each other's assertiveness training programs by serving as (a) models; (b) actors roleplaying the parts of significant others, such as co-workers or family members; (c) reinforcers; (d) feedback givers; and (e) evaluators. Group members are also involved in formulating behavioral assignments or "homework," which includes specifying behaviors to be performed between group sessions. Initially, the leader assumes major responsibility for giving behavioral assignments. As members increase their problem-solving skills, however, they take a more active role in structuring their own assignments as well as offering suggestions to others. In order to help them generalize their assertive responses, members rehearse them in the group, getting feedback and suggestions for improvement from each other and the leader.

Behavioral rehearsal is an essential component of an assertiveness training program. Some group members come with specific problems of assertiveness and can specify their desired assertive responses with minimal difficulty. They can then proceed to rehearse these assertive behaviors. Other members have general problems of assertiveness, requiring a variety of behavioral rehearsals to give them opportunities to practice a range of assertive responses to many different situations.

Evaluation

During the fifth and final session, the tasks of the group leader are (a) to help each member evaluate goal progress and (b) to provide additional suggestions for other assertiveness problems that were not addressed in the group. Group members use records of their behavioral assignments and their diaries in evaluating their progress. Members also help each other evaluate changes in assertive performances they have observed in role plays and other interactions in the group.

An evaluation of 110 individuals in 7 classes showed that 105 (95%) of the participants found the course helpful in solving their assertiveness problems and that 105 (95%) would recommend it to a friend. Courses of this type provide the opportunity to use small groups to influence significant numbers of individuals who identify themselves as having certain interpersonal difficulties. The course is an inexpensive, socially acceptable way for individuals to improve their communication skills without entering psychotherapy.

Conclusion

We have presented a time-limited behavioral group treatment model and described its components of assessment, planning, intervention, and evaluation. The model employs a problem-solving framework that applies behavior modification principles and small group theory in a systematic manner. Knowledge of group dimensions (for example, cohesiveness, communication patterns) and of related group management skills (for example, establishing and enforcing group norms) is used in directing group activities toward achievement of individual goals.

The model has been tested in a controlled study and has been applied to a variety of settings and populations. Adaptations of the model to train graduate students and to teach assertive behaviors have proved to be viable.

The systematic organization and focus of the model appeal to clients who prefer a structured approach to problem solving. Individuals with expectations for a nondirective leader, unstructured session plan, or looser norms for participation might find the model to be unsuitable. Such considerations are discussed with prospective clients individually during the intake session to determine their appropriateness for group membership.

Once the group has met, new members are not added. This helps maintain the continuity necessary for individual goal attainment. In addition, group members learn concepts related to assessment and treatment that build on information and skills obtained in earlier sessions. Groups that are open-ended in membership are typically less structured; that is, they allow members to attend as they wish, and new members may be added during the course of the group (e.g., Schopler & Galinsky, 1985). Further, open-ended groups may lack continuity from one session to the next, so that new members can participate without prior attendance. The groups may continue as long as the leader and members indicate that the group is serving its purpose.

Future research in the use of this model could focus on collecting evaluative data showing comparisons with other short-term group models, and determining the optimum composition and duration of groups for differing client populations and problems. Studies comparing the effects of single therapists versus cotherapists in time-limited groups would appear to be a valuable area of inquiry. Although the future of the time-limited treatment group appears to be linked to financial costs of treatment, its aims will continue to be the reduction of personal distress and the improvement of social functioning.

References

Alberti, R. E., & Emmons, M. L. *Your perfect right*. San Luis Obispo, Calif. Impact Publishers, 1974.

Budman, S. H. (Ed.). *Forms of brief therapy*. New York: Guilford Press, 1981.

Corey, G. *Theory and practice of group counseling*. Monterey, Calif. Brooks/Cole, 1981.

Flowers, J. V. Behavioral analysis of group therapy and a model for behavioral group therapy. In D. Upper & S. Ross (Eds.), *Behavioral group therapy*. Champaign, Ill.: Research Press, 1979.

Jakubowski, P., & Lange, A. J. *The assertive option: Your rights and responsibilities.* Champaign, Ill.: Research Press, 1978.

Lawrence, H., & Sundel, M. Behavior modification in adult groups. *Social Work,* 1972, *17*(2), 34–43.

Lawrence, H., & Sundel, M. Self-modification in groups: A student training method for social groupwork. *Journal of Education for Social Work,* 1975, *11*(2), 76–83.

Lawrence, H., & Walter, C. Testing a behavioral approach with groups. *Social Work,* 1978, *23*(2), 127–133.

Lazarus, A. A. *Behavior therapy and beyond.* New York: McGraw-Hill, 1971.

Lazarus, A. A. *Multi-modal behavior therapy.* New York: Springer-Verlag, 1976.

Lennard, H. L., & Bernstein, A. *Patterns in human interaction.* San Francisco: Jossey-Bass, 1970.

Miller, W. R. (Ed.). *The addictive behaviors: Treatment of alcoholism, drug abuse, smoking and obesity.* New York: Pergamon Press, 1980.

Rathus, S. A. A 30-item schedule for assessing assertive behavior. *Behavior Therapy,* 1973, *4,* 398–406.

Rose, S. *Treating children in groups.* San Francisco: Jossey-Bass, 1972.

Rose, S. *Group therapy: A behavioral approach.* Englewood Cliffs, N.J.: Prentice-Hall, 1977.

Rose, S. *A casebook in group therapy.* Englewood Cliffs, N.J.: Prentice-Hall, 1980.

Schopler, J. H., & Galinsky, M. J. The open-ended group. In M. Sundel, P. Glasser, R. Sarri, & R. Vinter (Eds.), *Individual change through small groups* (2d ed.). New York: The Free Press, 1985.

Sobell, M. B., & Sobell, L. C. *Behavioral treatment of alcohol problems.* New York: Plenum Press, 1978.

Sundel, M., & Lawrence, H. Time-limited behavioral group treatment with adults. *Michigan Mental Health Research Bulletin,* 1970, *4,* 37–40.

Sundel, M., & Lawrence, H. Behavioral group treatment with adults in a family service agency. In P. Glasser, R. Sarri, & R. Vinter (Eds.), *Individual change through small groups.* New York: The Free Press, 1974.

Sundel, M., & Lawrence, H. A systematic approach to treatment planning in time-limited behavioral groups. *Journal of Behavior Therapy & Experimental Psychiatry,* 1977, *8,* 395–399.

Sundel, M., & Sundel, S. *Behavior modification in the human services: A systematic introduction to concepts and applications* (2d ed.). Englewood Cliffs, N.J.: Prentice-Hall, 1982.

Sundel, S., & Sundel, M. *Be assertive: A practical guide for human service workers.* Beverly Hills, Calif.: Sage, 1980.

Sundel, M., & Sundel, S. S. Behavior modification with time-limited groups. In M. Sundel, P. Glasser, R. Sarri, & R. Vinter (Eds.), *Individual change through small groups* (2d ed.). New York: The Free Press, 1985.

Sundel, M., Glasser, P., Sarri, R., & Vinter, R. (Eds.). *Individual change through small groups* (2d ed.). New York: The Free Press, 1985.

Upper, D., & Ross, S. Behavioral group therapy: Emotional, avoidance, and social skills problems of adults. In M. Hersen, R. M. Eisler, & P. M. Miller (Eds.), *Progress in behavior modification* (Vol. 5). New York: Academic Press, 1977.

Upper, D., & Ross, S. (Eds.). *Behavioral group therapy.* Champaign, Ill.: Reserach Press, 1979.

Upper, D., & Ross, S. (Eds.). *Behavioral group therapy.* Champaign, Ill.: Research Press, 1980.

Upper, D., & Ross, S. (Eds.). *Behavioral group therapy.* Champaign, Ill.: Research Press, 1981.

Wilson, G. T. Behavior therapy as a short-term therapeutic approach. In S. H. Budman (Ed.), *Forms of brief therapy.* New York: Guilford Press, 1981.

2

A Review and Programmatic Model of Group Social Skills Training for Psychiatric Patients

PETER M. MONTI AND DAVID J. KOLKO

GENERAL INTRODUCTION

The literature on social skills training is so extensive as to preclude a comprehensive review in any one source. Although the field is quite new, its initially optimistic results have generated considerable analog and clinical research investigations. This chapter will provide a review of social skills training as well as a description of the programmatic model developed in our clinic. The chapter is divided into two sections reflecting each of these topics. The present discussion will focus on the historical development of the skills training model and its therapeutic application with both individuals and groups. The objective of this section is to describe the following content areas: (a) early work on the role of social competence and psychopathology; (b) paradigmatic operant research demonstrating the modifiability of social behavior; (c) an overview of clinical research applications emphasizing group training programs with various patient populations; and (d) a critique of research. In the second section, the content and characteristics of a group training program that has been employed at the Providence Veterans Administration (VA) Medical Center will be described.

SOCIAL SKILLS TRAINING PROGRAMS: AN INTRODUCTION AND REVIEW

SOCIAL COMPETENCE AND PSYCHOPATHOLOGY

Social skills deficits have figured heavily in the origins of psychopathology (Argyle, Trower, & Bryant, 1974). Early research on the role of social competence

PETER M. MONTI • Brown University and Veterans Administration Medical Center, Providence, Rhode Island 02908. DAVID J. KOLKO • Western Psychiatric Institute and Clinic and University of Pittsburgh School of Medicine, Pittsburgh, Pennsylvania 15260.

documented an association between degrees of social skills and various measures of psychosocial adjustment. For example, Zigler and Phillips (1960) reported a relationship between general measures of social effectiveness and particular groups of symptoms (e.g., avoidance of others, self-indulgence), a finding that was later corroborated by Phillips and Zigler (1961). Both studies found less pathological symptomatology in individuals functioning at higher levels of social competence. Similary, Zigler and Phillips (1962) found that the level of personal and social maturity was associated with the degree of overall disturbance found in psychiatric patients.

The results of more extensive investigations support the hypothesis that a positive relationship exists between premorbid social competence and prognosis (Phillips & Zigler, 1964; Zigler & Phillips, 1961); patients manifesting high levels of social competence were more likely to be released from the hospital, spent less time hospitalized, and were less likely to be rehospitalized than those who demonstrated low social competence. This early literature and more recent statements regarding the modification of social skills during psychotherapy (Frank, 1974; Gladwin, 1974) indicate that (a) individuals having greater social skills evidence less severe psychopathology; and (b) highly skilled patients are given better prognoses than those showing more severe skills deficits.

Perhaps the most comprehensive perspective on the social skills basis of psychopathology has been articulated by Phillips (1978). The author describes the changing views of traditional conceptual formulations of psychopathology and offers a skills-oriented approach as an alternative. In arguing for the relevance of social skills to clinical problems, Phillips (1978) states that (a) skills deficits are numerous and implicate behaviors that relate to peoples' interactions both flexibly and functionally; (b) a social skills conceptualization offers a parsimonious way of changing behavior and connects the inner (i.e., subjective experience) with the outer (i.e., social functioning) world; and (c) the social skills approach is a constructive, positive, and testable way of looking at social problems.

The assessment and methodological framework of the social skills model as highlighted by Phillips (1978) is based upon a number of empirical concerns. Of major emphasis are the following considerations: (a) the designation of specific and observable skills in reference to any given behavior; (b) a situationally specific definition of competence; (c) the direct measurement of changes in social skills; and (d) a concern for the conditions under which the behavior is demonstrated. Moreover, the implications of this approach seem to prompt certain assertions that bear upon its conceptual formulation and approach to individual behavior change; (a) social skills deficits may underlie psychopathology and can be changed through specifically programmed behavioral efforts; (b) the measurement and meaning of social skills are close to the empirical data as ascertained in research; and (c) the social skills approach fits well into those clinical activities that emphasize basic principles of learning, commonly described as behavior modification and therapy. Thus, the social skills model provides a learning-based, response-acquisition approach to the development of effective interpersonal functioning.

Paradigmatic Operant Research and the Modifiability of Social Behavior

Much of the early behavioral literature dealing with the modification of social and interpersonal behaviors focused upon the application of contingent reinforcement procedures. These classic studies were principally intended to demonstrate that social interaction and maladaptive behaviors could be strengthened or weakened, respectively, through explicit programming of response-contingent consequences. In successfully conditioning and maintaining social and cooperative behaviors, such efforts laid the groudwork for a basic social skills training technology.

In one of the earliest studies in this research area, Azrin and Lindsley (1956) showed that cooperation between young children could be developed and maintained when a single reinforcer was delivered for engaging in a cooperative response. This study demonstrated the acquisition of a complex social skill using reinforcement procedures. Ayllon and Haughton (1962) modified the social behavior (again, a cooperative response) of chronic schizophrenics using admission to the dining room as reinforcement. Not only was this cooperative social response learned, but also additional verbal and social behaviors occurred among other ward members. Ayllon and Azrin (1968) later used token reinforcement to condition adaptive and social-interaction behaviors. A host of appropriate behaviors involving social and self-care skills were strengthened after reinforcement was applied. Finally, cooperative and social responses have been shaped in schizophrenic children (Hingtgen & Trost, 1966). Following the application of a reinforcement program, the authors noted that eye contact increased, affect became more appropriate to the context, and the responses generalized to adults, both on the ward and at home.

Reinforcement procedures have likewise proven clinically useful in facilitating the appropriate verbal repertoires of mute psychotic patients (Isaacs, Thomas, & Goldiamond, 1960; Sherman, 1963, 1965; Wilson & Walters, 1966). These studies documented consistent improvements in imitative verbal behaviors by shaping behavioral approximations to a model's responses. As but one illustration, the study by Wilson and Walters (1966) demonstrated the effectiveness of modeling and reinforcement with pennies or modeling along in increasing verbal output in several adult patients, although limited generalization to the ward setting was found.

These initial studies convincingly demonstrated the positive effects of reinforcement in conditioning social and cooperative behaviors, considered as important rudimentary interpersonal skills (Hersen & Bellack, 1976). In the case of the psychiatric patient, reinforcement programs indeed suggested a judicious approach to the modification of symptomatic behavior by concentrating upon positive desirable behaviors. However, the use of reinforcement procedures *per se* is more feasible and cost-effective with those individuals who have already acquired rudimentary social skills repertoires (Eisler, Hersen, & Miller, 1973; Eisler, Miller, & Hersen, 1973). In addition, these procedures are quite time consuming (Combs & Slaby, 1977). Insofar as many individuals were found not to possess the appropriate social skills in their behavioral repertoire (Hersen & Bellack, 1976), greater attention was eventually paid to a broader social learning approach to the acquisition and development of these skills that has been generally referred to as *social skills training* (Curran & Monti, 1982). The historical background and procedural underpinnings of this novel behavioral approach will be briefly outlined before reviewing its empirical evidence.

Applications with Psychiatric Patients

The past decade has witnessed growing application of the social skills model in the treatment of a variety of psychiatric disorders and interpersonal difficulties (Bellack & Hersen, 1979; Twentyman & Zimering, 1979). The range of clinical populations that have benefited from behavioral training extends from chronic schizophrenics and other psychiatric patients to unassertive college students, sexual deviants, and distressed spouses (Heimberg, Montgomery, Madsen, & Heimberg, 1977). The suitability of these client groups for treatment has been largely determined on the basis of their lack or inefficient use of social and interpersonal skills. Therefore, training has encompassed the development of specific responses for use in certain situations or the acquisition of a more global social repertoire.

From a historical perspective, social skills training has most often been directed toward the modification of individual assertive behavior (Serber & Nelson, 1971; Weinman, Gelbart, Wallace, & Post, 1972; Wolpe, 1973), although group programs have been reported as well (Rathus, 1972, 1973). A variety of treatment strategies including behavioral rehearsal or role playing, modeling, feedback, instructions, coaching, discussion, social reinforcement, and *in vivo* homework assignments have been employed to teach and facilitate the expression of appropriate assertive responses. With an emphasis upon the systematic use of these procedures, assessment and treatment have typically focused upon the more objective elements of social interaction (Eisler, Hersen, & Miller, 1973; Hersen, Eisler, & Miller, 1973). For example, Eisler, Miller, & Hersen (1973) described one of the first empirically derived role-play tests for the behavioral assessment of social skills, focusing upon such component behaviors as looking, smiling, speech duration, and questions. Assessment devices of this sort have been widely used to identify skills deficits and evaluate program effectiveness (Bellack, 1983).

The broad appeal enjoyed by the construct of social skills has resulted in training programs for the development of interpersonal skills, social problem solving, emotional expressiveness, and personal effectiveness (Curran, 1979; Hersen, 1979). Further empirical extensions of this approach have related skills deficits to a host of diagnostic entities, including schizophrenia (Jaffe & Carlson, 1976), depression (Hersen, Bellack, & Himmelhoch, 1980), juvenile delinquency (Freedman, Rosenthal, Donahoe, Schlundt, & McFall, 1978; Kolko, Dorsett, & Milan, 1981), and sexual deviation (Barlow, Abel, Blanchard, Bristow, & Young, 1977). As attested to by several recent handbooks (Bellack & Hersen, 1979; Curran & Monti, 1982; Eisler & Frederiksen, 1980; Kelly, 1981), the relevance of social skills training procedures has been widely documented across varying contexts and populations. Indeed, although the social skills approach is still in its infancy, the interest and encouraging trends that it has generated argue for its consideration as a viable treatment alternative with a diverse range of clinical problems. What follows is a critical overview of skills training programs for patient populations conducted in a group context. However, a number of select individual training programs will be briefly described first in order to highlight the many empirical and therapeutic contributions made by these preliminary efforts (Eisler, 1976).

Individual Training Programs

Concurrent with the preliminary evaluation of behavioral training procedures designed to teach assertion to college students (Heimberg *et al.*, 1977), numerous experimental studies of skills training strategies were conducted with psychiatric patients in individual treatment analog situations. These studies generally involved brief treatment programs and the investigation of particular conceptual questions, but did not constitute conclusive clinical outcome trials (Hersen, 1979). Eisler, Hersen, and Miller (1973) were among the first to compare the effects of modeling, response practice, and no treatment on acquisition of different behavioral components of assertiveness (Eisler, Miller, & Hersen, 1973). Significant pre-post differences on five of eight behaviors (e.g., voice volume, eye contact) were found for the modeling group only, suggesting that this strategy was more effective than either practice or no treatment at all.

Hersen, Eisler, Miller, Johnston, and Pinkston (1973) extended the work of Eisler, Hersen, and Miller (1973) by comparing the effects of practice, instructions, and modeling (both alone and in combination), modeling plus instructions, and no treatment. The results indicated that subjects in the combined group received higher ratings on five of seven assertion skills components, whereas instructions and modeling alone produced the most gains in assertiveness on the remaining two components. These same three training procedures with the addition of generalization instructions were employed by Hersen, Eisler, and Miller (1974). The modeling plus instructions group showed the greatest improvement on seven of eight training and five of eight generalization role-play situations. Minimal transfer of training was obtained in a simulated, *in vivo* task in which clients were "shortchanged." Likewise, the generalization instructions failed to produce significant incremental effects. Goldstein, Martens, Hubben, van Belle, Schaaf, Wiersma, and Goedhart (1973) also found that subjects exposed to modeling, instructions, or rehearsal improved relative to controls. However, no differences were found between the experimental groups. Differences in the duration of training and target behaviors selected for training may account for the discrepancy between these results and those of Hersen, Eisler, and Miller (1973).

Goldsmith and McFall (1975) compared an interpersonal skills training program (rehearsal, modeling, coaching, response playback, feedback) based upon treatment scenes derived from the behavior-analytic method with two control groups (pseudotherapy, assessment only). The results pointed to the superiority of the skills training group over the other groups on self-report and behavioral measures obtained in an analog situation and during an *in vivo* simulation. An 8-month follow-up revealed a slight reduction in recidivism rates for the skills training program. In general, these preliminary findings suggested that skills training procedures showed promise in the treatment of assertion and general social skills deficits in psychiatric patients.

The encouraging outcomes described in early analog studies led to numerous clinical applications with unskilled patients. In an early uncontrolled case study, Serber (1972) discussed the shaping and teaching of nonverbal assertive behaviors in a case example of an inpatient who was unable to stand up for himself. The client was instructed through the use of instructions, modeling, role playing, and feedback to deny invalid charges made against him. The author reported anecdotally that some behavioral improvements were made (e.g., facial expression, eye contact). Eisler, Hersen, and Miller (1974) demonstrated the efficacy of instructions and feedback in shaping four assertive responses in two male inpatients. The improvements were confirmed by higher ratings of overall assertiveness after training. A follow-up inquiry indicated some transfer of skills to novel situations (e.g., work, home).

Turning to studies with schizophrenics, Hersen, Turner, Edelstein, and Pinkston (1975) employed social skills training consisting of instructions, rehearsal, feedback, and modeling with an extremely withdrawn and socially primitive patient. Using a multiple-baseline design, improvements were documented in all targeted behaviors that were reflected in ward ratings of social appropriateness and skill. Improvements were also observed for three untrained component behaviors, suggesting generalization across behaviors. As a result of these improvements, the client was able to benefit from vocational counseling and a job placement. The client was gainfully employed for the first time in 3 years at a 22-month follow-up. In a similar study, Edelstein and Eisler (1976) found that modeling alone produced few improvements in target behaviors with a paranoid schizophrenic. However, the combination of modeling, instructions, and feedback effected desired changes that generalized to novel role-play situations and interactions. No follow-up data were reported to suggest whether these improvements were maintained.

The use of single-case experimental designs has also been reported in an additional series of studies concerned with documenting the clinical efficacy of individual social skills training programs and follow-up maintenance of their effects (Bellack, Hersen, & Turner, 1976; Hersen & Bellack, 1976). Hersen and Bellack (1976) observed improvements in four identified skills of two chronic schizophrenics that were reflected in marked increases in global ratings of overall assertiveness. The improvements were maintained at a 2, 4, 6, and 8-week follow-up assessment. Bellack *et al.* (1976) found that a program consisting of instructions, modeling, and feedback was associated with considerable skills improvement in two female schizophrenics, but only modest improvement in a male schizophrenic. The two female patients also transferred the seven skills learned during training to a series of generalization and novel role-play situations and maintained their treatment gains at a 2, 4, and 10-week follow-up assessment. The authors suggest that the male patient's mixed results may have been attributed to a subtherapeutic medication regimen.

In a subsequent group comparison investigation, Eisler, Blanchard, Fitts, and Williams (1978) compared individual social skills training (role playing coaching, feedback) with and without modeling with schizophrenic and non-psychotic psychiatric patients. On all but one behavioral measure, significant treatment gains were observed for all groups. However, modeling was required for the schizophrenic patients only. For both groups, the skills acquired during training generalized to simulated interactions on the psychiatric ward. Similarly impressive data indicating the efficacy of a comprehensive program (role playing, modeling, feedback, instructions, and general suggestions) in improving skillful performance and facilitating generalization have been reported by Matson and Stephens (1978) who also noted corresponding reductions in aggressive behavior and increases in prosocial and self-care skills. These latter studies were well conducted from both therapeutic and methodological perspectives.

Group Training Programs

The transfer of behavioral procedures from an individual to a group context for the treatment of such problems as phobias (Paul & Shannon, 1966) and sexual dysfunction (Lazarus, 1968) was likewise evident in the case of assertion and social skills difficulties. Drawing upon proposed benefits associated with the naturalistic, reinforcing, supportive, and therapy-enhancing characteristics of a group situation, investigators have examined the feasibility of applying behavioral procedures previously employed with socially unskilled individuals to therapy groups (Kelly, 1981; Upper & Ross, 1977). To facilitate a critical appraisal of this literature, several therapeutic and empirical aspects of each program are summarized in Table 1.

Group assertion training programs were initially reported by Lomont, Gilner, Spector, and Skinner (1969) and Percell, Berwick, and Beigel (1974). Lomont *et al.* (1969) compared group insight therapy with assertion training consisting of coaching, feedback, modeling, rehearsal, and discussion with chronic inpatients. The assertion training group showed a reduction on the Depression and Psychasthenia scales of the Minnesota Multiphasic Personality Inventory (MMPI), although no differences were found on the Leary Interpersonal Check List. Percell *et al.* (1974) found that outpatients who rehearsed and then discussed the impact of certain component skills rated themselves as more assertive, self-accepting, and less anxious than those in a relationship control group that only discussed the skills. Participants in the training group were also rated as more assertive, aggressive, empathic, spontaneous, and outgoing, and as less anxious overall. However, no specific behavioral measures or index of generalization and maintenance were reported in either of these studies.

Working with a mixed group of outpatients and inpatients, Argyle *et al.* (1974) employed modeling, role playing and role reversal, coaching, verbal and videotape feedback, and social reinforcement to increase both verbal and non-

TABLE 1. General Characteristics of Group Training Programs[a]

Authors	Patients	Design	Measures	Treatment (sessions)	Results	Generalization	Follow-up	Comments
Lomont, Gilnes, Spector, & Skinner	12 chronic schizophrenics	Pre-post group comparison	(1) MMPI; (2) Leary Inter-Personal Check List	(1) AT—C, M, R, F, D (30) (2) group insight therapy	(1) AT group showed improvements on D & Pt scales of MMPI	None	None	(1) No behavioral measures or individual data
Booraem & Flowers (1972)	14 psychotic inpatients	Pre-post group comparison	(1) Spielberger Self-Evaluation Questionnaire; (2) verbal and nonverbal measures of personal space	(1) AT—RP, M, C, SR, HW plus milieu therapy (12); (2) milieu therapy only	(1) No significant group differences (more improvements noted for AT group)	None	Patients in AT group released earlier	(1) No behavioral measures or individual data; (2) poor description of program content
Bloomfield (1973)	8 chronic schizophrenics	Case study	(1) Anecdotal reports	(1) AT—M, R, RR, F, SR, I (?)	(1) Decrease in compliance and aggression; increased assertiveness	None	None	(1) No data presented; (2) no controls
Gutride, Goldstein, & Hunter (1973)	87 inpatients	Group comparison (ANOVAs)	(1) Self-report inventories (POMS, FIRO); (2) standardized role play; (3) naturalistic	(1) SLT—D, M, RP, F, SR plus psychotherapy (12); (2) SLT only; (3) Psychotherapy only	(1) SLT plus psychotherapy better than psychotherapy only on POMS	None	None	(1) Good methodology; (2) multiple behaviors were assessed

			interaction; (4) global ratings		and ratings of naturalistic interaction; (2) SLT better than no SLT POMS, ratings of naturalistic interaction, and global ratings			
Argyle, Trower, & Bryant (1974)	4 outpatients; 2 inpatients	Pre-post individual comparison	(1) Self-report inventories (Repertory Grid Test); (2) role-play measure (speeches); (3) global skill ratings	(1) SST—R, RP, F, SR, RR, M (6)	(1) 2/5 pts. given higher skill ratings after training; (2) 1/5 pts. reported change from real to ideal self on Repertory Grid Test	None	None	(1) No behavioral data or reliability on global ratings presented; (2) good description of content of program
Gutride *et al.* (1974)	120 chronic inpatients	Group comparison (ANOVAs)	(1) Self-report inventories (POMS, FIRO); (2) standardized role play; (3) naturalistic interaction;	(1) SLT—D, M, RP, F, SR (15); (2) SLT—same as #1 (21); (3) SLT—same as #1 plus on-site	(1) SLT groups better than both control groups on role play and naturalistic measures; (2) SLT plus	None	None	(1) Good use of *in vivo* training procedure; (2) limited description of methodology

(*continued*)

TABLE 1 (*Continued*)

Authors	Patients	Design	Measures	Treatment (sessions)	Results	Generalization	Follow-up	Comments
			(4) global ratings	transfer training (15); (4) social therapy control (meet with student companions); (5) No-treatment control	transfer training was best SLT group			
Percell, Berwick, & Beigel (1974)	24 outpatients	Pre-post group comparison	(1) Self-report inventories (Self-Acceptance Scale of CPI, TMAS) (2) global ratings	(1) AT—R, D (8); (2) discussion control	(1) AT group rated selves as more assertive and self-accepting and less axious; (2) AT group rated by judge as more assertive, aggressive, empathic, spontaneous, and outgoing, and less anxious	None	None	(1) No component behaviors or reliability on global ratings presented

Clark (1975)	36 Viet Nam veteran inpatients	Pre-post group comparison	(1) Self-reported improvements during role plays; (2) trained and untrained role plays; (3) global ratings	(1) SST—R, C, M, F (?); (2) dynamic role-play therapy; (3) didactic lecture control	(1) SST pts. reported greater improvements in performance; (2) SST received higher scores on all trained role plays; (3) SST rated more socially skilled, attractive, involving, and appropriate	SST led to higher scores on 3/4 categories of untrained situations	SST associated with more employment and less recidivism	(1) Good use of multiple measures
Doty (1975)	56 inpatients	Pre-post group comparison (repeated measures)	(1) Ward behavioral observations; (2) behavioral observations of social responsiveness in a group	(1) SST—I, RP, F (4); (2) incentive (monetary payoff for social interaction); (3) SST plus incentive; (4) nonspecific control; (5) no-treatment control	(1) Incentive groups showed most change in both measures; (2) incentive component better than role playing in increasing appropriate social behavior	Transfer of training to a group discussion	None	(1) Good description of methodology; (2) no reliability or individual data presented

(continued)

TABLE 1 (*Continued*)

Authors	Patients	Design	Measures	Treatment (sessions)	Results	Generalization	Follow-up	Comments
Field & Test (1975)	10 chronic schizophrenics (outpatients)	Pre-post group comparison	(1) Role-play measures	(1) SST—D, M, R, F, SR, tokens (12); (2) control (same as 1, but with no training on role plays used for assessment)	(1) SST showed greater improvements in compliance content and latency/ disruptive pauses	None	(10 mo): 4/5 pts. still showed gains; (6 mo): 8/10 employed; 9/10 lived in community; no relapses	(1) Good description of methodology; (2) no reliablity or individual data presented
Falloon, Lindley, McDonald, & Maxes (1977)	51 outpatients	Pre-post group comparison	(1) Self-report ratings of target social problems, anxiety avoidance, leisure activities, self-image, & mood); (2) global ratings of work, social, and general adjustment, social skill,	(1) SST—M, R, D (10); (2) SST plus structured HW assignments; (3) goal-directed group discussion	(1) SST showed greater improvements in target problem frequency and expressiveness compared to discussion only; (2) SST plus HW showed greater improvements in target problem fre-	None	SST given higher work adjustment ratings than discussion at 6-mo FU; gains were maintained by all groups at 12–24 mo FU	(1) Multiple measures assessed (2) good evaluation of homework assignments

			self-image, and expressiveness		quency and anxiety, unhappiness, social anxiety, and self-image than SST alone			
Finch & Wallace (1977)	16 schizophrenic outpatients	Pre-post group comparison	(1) Wolpe–Lazarus Questionnaire; (2) behavioral measures in role plays and spontaneous interactions	(1) SST—M, R, I, C, F, HW, attention focusing skills (12); (2) no-treatment control	(1) SST better than control on all measures	Improvements found on untrained and spontaneous role plays; nurses reported increase grooming and interaction	None	(1) Good use of different role plays and attention-focusing skills; (2) good reliability
Williams, Turner, Watts, Bellack, & Hersen (1977)	4 chronic schizophrenics	Multiple baseline across behaviors	(1) Behavioral measures in training, generalization, and novel role plays	(1) SST—M, I, R, F, SR (30)	(1) Improvements on training role plays after SST; (2) slight increase in ratings of assertiveness	Modest improvement on generalization and novel role plays	None	(1) Authors report savings of 70 hours from individual training format

(continued)

TABLE 1 (*Continued*)

Authors	Patients	Design	Measures	Treatment (sessions)	Results	Generalization	Follow-up	Comments
Trower, Yardley, Bryant, & Shaw (1978)	20 unskilled pts. (primary); 20 social phobics (secondary)	Pre-post group crossover comparison	(1) Social Situation Questionnaire; (2) behavioral measures in standardized interaction (3) clinical ratings	(1) SST—C, M, R, F, HW (?); (2) systematic desensitization	(1) Unskilled pts. showed greater improvements on all measures after SST; (2) phobics showed fewer but similar improvements after both treatments	None	None	(1) No-control group used; (2) no reliability reported; (3) different therapists in each group

[a]Abbreviations are as follows: AT = assertion training; SST = social skills training; R = behavioral rehearsal; RR = role reversal; RP = role playing; M = modeling; C = coaching; SR = social reinforcement; HW = homework; F = feedback; D = discussion; I = instructions; MMPI = Minnesota Multiphasic Personality Inventory; POMS = Psychiatric Outpatient Mood Scales; FIRO = Fundamental Interpersonal Relations Orientation-Behavior; TMAS = Taylor Manifest Anxiety Scale; CPI = California Psychological Inventory; FU = follow-up; pts = patients.

verbal skills. Such skills as self-disclosure and being rewarding in conversation complemented the wide range of trained behaviors. However, pre- and post-training global ratings of social skills by expert judges indicated improvements in only two of five subjects, which were reflected in similar changes on a self-report measure (Repertory Grid Test). No changes were reported in the only behavioral measure assessed—number of speeches made during training—and there was no follow-up assessment. Argyle *et al.* (1974) noted several advantages of a group training format, including its natural and real-life characteristics, cost-effectiveness, and empathic quality.

A heterogeneous group of outpatients was also described in a comprehensive study by Falloon, Lindley, McDonald, and Marks (1977). Patients were randomly assigned to one of three groups: (a) goal-directed group discussion; (b) modeling, rehearsal, and discussion; and (c) modeling, rehearsal, structured daily homework assignments, and discussion. Training for the latter two groups was directed toward a number of basic and more complex behavioral components of interpersonal interaction. Pre-post comparisons showed that all three groups produced significant improvements in self-report and behavioral measures, and in global ratings. In terms of individual groups, modeling and rehearsal led to greater improvements in the frequency of target problems and in expressiveness as rated by an assessor in a short interview. The addition of homework to rehearsal and modeling was associated with the same improvements along with increases in reported social leisure activities and ratings of both work and general adjustment.

Relative to the rehearsal and modeling group, the rehearsal, modeling, and homework group reported significant decreases in target problem anxiety and frequency, unhappiness, and social anxiety, and improved self-image at posttreatment and 6-month follow-up. However, a comparison of pretreatment and 6-month follow-up assessments revealed only one statistically significant difference (work adjustment) between the discussion group and the rehearsal and modeling group. It was reported that a greater percentage of patients in the two rehearsal groups were employed at follow-up. A long term follow-up (12 to 24 months posttreatment) indicated the maintenance of gains for all groups. In addition to assessing changes in a broad range of dependent measures, the authors give extensive consideration to a discussion of salient procedural variables, prognostic factors, and group treatment effects.

Trower, Yardley, Bryant, and Shaw (1978) investigated the effectiveness of social skills training (coaching, modeling, rehearsal, feedback) in the treatment of two forms of social failure, one due to skills deficits (primary) and the other due to inhibition or anxiety (secondary). The authors hypothesized that primary failure would be amenable to social skills training, whereas secondary failure would respond to an anxiety-alleviating treatment, namely desensitization. On the basis of pre-post comparisons, both groups of clients showed improvements in clinical, self-report, and behavioral measures, with the primary group responding in part as predicted. However, the secondary group responded similarly to both treatment methods. The authors suggested that skills training may facilitate the acquisition of behavioral skills while reducing anxiety as well. No control groups were employed, different therapists were assigned to the two groups, and no measures of generalization or maintenance were obtained.

Experimental investigations of social skills training have also been conducted in a group context with psychotic and schizophrenic patients (Booraem & Flowers, 1972). Working with psychotic inpatients, Booraem and Flowers compared an assertion training group consisted of coaching, modeling, role playing, social reinforcement, and homework assignments with the milieu therapy control group. No statistically significant differences between groups were found on a self-report measure of anxiety and behavioral measures of personal space, although the experimental group showed more improvement on both measures. The experimental group was also discharged earlier from the hospital.

Bloomfield (1973) found that assertion training composed of modeling, instructions, behavioral rehearsal and role reversal, feedback, and social reinforcement reduced social inhibition and facilitated development of interpersonal skills with a group of schizophrenics. The author reported the progress of one group member who showed increases in interpersonal skill and self-confidence as an example of the feasibility of a group training format. However, no formal data were reported, thus obscuring conclusions regarding the utility of the program.

In two more sophisticated empirical studies, Gutride, Goldstein, and Hunter (1973) and Gutride, Goldstein, Hunter, Carril, Clark, Furia, and Lower (1974) investigated the effects of Structured Learning Therapy (SLT; Goldstein, 1973), consisting of modeling, discussion, role playing, feedback (group and videotape), and social reinforcement. Working with an inpatient population, Gutride *et al.* (1973) found that SLT was associated with improvements on a self-report measure (Psychiatric Outpatient Mood Scales), in global ratings of social behavior, and in measures of a variety of target behaviors assessed during a naturalistic interaction. The addition of psychotherapy to SLT produced few incremental effects over SLT alone. In the Gutride *et al.* (1974) investigation, the following groups were compared: (a) standard SLT (15 sessions); (b) extended SLT (21 sessions); (c) SLT plus on-site transfer training (verbal prompts and social reinforcement at mealtime); (d) a social therapy control group (meetings with student companion therapists); and (e) a no-treatment control group. All three SLT groups showed greater improvement on target behaviors assessed in a standardized role-play and naturalistic interaction. The SLT plus on-site transfer training group was the most effective treatment group. This is one of the few group studies to assess the incremental benefits of *in vivo,* therapy enhancement procedures.

Field and Test (1975) investigated the benefit of receiving training on specific role-play situations later used for assessment purposes with two treatment groups composed of chronic schizophrenics. One group employed therapist and group feedback, discussion, modeling, rehearsal, reinforcement (social, token), and video playback with the same role plays on which the participants were evaluated. The other group received the same program without training on the role-play situations used for assessment. Greater improvement on behavioral measures of compliance, response latency, and disruptive pauses was found for the group receiving training on the role-play situations used for evaluation, suggesting limited generalization of skills to untrained scenes in the second group that did not receive exposure to these situations. Although no formal measures of generalization to novel settings were obtained, a 10-month follow-up revealed the maintenance of all gains in four of five patients in the first training group. Moreover, it was reported that none of the patients had been hospitalized, that nine patients had been living independently, and that eight patients were employed at 6-month follow-up. It must be added, however, that patients were exposed to different treatments once social skills training was completed.

Additional group training programs have provided more extensive evaluation of the efficacy of treatment while reporting certain procedural innovations. Psychiatrically hospitalized Viet Nam veterans participated in a novel program designed to train interpersonal responses to problem situations initially generated by the group involving assertion, heterosocial interaction, and job interview skills (Clark, 1975). Before the program began, the veterans gave preliminary responses to these situations that were evaluated in terms of social competence by persons in their immediate environment. The training program consisted of coaching, modeling, rehearsal, and feedback, and its content included those responses that had been judged highest in social competence. Compared to a dynamic role-play and didactic lecture control group, participants in the training program reported greater improvements on all training situations, which was confirmed by behavioral role-play measures of the training situations and on three of four categories of untrained situations. In an interaction with a female confederate, the training group was rated as more socially skilled, attractive, involving, and appropriate. At discharge, 11 of 12 training participants were employed, compared to 7 of 12 in each of the control groups. Two patients in the training group and 5 from each of the control groups were described as recidivists at 1-year follow-up.

Doty (1975) compared social skills training (instructions, role playing, feedback), an incentive condition (monetary payoff for social interaction), and a combined skills training incentive group, with nonspecific and no-treatment control groups. The incentive groups showed greatest change in ward behavior observations and in behavioral observations of social responsiveness during a group discussion (e.g., silences, responses to questions), which was suggestive of generalization of skills use across settings. No follow-up data were presented to shed light on the maintenance of these skills. The author's thorough description of the methodology employed facilitates an accurate appraisal of the integrity of this training program.

Finch and Wallace (1977) described a program for 16 nonassertive schizophrenics consisting of modeling both appropriate and inappropriate behaviors, rehearsal, instructions and coaching, and group as well as individual feedback. In addition, patients were trained in "attention-focusing" skills, and dyads were formed and given *in vivo* homework assignments to complete in order to enhance training effectiveness. In comparison to a matched control group, subjects in the interpersonal skills group exhibited greater improvement on behavioral measures of voice volume, fluency, latency, eye contact, and content, and they rated themselves as more assertive on the Wolpe–Lazarus Questionnaire. Moreover, the effects of training generalized to a series of untrained and inpromptu role-play scenarios. Two additional findings merit discussion in highlighting the beneficial impact of the program. Nursing staff reported improvements in grooming and social interaction on the ward. Moreover, five of the eight patients in the training program were discharged within 3 months, compared to only one patient in the control condition. Of five patients available for follow-up evaluation, three were employed, and one was in a vocational training program.

A similar program by Williams, Turner, Watts, Bellack, and Hersen (1977) provides further information regarding the generalized effects of a group training program as well as its cost-effectiveness. Four chronic schizophrenics received instructions, rehearsal, modeling, feedback, and verbal reinforcement. Using a multiple-baseline across-behaviors design, the authors observed sequential improvements on trained role plays in behavioral measures of eye contact, number of words, appropriate intonation, smiles, and physical gestures, and in ratings of overall assertiveness. Only moderate generalized training effects were obtained on untrained and novel role-play situations, and no follow-up data were reported. Regarding cost-effectiveness, it was concluded that a group training program requires 70% less treatment time (i.e., only 30 hours over 10 weeks) than is required by an individual training program.

In summary, the aforementioned investigations highlight the clinical utility of assertive and general social skills training with psychiatric populations. Dramatic improvements in targeted skills were observed in most studies and were reflected in overall changes in judged assertiveness and social competence. Further, generalization of training to extratherapy contexts and situations was documented in certain studies, although such measures were generally neglected in early studies.

Other Applications

Extensions of the skills training model to nonpsychiatric populations have recently been reported that have incorporated many of the procedures described herein in a group format. Rimm (1977) described a group assertion training program for the treatment of antisocial aggression that emphasized modeling rehearsal, group feedback, and social reinforcement. Although he did not report specific data, the author provided a coherent theoretical approach to and rationale for a group training format for problems involving anger expressiveness and aggression. Group skills training involving modeling, role playing, feedback, and homework assignments has also been applied with hospitalized male arsonists (Rice & Chaplin, 1979). In this study, two groups of patients received skills training and nondirective group psychotherapy in counterbalanced order. In comparison to group psychotherapy, the skills training program effected significant improvements on behavioral role-play assessment measures. Although formal measures of generalization were not obtained, no further firesetting incidents were reported for any patient at 1-year follow-up. A comparable program for male adult offenders residing in a state correctional facility resulted in increased effectiveness on training and generalization items in an interpersonal behavior role-play test compared to a wait-list control group (Bornstein, Winegardner, Rychatrik, Paul, Naifeh, Sweeney, & Justman, 1979).

Group social skills training has most recently been applied in the area of behavioral medicine. Dunn, van Horn, and Herman (1980) developed a program consisting of lectures, role playing, group and videotape feedback, and discussion to teach alternative interpersonal responses to spinal cord injury patients. Compared to control and educational-film-only groups, the skills training group was effective in increasing noncompliance to unreasonable requests and overall assertiveness. However, no generalization or follow-up data were reported. Similar results have been reported by Chaney, O'Leary, and Marlatt (1978) with a group of chronic alcoholics; participants in a skills training group involving instructions, modeling, rehearsal, and coaching showed greater improvement on a verbal situational competency test and a lower rate of relapse than a control group, and these improvements were maintained at 1-year follow-up. Finally, smoking modification groups emphasizing modeling and discussion have trained both actively smoking and at-risk adolescents to resist those social pressures that encourage polydrug use (McAlister, Perry, Killen, Slinkard, & Maccoby, 1980; Perry, Killen, Telch, Slinkard, & Danaher, 1980). After learning several interpersonal coping skills, participants in such schoolwide group programs have reported significant reductions in smoking incidence relative to controls, which have been confirmed by reduced carbon monoxide levels. These few programs suggest the feasibility and potential utility of group programs for the remediation of other medical problems.

Critique of Research

In summary, the overall findings from the studies reviewed here provide empirical documentation of the efficacy of group social skills training programs in facilitating the acquistion of a more effective interpersonal repertoire. Various psychiatric as well as medical patient populations have benefited from such programs. Nevertheless, methodological inadequacies preclude deriving any firm conclusions regarding the specific outcomes and long-term benefits associated with skills training programs.

One major limitation involves the assessment procedures employed to evaluate skills deficits (see Bellack, 1983). Several studies and early clinical reports failed to provide an objective, performance-based evaluation of the patients' relative strengths and weaknesses prior to training, or included only self-report data to establish treatment effectiveness (Bloomfield, 1973; Lomont *et al.*, 1969). In certain studies, the psychometric adequacy of assessment measures was not established (Booream & Flowers, 1972). Consequently, the utility of this assessment information in identifying skills deficits and empirically illustrating the effects of training have not been clearly determined. Future training efforts must establish empirically obtained improvements to support claims of therapeutic potency.

A comparable practical limitation deals with the fact that early studies trained participants in a restricted range of component skills. As the knowledge and empirical base of social skills curricula is refined and extended, a more diverse array of skillful behaviors will be required to ensure the comprehensiveness of training programs. The assessment of treatment gains obviously will be greatly facilitated through the use of validated evaluation procedures, such as the behavior-analytic model (Goldfried & D'Zurilla, 1969) and multiple component behaviors targeted for modification. By using a range of skills for measurement purposes, training programs can proceed sequentially across relevant behaviors both within and across participants, thereby permitting the demonstration of experimental control in terms of functional effectiveness at the level of the individual (Eisler *et al.*, 1978). The expanded focus of training will most likely result in more sufficient and enduring treatment outcomes.

A third concern involves transfer of training effects. Numerous investigators have reported moderate generalization of learned skills to untrained role-play situations, simulated or staged interactions, hospital wards, or naturalistic situations outside the hospital (Finch & Wallace, 1977; Trower *et al.*, 1978), although this information has not been routinely obtained. Subsequent research should be directed toward enhancing and empirically documenting the generalization of training effects as well as developing naturalistic measures of *in vivo* performance. *In vivo* therapy enhancement procedures have begun to receive therapeutic application in group (Finch & Wallace, 1977; Falloon *et al.*, 1977; Gutride *et al.*, 1974) and individual programs (Matson & Zeiss, 1979). Recent work by Firth, Schneider, Conger, & Higbee (1981) has also been helpful in addressing the psychometric adequacy of naturalistic assessments with heterosocially unskilled college students, which may be of relevance to programs for psychiatric patients. The fact that greater attention is being paid to extratherapy assessment and training suggests that generalization across settings (e.g., on the ward, in the therapy situation) and people (e.g., confederates, spouses) will continue to serve as one of the principal indications of training effectiveness.

The long-term benefits associated with skills training programs also deserve more rigorous empirical evaluation. Although follow-up data are thus far encouraging, very few studies have reported formal follow-up assessments for periods longer than 1 or 2 months posttreatment. As convincingly argued by Curran (1979), the assessment of the maintenance of treatment effects must become a priority in subsequent studies. Such research will aid in determining the length and conditions of follow-up and those follow-up measures that should be typically employed (e.g., relapse, rehospitalization). It is clear that program developers should be apprised of the impact of a training program on patient's psychosocial adjustment. Statements of this nature would shed light on the social validity and overall cost-effectiveness of a given program (Kazdin, 1977). In terms of clinical practice, maintenance effects might be facilitated if training is extended for longer periods of time and involves a wide range of training situations (Bellack, 1983). The inclusion of significant others during treatment may be one additional procedural innovation likely to enhance the impact of a treatment program.

Three additional considerations are in order. Subject selection procedures should clearly outline the inclusion and exclusion criteria of each sample studied, including control groups. This will permit more conclusive statements regarding the specificity of treatment effects for specific subject populations. Along with a clearer description of subject selection procedures, investigators should describe in greater detail the characteristics of their programs, such as the number of sessions, session duration, therapist training, group assignment, and session content. Wide differences in these parametric variables may produce differential effects on performance that could obscure accurate comparisons across studies. As but one example of this diversity, the number of treatment sessions represented herein has varied from 4 (Doty, 1975) to 30 (Williams *et al.*, 1977). Other procedural differences would certainly compound the difficulty inherent in drawing accurate conclusions based on this research literature.

A final issue concerns the specification of treatment procedures under the general rubric of *social skills training*. Various component procedures have been described across studies and, in many cases, without sufficient detail. Inadequate descriptions may not permit the conduct of needed experimental evaluations of individual procedures. In addition to verification of the validity of such procedures, of particular importance is the development of a skills training technology to assist in the standardization of training protocols and the procedures upon which the social skills model is based. A systematic skills training program refined across treatment outcome studies would begin to address the need for a standardized skills training technology that has only just begun to realize its therapeutic potential.

A Programmatic Model

Patient Population and Referral Process

Having reviewed the group social skills training literature that has been conducted with psychiatric patients, let us now turn our attention to the social skills training program that we have developed over the past 7 years at the Providence VA Medical Center.

The patients served by our training program are typically either hospitalized patients or outpatients participating in our Day Hospital Program. The patients who participate in this program are not selected on the basis of diagnostic category. Rather, they are considered for our skills training groups on the basis of a recommendation from the clinical treatment team, irrespective of the patient's diagnosis. Though there may be advantages to assigning patients to skills groups on the basis of diagnostic criteria, patient flow through our treatment units to date has precluded our assigning patients to treatment groups on this basis.

Upon referral, all patients are given a standard interview (Monti, 1983) by a member of our staff who is likely to be one of the group co-therapists. The interview is initially focused on building rapport with the patient and getting a social/developmental history. Another major focus is on the particular strengths and deficits of each candidate. Careful attention is paid to situational factors that seem to influence the patient's skills level. Extensive notes are taken during this interview, and a standard format is followed. Although the social skills interview is only a small part of a larger assessment protocol (see Curran, 1982, for details concerning our assessment battery), it is nonetheless a very important part of the process of conducting a social skills training program.

Therapists

The co-therapists who lead our groups are highly trained and are closely supervised. A series of therapist training videotapes as well as a training manual provide the basis for therapist training. Although every attempt is made to have opposite-sex co-therapists lead a particular group, an equally important matching variable is the experience level of the co-therapist regarding skills training. All potential co-therapists, regardless of general level of clinical sophistication, observe at least one complete group prior to serving as co-therapist. Following therapist training and group observation, novice therapists are always paired with more senior therapists while leading their first few groups.

Although most of our therapists have held advanced degrees in psychology, we have extended our training program to interested members of our nursing staff. The incorporation of nursing staff into our therapist training program has enhanced the relationship between our clinical units and our research team. Furthermore, it has facilitated the referral of patients, provided for better continuity of care, and at the same time has been very cost-effective. In addition, as has been anecdotally reported in other areas of clinical research, the introduction of our research program to our clinical units has improved the overall quality of care received by our patients, and the incorporation of clinical staff into our program has facilitated this effect.

The use of co-thearpists in our groups has worked well for several reasons. In addition to providing a training opportunity for the less experienced therapists, each co-therapist alternates between two distinct roles. In any given session, one therapist is responsible for presenting the content of the day's lesson, whereas the other therapist is responsible for attending to group dynamics and serving as a role-play partner. The therapists switch roles on alternate days so that the group members become comforable with therapists in either role. The fact that the co-therapists are of opposite sexes makes sex-relevant role plays more realistic. Finally, the use of two therapists insures continuity of treatment when one of the therapists cannot be at a particular session.

Format Characteristics: Program Structure

Each group session is followed by a debriefing session during which the co-therapists review the group. Group supervisors sit in on sessions at least weekly and meet with the co-therapists for an extended debriefing session at this time. Co-therapists are in regular daily contact with patients' ward or day hospital treatment teams. This contact is either in the form of a progress note or attendance at staff meetings. Such frequent contact insures the timeliness of relevant clinical information while at the same time fostering the relationship between the clinical and research teams.

Our social skills training groups usually run for 1 hour daily, 5 days per week, for 4 consecutive weeks. For several reasons, this schedule has worked well for both our inpatient and day hospital populations. By conducting sessions on a daily basis, patients are able to complete homework assignments that constitue an important component of our program. Inpatients typically do assignments with either nursing staff, visitors, or other patients. Day hospital patients usually practice homework assignments when they return home in the evening. The 3 weekends that bridge the treatment weeks provide additional extended opportunities for homework completion. For inpatients who receive weekend passes, the weekends provide a unique opportunity to practice assignments out of the hospital environment.

An additional advantage of scheduling daily sessions is the continuity it provides both with respect to the content of the program and the patients' schedules of other treatment activities. We typically start a new group on the first Monday of every month, having found that the predictability that this schedule offers the various treatment teams that refer patients to us has resulted in an increase in referrals to our groups.

As is evident from the description of our training program thus far, we feel that it is very important that the training groups, co-therapists, and research team in general are well integrated into the clinical activities and daily routine of the clinical unit that the group serves. Though initially requiring much careful negotiation and flexibility with nursing staff, unit chiefs, and hospital administrators, the successful functioning of our program has made the initial time an effort well invested.

Component Procedures

Having presented descriptions of our patient population, referral system, co-therapists, and basic program structure, we will now summarize the basic component procedures that constitute our skills training program. Although most procedures are used in every session, as has been described in detail elsewhere (Monti, Corriveau, & Curran, 1982), for illustrative purposes we will use an example of the first training session to demonstrate what the basic procedures are and how they may be employed.

A description of the first training session would be incomplete without mentioning a *group-building* exercise with which we routinely begin this session. After introductions between patients and co-therapists, the co-therapists make several general comments outlining that the major objectives of social skills training will be to increase the participants' social competencies in interpersonal situations. Next, the co-therapists introduce the notion that the group itself is an interpersonal situation that will serve as a forum for skills training work to be done during the program. This notion sets the stage for the group-building exercise that usually consists of the therapists going around the group circle assigning the letters *A* or *B* alternately to each member, starting with one therapist. Next, the therapists request that during the following 5 minutes each person assigned the letter *A* initiate a conversation with his or her *B*-lettered neighbor. It is further explained that the major purpose of this conversation is for Person A to get to know Person B so that he can share something interesting about Person B with the rest of the group. After 5 minutes, *A* and *B* partners are asked to reverse roles, and the procedure is repeated. After the second 5-minute interaction, each Person A is asked to share something interesting about his or her partner with the members of the group. *B*-lettered partners immediately follow their respective *A*-partner's report. The *A*-lettered co-therapist leads off by reporting on the first *B*-lettered patient, and the procedure is followed until all *A-B* partnerships have reported.

This group exercise serves several very useful functions. Most importantly, it helps the group members get to know each other as well as their therapists in the context of what usually turns out to be a fun experience. The group-building function that this exercise serves is an often underemphasized aspect of conducting group social skills training. We feel that the group process that is set in motion through this exercise is a key aspect of doing skills training in a group setting and, to the extent that this exercise accomplishes this goal, it will set a positive tone for the many exercises and/or role plays that follow.

Another important point that is made on the basis of this exercise relates to the interpersonal nature of what the group is all about. The turn-taking and information-gathering aspects of the interaction, which are modeled by the *A*-therapist, set the stage for the modeling and role playing that are so heavily emphasized in later sessions. Indeed, this exercise is the first simple modeling exercise in the group. More complex modeling usually follows at some later point when the co-therapists may be attempting to contrast several different ways of handling a given situation.

An important feature of group social skills training that is related to the group interaction aspect mentioned previously is that group training may have some benefits that go beyond individual skills training. Apart from the obvious savings in therapists' time and effort, group training offers greater opportunities for behavioral modeling that is likely to provide the opportunity for vicarious learning (Upper & Ross, 1977). Indeed, as Upper and Ross (1977) point out with respect to behavioral groups in general, group situations may also offer unique opportunities through which generalization can be facilitated because of differences among the patients with whom any members can practice alternative ways of responding. These authors further note that additional benefits derived from a group situation are the increased opportunity for social reinforcement and motivational stimulation. They state:

> Just as group pressure motivates the client to attempt new behaviors, group approval serves as a powerful reinforcer of those behaviors, further increasing the probability that it will be repeated and will generalize to other situations. (p. 153)

There are other important benefits derived from the group situation. To the extent that other patients in the group have had similar experiences in social situations, this is likely to promote empathy and to facilitate communication. Another benefit is that in a group setting there is a greater availability of ideas and perspectives as to how to approach problem social situations. Indeed, patients' suggestions may have greater social validity than those of the therapists in that patients may share more common experiences. An additional point is that in a group setting patients get *in vivo* practice in some aspects of the treatment package. One example may be in giving and receiving criticism through role-play feedback. In general, the conduct of social skills training in a group context makes much sense from both a conceptual and practical point of view.

The important components of *reinforcement* and *shaping* may be illustrated by the group-building exercise mentioned previously. Therapists selectively reinforce (with praise) those aspects of a patient's response that are directed at the target question (i.e., those comments that reveal something interesting about one's partner) and do not reinforce irrelevant or misdirected comments. The selective application of reinforcement (shaping) is as critical in the initial stages of skills training as it is in any other learning situation. However, it is important that the major objective of the therapist is to encourage participation during this first exercise. Shaping appropriateness should be of secondary importance and special care should be taken not to punish any patient who is struggling to at least say something.

Patient responsiveness to this first exercise provides the co-therapists with valuable baseline data on both patients involved in each interaction. These data are of particular importance and should help the therapists in setting goals and objectives for each participant. The use of observational data collected in session is an important focal point of the postgroup debriefing.

A major treatment component and one that features prominently in the first session is that of *information*, or *instruction*. Information is presented through live role plays and discussions and on written forms or "handouts," blackboards, or videotapes. Though the type of information being presented may govern the manner of presentation, the same information is sometimes presented in several different ways. One example of information presented in the first session is the distinction between *assertive*, *aggressive*, and *passive* behavior. Information relevant to these three response styles is first presented in the context of three role plays involving the same situation. The co-therapists first model a passive, then an aggressive, and finally an assertive response to a particular interpersonal situation. Each role play is followed by group discussion that is prompted by the co-therapists. Every attempt is made to incorporate as many patients as possible in this feedback process. The labels for the three response styles are written on the blackboard and also appear on handouts that the patients are encouraged to take with them when they leave the session.

Although the use of videotaped instruction or information is usually not possible during our first session due to time limitations, an example of its use in our groups might involve different role models enacting each response style (passive, aggressive, and assertive) in a situation other than that portrayed by the co-therapists. The use of videotaped instructions or information offers several advantages when compared to instruction by live models. One such advantage is the standardization that it offers beyond that obtainable with live models. Another advantage, most salient on days when the co-therapists are particularly busy in session, is that it gives the therapists somewhat of a break. Finally, videotaped instructions are particularly useful when one therapist must lead the group alone. On the negative side, video instruction can be somewhat confusing. This is especially likely if the material is presented either too technically or too rapidly. To counteract this potentially negative effect, we present relatively short video segments and follow them up with additional information and coaching by our therapists. Careful monitoring of patients' reception of information is especially important when using videotaped instruction.

The *modeling* procedure that is involved in demonstrating passive, aggressive, and assertive response styles during our first session is very representative of that that occurs throughout our training program. Modeling is used whenever a new skill is introduced to the group. Contrasting response styles (e.g., assertive vs. aggressive) are demonstrated, and their respective consequences are discussed. As mentioned before, videotaped role-play models may be used to give patients exposure to models other than the co-therapists. When live modeling is done, therapists usually model behaviors with each other, and then they pair up with different patients. After modeling a particular set of behaviors, therapists and patients do a role reversal, and the patient is expected to perform in the role just played by the therapist. Based on the patient's performance, additional modeling may be done on the same situation.

Practice or behavioral rehearsal is employed after patients have been given information and modeling on a particular skill. Initially, rehearsal is done between therapist and patient until patients learn the technique. These initial behavioral rehearsals are done on prepared role plays. After the behavioral rehearsal technique is learned, patients are encouraged to practice with each other while receiving feedback from the therapists. Ultimately, the technique of behavioral rehearsal is done with situations that are particularly relevant to a given patient. Indeed, patients are encouraged to develop their own situationally relevant role plays. These are first conducted with co-therapists and then with other patients. Though the technique of behavioral rehearsal is discussed in the context of the first session, the quantity of information presented usually precludes the conduct of any rehearsals. Subsequent sessions devote a large proportion of time to role plays. Besides providing practice, these role plays also provide opportunities for observational learning from a coping model perspective.

Homework is a component procedure that is emphasized throughout our training program. It is the vehicle through which skills learned in session are practiced in the "natural environment." We feel that the generalization of our treatment effects can be most enhanced through the use of homework. The groundwork for delineating the role that homework plays in our program is firmly laid during the first session. The concept of homework is described, and its relevance for our training program is explained. Though this description occurs at the end of the first session, therapists are encouraged to leave adequate time to insure that the importance of doing homework is understood. Following these general comments, the homework assignment for the first session is clearly presented. Homework sheets are distributed, the assignment is explained in detail, and questions are solicited and answered.

With the exception of the first session, the first 15 minutes of every session are spent reviewing the previous homework sheets. The therapists then go around the room asking each patient to summarize his or her particular experience in doing (or not doing) the assignment. Patients are always reinforced for having attempted a particular assignment, regardless of the outcome. If a patient has not done the homework, the circumstances surrounding his or her not doing it are discussed, and alternative solutions as to how it might get done in the future are suggested. At the discretion of the co-therapists, the patient who has not done the assignment may be asked to do it in the group session itself.

Homework sheets or handouts provide both a written summary of the assignment and a place where patients are expected to write a brief written response. These sheets seem to serve both as a discriminative stimulus for doing the assignment and a way for therapists to check and see if patients at least attempted a written response. Upon completion of the homework review, all homework sheets are collected and filed by the therapists.

As mentioned earlier, patients are encouraged to do their assignments in their natural environment, that is, either at home or work when possible, or on their clinical units. Patients' reports of these experiences provide therapists with much information that is utilized in further identifying patients' strengths and weaknesses. Practicing social skills in a group setting is very different from performing in the real world, and homework assignments are designed to help bridge this gap.

Another technique that we have developed to promote transfer of training is that of *adjunct role playing*. Adjunct role players (ARPs) are individuals, other than the co-therapists, who are brought into the group for the primary purpose of providing new and different people for the patients to practice with. Whenever possible we use therapists-in-training as ARPs, thereby serving both their need to observe and the patients' need to practice with different models. So as to minimize confusion, we do not introduce ARPs until after the third session. Although we have no data on the subject, we feel that the more similar the ARP is to the significant others in the patient's environment, the more likely is the transfer of training to those individuals.

Content of Training Curriculum

As we have previously mentioned, our treatment groups typically run for 20 sessions. Accordingly, we have developed a treatment manual that parallels this structure. Our manual consists of 10 lessons in addition to the introductory session previously described. Each lesson deals with specific skills and is the subject of approximately two sessions. Because we have recently presented the basic skills discussed in each chapter elsewhere (Monti *et al.* 1982), here we will merely present an outline of the lesson titles followed by a detailed example of how our therapists progress through a representative lesson.

An outline of our lesson titles that reflects the basic skills taught in our program can be found in Table 2. As is evident from this table, we cover a wide range of material in our treatment program. The content of the manual has evolved over our years of clinical experience with several different patient populations. These have included both in- and outpatients at the Providence VA Medical Center as well as inpatients at a private psychiatric hospital here in Providence. In addition, the social skills training literature for psychiatric patients (e.g., Hersen, 1979) has been an important influence on what is and is not included in our treatment program. Because we agree with Goldsmith and McFall (1975) that the content of treatment is extremely important, our training manual has undergone several revisions over the years of experience using it.

Each training lesson has a basic theme as is reflected in its title. After discussing the importance of a particular theme, with respect to its impact on the patient's general functioning and satisfaction, therapists discuss relevant aspects of the behavior(s) to be covered. An important part of the rationale for any lesson is to tie in skill with overall adjustment. For example, it may be pointed out that by increasing skill, one may make friends more easily and thereby decrease loneliness and boredom, while at the same time increasing self-esteem and feeling good. The connection between skill and general functioning is made in a nonthreatening fashion by using positive examples.

Let us take Lesson 1, Starting Conversations, as an example of how a lesson is conducted. In the first session on this lesson therapists talk about the importance of choosing a good time and place to start a conversation with someone. Several examples are given as to what is meant by a good time and place.

When the therapists judge that the patients have understood this concept, they move on to a discussion of relevant topics for starting conversations. As is the case with much of the content of our training manual, many patients have misconceptions about what are good topics for starting conversations. Many patients feel that they do not have anything "intelligent" to talk about and that "small talk" is stupid and boring. Some time is usually spent on clarifying the

TABLE 2. Lessons of the Social Skills Training Manual

Lesson 1:	Starting conversation
Lesson 2:	Nonverbal behaviors
Lesson 3:	Giving and receiving compliments
Lesson 4:	Negative thoughts and self-statements
Lesson 5:	Giving criticism
Lesson 6:	Receiving criticism
Lesson 7:	Listening skills and "feeling talk"
Lesson 8:	Being assertive in business situations
Lesson 9:	Close relationships
Lesson 10:	Intimate relationships

role of small talk in starting conversations. A very workable aspect about patient-generated beliefs such as these is that because they come from the group members the patients are usually interested and motivated to discuss them.

Following what usually turns out to be a lively discussion about how to start a conversation, the therapists introduce the issue of self-disclosure in interpersonal interactions. The major point here is that the level of self-disclosure should be governed by the nature of the relationship. In starting a conversation with a stranger, too much self-disclosure could be problematic. On the other hand, aloofness should be avoided at the other extreme. This point is usually followed by modeling by the therapists on starting conversations. Because we want to emphasize the importance of the nature of the relationship and how this interacts with other points to be remembered in starting a conversation, clearly setting the context for the role plays is very important here.

After several successful role plays or modeling scenes demonstrating successful conversations, the therapists model what can happen when one uses closed-ended statements in conversations, and then this is discussed by the group. Finally, the therapists roleplay various ways of ending a conversation.

After description and/or modeling of each of the preceding points, the main lesson topics are summarized and written on the blackboard as follows:

1. Choosing a good time and place
2. The appropriateness of the topic
3. The role of self-disclosure
4. The pitfalls of using closed-ended statements
5. The importance of how one ends a conversation

Following the presentation of this outline, the therapists model another conversational interaction, this time incorporating all of the preceding elements. A discussion of the performance and review of the points follows immediately. Depending on how the patients appear to be incorporating the material (as determined by questions and answers), what follows next are either patient–therapist or patient–patient role plays modeled after those demonstrated by the therapists.

These role plays are videotaped and immediately played back to the group for evaluation and feedback. Special care is taken to direct attention to those lesson elements that the patients incorporated into their performance. A particular role play may be repeated and videotaped several times until the therapists and patients are satisfied with the performance. Reinforcement and constructive feedback are solicited from the group members.

As is the case with the first session of most lessons, relatively few patient role plays are conducted before the therapists must stop to discuss the homework assignment for that night. For Session 1, the homework usually involves the patients starting conversations both with someone they know and a stranger. Homework sheets are distributed, and questions are entertained before patients leave the session.

Session 2 of all lessons starts with a review of the previous night's homework assignment. As was previously discussed, a major objective here is to reinforce those patients who have at least attempted the assignment. Those patients who may not have completed the assignment serve as the first role players of the day by conducting their assignments in sessions. In reviewing the work of all the patients, both those who completed the homework out of session and those who did not, the therapists can evaluate the performance of all participants on a given content area. The majority of Session 2 is spent on roleplaying with all group members participating. Special emphasis is given to those patients whom the therapists identify as being in need of more role-play practice. By the end of Session 2 of any lesson, all patients should have had some videotaped role-play experience on that lesson. Indeed, role playing followed by video and group feedback is the most salient treatment component of the second session of all treatment lessons, and its importance cannot be overemphasized.

Treatment Outcome

Given the philosophy we share with Paul (1969) that good treatment demands good assessment, we have invested much time and energy over the years into the evaluation of our social skills training program. This evaluation has taken the form of several treatment outcome studies (e.g., De Lancey, 1979; Monti, Curran, Corriveau, De Lancey, & Hagerman, 1980; Monti, Fink, Norman, Curran, Hayes, & Caldwell, 1979). Because a review and synthesis of these studies and others from our treatment outcome group have recently been done elsewhere (Monti *et al.*, 1982), we will not present a detailed review here. Rather, we will highlight some of the more salient aspects of our treatment outcome research program.

Because the development of our treatment outcome research has paralleled not only the development and refinement of our basic treatment program but also the development of our social skills and social anxiety assessment technology (e.g., Curran, 1982; Monti, Wallander, Ahern, Abrams, & Munroe, 1983), the tests of our treatment program have become more rigorous from an experimental design perspective over time. For example, our first treatment outcome study merely compared our skills training package to the "typical outpatient treatment" usually received by patients in the Mental Hygiene Clinic (Monti *et al.*, 1982). Although patients were randomly assigned to either treatment groups or to routine individual treatment, this study's design clearly did not control for variables such as therapist and/or group contact time. In another study (Monti *et al.*, 1980), after we had suggestive evidence that our basic treatment was effective, we introduced proper control procedures for both therapist and contact time. In the context of this more sophisticated design we, once again, demonstrated the efficacy of our skills training program.

The development of our level of sophistication in asking questions about our treatment program is also reflected along another dimension of complexity. This has involved asking questions relevant to whether adding or subtracting components to and from our basic treatment program makes for differential treatment effectiveness. For example, in one study (Monti *et al.*, 1979) we determined that group contact was a significant component above and beyond simply presenting patients with instruction. In another study (De Lancey, 1979), one of our colleagues demonstrated that the addition of a cognitive covert reinforcement procedure did not enhance social skills. Our basic treatment program, as described earlier, reflects what has "tested out" as being the best general "package" that we have developed to date.

Overall, the results of our treatment outcome studies have suggested that our basic treatment program is effective as measured by pre- and posttreatment comparisons of experimental and control groups. Such comparisons have usually been made on both self-report and behavioral measures of social skills and social anxiety. Indeed, the use of one particular behavioral assessment measure of the skills and anxiety constructs has been a kind of hallmark of our program. This assessment instrument, known as the Simulated Social Interaction Test (SSIT), is basically a behavioral role-play test. Curran (1982) reviews several studies conducted in our laboratory that document the reliability and validity of the SSIT. Results on our treatment outcome studies have routinely shown significant improvement on both the SSIT and on a variety of self-report measures (Monti *et al.*, 1979; Monti *et al.*, 1980).

Another finding consistent across our treatment studies is that treatment effects seem to be holding up for at least as long as we have systematically measured them. Our follow-up periods across several studies have ranged from 6 to 24 months. Although the assessment measures we used at follow-up have somewhat depended on the aims of a particular study, we have systematically used the SSIT across studies and have found that improvement on this measure has been maintained at follow-up for both anxiety and social skills indexes (Monti *et al.*, 1980).

We have also been very concerned about assessing the generalization of the effects of our treatment. As pointed out earlier, we attempt to systematically program transfer of training through the use of adjunct role players and extensive use of homework assignments. On the assessment side of the generalization problem, we have attempted to measure transfer of training both within our role-play test and through more naturalistic measures. In the context of role plays, we studied performance on both trained (role plays that have been practiced in groups) and untrained role plays. We have also studied performance in an *in vivo* generalization task as well as on a structured interview given at follow-up (the Clinical Outcome Criteria Scale; Strauss & Carpenter, 1972). This structured interview is designed to study outcome variables such as quality and number of social relationships, employment history, job satisfaction, and so forth. In general, we found that our treatment effects did significantly generalize to some extent, particularly when measured by untrained role-play scenes and by the Clinical Outcome Criteria Scale. Although we have been encouraged by the apparent generalization that our treatment seems to have, we are not yet satisfied, and we continue to work at studying both the generalization of our treatment effects and the generalizability of our assessment measures (e.g., Curran, 1982; Monti *et al.*, 1983).

Conclusions

The group social skills training research that we have just summarized has attempted to study the efficacy of this type of group treatment with a heterogeneous group of skills deficient psychiatric patients. A stength of this research is that the treatment program has remained essentially consistent across several studies, thus permitting comparisons to be made across studies as well as facilitating the use of the treatment program in other settings. This notion of the portability of our treatment program is especially important because, with one exception (Monti *et al.*, 1980), our program has been studied only with VA psychiatric patients. Though we are optimistic regarding the applicability of our treatment to other populations, further research is needed to substantiate this optimism.

In addition to consistently applying our basic treatment package, we have been equally systematic in using at least one consistent measure across treatment outcome studies, namely the SSIT. The systematic use of a behaviorally based assessment instrument in group training work is clearly the exception, not the rule. The use of the SSIT across treatment studies has enabled us further to develop this assessment instrument and to assess its psychometric properties (Monti, *et al.*, 1983) while at the same time allowing for cross-study comparisons.

Another hallmark of our treatment/research program has been the incorporation of both follow-up and generalization data. As pointed out in the first section of this chapter, systematic collection of these data is rare in most group skills training research programs. Though we have collected data on relatively long follow-up intervals, we feel that our follow-up intervals should be lengthened further and that greater effort should be expended on obtaining data on more of the original subjects at follow-up intervals. Perhaps we could learn something from our epidemiologically oriented colleagues with respect to collection and reporting of long-term follow-up data.

Although we have attempted to collect data reflecting the generalization of our treatment effects and have been somewhat satisfied with the results of these efforts, we feel that it would be productive to further program generalization into our treatment package. As mentioned earlier, the techniques of using adjunct role players and extensive homework assignments do seem to facilitate transfer of training. Consistent with the apparent effects of these techniques and with the recent suggestions of Scott, Himadi, and Keane (1984), we presently are conducting a pilot investigation to study the feasibility of working with family members themselves in the context of our skills groups. Though the logistical challenges of conducting such a skills group have been formidable, our clinical experience suggests that the incorporation of significant others has a major impact on both the group experience and treatment effectiveness. We are enthusiastic about the effects that such a treatment component might have with respect to promoting transfer of training and possibly enhancing the ultimate outcome of our treatment program.

In conclusion, the general literature on group social skills training provides considerable optimism for improving the social and interpersonal functioning of chronic psychiatric patients. A growing interest in this form of behavioral treatment has resulted in the development and continued refinement of a technology for evaluating and modifying one's social skills repertoire. However, the clinical relevance and empirical adequacy of research findings in the area have not been sufficiently demonstrated to permit firm conclusions. As reflected in the program model currently in use at the Providence VA Medical Center, greater attention should be paid to the development of comprehensive training curricula, methodologically sophisticated assessment measures, and strategies for the enhancement of generalization and maintenance of treatment gains. These advancements, we hope, will ensure utilization and evaluation of the most cost-effective behavioral group training programs.

ACKNOWLEDGMENT

The authors would like to thank Jody Binkoff for her helpful comments on an earlier draft of this chapter.

REFERENCES

Argyle, M., Trower, P., & Bryant B. Explorations in the treatment of personality disorders and neuroses by social skills training. *British Journal of Medical Psychology*, 1974, *47*, 63–72.

Ayllon, T., & Azrin, N. H. *The token economy: A motivational system for therapy and rehabilitation*. New York: Appleton-Century-Crofts, 1968.

Ayllon, T., & Haughton, E. The control of behaviour of schizophrenic patients by food. *Journal of the Experimental Analysis of Behavior*, 1962, *5*, 343–352.

Azrin, N., & Lindsley, O. The reinforcement of cooperation between children. *Journal of Abnormal and Social Psychology*, 1956, *52*, 100–102.

Barlow, D. H., Abel, G. G., Blanchard, E. B., Bristow, A. R., & Young, L. D. A heterosocial skills behavior checklist for males. *Behavior Therapy*, 1977, *8*, 229–239.

Bellack, A. S. Recurrent problems in the behavioral assessment of social skills. *Behaviour Research and Therapy*, 1983, *21*, 29–41.

Bellack, A. S., & Hersen, M. (Eds.). *Research and practice in social skills training*. New York: Plenum Press, 1979.

Bellack, A. S., Hersen, M., & Turner, S. M. Generalization effects of social skills training in chronic schizophrenics: An experimental analysis. *Behaviour Research and Therapy*, 1976, *14*, 391–398.

Bloomfield, H. H. Assertive training in an outpatient group of chronic schizophrenics: A preliminary report. *Behavior Therapy*, 1973, *4*, 277–281.

Booraem, C. D., & Flowers, J. V. Reduction of anxiety and personal space as a function of assertion training with severely disturbed neuro-psychiatric inpatients. *Psychological Reports*, 1972, *30*, 923–929.

Bornstein, P. H., Winegardner, J., Rychatrik, R. G., Paul, W. P., Nafeh, S. J., Sweeney, T. M., & Justman, A. Interpersonal skills training: Evaluation of a program with adult male offenders. *Criminal Justice and Behavior*, 1979, *6*, 119–132.

Chaney, E., O'Leary, M., & Marlatt, G. A. Skill training with alcoholics. *Journal of Consulting and Clinical Psychology*, 1978, *46*, 1092–1104.

Clark, K. W. Evaluation of a group social skills training program with psychiatric patients: Training Viet Nam era veterans in assertion, heterosexual, and job interview skills. (Doctoral Dissertation, University of Wisconsin-Madison, 1974). *Dissertation Abstracts International*, 1975, *35*, 4642B. (University Microfilms No. 74–28, 795)

Combs, M. L., & Slaby, D. A. Social-skills training with children. In B. B. Lahey & A. E. Kazdin (Eds.), *Advances in clinical child pychology* (Vol. 1). New York: Plenum Press, 1977.

Curran, J. P. Social skills: Methodological issues and future directions. In A. S. Bellack & M. Hersen (Eds.), *Research and practice in social skills training*. New York: Plenum Press, 1979.

Curran, J. P. A procedure for the assessment of social skills: The Simulated Social Interaction Test. In

J. P. Curran & P. M. Monti (Eds.), *Social skills training: A practical handbook for assessment and treatment*. New York: Guilford Press, 1982.

Curran, J. P. & Monti, P. M. (Eds.), *Social skills training: A practical handbook for assessment and treatment*. New York: Guilford Press, 1982.

De Lancey, A. *The effects of covert reinforcement and social skill training with psychiatric patients*. Unpublished doctoral dissertation, Boston College, 1979.

Doty, D. W. Role playing and incentives in the modification of the social interaction of chronic psychiatric patients. *Journal of Consulting and Clinical Psychology*, 1975, *43*, 676–682.

Dunn, M., Van Horn, E., & Herman, S. H. Social skills and spinal cord injury: A comparison of three training procedures. *Behavior Therapy*, 1980. *12*, 153–164.

Edelstein, B. A., & Eisler, R. M. Effects of modeling and modeling with instructions and feedback on the behavioral components of social skills. *Behavior Therapy*, 1976, *7*, 382–389.

Eisler, R. M. The behavioral assessment of social skills. In M. Hersen & A. S. Bellack (Eds.). *Behavioral assessment: A practical handbook*. New York: Pergamon Press, 1976.

Eisler, R. M., & Frederiksen, L. W. *Perfecting social skills: A guide to interpersonal behavior development*. New York: Plenum Press, 1980.

Eisler, R. M., Hersen, M., & Miller, P. M. Effects of modeling on components of assertive behavior. *Journal of Behavior Therapy and Experimental Psychiatry*, 1973, *4*, 1–6.

Eisler, R. M., Miller, P. M., & Hersen, M. Components of assertive behavior. *Journal of Clinical Psychology*, 1973, *29*, 295–299.

Eisler, R. M., Hersen, M., & Miller, P. M. Shaping components of assertiveness with instructions and feedback. *American Journal of Psychiatry*, 1974, *131*, 1344–1347.

Eisler, R. M., Blanchard, E. B., Fitts, H., & Williams, J. G. Social skill training with and without modeling on schizophrenic and non-psychotic hospitalized psychiatric patients. *Behavior Modification*, 1978, *2*, 147–172.

Falloon, I. R. H., Lindley, P., McDonald, R., & Marks, I. M. Social skills training of out-patient groups: A controlled study of rehearsal and homework. *British Journal of Psychiatry*, 1977, *131*, 599–609.

Field, G. D., & Test, M. A. Group assertive training for severely disturbed patients. *Journal of Behavior Therapy and Experimental Psychiatry*, 1975, *6*, 129–134.

Finch, B. E., & Wallace, C. J. Successful interpersonal skills training with schizophrenic inpatients. *Journal of Consulting and Clinical Psychology*, 1977, *45*, 885–890.

Firth, E. A., Schneider, P. A., Conger, J. C., & Higbee, G. H. *An exploration of naturalistic interactions for the assessment of heterosocial skills*. Paper presented at the Annual Meeting of the Association for Advancement of Behavior Therapy, Toronto, 1981.

Frank, J. D. Therapeutic components of psychotherapy: A 25-year progress report of research. *Journal of Nervous and Mental Disease*, 1974, *159*, 325–342.

Freedman, B. J., Rosenthal, L., Donahoe, C. P., Schlundt, D. G. & McFall, R. M. A social behavioral analysis of skill deficits in delinquent and nondelinquent adolescent boys. *Journal of Consulting and Clinical Psychology*, 1978, *46*, 1448–1462.

Gladwin, T. Social competence and clinical practice. *Psychiatry*, 1974, *30*, 30–43.

Goldfried, M. R., & D'Zurilla, T. J. A behavioral-analytic model for assessing competence. In C. D. Spielberger (Ed.), *Current topics in clinical psychology* (Vol. 1). New York: Academic Press, 1969.

Goldsmith, J. B., & McFall, R. M. Development and evaluation of an interpersonal skill-training program for psychiatric inpatients. *Journal of Abnormal Psychology*, 1975, *84*, 51–58.

Goldstein, A. P. *Structured learning therapy*. New York: Academic Press, 1973.

Goldstein, A., Martens, J., Hubben, J., van Belle, H., Schaaf, W., Wiersma, H., & Goedhart, A. The use of modeling to increase independent behavior. *Behaviour Research and Therapy*, 1973, *11*, 31–42.

Gutride, M. E., Goldstein, A. P., & Hunter, G. F. The use of modeling and role playing to increase social interaction among asocial psychiatric patients. *Journal of Consulting and Clinical Psychology*, 1973, *40*, 408–415.

Gutride, A., Goldstein, A., Hunter, G., Carroll, S., Clark, L., Furia, R., & Lower, W. Structured Learning Therapy with transfer training for chronic inpatients. *Journal of Clinical Psychology*, 1974, *30*, 277–279.

Heimberg, R. G., Montgomery, D., Madsen, C. H., & Heinberg, J. S. Assertion training: A review of the literature. *Behavior Therapy*, 1977, *8*, 953–971.
Hersen, M. Modification of skill deficits in psychiatric patients. In A. S. Bellack & M. Hersen (Eds.), *Research and practice in social skills training*. New York: Plenum Press, 1979.
Hersen, M., & Bellack, A. S. Social skills training for chronic psychiatric patients: Rationale, research findings, and future directions. *Comprehensive Psychiatry*, 1976, *17*, 559–580.
Hersen, M., & Bellack, A. S. Assessment of social skills. In A. R. Ciminero, K. S. Calhoun, & H. E. Adams (Eds.), *Handbook for behavioral assessment*. New York: Wiley, 1977.
Hersen, M., Eisler, R. M., & Miller, P. M. Development of assertive responses: Clinical, measurement and research considerations. *Behaviour Research and Therapy*, 1973, *11*, 505–521.
Hersen, M., Eisler, R. M., Miller, P. M., Johnson, M. B., & Pinkston, S. G. Effects of practice, instructions, and modeling on components of assertive behavior. *Behaviour Research and Therapy*, 1973, *11*, 443–451.
Hersen, M., Eisler, R. M., & Miller, P. M. An experimental analysis of generalization in assertive training. *Behaviour Research and Therapy*, 1974, *12*, 295–310.
Hersen, M., Bellack, A. S., & Himmelhoch, J. M. Treatment of unipolar depression with social skills training. *Behavior Modification*, 1980, *4*, 547–556.
Hersen, M., Turner, S. M., Edelstein, A. B., & Pinkston, S. G. Effects of phenothiazines and social skills training in a withdrawn schizophrenic. *Journal of Clinical Psychology*, 1975, *31*, 588–594.
Hingtgen, J. N., & Trost, F. C. Shaping cooperative responses in early childhood schizophrenics: II. Reinforcement of mutual physical contact and vocal responses. In R. Ulrich, T. Strachnik, & J. Mabry (Eds.), *Control of human behavior*. Chicago: Scott, Foresman, 1966.
Isaacs, W., Thomas, J., & Goldiamond, I. Application of operant conditioning to reinstate verbal behavior in psychotic patients. *Journal of Speech and Hearing Disorders*, 1960, *25*, 8–12.
Jaffe, P. G., & Carlson, P. M. Relative efficacy of modeling and instructions in eliciting social behavior from chronic psychiatric patients. *Journal of Consulting and Clinical Psychology*, 1976, *44*, 200–207.
Kazdin, A. E. Assessing the clinical or applied importance of behavior change through social validation. *Behavior Modification*, 1977, *4*, 427–452.
Kelly, J. A. *Social-skills training*. New York: Springer, 1981.
Kelly, J. A. Group training of social skills: Clinical applications and procedures. In D. Upper & S. M. Ross (Eds.), *Behavioral group therapy: An annual review*. Champaign, Ill.: Research Press, 1981.
Kolko, D. J., Dorsett, P. G., & Milan, M. A. A total-assessment approach to the evaluation of social skills training: The effectiveness of an anger control program for adolescent psychiatric patients. *Behavioral Assessment*, 1981, *3*, 383–402.
Lazarus, A. A. Behavior therapy in groups. In G. Gazda (Ed.), *Basic approaches to group psychotherapy and group counseling*. Springfield, Ill.: Charles C. Thomas, 1968.
Lomont, J. R., Gilner, F. H., Spector, N. J., & Skinner, K. K. Group assertion training and group insight therapies. *Psychological Reports*, 1969, *25*, 463–470.
Matson, J. L., & Stephens, R. M. Increasing appropriate behavior of explosive chronic psychiatric patients with a social-skills training package. *Behavior Modification*, 1978, *2*, 61–76.
Matson, J. L., & Zeiss, R. A. The buddy system: A method for generalized reduction of inappropriate interpersonal behavior of retarded psychiatric patients. *British Journal of Social and Clinical Psychology*, 1979, *18*, 401–405.
McAlister, A., Perry, C., Killen, C., Slinkard, L. A., & Maccoby, N. Pilot study of smoking, alcohol and drug abuse prevention. *American Journal of Public Health*, 1980, *70*, 719–721.
Monti, P. M. The social skills intake interview: Reliability and convergent validity assessment. *Journal of Behavior Therapy and Experimental Psychiatry*, 1983, *14*, 305–310.
Monti, P. M., Fink, E., Norman, W., Curran, J. P., Hayes, S., & Caldwell, A. The effect of social skills training groups and social skills bibliotherapy with psychiatric patients. *Journal of Consulting and Clinical Psychology*, 1979, *47*, 189–191.
Monti, P. M., Curran, J. P., Corriveau, D. P., De Lancey, A., & Hagerman, S. M. Effects of social skills training groups and sensitivity training groups with psychiatric patients. *Journal of Consulting and Clinical Psychology*, 1980, *48*, 241–248.
Monti, P. M., Corriveau, D., & Curran, J. P. Social skills training for psychiatric patients: Treatment

and outcome. In J. P. Curran & P. M. Monti (Eds.), *Social skills training: A practical handbook for assessment and treatment*. New York: Guilford Press, 1982.

Monti, P. M., Wallander, J. L., Ahern, D. K., Abrams, D. B., & Munroe, S. M. Mutli-modal measurement of anxiety and social skills in a behavioral role-play test: Generalizability and discriminant validity. *Behavioral Assessment*, 1983, *6*, 15–26.

Paul, G. L. Behavior modification research: Design and tactics. In C. M. Franks (Ed.), *Behavior therapy: Appraisal and status*. New York: McGraw-Hill, 1969.

Paul, G. L., & Shannon, D. T. Treatment of anxiety through systematic desensitization in therapy groups. *Journal of Abnormal Psychology*, 1966, *71*, 124–135.

Percell, L. P., Berwick, P. T., & Beigel, A. The effects of assertive training on self-concept and anxiety. *Archives of General Psychiatry*, 1974, *31*, 502–504.

Perry, C., Killen, J., Telch, M., Slinkard, L. A., & Danaher, B. G. Modifying smoking behavior of teenagers: A school-based intervention. *American Journal of Public Health*, 1980, *70*, 722–725.

Phillips, E. L. *The social skills basis of psychopathology*. New York: Grune & Stratton, 1978.

Phillips, L., & Zigler, E. Social competence: The action–thought parameter and vicariousness in normal and pathological behaviors. *Journal of Abnormal and Social Psychology*, 1961, *63*, 137–146.

Phillips, L., & Zigler, E. Role orientation, the action–thought dimension and outcome in psychiatric disorder. *Journal of Abnormal and Social Psychology*, 1964, *68*, 381–389.

Rathus, S. A. An experimental investigation of assertive training in a group setting. *Journal of Behavior Therapy and Experimental Psychiatry*, 1972, *3*, 81–86.

Rathus, S. A. Instigation of assertive behavior through videotape mediated assertive models and directed practice. *Behaviour Research and Therapy*, 1973, *11*, 57–65.

Rice, M. E., & Chaplin, T. C. Social skills training for hospitalized male arsonists. *Journal of Behavior Therapy and Experimental Psychiatry*, 1979, *10*, 105–108.

Rimm, D. C. Treatment of antisocial aggression. In G. G. Harris (Ed.), *The group treatment of human problems*. New York: Grune & Stratton, 1977.

Serber, M. Teaching the nonverbal components of assertive training. *Journal of Behavior Therapy and Experimental Psychiatry*, 1972, *3*, 179–183.

Serber, M., & Nelson, P. The ineffectiveness of systematic desensitization and assertive training in hospitalized schizophrenics. *Journal of Behavior Therapy and Experimental Psychiatry*, 1971, *2*, 107–109.

Scott, R. R., Himadi, W., & Keane, T. M. A review of generalization in social skills training: Suggestions for future research. In M. Hersen, R. Eisler, & P. Miller (Eds.), *Progress in behavior modification*. San Diego: Academic Press, 1984.

Sherman, J. A. Reinstatement of verbal behavior in a psychotic by reinforcement methods. *Journal of Speech and Hearing Disorders*, 1963, *25*, 8–12.

Sherman, J. A. Use of reinforcement and imitation to reinstate verbal behavior in mute psychotics. *Journal of Abnormal and Social Psychology*, 1965, *70*, 155–164.

Strauss, J., & Carpenter, W. The prediction of outcome in schizophrenia: I. Characteristics of outcome. *Archives of General Psychiatry*, 1972, *27*, 739–746.

Trower, P., Yardley, K., Bryant, B. M., & Shaw, P. The treatment of social failure: A comparison of anxiety-reduction and skills-acquisition procedures on two social problems. *Behavior Modification*, 1978, *2*, 41–60.

Twentyman, C. T., & Zimering, R., Behavioral training of social skills: A critical review. In M. Hersen, R. M. Eisler, & P. M. Miller (Eds.), *Progress in behavior modification* (Vol. 7). New York: Academic Press, 1979.

Upper, D., & Ross, S. M. Behavioral group therapy. In M. Hersen, R. M., Eisler, & P. M. Miller (Eds.), *Progress in behavior modification* (Vol. 5). New York: Academic Press, 1977.

Weinman, B., Gelbart, P., Wallace, M., & Post, M. Inducing assertive behavior in chronic schizophrenics: A comparison of socioenvironmental, desensitization, and relaxation therapies. *Journal of Consulting and Clinical Psychology*, 1972, *39*, 246–253.

Williams, M. T., Turner, S. M., Watts, J. G., Bellack, A. S., & Hersen, M. Group social skills training for chronic psychiatric patients. *European Journal of Behavioural Analysis and Modification*, 1977, *1*, 223–229.

Wilson, F. S., & Walters, R. H. Modification of speech output of near mute schizophrenics through social learning procedures. *Behaviour Research and Therapy*, 1966, *4*, 59–67.

Wolpe, J. *The practice of behavior therapy* (2d ed.). New York: Pergamon Press, 1973.

Zigler, E., & Phillips, L. Social effectiveness and symptomatic behaviors. *Journal of Abnormal and Social Psychology*, 1960, *61*, 231–238.

Zigler, E., & Phillips, L. Social competence and outcome in psychiatric disorder. *Journal of Abnormal and Social Psychology*, 1961, *63*, 264–271.

Zigler, E., & Phillips, L. Social competence and the process-reactive distinction in psychopathology. *Journal of Abnormal and Social Psychology*, 1962, *65*, 215–222.

3

Preparing Clients for Behavioral Group Therapy

NANCY B. COHN AND NEAL H. MAYERSON

INTRODUCTION

Group therapy is a process that is presumed to be facilitated by specific types of client behaviors. For example, Yalom (1975) described a number of "curative factors" in interactional group therapy, including processes such as (a) learning that others have similar kinds of problems and feelings (universality); (b) emotional catharsis; and (c) learning how one's behavior affects people. Certain client behaviors, such as self-disclosure of problems and feedback to other group members, serve to promote these "curative factors."

Behavioral group therapy may be conceptualized as therapy implemented *by* a group (Goldstein, Heller, & Sechrest, 1966) that utilizes learning principles as the basis for intervention. Consequently, the types of appropriate client behaviors that might facilitate group process and subsequent outcome are defined by learning theory. For example, Flowers (1979) noted that *why* questions (i.e., those that elicit speculations regarding motivation underlying behavior) were less appropriate to behavioral groups than questions asking *what* (e.g., questions appropriate to a functional analysis of behavior; cf. Kanfer & Saslow, 1969). In his theoretical model, Flowers (1979) also emphasized that, to qualify as behavioral group therapy, an intervention must be systematic and assessable (i.e., target problems are operationally defined and measurable). Therefore, content-specific groups typically thought of as behavioral (e.g., weight control groups, assertion training models) would be considered behavioral group therapy only if treatment were administered *through* the group using systematic interventions based on learning principles. For a client, who is typically naive to these principles and to psychotherapy in general, becoming a viable member of a behavioral

NANCY B. COHN • Veterans Administration Medical Center, Salt Lake City, Utah 84148. NEAL H. MAYERSON • Behavioral Medicine Associates, Salt Lake City, Utah 84148.

therapy group may be an anxiety-provoking challenge. If therapeutic progress depends to a large degree on certain specifiable client behaviors, then it may be argued that it is desirable to specify these behaviors and assist clients to engage in them.

The issue of preparing clients for behavioral group therapy, as opposed to individual therapy, is especially cogent. The central role played by the therapist in individual therapy results in a higher degree of control over the nature of interactions than is true for group modalities. In contrast, behavioral group therapies consist of a high proportion of client–client interactions, and consequently, control over the nature of the interactions is determined largely by the clients themselves. Because a high proportion of client–client interactions is reportedly related to treatment outcome (Flowers & Booraem, 1976), it would seem that preparing clients to engage "appropriately" in interactions with other group members *prior* to therapy onset might further enhance outcome.

Additionally, clients may approach group therapy with heightened and unique fears and anxieties. These fears are related to sharing issues with a group of strangers, negative past experiences with groups, concerns over "getting worse" from observing and listening to other people's problems, concern about receiving sufficient personal attention, and anxiety about confidentiality. These fears may be related to treatment attrition as is suggested by evidence that patients who do not understand the rationale of therapeutic procedures tend to withdraw from treatment (Baekeland & Lundwall, 1975; Frank, 1974). Similarly, group member confusion or ambiguity about expected group behavior may hamper the creation of group cohesiveness, an important component of the therapeutic process (Yalom, 1975).

"Appropriate" group member behaviors are generally developed during the course of therapy, often modeled or reinforced by therapists. Consequently, some members develop, at different rates, into "good" group members, whereas others have difficulty discriminating appropriate behaviors and becoming motivated to enact them. Difficulties associated with the development of appropriate client participation may not only decrease the likelihood that such members will benefit from the group experience but can also negatively affect other group members. For instance, much group time can be unproductively consumed in addressing a member's defensiveness, with the group's becoming disrupted by premature terminations and irregular attendance. This is especially true when unusual techniques, for example, the use of tokens described by Flowers and Booraem (1976), are implemented.

An alternative approach to developing behavioral norms within the context of the group session is to do so more explicitly and formally before the first group therapy session. Pretherapy training, that is, an "intervention" prior to the onset of treatment, may enhance or accelerate the therapeutic process (Bednar, Weet, Evensen, Lanier, & Melnick, 1974; Heitler, 1973). However, there is a paucity of literature bearing on this issue. The remainder of this chapter will review the client preparation literature from both individual and group perspectives and suggest guidelines for preparing behavioral group therapy clients.

Pretherapy Training

Pretherapy training has typically served three roles: to communicate a therapy rationale, provide client-role expectations, and set positive outcome expectation. Although these may, of course, occur over the natural course of therapy, pretraining aims to systematically make explicit these three points. As Bandura (1977) proposed, the probability of a person's engaging in a particular behavior depends upon "self-efficacy" and "outcome" expectations, that is, the belief that a set of behaviors *can* be executed and will result in an outcome that is positively valued. It might be predicted, therefore, that active participation in the group therapy process would be promoted by (a) understanding of the "client role" (e.g., behaviors in which a client is expected to engage, such as self-disclosure); (b) belief that this role can be adequately fulfilled; and (c) anticipation that role-congruent behaviors will not be unduly aversive (short-term outcome) and will lead to positive long-term outcome.

The preponderance of client preparation methods may be conceptualized as either oral and/or written (verbal) persuasion procedures, modeling (vicarious learning) procedures, or a combination of these two formats. Attempts at verbal persuasion have been presented via flexible, individual interviews, more structured lecture formats, standardized written, didactic materials, and audiotaped or videotaped presentations. Verbal persuasion procedures typically address some combination of the three points mentioned before. Most communicate a rationale and at least points related to client role. In contrast, modeling procedures provide examples of desirable group behavior via audiotape or videotape. Combination procedures employ both verbal persuasion and modeling methods.

In addition to different methods of pretherapy training, there has been a wide diversity of variables that investigators have expected to be affected as a function of client preparation. These have included process variables such as client expectations, ingroup verbal behavior, client satisfaction, attendance and attrition as well as a variety of outcome measures (see Table 1 for a summary of studies by variables). The following will summarize much of the existing individual and group preparation research according to the type of procedure and the measures investigated.

Individual Therapy Preparation

Verbal Persuasion Methods

An early investigation of client preparation (Hoehn-Saric, Frank, Imber, Nash, Stone, & Battle, 1964) used a role-induction interview based on procedures outlined by Orne and Wender (1968). The interview was designed to provide a treatment rationale, define appropriate role behavior, and set expectations for improvement. Hoehn-Saric *et al.* (1964) found that pretherapy training positively affected both behavior in therapy and attendance. Therapists also

TABLE 1. Summary of Pretherapy Training Studies

Study	Training method	Dependent variables/outcome: Significant	Dependent variables/outcome: Nonsignificant
		Individual therapy	
Craigie & Ross, 1980	Combination	Outcome (treatment seeking)	
Frank, 1974	Verbal persuasion (role induction)	Ingroup behavior[a] Outcome[a]	
Hoehn-Saric *et al.*, 1964	Verbal persuasion (role induction)	Ingroup behavior[b] Attendance Outcome[b,c]	
Krumboltz, Varenhorst, & Thoresen, 1967	Modeling	Outcome (job-seeking behavior)	
Lieberman *et al.*, 1972	Follow-up of Hoehn-Saric *et al.*		Outcome (5-year between-groups difference)
Parrino, 1971	Verbal persuasion (written didactic)	Outcome (anxiety decrease; snake-approach increase)	
Rague, 1974	Modeling	Ingroup behavior[d]	
Sloane, Cristal, Pepernick, & Staples, 1970	Verbal persuasion (role induction)	Outcome[b]	Attendance
		Group therapy	
Annis & Perry, 1977, 1978	Modeling	Ingroup behavior[e]	
Bugan, 1977	Verbal persuasion (lecture)		Cohesion[c]
Cartwright, 1976	Modeling	Client expectations	
Curran, 1978	Combination	Outcome[b,c]	Outcome[b,c]
Garrison, 1978	Verbal persuasion, oral/written	Ingroup behavior[f] Attendance Attrition	Client expectations Ingroup behavior[b]
Heitler, 1973	Verbal persuasion (interview)	Ingroup behavior[e]	Client satisfaction

(*continued*)

TABLE 1 (*Continued*)

Study	Training method	Dependent variables/outcome: Significant	Dependent variables/outcome: Nonsignificant
Jacobs, Trick, & Withersty, 1976	Verbal persuasion (lecture)		Ingroup behavior[a] Client attitudes[c] Client satisfaction
Piper, Debanne, Garant, & Bienvenu 1979	Verbal persuasion (lecture)	Attendance	Dropout
Silver & Conyne, 1977	Modeling and direct experience	Attraction to group	
Strupp & Bloxom, 1973	Modeling and verbal persuasion (interview)	Ingroup behavior[b] Client satisfaction[c] Client motivation[b]	Attendance Outcome[b,c]
Truax & Carkhuff, 1965; Truax & Wargo, 1969	Modeling	Outcome[g]	
Truax, Wargo, Carkhuff, Kodman, & Moles, 1966; Truax, Shapiro, & Wargo, 1968; Truax, Wargo, & Volksdorf, 1970	Modeling		Outcome[c]
Whalen, 1969	Combination, modeling, & verbal persuasion	Ingroup behavior[f,h]	Ingroup behavior[g,i] Ingroup behavior[g,i]
Wogan, Getter, Amdur, Nichols, & Okman, 1977	Verbal persuasion and experiential exercise		Outcome[c] Ingroup behavior[a]
Yalom, Houts, Newall, & Rand, 1967	Verbal persuasion (interview)	Ingroup behavior[i]	Attendance, cohesion, mood, & progress[c]

[a]Unspecified.
[b]Therapist ratings.
[c]Client ratings.
[d]Expression of feelings.
[e]"Self-exploratory" verbalizations.
[f]Self-disclosure.
[g]MMPI measures.
[h]Verbal feedback.
[i]Group-oriented statements.

rated clients who had participated in the role-induction procedure as more improved than clients in a control group. Similar findings were obtained by Schonfield, Stone, Hoehn-Saric, Imber, and Pande (1969). A 5-year follow-up (Liberman, Frank, Hoehn-Saric, Stone, Imber, & Pande, 1972) indicated that between-group outcome effects had disappeared, suggesting that although pretherapy induction may be useful in affecting behavior within the therapeutic context, it is probably only one of many equally potent factors that influence long-term outcome. Frank (1974) similarly investigated the effect of a pretherapy role-induction interview with outpatients prior to the onset of individual therapy. Although the measures employed in the study are unclear, it was reported that prepared clients demonstrated more appropriate behavior in therapy and "better outcome."

Sloane, Cristal, Pepernick, and Staples (1970) investigated the efficacy of the role-induction interview employed by Hoehn-Saric *et al.* (1964). Four conditions were included: (a) an "anticipatory socialization" condition in which client role was defined; (b) outcome expectation only; (c) an anticipatory socialization *plus* outcome expectation condition; and (d) a no-pretreatment control group. Unfortunately, Sloane *et al.* (1970) failed to analyze the four groups individually and instead collapsed the two anticipatory socialization groups and compared them to the outcome expectancy and no-treatment control combined. Pretreatment clients were rated by their therapists as significantly more improved on a total adjustment measure than were controls. Although attendance did not differ between pretraining and control clients, there was a substantially higher, unexplained attrition rate among pretrained clients!

Parrino (1971) appeared to concentrate on treatment rationale and role expectancy in preparing snake phobic clients for therapy. Subjects were given written didactic material on learning theory prior to an operant conditioning intervention. Pretherapy clients demonstrated greater snake-approach scores and self-reported anxiety reduction than did controls. It is unclear whether the preparation procedure affected other variables such as client satisfaction or therapy attendance.

Modeling Procedures

There is an extensive literature on the efficacy of naturalistic and therapeutic modeling procedures in learning new behaviors (see Bandura, 1977). It might be expected that acquisition of desirable intherapy behavior would be facilitated by a pretherapy vicarious learning process. It is surprising that there is a dearth of research on the use of modeling techniques alone in preparing clients for individual therapy. One unpublished study (Rague, 1974) indicated that university students who were exposed to a videotape of appropriate therapy behavior (expression of feelings) emitted higher rates of this behavior across three initial therapy sessions than did control clients. Another investigation utilizing modeling procedures presented job-seeking high school students with a videotaped model engaging in desirable job-seeking behaviors prior to vocational counseling interviews (Krumboltz, Varenhorst, & Thoresen, 1967). It was found that experimental subjects demonstrated more job information-seeking behavior than did control subjects who received encouragement from a counselor to engage in information-seeking behavior.

Combination Procedures

In a unique pretherapy study, Craigie and Ross (1980) investigated the efficacy of a combination procedure in increasing treatment-seeking behavior of detoxifying alcoholics. A videotape consisting of treatment-seeking behaviors (e.g., "I have an alcohol problem and need to get help") and vignettes of therapy procedures was shown to experimental subjects with subsequent discussion to further clarify procedural issues in psychotherapy. A comparison procedure consisted of videotaped alcohol education films and a more general discussion. The results indicated that experimental subjects made more requests for treatment referrals and made more initial treatment contacts than did comparison subjects.

In summary, pretherapy training of clients for individual treatment has used verbal presuasion, modeling, and combination techniques with modest success in positively affecting both intherapy behavior and outcome. However, conclusions drawn from this literature are subject to the same limitations that apply to the group therapy literature to be discussed next.

Group Therapy Preparation

Verbal Persuasion Procedures

Yalom and his colleagues (Yalom, Houts, Newell, & Rand, 1967) empirically investigated a verbal persuasion procedure designed to orient outpatients to appropriate group therapy behavior. All three aspects of pretherapy training were addressed. A detailed history and rationale of group therapy was provided, appropriate group member behavior was made explicit, and outcome expectations were set by delineating the kinds of personal changes that people make over time in group therapy. Yalom *et al.* (1967) assessed several process variables, including ingroup verbal behavior, faith in therapy, attendance, and attrition. They demonstrated that prepared group members only differed from nonprepared members on ingroup verbal behavior.

Another study that prepared clients for group therapy used detailed instructional procedures, administered to groups, that actually comprised the initial three intervention sessions (Jacobs, Trick, & Withersty, 1976). Group therapy philosophy, rationale, and procedures were provided; desirable therapy behavior was specified (e.g., discussing feelings in the here and now, disclosing feelings, giving and receiving feedback) as was inappropriate therapy behavior (e.g., asking questions other than those requiring feedback). Outcome expectations were addressed by describing how treatment would help with personal problems. A questionnaire that measured acquisition of didactic material indicated that pretrained subjects understood this material better than subjects who had no exposure to pretherapy procedures. Ingroup verbal behavior, client attitude, and satisfaction were assessed, with no differences demonstrated between prepared and nonprepared group members.

A similar study that also used multiple preparatory sessions but reported more positive results was conducted by Piper and his associates (Piper, Debanne, Garant, & Bienvenu, 1979). They exposed clients to conceptual didactic material and then provided an "experience about the concept and an opportunity to link the cognitive material with the experience" (p. 1253). The rationale for the structure of group therapy was provided, and specific behaviors were illustrated (e.g., reporting feelings in the here and now). Outcome expectancies were not addressed in pretraining sessions. Individuals attended pretherapy training sessions with the same clients that comprised their subsequent therapy group. Piper *et al.* did not measure interactive process variables or therapeutic outcome but reported the effect of client preparation on attendance and attrition. Groups that experienced preparatory procedures demonstrated a significantly higher attendance rate and tended to have a lower attrition rate than nonprepared groups. It would be interesting to determine the effect of attending a classroomlike preparatory group on subsequent verbal behavior in group; however, to date this has not been investigated.

Bugen (1977) attempted to promote cohesion with graduate students in "growth groups" via a verbal preparatory procedure. The prepared groups were oriented prior to the first meeting with a message emphasizing here-and-now thoughts and feelings and the interactive nature of group process. Preparation had no effect on the results of a questionnaire designed by Liberman, Yalom, and Miles (1973) that was used to assess cohesion. It is unclear whether other indicators of cohesion (see later discussion) may in fact have been affected.

Cohesion was also purportedly the focus of a study employing a combined verbal persuasion procedure and experiential exercise (Wogan, Getter, Amdur, Nichols, & Okman, 1977). College-aged outpatients were exposed to one of four experimental conditions: (a) a cognitive experiential pretraining group, consisting of a rationale for group therapy, instructions to give interpersonal feedback, and a "chance to practice" (p. 26); (b) a T-group condition comprised of structured exercises; (c) an attention control group that met with no instructions other than to remain together for 1 hour; and (d) a control group that simply began therapy on the first meeting. Wogan *et al.* (1977) employed both process and outcome measures and stated that cohesion was "measured only indirectly, through the rated improvement measure" (p. 43). Their results, although difficult to interpret, suggested that therapist characteristics had greater impact on process and outcome than did preparatory procedures.

A study of pretherapy training with low-income psychiatric inpatients was conducted by Heitler (1973). Using the anticipatory socialization interview employed by Hoehn-Saric *et al.* (1964) with individuals and by Yalom *et al.* (1967) with groups, Heitler (1973) essentially focused on client role expectations and both short- and long-term outcome expectations. Direct behavioral observation was used at several points in therapy to measure a variety of ingroup verbal behaviors, including self-exploratory communications, verbal initiative, and talk time.

It was demonstrated that early in therapy, prepared clients engaged in more of the targeted verbal behaviors than did nonprepared clients. In addition, therapists rated prepared clients more favorably than nonprepared clients on dimensions of involvement in group and prognosis. Preparation did not affect therapist perceptions of client likeability or anxiousness, and ratings made by clients did not differ as a function of preparation.

The relative efficacy of verbal versus written persuasion procedures was investigated with community mental health outpatients (Garrison, 1978). Experimental subjects received either verbal or written preparatory interviews; control subjects simply received a routine client interview. In the preparatory conditions, client role expectation was defined, and outcome expectation was addressed both by delimiting potential difficulties in group therapy and by establishing positive expectations about long-term therapeutic gains as a function of group therapy. Client expectations were measured prior to therapy and following early sessions. Therapist ratings of ingroup verbal behavior were obtained following the first therapy session, and attendance and attrition measures were collected through Session 6. Prepared clients did not differ from nonprepared clients in their expectations of therapy. However, both experimental groups demonstrated significantly greater rates of desirable ingroup verbal behavior than did the control group. Attendance was also significantly more frequent for the experimental than for the control groups.

Pretherapy preparation employing verbal persuasion procedures appears to be beneficial in effecting more rapid development of appropriate ingroup verbal behavior (Garrison, 1978; Heitler, 1973; Yalom *et al.*, 1967;). These differences may only be apparent early in the course of therapy (Heitler, 1973), suggesting, perhaps, that the effect of pretherapy training on ingroup verbal behavior is accelerative; it serves to bring about desirable verbal behavior more quickly than otherwise develops naturally over the group life span. Jacobs *et al.* (1976) suggested that their failure to demonstrate changes in verbal behavior as a function of preparation may have in part been accounted for by heightened client anxiety about saying the "wrong" thing. Procedural issues including the length of preparation (three sessions) and the concurrent nature of the procedure and therapy *per se* are other likely sources of the negative results of Jacobs *et al.* (1976). It may be that the natural development of appropriate role behaviors "catches up" with the preparation-induced quite early in therapy. Verbal persuasion procedures may also increase member attendance (Garrison, 1978; Piper *et al.*, 1979), thereby providing for greater opportunity to develop behavior facilitative to the group process.

Modeling procedures

Truax and his colleagues (Truax & Carkhuff, 1965; Truax, Shapiro, & Wargo, 1968; Truax & Wargo, 1969; Traux, Wargo, Carkhuff, Kodman, & Moles, 1966; Truax, Wargo, & Volksdorf, 1970) researched the efficacy of pretherapy training using a modeling procedure. An audiotape of actual group therapy segments illustrating desirable group therapy behaviors was played for experimental subjects prior to the first group session. Each of the Truax studies investigated the effect of pretraining on outcome, employing a variety of measures including the Minnesota Multiphasic Personality Inventory (MMPI) and client and therapist reports. Exposure to the audiotape was related to changes on MMPI Scales 7 (Truax & Carkhuff, 1965; Truax & Wargo, 1969), 8 (Truax & Carkhuff, 1965), 2, and 3 (Truax & Wargo, 1969). No process variables were included in any of the Truax studies. The authors noted (Truax *et al.*, 1968) that these studies consisted of groups led by therapists of various theoretical orientations, whereas the modeling tape was consistently presented to all subjects. It is difficult to evaluate this series of studies because the content of the tape was not specified.

Strupp and Bloxom (1973) investigated the relative merits of verbal persuasion and modeling preparatory procedures. The verbal persuasion procedure consisted of a role-induction interview as described by Orne and Wender (1968). The modeling condition employed a role-induction film that portrayed a case example, complete with an individual problem, group therapy sessions, and positive outcome. In general, the film communicated a therapy rationale via depiction of group sessions, established appropriate client behaviors, and set outcome expectations by illustrating the model's improvement over the course of therapy. A control group viewed a film on the topic of early marriage. Four therapy groups were exposed to each condition, and preparation procedures were presented in the group format. Both preparatory procedures were effective in a number of areas. Therapists indicated that prepared clients demonstrated more appropriate ingroup behavior than did nonprepared clients, with the modeling procedure more effective than the interview. Client satisfaction with the group, satisfaction with their own progress, and general interpersonal relationships were enhanced for both preparatory conditions. Again, the modeling condition exceeded the interview. Prepared and nonprepared clients did not differ in attendance, nor did therapist-rated outcome differ between the groups.

Cartwright (1976) investigated the effect of a modeling film on client expectations about group therapy. Compared to a group that received no exposure to group therapy concepts, prepared subjects demonstrated more accurate expectations about the structure and process of group therapy.

An analog study examining attraction to sensitivity groups (Silver & Conyne, 1977) employed a modeling film, which was compared with direct experience with structured T-group exercises and a no-preparation control group. Both experimental conditions produced greater attraction to sensitivity groups, with direct experience significantly more effective than modeling.

Another analog study investigated the effect of a modeling procedure administered prior to the onset of a brief laboratory interaction group (Annis & Perry, 1978). The target behavior—self-disclosure—was modeled for the experimental groups either by audiotape or videotape; the control group simply participated in their discussion groups without initial exposure to models engaging in self-disclosure. Both experimental groups demonstrated more depth of self-disclosure than did the control group. The results of this study provide further support for the efficacy of pretherapy preparation for specific, measurable ingroup verbal behaviors.

In general, modeling procedures to prepare clients for group therapy have demonstrated moderate utility in both analog and clinical studies. By providing a rationale for therapy, delimiting specific, desirable behaviors in group, and setting outcome expectations, positive impact has been reported in areas including client expectations (Strupp & Bloxom, 1973), ingroup verbal behavior (Annis & Perry, 1978; Strupp & Bloxom, 1973; Whalen, 1969), client satisfaction (Strupp & Bloxom, 1973), and outcome (Strupp & Bloxom, 1973; Truax *et al.*, 1965; 1969). However, negative results have also been obtained for ingroup verbal behavior (Whalen, 1969), attendance (Strupp & Bloxom, 1973), and outcome (Strupp & Bloxom, 1973; Truax *et al.*, 1966, 1968, 1970). Possible explanations of these equivocal findings will be presented in the discussion section of this chapter.

Combination Procedures

Whalen (1969) studied the differential effects of three preparatory procedures on subsequent group member behavior. The procedures, a modeling film, an audiotaped verbal instruction procedure, and a combination of the two, were employed in an analog study using male college students who engaged in a single, nonclinical leaderless discussion group. The modeling film illustrated both inappropriate group member behavior (e.g., discussing biographical information) and appropriate behavior (members discussing feelings, giving and receiving interpersonal feedback). The verbal instruction procedure briefly described the purpose of the group, defined appropriate role behaviors (as depicted in the film), and stated that personal learning from the group depended upon enactment of the prescribed behaviors. A combination procedure employed both methods, and a control group received only minimal instructions to interact as a group. Each preparatory condition, therefore, defined role behavior for the participants. Outcome expectations were also set by informing members of the behaviors necessary for learning during group participation.

Continuous direct observation ratings of verbal responses were obtained. Three classes of responses were measured: (a) self-disclosure of personal material; (b) feedback to others; and (c) superficial discussion. Whalen's (1969) results indicated that combined verbal instruction and modeling procedures produced significantly more self-disclosure and feedback and significantly less impersonal discussion than either of the single procedures or no preparation. Whalen (1969) suggested that the relatively minimal impact of either preparatory procedure alone was greatly increased when they were combined.

A similar study (Curran, 1978) examined the effects of a combined verbal persuasion/modeling preparatory procedure in an actual clinical setting. The experimental group was pretested and subsequently reviewed a modeling videotape that depicted the procedures employed in group sessions, demonstrated appropriate client behaviors (e.g., giving and receiving positive and negative feedback), and presented a rationale regarding the efficacy of the treatment procedure. Following the presentation of the modeling tape, a modified version of the role-induction interview (Orne & Wender, 1968) was administered. Two control conditions were employed, a no-pretest–preparation group and a no-pretest–no-preparation group. The dependent variables were all outcome measures and included client ratings of motivation to change, specific behavioral changes, and goal attainment. Posttreatment therapist ratings of client functioning in five social interaction areas were also collected. Results indicated that prepared clients were significantly more motivated to change than control subjects. Therapists rated prepared clients as more improved than nonprepared clients in family functioning and primary goal attainment. Posttreatment client ratings demonstrated greater attainment of primary and secondary goals by the experimental preparatory group; the no-pretest–preparation group reported attaining significantly more tertiary goals than the other groups. Client ratings of specific behavioral changes did not differentiate the groups.

In a somewhat different manner, Conyne and Silver (1980) investigated the effects of a variety of pretherapy procedures on attitudes toward group therapy. They compared direct participation in interactive exercises with vicarious participation, vicarious participation combined with subsequent discussion, and no participation. In was reported that direct experience with interactive process enhanced positive attitudes toward group therapy. Direct experience also resulted in a greater desire to participate in group process than did vicarious experience. Actual ingroup behavior was not assessed nor were outcome measures obtained.

Combination procedures to prepare clients for group therapy, as with individual therapy, appear to be at least as successful as the use of either verbal persuasion or modeling procedures alone. Whalen (1969) noted that appropriate verbal behavior was increased *only* with combined procedures, and a number of outcome measures have also been significantly affected by combination preparatory procedures (Curran, 1978). Bandura (1977) discussed the relative potencies of the various sources of expectations (i.e., performance accomplishments, vicarious experience, verbal persuasion, and emotional arousal). He suggested that verbal persuasion is relatively less effective in setting positive expectations than is direct or vicarious experience. Thus, there is some reason to believe that a combination procedure might prove more powerful than a verbal persuasion procedure alone, but this has yet to be established empirically.

Discussion

In general, the pretherapy training literature yields mixed results. The three pretraining procedures discussed previously—verbal persuasion techniques, modeling procedures, or some combination—have each yielded both positive and negative results, with some procedures perhaps more effective with specific behaviors than others. Further, each of the categories of pretherapy training variables delineated earlier in this chapter (client expectations, ingroup verbal behavior, client satisfaction, attendance and attrition, and therapy outcome) seem equivocally related to pretherapy training procedures.

Although the positive findings are encouraging, conclusions regarding pretherapy training must be tentative due to statistical limitations. One of the most serious problems is related to conceptual weakness that is apparent in the client preparation literature. In addition to the variety of pretraining procedures employed, a plethora of dependent measures has been investigated. It appears as if investigators are unsure of the effects the procedures might produce. Consequently, so-called *data snooping* is employed in the hope of discovering some relationship among the many variables of interest. Statistically, this process inflates the probability of obtaining spurious positive results (Tatsuoko, 1980). Also resulting in overestimations of positive results is the tendency of investigators to employ the same statistical procedures to group therapy research as is appropriate for research with individual subjects. Briefly, when treating scores for individual group members as independent, that is, obtaining the error term and degrees of freedom from number of individuals rather than groups, F values may be artificially inflated. Consequently, significance tests are inappropriately liberal, resulting in a higher frequency of Type I error (for an excellent discussion of both statistical issues and remediation, see Anderson & Ager, 1978; Bednar & Moeschl, 1981). Further complicating the interpretation of pretherapy training research is the tendency for positive results to be overrepresented in the general research literature, that is, more frequently published than negative results. Thus, there is justified concern that there are at least as many nonsignificant as significant treatment effects found in client preparation studies because many of the statistical problems described before raise questions regarding the true frequency of positive results. Conclusions regarding the value of pretherapy training, based upon experimental evidence, must be interpreted cautiously at best. We may, however, broaden our approach to group therapy preparation and consider the research heretofore as descriptive or exploratory. It is then important to determine the process and outcome variables that are most affected (either theoretically or empirically) by client preparation for group therapy and to devise a strategy for systematic application of procedures to train clients to some specified criterion. General trends apparent in the literature may provide a direction for clinicians interested in preparing clients for behavioral group therapy.

Verbal persuasion preparatory procedures appear to be at least modestly useful in effecting more accurate client expectations *prior to the onset of therapy*. That is, group members who are exposed to didactic material regarding the nature of group therapy, client roles, and other, similar information tend to better understand this kind of information compared to nonexposed individuals (Jacobs *et al.*, 1976; Strupp & Bloxom, 1973). These results, however, are by no means definitive (Garrison, 1978). Modeling procedures are at least as effective as verbal persuasion (Cartwright, 1976; Conyne & Silver, 1980) and possibly more so (Strupp & Bloxom, 1973).

The training of appropriate ingroup verbal behaviors such as self-disclosure and feedback delivery makes heuristic sense and has in fact been positively affected by verbal persuasion (Garrison, 1978; Heitler, 1973, Strupp & Bloxom, 1973; Yalom *et al.*, 1967), modeling (Annis & Perry, 1977, 1978) and combination procedures (Whalen, 1969). Again, negative results have also been reported within each training modality (Jacobs *et al.*, 1976; Whalen, 1969; Wogan *et al.*, 1977). However, the number of positive findings considerably outweighs the negative results, with statistical strength of the positive results (see Hays, 1973; Mayerson, 1984) supporting the utility of further research in this area.

Attendance and attrition are obvious issues of concern to group therapists because they may affect a number of other variables related to outcome, for example, self-disclosure, group stability, and cohesion (Yalom, 1975). As is true of so many group therapy variables, attendance and attrition may be affected by a variety of factors, including both those addressed by pretraining procedures and other, extraneous factors such as symptomatic relief. Consequently, attendance and attrition may not necessarily reflect effectiveness of group therapy preparation procedures. Verbal persuasion methods used to affect attendance have produced both positive (Garrison, 1978; Piper *et al.*, 1979) and negative results (Strupp & Bloxom, 1973; Yalom *et al.*, 1967).

Client satisfaction is an equally complex variable that is influenced by many factors. It may derive from an individual's perceptions regarding the group, for example, degree of discomfort experienced and amount of perceived cost to perceived benefit, or may, as suggested by Flowers and Booraem (1980), be critically tied to a "group" variable such as cohesion. Conceptually, therefore, client satisfaction is not necessarily a direct measure of preparatory procedure efficacy. Of the group therapy studies reviewed addressing client satisfaction, only one (Strupp & Bloxom, 1973) reported facilitation of client satisfaction through preparation. Additionally, it might be premature to assess some global measure of *satisfaction* before treatment outcome is apparent. The validity of *enhanced satisfaction* becomes questionable when it is not tied to some other, more concrete, and specified variable. It would perhaps be more clinically meaningful to assess, as did Flowers and Booraem (1980), variables underlying satisfaction that can be directly manipulated. Group cohesion appears to be one of these variables.

Cohesion, loosely defined, is the attraction of a group for its members (Liberman, 1971), that which "binds the individual to the group" (Lieberman, Lakin, & Whitaker, 1968, p. 30). It is unique to group, rather than individual, therapy and may be essentially related to therapeutic outcome (Bednar & Lawlis, 1971; Yalom, 1975). Members of cohesive groups are reportedly more productive, more open to giving and receiving feedback (Bednar & Lawlis, 1971), report greater satisfaction, and trust more group members than do individuals in less cohesive groups (Flowers & Booraem, 1980). A number of discrete behavioral components of cohesion have been summarized (Flowers & Booraem, 1980; Krumboltz & Potter, 1973). These include increased attention to the speaker, increased problem disclosure, increased proportion of negative feedback dispersed equitably among group members, decreased frequency of group members giving or receiving disproportionate amounts of negative feedback, and high rates of interactions between group members as compared to between therapist and member. These empirically determined components seem an appropriate focus for behavioral group therapy preparation.

Ultimately, the measure of treatment efficacy and speculatively pretreatment procedures is outcome. Measures of group therapy outcome have included variables as diverse as subjective ratings (see Bednar & Lawlis, 1971) and ratings by others, including therapists (e.g., Curran, 1978) and significant others (Flowers, 1979). Although the latter has not been employed in pretherapy training research, it has been successfully used with a number of patient populations and might be considered for future clinical and research purposes. In general, there are many problems associated with outcome research (Bergin & Lambert, 1978), a discussion of which far exceeds the scope of this chapter. As might be expected, outcome-related measures of preparatory procedure efficacy have yielded equivocal results. Client-rated outcome of verbal persuasion procedures has been both positive (Strupp & Bloxom, 1973) and nonsignificant (Jacobs *et al.*, 1976; Yalom *et al.*, 1967). Modeling procedures have also yielded mixed outcomes, with reports of significant client ratings (Truax *et al.*, 1965, 1969), nonsignificant client ratings (Truax *et al.*, 1966, 1968, Truax 1970), and nonsignificant therapist ratings (Truax *et al.*, 1970). Combination procedures have also failed to effect significant differences between prepared and nonprepared clients on outcome measures (Curran, 1978; Wogan *et al.*, 1977).

It is clear that it is not possible to definitively assess the impact of group therapy pretraining on therapeutic outcome. In order to more effectively determine the relationship between pretherapy training and therapeutic outcome, the theoretical and empirical relationships between pretraining and group process and group process and outcome must be specified. It may be the case that pretherapy training affects outcome only indirectly, through its effect on group process; to treat the group therapy process *per se* as a "nuisance" variable makes little sense. Furthermore, pretherapy training may effect the *rate* of development of targeted behaviors. Assessing the effects of client preparation on group process at various points in the life of the group should clarify further the relationships between pretherapy training, process, and outcome. It is also essential that outcome variables measure behaviors that relate in some way to behaviors that are addressed therapeutically; few would be surprised at nonsignificant changes in MMPI scales at the end of a group designed to alleviate snake phobia.

Suggestions for Behavioral Group Therapy Pretraining

The initial task in developing a standardized set of pretherapy preparatory procedures is, as described before, to communicate a general therapy rationale. In preparing clients for behavioral group therapy, it would be useful to first convey basic principles. For example, it may be communicated that

1. Behavioral group therapy offers a unique opportunity to provide an understanding of how we behave in relation to other people (Goldstein & Wolpe, 1972). It is a supportive environment where one can try new behaviors and get feedback in ways not usually available in daily living.
2. Our behavior, including feelings, is acquired, changed, or maintained by its consequences; behavior that is followed by positive responses tends

to be maintained or increased, whereas behavior that is followed by negative responses tends to decrease.

3. One important way in which we learn to behave in new, more adaptive ways is by observing and imitating others. Behavioral group therapy consists of interactions between multiple models, a potent method of changing behavior (Sansbury, 1979).
4. When other people view our progress, we are more motivated to do well and try new behaviors (Sansbury, 1979).

A second goal of pretraining clients is to delineate appropriate ingroup behavior, that is, set role expectations. If the therapist is unclear about desirable client behaviors, it is unlikely that clients will engage in activity related to positive outcome. Flowers and his colleagues (Flowers, 1979; Flowers & Booraem, 1976, 1980; Flowers, Booraem, Brown, & Harris, 1974; Flowers, Booraem, & Hartman, 1981; Flowers, Booraem, & Seacat, 1974) have specified a variety of client behaviors related to increased group cohesion and more positive outcome. These include (a) a high percentage of valenced (positive and negative) interactions between group members; (b) high levels of interactions between group members, rather than between a member and the therapist; (c) a proportionate amount of negative feedback dispersed across *all* group members, that is, no group member is singled out for negative feedback; (d) feedback given as alternatives or instructions rather than advice; and (e) client flexibility (i.e., changes) across group sessions with respect to kinds of feedback given and received, activity level, and "role" adopted (see Flowers, 1979). Additional client behaviors directly related to cohesion include looking at the group member speaking and high rates of self-disclosure.

In preparing clients for behavioral group therapy, both desirable and prohibited behaviors should be specified. The following points may be made to the client to set role expectations. In the course of delineating appropriate role behavior, expectations for positive outcome may also be set:

1. To maximize learning in group therapy, it is important to share personal information about yourself. It is also important to pay attention to other group members when they are talking about themselves.
2. Behavioral therapy groups focus on what is happening "here and now." We generally do not talk about our past histories during therapy sessions.
3. In group, there is usually a lot of both positive and negative feedback exchanged between group members. Some people may talk more than or less than other group members at any given point in time, or they may be about average. Over the long run, the amount of time people talk in group tends to average out.
4. Those members who change the amount of time they spend talking from session to session seem to do well in group. Group members also take different perspectives at different times in the group. Sometimes they are in a position to give feedback to others; sometimes they receive more feedback than they give; and at times feedback is both given and received

during a group session. Being flexible about giving and receiving feedback is typical and desirable for group therapy members.

Bandura (1977) noted that self-efficacy, that is, understanding what is expected of one and believing that such a role *can* be fulfilled, and outcome expectations, that is, believing that behaving in a role-congruent manner will result in a desired outcome, are powerful determinants of behavior. The second and third goals of pretraining clients—providing role expectations and setting positive outcome expectations—may be achieved via the same strategies discussed previously and delineated by Bandura's (1977) self-efficacy theory. These would include preparing clients for group therapy through verbal persuasion or vicarious experience, or additionally, via direct experience.

The initial phase of the preparatory program described previously may consist of a verbal presentation. There is evidence that a flexible interview (Orne & Wender, 1968) may be more effective than a noninteractional lecture or monologue. Included in this part of the program would be procedural issues (e.g., frequency and duration of sessions, number of therapists, confidentiality issues, size of group, etc.) as well as group therapy rationale, client role, and outcome expectancies. Subsequently, a prospective group member might be exposed to a videotaped or filmed presentation of an actual or role-played group. A time-elapsed format, ranging from pretherapy to posttherapy (used by Strupp & Bloxom, 1973), may be implemented to provide models of clients coping with improvement of appropriate role behaviors over time. In constructing such a presentation, attention should be paid to the many important modeling variables that have been empirically identified, such as model–observer similarity, complexity of target behaviors, use of multiple models, coping or mastery presentation as well as others (see Thelen, Fry, Fehrenbach, & Frautschi, 1979, for a review). Additionally, filming techniques may be employed that highlight desirable group therapy behaviors, perhaps promoting vicarious learning. This phase of pretherapy training may be administered to one client, to a group of clients simultaneously, or it may be self-administered.

Along with verbal persuasion and modeling procedures, clients may be prepared for behavioral group therapy through direct experience. After being administered the procedures described previously, a client and therapist might roleplay the behaviors described by the training procedures as role appropriate (e.g., giving or receiving valenced feedback) and additionally anticipate and rehearse anxiety-provoking situations to decrease the potential for negative emotional reactions early in therapy. During pretherapy training, self-instructional strategies (Meichenbaum, 1976) may be given to clients to facilitate better coping with behaviors, for example, self-disclosure, which may elicit anxiety. For instance clients may be taught to verbalize subvocally that

> I'm really nervous about sharing with this group. First I need to take a few deep breaths and calm down. To get what I want out of group I need to participate and talk about myself. The group will be supportive of my disclosing behavior.

Role-playing may also be beneficial in preparing clients for participation in special analog or communication techniques employed in some behavioral groups (e.g., tokens to monitor valenced feedback; Flowers, 1979). It has been suggested (Flowers, personal communication, 1979) that using tokens to accompany feedback in behavioral group therapy is initially uncomfortable and unwieldy, with a reduction in discomfort after 1 to 2 sessions. It could be interesting to determine the effect of pretherapy training, including direct experience with the token exchange procedure, on comfort and competence with the procedure.

The client preparation program outlined in this chapter requires approximately 1 to 2 hours of therapist time and, if tapes or written material are given to the client 2 to 3 hours of client time. Such time would be included as a condition of treatment. The program is addressed primarily to training verbal behaviors appropriate to behavioral group therapy and to the development of cohesion as has been empirically determined (Flowers & Booraem, 1980). Thus, assessment of the utility of this program should focus specifically on these variables. Therapy outcome is, of course, of experimental and, especially, of clinical interest. However, it must be remembered that outcome largely reflects not only preparatory procedures but the efficacy and execution of the therapeutic model itself.

References

Anderson, L., & Ager, J. Analysis of variance in small group research. *Personality and Social Psychology Bulletin*, 1978, *4*, 341–345.

Annis, L. V., & Perry, D. F. Self disclosure modeling in same-sex and mixed-sex unsupervised groups. *Journal of Counseling Psychology*, 1977, *24*, 370–372.

Annis, L. V., & Perry, D. F. Self disclosure in unsupervised groups: Effects of videotaped models. *Small Group Behavior*, 1978, *9*, 102–108.

Baekeland, F., & Lundwall, L. Dropping out of treatment: A critical review. *Psychological Bulletin*. 1975, *82*, 738–783.

Bandura, A. Self-efficacy: Toward a unifying theory of behavioral change. *Psychological Review*, 1977, *84*, 191–215.

Bednar, R. L., & Lawlis, G. F. Empirical research in group psychotherapy. In A. E. Bergin & S. L. Garfield (Eds.), *Handbook of psychotherapy and behavior change; An empirical analysis*. New York: Wiley, 1971.

Bednar, R. L., & Moeschl, M. J. Conceptual and methodological considerations in the evaluation of group psychotherapies. In P. McReynolds (Ed.), *Advances in psychological assessment* (Vol. 5). San Francisco: Jossey-Bass, 1981.

Bednar, R. L., Weet, C., Evensen, P., Lanier, D., & Melnick, J. Empirical guidelines for group therapy: Pretraining, cohesion and modeling. *Journal of Applied Behavioral Science*, 1974, *10*, 149–165.

Bergin, A. E., & Lambert, M. J. The evaluation of therapeutic outcomes. In A. E. Bergin & S. L. Garfield (Eds.), *Handbook of psychotherapy and behavior change*. New York: Wiley, 1978.

Bugen, L. A. Composition and orientation effects on group cohesion. *Psychological Reports*, 1977, *40*, 175–181.

Cartwright, M. H. A preparatory method for group counseling. *Journal of Counseling Psychology*, 1976, *23*, 75–77.

Conyne, R. K., & Silver, R. J. Direct, vicarious, and vicarious-process experiences: Effects on increasing therapeutic attraction. *Small Group Behavior*, 1980, *11*, 419–429.

Craigie, F. C., & Ross, S. M. The use of a videotape pretherapy training program to encourage treatment-seeking among alcohol detoxification patients. *Behavior Therapy*, 1980, *11*, 141–147.

Curran, T. Increasing motivation to change in group treatment. *Small Group Behavior*, 1978, *9*, 337–348.

Flowers, J. V. Behavioral analysis of group therapy and a model for behavioral group therapy. In D. Upper & S. M. Ross (Eds.), *Behavioral group therapy 1979: An annual review.* Champaign, Ill.: Research Press, 1979.

Flowers, J. V., & Booraem, C. D. The use of tokens to facilitate outcome and monitor process in group therapy. *International Journal of Group Psychotherapy*, 1976, *26*, 191–201.

Flowers, J. V., & Booraem, C. D. Three studies toward a fuller understanding of behavioral group therapy: Cohesion, client flexibility, and outcome generalization. In D. Upper & S. M. Ross (Eds.), *Behavioral group therapy, 1980: An annual review.* Champaign, Ill.: Research Press, 1980.

Flowers, J. V., Booraem, C. D., & Seacat, G. F. The effect of positive and negative feedback on members' sensitivity to other members in group therapy. *Psychotherapy: Theory, Research and Practice*, 1974, *11*, 346–350.

Flowers, J. V., Booraem, C. D., Brown, T. R., & Harris, D. E. An investigation of a technique for facilitating patient-to-patient interactions in group therapy. *Journal of Community Psychology*, 1974, *2*, 39–42.

Flowers, J. V., Booraem, C. D., & Hartman, K. A. Client improvement on higher and lower intensity problems as a function of group cohesiveness. *Psychotherapy: Theory, Research and Practice*, 1981, *18*, 246–251.

Frank, J. D., Therapeutic components of psychotherapy. *Journal of Nervous and Mental Disease*, 1974, *5*, 325–342.

Garrison, J. Written vs. verbal preparation of patients for group psychotherapy. *Psychotherapy: Theory, Research, and Practice* 1978, *15*, 130–134.

Goldstein, A. F., Heller, K., & Sechrest, L. B. *Psychotherapy and the psychology of behavior change.* New York: Wiley, 1966.

Goldstein, A., & Wolpe, J. Behavior therapy in groups. In H. I. Kaplan & B. Sadock (Eds.), *New models for group therapy.* New York: Jason Aronson, 1972.

Hays, W. L. *Statistics for the social sciences* (2d ed.). New York: Holt, Rinehart & Winston, 1973.

Heitler, J. Preparation of lower-class patients for expressive group psychotherapy. *Journal of Consulting and Clinical Psychology*, 1973, *41*, 251–260.

Hoehn-Saric, R., Frank, J., Imber, S., Nash, E., Stone, A., & Battle, C. Systematic preparation of patients in psychotherapy: I. Effects on therapy behavior and outcome. *Journal of Psychiatric Research*, 1964, *2*, 267–281.

Jacobs, M., Trick, O. L., & Withersty, D. Pre-training psychiatric inpatients for participation in group psychotherapy. *Psychotherapy: Theory, Research, and Practice*, 1976, *13*, 361–367.

Kanfer, F. H., & Saslow, G. Behavioral diagnosis. In C. M. Franks (Ed.), *Behavior therapy: Appraisal and status.* New York: McGraw-Hill, 1969.

Krumboltz, J. D., & Potter, B. Behavioral techniques for developing trust, cohesiveness and goal accomplishment. *Educational Technology*, 1973, *13*, 26–30.

Krumboltz, J. D., Varenhorst, B. B., & Thoresen, C. E. Non-verbal factors in the effectiveness of models in counseling. *Journal of Counseling Psychology*, 1967, *14*, 412–418.

Liberman, B. L., Frank, J. D., Hoehn-Saric, R., Stone, A. R., Imber, S. D., & Pande, S. K. Patterns of change in treated psychoneurotic patients: A five-year follow-up investigation of the systematic preparation of patients for psychotherapy. *Journal of Consulting and Clinical Psychology*, 1972, *38*, 36–41.

Lieberman, M. A., Lakin, M., & Whitaker, D. S. The group as a unique context for therapy. *Psychotherapy: Theory, Research and Practice*, 1968, *5*, 29–36.

Lieberman, M. A., Yalom, I. D., & Miles, M. B. *Encounter groups: First facts.* New York: Basic Books, 1973.

Liberman, R. Reinforcement of cohesiveness in group therapy: Behavioral and personality changes. *Archives of General Psychiatry*, 1971, *25*, 168–177.

Mayerson, N. H. Preparing clients for group therapy: A critical review and theoretical formulation. *Clinical Psychology Review*, 1984, *4*, 191–213.

Meichenbaum, D. A self-instructional approach to stress management: A proposal for stress inoculation training. In C. Spielberger & I. Sarason (Eds.), *Stress and anxiety in modern life.* New York: Winston & Sons, 1976.

Orne, M., & Wender, P. Anticipatory socialization for psychotherapy: Method and rationale. *American Journal of Psychiatry*, 1968, *124*, 88–98.

Parrino, J. J. Effect of pretherapy information on learning in psychotherapy. *Journal of Abnormal Psychology*, 1971, *77*, 17–24.

Piper, W. E., Debbane, E. G., Garant, J., & Bienvenu, J. Pretraining for group psychotherapy: A cognitive-experiential approach. *Archives of General Psychiatry*, 1979, *36*, 1250–1256.

Rague, D. W. The effects of a videotaped pre-therapy training program on the behavior of clients during their initial therapy sessions. *Dissertation Abstracts International*, 1974, 34(9B), 4673.

Sansbury, D. L. The role of the group in behavioral group therapy. In D. Upper & S. M. Ross (Eds.), *Behavioral group therapy, 1979: An annual review*. Champaign, Ill.: Research Press, 1979.

Schonfield, J., Stone, A. R., Hoehn-Saric, R., Imber, S. R., & Pande, S. Patient–therapist convergence and measures of improvement in short-term psychotherapy. *Psychotherapy: Theory, Research, and Practice*, 1969, *6*, 267–272.

Silver, R., & Conyne, R. Effects of direct experience and vicarious experience on group therapeutic attraction. *Small Group Behavior*, 1977, *8*, 83–92.

Sloane, R., Cristal, A., Pepernick, M., & Staples, F. Role preparation and expectancy of improvement in psychotherapy. *Journal of Nervous and Mental Disease*, 1970, *150*, 18–26.

Strupp, H., & Bloxom, A. L. Preparing lower class patients for group psychotherapy: Development and evaluation of a role induction film. *Journal of Consulting and Clinical Psychology*, 1973, *41*, 373–384.

Tatsuoko, M. M. *Multivariate analysis: Techniques for educational and psychological research*. New York: Wiley, 1980.

Thelen, M. H., Fry, R. A. Fehrenbach, P. A., & Frautschi, N. M. Therapeutic videotape and film modeling: A review. *Psychological Bulletin*, 1979, *86*, 701–720.

Truax, C. B., & Carkhuff, R. Personality change in hospitalized mental patients during group psychotherapy as a function of the use of alternate sessions and vicarious therapy pretraining. *Journal of Clinical Psychology*, 1965, *21*, 225–228.

Truax, C. B., & Wargo, D. B. Effects of vicarious therapy pretraining and alternate sessions on outcome in group psychotherapy with outpatients. *Journal of Consulting and Clinical Psychology*, 1969, *33*, 440–447.

Truax, C., Shapiro, J., & Wargo, D. The effects of alternate sessions and vicarious therapy pretraining on group psychotherapy. *International Journal of Group Psychotherapy*, 1968, *18*, 186–198.

Truax, C. B., Wargo, D. G., Carkhuff, R. R., Kodman, J., & Moles, E. A. Changes in self-concepts during group psychotherapy as a function of alternate sessions and vicarious therapy pretraining in institutionalized mental patients and juvenile delinquents. *Journal of Consulting Psychology*, 1966, *30*, 309–314.

Truax, C., Wargo, D., & Volksdorf, N. Antecedents to outcome in group counseling with institutionalized juvenile delinquents: Effects of therapeutic conditions, patient self-exploration, alternate session, and vicarious therapy pretraining. *Journal of Abnormal Psychology*, 1970, *76*, 235–242.

Whalen, C. Effects of a model and instructions on group verbal behaviors. *Journal of Consulting and Clinical Psychology*, 1969, *33*, 509–521.

Wogan, M., Getter, H., Amdur, M. J., Nichols, M. F., & Okman, G. Influencing interaction and outcomes in group psychotherapy. *Small Group Behavior*, 1977, *8*, 25–46.

Yalom, I. D. *The theory and practice of group psychotherapy*. New York: Basic Books, 1975.

Yalom, I. D., Houts, P. S., Newell, G., & Rand, K. H. Preparation of patients for group therapy: A controlled study. *Archives of General Psychiatry*, 1967, *17*, 416–427.

4

Teaching Problem-Solving Skills to Chronic Psychiatric Patients

JEFFREY R. BEDELL AND DIANN DEE MICHAEL

INTRODUCTION

Recent developments in psychological treatment are built upon the concept that pathological behavior is best modified through the application of the empirical and scientific approach to clinical treatment. Consistent with this approach, significant advances in treatment have occurred when behavior was objectively observed, manipulated, and evaluated. The foundations of many of these modern treatments are found in learning theory that were originally based on laboratory data generated from research with animals and were later successfully applied to human behavior (e.g., Watson & Rayner, 1920). Although some of the mechanistic assumptions required for the functional analysis of behavior have been criticized on humanistic grounds, the heuristic contributions of these theories in the development and refinement of treatment techniques must be acknowledged. As learning theory has been applied in psychological and educational settings, differing procedural approaches have developed. Educational applications have emphasized procedures that led to cognitive awareness, understanding, and mental development. Psychological applications of learning theory, especially in areas of mental health treatment, have emphasized procedures leading to behavioral change and enhanced performance. Most recently, the techniques of psychological and educational practice have been brought together, and this has lead to effective programs of psychoeducational treatment (Bedell, Archer, & Marlowe, 1980; Bedell & Weathers, 1979). This approach to theory allows the potential to borrow the most effective procedures from psychology and education, creating a powerful behavior change tool.

The emphasis on psychoeducational programming is also based, in part, on a philosophy of treatment that attempts to build on individual strengths rather than emphasizing weakness and pathology. There have been a number of at-

JEFFREY R. BEDELL and DIANN DEE MICHAEL • University of South Florida and Florida Mental Health Institute, Tampa, Florida 33612.

tempts to develop concepts of competency. Some focus on achievements (Phillips & Cowitz, 1953; Richards, Holland, & Lutz, 1966), whereas others look for internal antecedents of effective behavior (Doll, 1953; Foote & Cattrell, 1955). These definitions of compentency do not fit into a behavioral program, however. The definition based on achievement emphasizes the *external products* of effective behavior rather than the behavior itself. Similarly, definitions of competency based on the *internal antecedents* of effective behavior focus on nonbehavioral phenomenon such as attitudes, motives, and traits.

A more operational approach to defining competence focuses on behavior–environment interactions and is more consistent with current psychological and educational practices. Such definitions of competence have led to a focus on the development of specific skills such as problem-solving ability.

An excellent example of this approach was presented by Goldfried and D'Zurilla (1969) who focused on problem solving and proposed a behavioral definition of competence that identifies the *effective response* as the basic unit. They define *effective behavior* as behavior that has the desired influence on the environment. They further apply the definition of competence to situations that are "problematic" and require a solution. According to these authors, problem solving is required in situations in which present difficulties are caused by the failure of previously effective responses. Goldfried and D'Zurilla consider problem-solving ability to be fundamental to effective behavior. They define *problem-solving ability* as a behavioral process that generates a variety of alternatives to solving a problem and increases the probability of selecting and using an effective alternative. Their schema for evaluating effective behavior conceptualizes both competence and problem-solving behavior in a way that is consistent with a stimulus-response (S-R) paradigm.

Assessing Problem-Solving Ability

Goldfried and D'Zurilla (1969) distinguish among three methods of evaluating problem-solving ability. The first is the *naive empirical* approach, in which measurement instruments are devised according to their ability to predict certain criterion behaviors. The second is the *global* approach that focuses on the clinical interpretation of data to infer personality characteristics. The third method is the *analytic* approach that focuses on a criterion analysis and attempts to identify the personality characteristics of an "effective individual" in a particular environment and then assesses the extent to which specific individuals possess these characteristics. Goldfried and D'Zurilla cite the shortcoming of these approaches and suggest a fourth method that they call the *behavior-analytic* approach. This model utilizes the behavioral analysis approach of Kanfer and Saslow (1965) and also includes the analytic approach outlined by Stern, Stein, and Bloom (1956).

Moreover, the behavioral-analytic model proposes that a comprehensive and detailed criterion analysis be carried out separately for the problematic situation and for the various potential responses to the situation. Goldfried and

D'Zurilla emphasize the importance of assessing the various possible behavior-environment interactions. They also suggest the development of measurement instruments based specifically on those behavior–environment interactions rather than using the traditional assessment tools of clinical psychology.

Specific steps presented in the behavioral-analytic approach include (a) situational analysis; (b) response enumeration; (c) response evaluation; (d) development of measurement instruments; and (e) evaluation of this measure. As part of the situational analysis, Goldfried and D'Zurilla emphasized a thorough survey of the relevant situations with which the individual must cope. This component is proposed to be the basis of the behavioral-analytic approach. They suggest techniques such as naturalistic observation, interviews with persons who often observe the problematic situation occurring, and self-report as methods of conducting the situational analysis.

In the process of response enumeration, these authors suggest that it is necessary to develop an array of possible responses to the identified problem. This can be done by direct observation, role playing, interview, or using questionnaires. They further emphasize that each of the possible responses must be described in detail so that its general nature is clear as to the way the response will be implemented.

In the response evaluation step, each possible response must be evaluated according to its degree of effectiveness and its possible consequences. Goldfried and D'Zurilla suggest that these decisions can be assisted by the client's significant others, and that some consensus among those significant others regarding these judgments should be established.

Goldfried and D'Zurilla (1969) suggest a "behaviorally oriented" criterion analysis to help specify the content of the items in the measuring instrument to be employed and defer standards for the evaluation of the measurement tool to those set forth in the APA Standards for Educational and Psychological Tests and Manuals (American Psychological Association, 1966).

The Psychoeducational Model

As mentioned earlier, the combination of various techniques derived from both educational and psychological practice has been called the *psychoeducational approach* to skills training. This model of treatment has been applied to the work of Goldfried and D'Zurilla in an attempt to develop an effective program to teach problem-solving skills, or "effective behavior." Bedell and Weathers (1979) presented a psychoeducational model characterized by the modified roles of the therapist and the client, and the instructional style of the therapy group. The therapist's role was defined to be therapist-as-educator, and the client assumed an active participant role, in contrast with the traditional passive role as recipient of treatment. They suggested that the psychoeducational model was most effective when presented in a group format, which lends itself well to the instructional presentation of material, vicarious learning opportunities from watching other participants, and additional information sharing and feedback derived from the interactional opportunities in the group format.

The psychoeducational model is schematically represented in Figure 1. This model can function as a guide to the therapist and summarizes four major sequential stages of treatment: (a) definition of the skill to be trained; (b) awareness training; (c) skill enhancement; and (d) generalization training. Each step is sequential, and evaluation points are included in the program to allow the clients' skills to be assessed at each step and parts of the program to be repeated if necessary.

The initial step of the program involves defining the skill to be trained. This skill is usually defined by a functional analysis of the client's strengths and weaknesses. After choosing the particular skill to be trained (such as problem solving), the components of that skill are identified, specified, and opera-

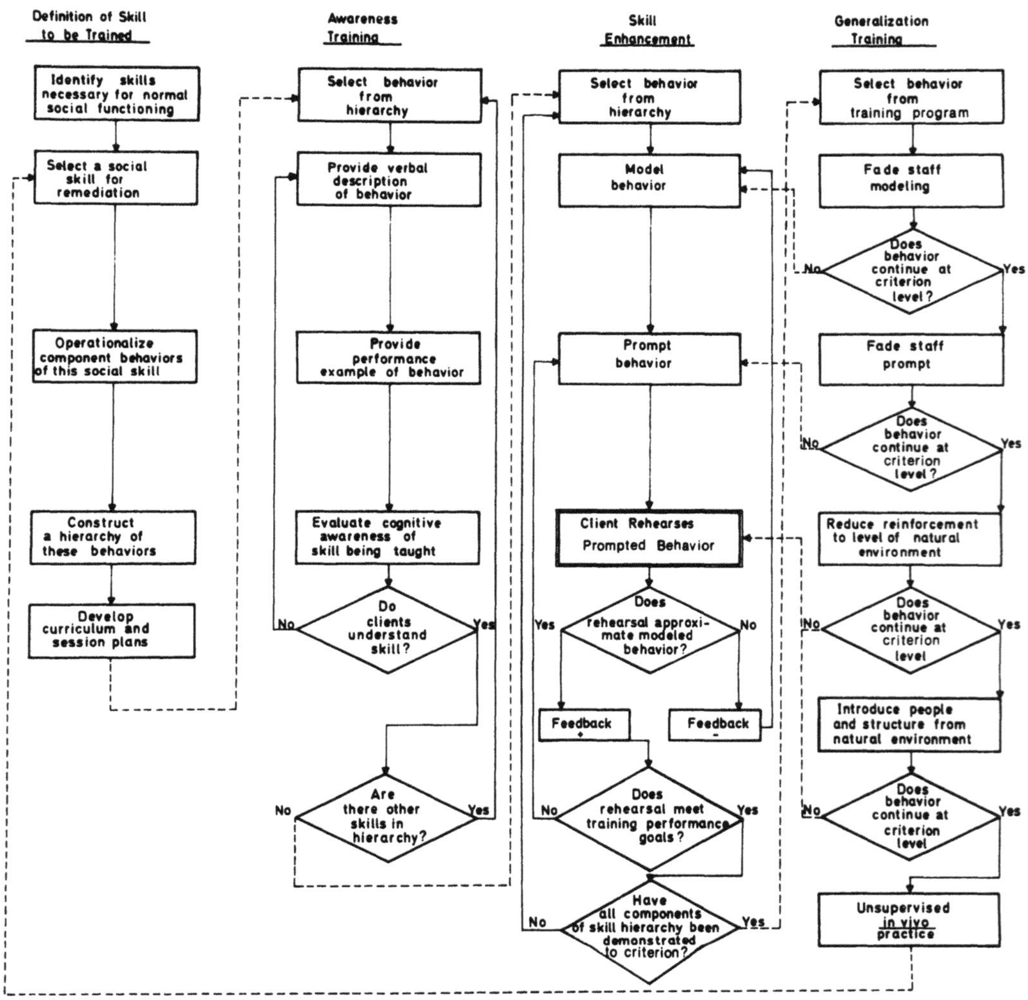

FIGURE 1. A model for psychoeducational programs.

tionalized. In the present case, these components were adapted from Goldfried and D'Zurilla and include problem identification, alternative generation, and the like. These operationalized component behaviors are then organized hierarchically from the most simple and fundamental to the more sophisticated. Bedell and Weathers (1979) emphasized that the skill definition section of the program is essential and is well grounded in educational technology. It is a step often overlooked in most therapy groups.

The process of acquainting the clients to the scope and content of the behaviors to be learned is termed *awareness training*. This technique is similar to what is referred to elsewhere in this volume as *pretherapy training*. These two techniques are similar in that they lay the groundwork for behavioral change and skills acquisition. These methods rely primarily on didactic educational techniques, and clients are presented with descriptions and examples of the desired skills behaviors. An attempt is made to produce an understanding of the cognitive components of the skills to be learned by the client.

Training the clients how to perform the new behaviors is referred to as *skill enhancement* and relies heavily on behavior modification techniques. The therapist models the behavior, then prompts the clients to perform the behavior (rehearsal), with feedback provided on their performances. Each behavior targeted from the hierarchy is repeated until performance reaches criterion standards, and then another behavior is learned.

Techniques from behavior therapy are also employed in the generalization training stage, which focuses on the transfer of the skills attained in the sheltered setting to the natural environment. In this phase, the artificially structured aspects of the group, such as staff modeling and staff prompting, are reduced and eliminated. Reinforcement of the performance of the new behaviors is reduced to levels that are more consistent with those in the natural environment, and the use of homework assignments integrates natural reinforcers into the behavior chain.

As may be seen, the educational and psychological procedures complement each other and work together to create the various cognitive and behavior changes desired. The actual program that has been developed that applies this approach to the work of Goldfried and D'Zurilla will be presented later in this chapter. In order to understand the psychoeducational adaptation of the problem-solving process, however, a brief review of the approach of Goldfried and D'Zurilla will be presented first.

Facilitating Competence: The Stony Brook Approach

In the report of their work conducted at Stony Brook, Goldfried and D'Zurilla (1969) applied the behavioral-analytic approach to the assessment of competence in college freshmen. In the situational analysis, they collected descriptions of a sample of the problematic situations likely to confront male college freshmen during their first semester in college. They utilized several sources in collecting these descriptions, including self-observations by the students, observations by the resident assistants, interviews with faculty and staff, and a survey of the clinical folders of male freshmen applying for treatment at the university psychology center. Using this process, they identified 181 problematic situations such as academic work and dormitory relationships that had a high probability of occurring for male freshmen.

In the response enumeration phase, Goldfried and D'Zurilla (1969) sought to identify possible effective responses to the 181 problem situations. They only considered a subset of the situations for study, using the following method. First, they presented problematic situations to their subjects and asked them to give all of their possible reactions to each situation. Using this procedure, they obtained approximately 20 different responses to each situation. The range of effectiveness of each response was rated by two independent judges. Based on a process of selecting problem situations with response alternatives that potentially could be carried out, a group of 88 problems remained.

Response evaluation involved obtaining ratings from faculty, dormitory counselors, and "significant others" on the effectiveness of the various alternatives generated for each problematic situation. Effectiveness was defined by asking the raters which response would best resolve the problematic nature of the situation and would maximize other positive consequences.

Based on this process of response enumeration, simulations of problematic situations were developed. Subjects were asked to respond to these simulations with detailed discriptions of their likely responses. Comparing these responses to those considered to be effective, the researchers identified students who were potentially ineffective problem solvers. These individuals were then presented with a preventative treatment program. The primary goal of which was problem-solving training. The program attempted to develop an awareness of the most effective responses to problematic situations, thus establishing a process of self-control wherein the individual could become more effective by manipulating external stimuli and internal thought operations. D'Zurilla and Goldfried (1971) conceived problem solving as the first phase in the process of developing self-control, and this self-control would in turn lead to effective or competent behavior. They suggested a variety of training techniques that would be useful in facilitating competency through the training of the problem-solving process. Techniques that were suggested included verbal instructions and discussion, behavioral rehearsal, programmed texts, and computer-aided teaching machines.

Training Problem-Solving Processes: The Florida Mental Health Institute Approach

Building on the work of D'Zurilla and Goldfried (1971), a problem-solving program was developed at the Florida Mental Health Institute. Although in many respects the specific procedures used to train the problem-solving behaviors are innovative, the underlying process is adapted from D'Zurilla and Goldfried. As described previously in this chapter, these researchers developed and presented a problem-solving model that resulted from extensive analysis of the problem-solving process. They defined problem solving as

> a behavioral process, whether overt or cognitive in nature, which (a) makes available a variety of potentially effective response alternatives for dealing with the problematic situation, and (b) increases the probability of selecting the most effective response from among these various alternatives. (p. 108)

After an extensive review of the literature and a critical analysis of the components of the problem-solving process, they concluded that there was much agreement with regard to the general aspects of the effective problem-solving process. They proposed the following five stages as representing a general consensus of the literature: (a) general orientation ("set" and attitude); (b) problem definition and formulation; (c) generation of alternatives; (d) decision making; and (e) verification.

Bedell, Archer, and Marlowe (1980) reported on an adaption of this model as the foundation of a problem-solving skills training program. The program had 12 sessions, each divided into sections focusing on either awareness training or skill enhancement/generalization training. In the awareness training section, the clients are presented with the problem-solving model that includes (a) problem recognition; (b) problem definition; (c) alternatives generation; and (d) alternative evaluation and decision. The clients apply the model in the skill enhancement/generalization training section by practicing each of the four phases of problem solving separately, then employing them sequentially as a completed process. The training program also included the use of client journals and homework assignments. Clients practiced utilizing the problem-solving model with hypothetical problems through role playing and later applied the model to their own personal real-life problems.

As can be seen, Bedell, Archer, and Marlowe (1980) adapted the problem-solving skills that were the focus of their program from the model presented by D'Zurilla and Goldfried (1971). Four major processes of problem solving were identified for training: (a) problem recognition; (b) problem definition; (c) alternatives generation; and (d) alternatives evaluation and decision. Of particular interest was the breakdown of fourth process—alternatives evaluation—into subskill areas that involved (a) predicting possible outcomes of alternative solutions; (b) determining the likelihood of each outcome; (c) determining the desirability of each outcome; (d) rankordering alternative solutions; and (e) making a decision.

The Problem Solving Skills Training program utilized didactic lectures, structured role play, journals, psychotherapeutic games, and homework as methods of presenting material and establishing the behaviors necessary to successful problem solution.

The problem recognition step involved acknowledging the problem, identifying and specifying it, and accepting responsibility for the problem. This step was essential and basic to the remainder of the process. After establishing the recognition and specification of the problem, problem definition involved breaking it into workable units and stating the problem in a solvable form.

The alternatives generation step was trained through brainstorming, changing the frame of reference, adapting solutions from similar problems, and using an idea checklist or drawing a problem diagram.

The generalization training step utilized homework assignments as the primary mechanism for encouraging the use of newly learned skills in the natural environment. Client journals were employed in conjunction with homework, and journal entries were brought back into the therapy group for discussion. Thus, it may be seen that the Florida Mental Health Institute (FMHI) problem-solving program was highly structured and sequential. Procedures for presenting the various stages of the problem-solving process were based on educational and psychological procedures and were heavily influenced by the Stony Brook approach. The program presented in this chapter is a further development of the FMHI approach to problem-solving skills training and illustrates the usefulness of the psychoeducational model as a set of guidelines for program development. Also, the present program was specifically designed for application in a mental health setting with clients having significant deficits in social skills areas of functioning.

Evaluation of Problem-Solving Programs

Assessment in problem solving is a relatively recent area of inquiry, as several researchers have noted (Heppner, 1978; Horan, 1979). A few of the more representative reports dealing with the evaluation of problem-solving ability will be reviewed here. As will be seen, there has not been a vast amount of research in this area, and much remains to be done. A review of these important studies will, however, provide the reader with a sense of the current status of this area.

Platt and Spivack (1972a, 1972b) developed a *means–ends–problem-solving procedure* with which they have since investigated the problem-solving processes of adolescents (Platt, Spivack, Altman, Altman, & Peizer, 1974). Shure and Spivack (1972, p. 348) define *means–ends thinking* as

> the ability to carefully plan, step by step, means to reach a stated goal. Such planning includes insight and forethought to forestall or circumvent potential obstacles, and, in addition, having at one's command alternative routes if such an obstacle is realistically or psychologically insurmountable.

They suggest that certain subjects become "overwhelmed" by the environment and experience a narrowing of means–ends thinking through preoccupation with the end goal, rather than focusing on the means by which they may attain it.

Research in the area of means–ends thinking indicates that normal adolescents have a wider repetoire of means–ends thinking than do disturbed adolescents (Spivack & Levine, 1963), with similar results being found for normal adults and psychiatric patients (Platt & Spivack, 1970). Also, this pattern of narrowed means–ends thinking apparently emerges at an early age with less well-adjusted 4-year-olds who were found to provide fewer solutions and fewer categories of relevant and adaptable solutions than well-adjusted children of the same age (Shure & Spivack, 1970). Shure and Spivack (1972) found significant differences in the means–ends solutions employed by normal versus disturbed elementary students, regardless of social class and independent of IQ. In this study, they reported that normal children employed a broader spectrum of possibilities and a greater number of strategies of planning. Disturbed children also were found to employ alternatives that would be contrary to social codes, for example, physical aggression.

Heppner and Petersen (1982) investigated the dimensions underlying real-life, personal problem solving, utilizing a factor-analytic approach and developed a measure of problem solving. They describe a Problem Solving Inventory that consisted of a 6-point Likert-type format of 35 items, representing five problem-solving stages. They also utilizied a *Level of Problem-Solving Skills Estimate Form* (LPSSEF) (Heppner, 1979) and the *Rotter Internal-External* (I-E) *Locus of Control* (Rotter, 1966). The LPSSEF provided self-ratings of subjects' level of problem-solving skills on a 1–9 scale and their level of satisfaction or dissatisfaction (1–6) with their present level of problem-solving skills. Their results indicated three dimensions underlying the perceived problem-solving process as being (a) confidence in one's problem-solving ability; (b) an approach-avoidant style; and (c) personal control.

Assessment techniques applied to problem-solving skills training seem to fall into two categories. One technique involves the estimation of a subject's problem-solving ability, either by self-report, observation of teachers, co-workers, or significant others. The other technique obtains scores of problem-solving performance in response to case examples of problem situations. The subjects' selection of alternative choices is compared with some predetermined ideal to determine their appropriateness.

In general, there is much left to be done in the area of evaluation of problem-solving skills. Much of the difficulty of evaluation has to do with the complexity of the area of study and the indiosyncracies of problems.

One observation that guided the development of the problem-solving approach used by the FMHI was the importance of having a process for evaluating the various possible solutions to each individual problem. It was decided to emphasize this relatively neglected aspect of the problem-solving training. As will be noted later, the problem-solving process was expanded from that used previously to include an evaluation phase. In this phase, clients and significant others provide input regarding how effective the alternative behavior selected was in solving the problem situation.

Description of Problem-Solving Program

The following section of this chapter describes a problem-solving skills training program based on the psychoeducational model described previously by Bedell and Weathers (1979). This model provided a guide for developing and organizing group procedures so that both educational and psychological processes occurred. The combination of these procedures has been shown to enhance the effectiveness of social skills training programs for chronic mental patients.

The unique features of a psychoeducational program for training problem-solving skills are primarily related to its educational flavor. The therapist or group leader takes on the role of educator and trainer. He or she instructs at both the cognitive and behavioral levels using didactic presentations, "lesson plans," and other structured teaching methods. The overall content of the skills training program is defined by a written curriculum that sets both the performance goals of each training session and also the scope of the overall program. There are clearly specified goals for each group session as compared to the unstructured process of traditional group therapy where the therapist guides the content of the session according to his or her clinical judgment. This comparison does not imply that a psychoeducational program is inflexible and cannot be tailored to deal with the current issues of individual clients. On the contrary, the program is flexible and, as will be shown in the description of sessions to follow, currently relevant, and individualized material is the principal focus of treatment.

The client in a psychoeducational program also has a different role than in traditional group therapy. He or she is a student learning new concepts and behaviors. The goal of the program is skills enhancement rather than the identification of psychopathology. As a student, the client is expected to take an active role in the process of treatment and to take an interest in and responsibility for personal development. Clients in a psychoeducational program are not provided a cure by the trainer but join into an alliance in an effort to improve social functioning.

The use of the educationally oriented "curriculum" to both define and to set boundaries for each session and for the entire problem-solving program is fundamental to the present program. Using this approach facilitates the use of a variety of levels of staff and various disciplines. Staff are typically trained by someone experienced in the program, and once they reach proficiency, they can operate with minimal supervision. The material to be presented and the type of learning that is to occur is clear and objective. Nurses, social workers, and staff trained in other mental health disciplines have been able to conduct these programs with little difficulty arising from their differing professional orientations and training backgrounds.

The limited curriculum also helps to control costs and the length of stay in the program because the amount of gain expected of the client is controlled by the curriculum rather than each individual practitioner.

Comparison of Treatment Program to Other Psychoeducational Treatment

Programs similar to the present one have been developed at the Florida Mental Health Institute and have been described elsewhere (Bedell & Weathers, 1979; Bedell *et al.*, 1980). The present program represents a refinement of previous systems becuase it provides much greater flexibility and in many ways removes the major practical shortcoming of psychoeducationally oriented skills training programs (i.e., the difficulty adjusting to a constantly changing class composition).

In previous applications, each training session laid the groundwork for subsequent sessions, and later sessions built upon prior learning. This method or training is, of course, comparable to the traditional classroom situation where a certain number of classes are held over a period of time. In traditional educational programs, learning is progressive throughout an extended period of time, and material at the end of a course could not be learned without the knowledge gained in earlier classes. Because there is a large number of classes comprising each course, adjustments can be made if students have difficulty with a concept or if learning proceeds more quickly than expected. As long as attendance can be assured throughout the course, it can be expected that learning will occur. Also, everyone in the typical educational program begins and ends a course at the same time. If one cannot begin the course at its inception, then he or she must wait until the next term. Also, excessive absences would be likely to result in poor learning.

In mental health, it is very difficult to adhere to some of these fundamental premises that underlie the traditional classroom education system. Mental patients typically experience unplanned episodes of disturbance making it impossible for them to schedule the beginning of their treatment. Once a client becomes involved in the mental health system, there is a relatively brief period of time for some treatment to begin. It is not easy for the mental health system to hold clients for more than a few days before beginning treatment. Because of these circumstances, a treatment program will continuously receive referrals from other agencies and practitioners. If these referrals cannot be accommodated quickly, the pressing need for a placement will not be satisfied, and agencies may seek help elsewhere, or the client may be lost by the mental health system.

For these reasons, a psychoeducational program, in order to interface with the mental health system, must be able to accommodate continuous, even daily, additions of new "students" rather than the periodic startups of the typical school curriculum. At the same time, a sequential, building type of skills training program is desirable since this kind of program is consistent with the way people learn new skills. The present program has addressed this problem and has accommmodated it within the psychoeducational model. This issue will be addressed in more detail later in this chapter.

Target Group for Problem-Solving Skills Training

The Problem-solving program described in this chapter is designed and has been tested on low-functioning individuals generally considered chronically mentally handicapped. Most of the clients with which this program has been used have habitually received services from the public mental health system, and most have received treatment in state mental hospitals. The type of client on which this program has been tested has been referred to as the *new chronic* (Pepper & Ryglewicz, 1982). That is, a new chronic is an individual who is relatively young and has many short-term hospitalizations, between which he or she has maintained a borderline adjustment in the community.

Although this program was designed for the chronic mental patient, it also appears to have application for any group of individuals who would benefit from enhanced problem-solving ability. The present program is suitable, for example, for use in outpatient settings with a wide variety of client groups. It has also been adapted for use with "normal" adults interested in personal growth. Members of our staff have often indicated a sense of personal development as a function of being exposed to the program. Certainly, the application of the program is broad.

Objective of Program

Consistent with the psychoeducational model of skills training, goals were established for each treatment session and for the program as a whole. These goals specify the nature of the learning that is intended to occur. As mentioned before, it was also desirable to design a program for use with a group of clients that has almost daily changes in its composition. That is, the client group would have new members added, and older members leaving, on a daily basis. Each individual client, however, is expected to stay in the therapy group for an extended period of time. The amount of time each client takes to master the skills being taught is also expected to be variable because a heterogeneous group of people are typically receiving treatment. Some of the clients, for example, come to the program with good problem-solving skills and will be quick learners of the desired behaviors. These individuals only need a short time (perhaps 2 days) to master the requisite skills. On the other hand, some clients have very poor problem-solving skills and need a long period to master the basic skills.

This issue of group heterogeneity and transient composition represented a difficult program development issue. The solution to this problem has several aspects. First of all, it was decided that performance criteria would determine the rate of a client's advancement through the program. Thus, clients would move through the program at their own individual rates. If one client mastered a group in one session, he or she would move to the next treatment component. If criterion performance was not met and the session needed to be repeated, the client would stay at the same level until the material was mastered. Reference to Figure 1 will show the concept of evaluation and movement from one skill to another. However, if a client repeated a session (which was the general case), it would be boring and uninteresting for him or her to deal with the identical material that was presented in the first session. Therefore, variety was built into the sessions so that the same skills could be taught with different case examples and personal problems selected to which the skills being taught were applied. Thus, a large variety of lessons were developed that would vary in content but train the same skills.

Also, the overall problem-solving program was divided into two large segments. The goal of the first segment, Problem Solving I, focused on the awareness training aspects of the psychoeducational approach. The goal of this phase of training was to establish a cognitive awareness of the various aspects of the problem-solving model. In this segment, the problem-solving model was explained, and the behaviors to be learned were discussed. The client's vocabulary and understanding of problem-solving issues was the principal focus. The techniques employed to present this material were educational in nature, namely didactic lectures that were reinforced by examples and illustrations. Generally, the problem-solving model shown in Table 1 was presented to the group, and an understanding of this model and its various components is the goal of this segment of training.

Because the goal of Problem Solving I is understanding and awareness, examples of problems are kept simple so that more attention is focused on the process of problem solving than on the problem itself. At the Problem Solving I level, the clients begin to apply the problem-solving techniques to their own personal problems. They are instructed, however, to limit the type of problem used for practice to a short-term problem that has happened recently; that is, a

TABLE 1. An Outline of the Problem-Solving Process Taught in Problem Solving I and Which Was the Basis for Problem Solving II

- I. Identify the problem situation
  - A. Describe: who, what, when, where, objective, brief
  - B. Cues
    - 1. Feelings: happy, sad, anger, fear, love
    - 2. Behaviors: prior to or associated with the problem situation and feelings.
- II. Accept responsibility
  - A. Excuse: placing blame outside
  - B. Cause: "I" language
- III. Goal-directed statement
  - A. State problem in goal-directed form "how to"
- IV. Alternative generation
  - A. Brainstorm alternatives
  - B. Identify solution consequences
    - 1. Short-term consequences
      - a. Feelings
      - b. Behaviors
    - 2. Long-term consequences
      - a. Feelings
      - b. Behaviors
  - C. Evaluate solution consequences
    - 1. Positive
    - 2. Negative
- V. Decision
- IV. Evaluate Decision
  - A. Are the consequences positive?
  - B. What is the probability of success?
  - C. Did you act on your decision?
  - D. Did it move toward your goal?

problem that is relatively minor and of limited complexity that has occurred within 24 hours.

The process of Problem Solving I may be described as follows. First the client is presented the didactic material describing the problem-solving model. Next, he or she is required to begin to apply what has been presented. As mentioned before, he or she will first attempt to recognize and define a short-term problem. Next, feelings and thoughts associated with the problem are identified, and the individual learns to express personal responsibility for various aspects of the problem. Next, the problem is stated in such a way that it is solvable and goal directed. Various alternative solutions are generated next, using procedures such as brainstorming. Each possible solution is evaluated with regard to consequences, and a decision is made with regard to the course of action to take. At this point, the client evaluates the decision in terms of its probable workability, success, and effectiveness.

Certain decisions regarding the content of the didactic material presented were guided by characteristics inherent in the chronic psychiatric populations. For example, concrete problems occurring within 24 hours are emphasized to prompt specificity and accuracy in description as well as to avoid problems arising from memory deficits.

Also, five basic feelings are utilized in describing emotions to facilitate the use of common language, to aid communication among group members, and to reduce idiosyncratic responses. Clarity in the distinction between thoughts and feelings was emphasized to prompt awareness of mental processes as distinguished from emotional reactions. Clients were required to identity an *excuse* that was defined as a *blaming statement* in order to make this common deterrent to effective coping explicit and increase the clients' awareness of this process. A *cause* was clearly stated, which encouraged awareness of the *expectations* often implicit and basic to the clients' emotional reaction to events in their lives. Further, clients were to formulate a positive statement of what they want in the situation in a how-to statement. This statement operationalizes and defines their goal, aiding in the subsequent development of problem-solving alternatives. Clients were also prompted to evaluate each alternative for both short-term and long-term consequences with regard to feelings and behaviors for themselves and others. The specificity and concreteness of the content of the didactic presentation aided clients of even very low functional levels to identify a concrete problem situation and utilize common language, thus facilitating communication and problem-solving training.

The goals of the second section of the program (Problem Solving II) were oriented toward the skills acquisition phase of the psychoeducational program. Because the clients who have completed Problem Solving I have a good understanding of the problem-solving process and the various definitional issues, attention now can be focused on developing behavioral skills. The clients are provided the opportunity to apply the techniques to long-term, recurring personal problems. This is done by first focusing on simulations of real problems and then with actual problems the client is attempting to solve as part of his or her treatment. The program was structured to focus on the following topic areas:

(a) intimate and marital relationships; (b) friendship and social support; (c) family relationships; (d) employment; (e) housing; and (f) physical health. These categories were selected for attention because they are areas where problems warranting attention commonly develop. Focusing on these topics provides a structure that helps clients to focus attention to each of these critical areas of their lives and to facilitate improvement. These topics were also chosen to target personal and community adjustment and to facilitate the clients' active problem solving in their own discharge plans.

Generalization of the problem solving skills outside of the group therapy setting and to the natural environment was another central goal of Problem Solving II. This was accomplished by the use of structured homework assignments in which issues that surface in the therapy setting are carried over to free time and to out-of-group activities. The homework assignments are subsequently reviewed by the group and the therapist to provide support, feedback and so that success can be reinforced and difficulties in approach can be corrected.

Treatment and Training Procedures[1]

Example of Problem Solving I

Because this phase of the program is directed toward awareness training, the first portion of the training is a didactic lecture. A shortened example of the presentation follows

> We will be learning a problem-solving model that allows us to better deal with specific problem situations. In this group, we will identify our feelings and behaviors related to a problem situation. In order to solve a problem, we must take responsibility and develop a positive, goal-directed statement. In order to develop a plan for solution, we will generate and evaluate alternatives. Evaluating alternatives involves becoming aware of the consequences of each alternative, both for ourselves and others. After evaluating our alternatives, we must make a decision and act on it. Problem solving does not end with the decision, however, for we then need to review and evaluate our decision for its effectiveness.
>
> The first step to problem solving is acknowledging the existence of a problem situation and identifying it clearly. In identifying the situation we want to (a) specify our own and/or other's behavior (who and what); (b) make a statement of the situation that is free of feelings or judgments; (c) make a brief and objective statement of the situation; (d) specify a statement that has resulted in an emotional response; (e) describe a problem situation that has occurred within 24 hours (when); (f) specify the location where the problem situation occurred (where); and (g) describe one problem aspect only.

[1]The problem-solving groups described here were developed as a team effort of the Florida Mental Health Institute's Department of Adult Programs' staff and many individual staff members of the Intensive Residential Treatment Unit II made useful and significant contributions. We wish to acknowledge the staff members of IRT II and the following individuals for their collaboration in the development of the program: Kathy Penner, Barry Naster, Steve Hinrich, and Jan Harvey.

The leader then has a client put some examples of a problem situation on the board, and the group will correct the example until a brief, nonjudgmental statement of the situation indicates a *who, what, where,* and *when*. In summarizing the problem identification step of problem solving, the staff member stresses the following: (a) objectivity; and (b) briefness. Examples such as the following are used to aid in the process of problem identification.

WRONG: My boyfriend really makes me mad when he is inconsiderate and when we get in fights.
RIGHT: Last night at 5 P.M., my boyfriend called me on the phone and told me that he would pick me up at 7 P.M. at my house to go out.
WHO: Boyfriend and me.
WHAT: Boyfriend told me that he would pick me up at 7 P.M. to go out.
WHEN: He told me this at 5 P.M.
WHERE: He told me on the phone at my house.

The group leader calls on members to describe the situation as suggested by the model. Other members are asked to indicate agreement/disagreement and to discuss the member's description. The group leader seeks to ensure that the following are discussed. (This step may be repeated before proceeding.)

1. Are own and others' behaviors related to situation?
2. Is statement free of feelings and judgments?
3. Is statement objective and brief?
4. Does statement create an emotional response?
5. Is statement short term (specific time, when)?
6. Does statement have a specific location (where)?
7. Does statement describe the problem?

When we have a problem situation, there are feelings and behaviors that accompany the problem and function as cues for us. Our feelings and behaviors are cues, or signposts, that there is a problem that needs to be identified and solved. Thus, we can use our feelings and behaviors as cues that something is wrong and a situation needs attention. For example, if I slam my car door and snap at my friend when he says "hello," these behaviors are cues that there is a problem. I may be unaware of the problem, or I may be only partially aware of it. My friend may ask me what's wrong, thus aiding me in becoming more aware of my behavior. Behaviors are actions which are observable and audible, or may be actions which are not observable and audible (sit, listen), but always have accompanying body postures which can be observed or heard (sit, stand, lie down, talk).

The leader then has a client put an example of a behavior which accompanies a problem situation on the board and the group discusses it.

I may also become aware of my feelings, for example, being angry. Often if we stop to consider our feelings and behaviors, we can start to identify a problem objectively.

In order to specify our feelings, it is important to recognize the difference between feelings and thoughts. Feelings are emotional reactions that are accompanied by bodily sensations. For example, when we feel angry, we often get hot, tense, our blood pressure goes up, our stomach tightens, etc. There are two different types of feelings, physical and emotional. Examples of physical feelings are being tired, hungry, or thirsty. Emotional feelings have different intensities. I may feel "a little angry" or a "lot of anger." It is important to recognize the intensity of a feeling so that something can be done to work through the feeling if it is desired that the feeling not increase or decrease.

Thoughts are mental statements. Often we have thoughts that express desires, make comparisons, or are descriptions of feelings. These thoughts are not feelings. For example, there are thoughts such as "I want" [*mental statements of desire*], "I feel like" [*mental statement of a comparison*], "I feel anxious" [*mental statement of a feeling*]. What are some other statements that are thoughts and often are confused for feelings [*group discussion*]?

There are five basic feelings: happiness, sadness, anger, fear, and love. These are basic feelings in that they cannot be broken down further into simpler emotions. Often we use words like *grief* to express a feeling. Grief is a feeling, but it is complex and refers to several basic feelings such as anger and sadness, specifically regarding the loss of a loved one. Thus, grief is a combination of three of the basic feelings: love, sadness, and anger. Another example of a complex emotion is compassion. If you feel compassion, you may experience love, sadness, anger, happiness, etc., in relation to another person. Compassion is complex because you feel happy for the other person when things are going well for them and sad when things are going poorly for them. Compassion involves concern regarding another person's well-being and involves several of the basic emotions depending on the situation.

In order to problemsolve effectively you need to identify your basic feelings. Often we are aware of more than one basic feeling, and that is fine. All feelings are acceptable, and it is not a matter of "right" or "wrong" to have any feeling in regard to any situation.

There are *behavior cues* that are associated with our feelings, both before and after the situation occurred. Feelings and behavior cues help us to be aware of our feelings. For example, I may slam my car door and snap at my friend, thus cuing me that I am angry. Often, our behavior and feelings occur so close in time that we "act" before we are aware of our feelings. Thus, behaviors and feelings are cues that we are reacting to a problem situation. [*Clients are asked for examples of feelings prior to and during the situation that are written on the board and discussed by the group.*]

When we find ourselves in a problem situation, we often place blame outside ourselves, thus forming an "excuse." *Excuses* are statements that place the blame for a situation outside ourselves. For example, I may be angry because "the traffic was too heavy" or because my friend "didn't call and wake me in time." Excuses are thoughts that blame anyone or anything, including "self"—for example, "I was so stupid." These statements allow us to avoid taking responsibility for the problem situation. Only through accepting responsibility for the problem situation, for our own feelings, and for our own behaviors, can we make a constructive attempt to solve a problem.

Being aware of the *cause* of a problem situation is taking responsibility for one's contribution to the situation itself—your feelings, and your behaviors. The cause is a thought, and becoming aware of it involves identifying your loss or gain with regard to your expectations in the situation. Our feelings are reactions to whether the world fulfills our expectations. If we are losing something we expect to have available to us, we are afraid, angry, or sad. These emotions are all related to a *loss* in relation to our expectations. If we *gain* something in relation to our expectations, we are happy. The following are examples of expectations: "I expected my boyfriend to come over at 7 P.M. and he didn't," or "I expected my boyfriend to keep his promise and when he didn't, I thought I was not important to him, and I lost some self-esteem."

Our expectations are important in defining our feelings. We can change our expectations and thus deal with our feelings and/or behaviors in regard to a problem situation. This process of redefinition of our expectations in regard to the world may eliminate problems by restructuring our thinking about them. [*The leader asks for an example of an excuse and a cause from clients that related to their feelings during a situation and then writes it on the board for group discussion.*]

Once we have been very clear about defining our problem situation, feelings, behaviors, and "excuses," we can accept responsibility by owning the *cause* of the problem situation by defining the expectations we had. We are now ready to make a positive, goal-directed how-to statement regarding the situation and regarding our feelings. The how-to statement directs our solution by making a concrete, behavioral statement of what we want or need in the situation.

The alternatives we generate should relate to our goal-directed how-to statements. The how to can be global or specific and needs to be within your control; that is, "How to get Mary to clean up her mess" is not within my control, but "How to ask Mary to clean up the mess" is within my control. [*The leader asks the client to write a sample how-to statement on the board for group discussion.*]

In generating alternatives, any alternative that relates to the how-to statement is acceptable. In generating solutions, we try to "brainstorm" alternatives. Since any idea is a possible solution, all answers are acceptable for consideration. The following are some examples of ways to generate alternatives: (a) fantasize for solution ideas; (b) observe others for solution ideas; (c) use reference sources for solution ideas—books, magazines, movies, TV, etc.; (d) change frame of reference for solution ideas—imagine how others deal with similar situations; and (e) talk to others—ask for suggestions, etc. [*The leader asks for six alternatives to write on board for group discussion.*]

In order to evaluate the alternatives, we must be aware of the immediate, short-term consequences that each alternative will generate. Each alternative will have possible consequences in feelings and behaviors for ourselves and for others. The possible short-term consequences of an alternative may be different from the long-term consequences. Part of evaluating the effectiveness of a solution is to forecast your feelings and behaviors if the situation recurs in order to evaluate the long-term consequences for ourselves and for others.

While we can never be absolutely sure about how each alternative will work out, evaluating possible consequences of each alternative will aid us in solving problems. The alternative you choose must be socially appropriate and legal. [*The leader has a client write an example of the short- and long-term consequences of the problem on the blackboard and choose a socially acceptable and legal decision. The following issues are discussed*]:

1. The solution should relate to your how-to statement.
2. After we make a decision, we develop new expectations. Next, we base our feelings on whether our decision got us what we wanted [*expected*] or didn't get us what we wanted [*expected*]. If we start to become aware of this process, we will be more in control of feelings, as it is our choice to react to our losses and gains in a neutral manner, positively or negatively.
3. How will I feel if my decision does not meet my how-to goal?
4. In order to adequately evaluate your decision, you need to act on it. If you chose a decision you did not act on, perhaps another choice would have been preferable. We need to ask what happened as a result of your actions and how your decision moved you toward your goal in regard to the situation and your feeling.

Sometimes after evaluating a decision, we find another alternative to be useful and decide to apply it to the situation. Problem solving is a continual learning process of awareness, action, and reflection in moving toward meeting our needs and taking responsibility for ourselves.

Having been presented this material, the clients are then given a written case example so that they can apply what they have learned in the lecture. Using this case example, they apply the problem-solving model described in Table 1.

First, they work independently; then a client is selected to present his or her materials to the group. The group leader selects the client by asking for volunteers. If no one volunteers, then the trainer may discuss this issue to see if it is due to shyness or a lack of understanding of the material. Once this is rectified and if there still are no volunteers, the leader will use his or her judgment in selecting an appropriate client to present the materials to the group. This individual explains his or her problem-solving ideas to the group and writes on the blackboard how he or she applied the problem-solving model to the case example. Other clients and the leader comment and provide feedback about the approach taken. Erroneous ideas or content areas that are not understood are discussed and clarified, and this process continues until the client presents a solution that is consistent with the guidelines. Another client is then asked to present his or her solution, and discussion continues for approximately 30 minutes.

At this point, the clients are instructed to apply these same techniques and procedures to a short-term personal problem they have experienced lately. Each client identifies such a problem and applies the problem-solving model to it. The group leader assists where necessary. Clients are instructed that, as a homework assignment, they are to act on the decision made as a result of their problem-solving process. They will be asked later to explain how the decision worked out and generally to evaluate the outcome of their actions.

Later, this homework is evaluated, and points are assigned according to a standardized system for the successful completion of each component of the problem-solving model. If there are areas where performance is poor, these areas receive further attention and instruction. The client "passes" the Problem Solving I group when he or she demonstrates on the worksheets that 80% of the information is correct. Examples of questions on the worksheet are the description of a problem situation, the generation of alternative solutions, and selecting a decision.

If the client participates in the Problem Solving I group and a homework application of the material without meeting the criteria to "pass" the group, he or she will repeat the group. The materials presented the next time the group is held (it is conducted three times a week) are similar in task but different in specific content. The didactic material relating to the problem-solving model is, of course, the same, but the model is applied to a different case example in each session. There are 12 case examples that have been developed for the Problem Solving I module. Each case example deals with a different type of problem that is considered appropriate for this level of training. That is, the problem is not overly complex or highly emotionally charged but represents a prototype of a meaningful issue with which the clients can identify. The intent of the case example at this point is to encourage the application of material at the cognitive, or understanding, level. For example, one case to which the model is applied relates to an individual becoming frustrated and angry because he runs out of cigarettes and has no money to purchase more. Our experience has indicated this is a problem situation with which a majority of clients very readily identify. Another case example has to do with asking for a date and dealing with being turned down. Still another poses the problem of what to do with an overly sloppy roommate. Each case example is designed to provide a format for eliciting from the client what he or she understands about the problem-solving material being presented. Each application is different enough to keep clients who must repeat the session interested and were developed from situations that clients had often posed as being problematic for them. The program is designed so that a client could attend the Problem Solving I Group 12 times and each time have a new and different case example on which to apply his or her knowledge. As will be shown later, most clients complete Problem Solving I in less than five sessions.

This format also allows for new members to continuously join the group while others are leaving, by meeting the criteria for passing. As mentioned earlier, continuous admissions and discharges are typical of mental health treatment groups, and this situation represents a difficulty for the sequential psychoeducational program. A brief description of a typical session will serve to illustrate this programmatic innovation that adapts problem-solving training to continuously changing group membership.

On a given day, the Problem Solving I group has 10 to 12 participants. Several of these individuals are experiencing the group for the first time. Several will be repeating it for the second or third time, and several may be repeating it for the fourth time or more. Clients at each of these levels experience the group differently. The newcomers hear the information for the first time, apply it to a case example and to a homework problem. These individuals may reach criterion after the first presentation and move on the the skills-acquisition-oriented Problem Solving II group. Others who are present in the group have heard the presentation before, but for some reason did not reach criterion on the case example and the homework assignment. This time, they will already know some of the material but will be learning those aspects they failed to master during previous presentations. These clients apply the material to a new case example and work on a new homework problem.

Those clients who are repeating the group for the third, fourth, fifth, or more times are learning a little more from each presentation of the didactic lectures and applying what they have learned to a new case example and to their personal homework problem. The important point is that all these different clients can work side by side in this group without any difficulty or change in the group presentation. Each client works at his or her own level until reaching criteria for passing to Problem Solving II.

Individuals who learn fast or have a good awareness of problem solving on which to build may pass the group the first time. If they have a poor awareness and background, they can slowly build their understanding. In this format, the various levels of functioning can be blended without disruption of the training program. In fact, the good students can and do help those who are functioning at a lower level. By explaining to others what they understand of the model, clients not only help others, but they also reinforce and solidify their own understanding.

Clients who have difficulty with the problem-solving homework are identified after several sessions, and additional, structured homework assignments are developed for them to practice. If a client does not improve with additional practice homework, they review their homework with a staff member for additional sessions. Clients who have writing, reading, or sight difficulties receive help in filling out sheets, and individualized assignments are developed for clients with intellectual limitations, language deficits, or sensorimotor impairments. Thus, all clients can participate in group sessions, while specific performance deficits are identified and specialized individual training is provided such clients.

Example of Problem Solving II

Eventually, everyone masters the Problem Solving I material. At this point, they begin the Problem Solving II program. Problem Solving I and II are, of course, highly similar because they are based on the problem-solving model (see Table 1). Level II is, however, more oriented toward skills acquisition, whereas the first level emphasized awareness training. Our experience has shown that the skills-acquisition phase is facilitated by the fact that everyone is aware of and can apply the problem-solving model. Also, Problem Solving II addresses complex, multifaceted problems and emphasizes application of the model to out-of-group practice in order to facilitate generalization training. Consistent with its orientation, Problem Solving II specifically targets attention to what are considered to be central topics of life where problem solving is particularly relevant and necessary. These topics of attention will be illustrated later and consist of the following: (a) intimate and marital relationships; (b) friendships and social support; (c) family relationships; (d) employment; (e) housing; and (f) physical health. In order to "pass" the Problem Solving II module, proficiency in identifying and solving a personal problem in each of these six topics is required.

The process of the Problem Solving II group is similar to that described previously for the Level I program. Because the group members have demonstrated an understanding of the problem-solving model, little time is necessary for review of this material. Each group session targets one of the selected topics (for example, intimate and marital relationships) as the focus of that session.

Problem Solving II sessions consist of a didactic presentation and group discussion of the problem area under consideration, stressing the possible application of the problem-solving model to a particular area of life. Clients participate in the presentation by active discussion of the problems one encounters in dealing with these situations in life. Because all the clients have experienced problems in these life situations, active participation is usual and is encouraged. A case example that typifies this type of situation is presented, and the problem-solving model is applied to this example under the leadership of the staff member with participation from the group members. An important new concept of Problem Solving II involves the breaking down of complex problems into smaller workable units or parts.

After working with the case example, clients are guided to identify a personal problem in the targeted area to which they apply the model. They continue to work on this problem as a homework assignment. The worksheets that guide the breaking down of the problem and the application of the problem-solving process are subsequently scored, and areas of difficulty are identified and corrected.

Because the focus of Problem Solving II is on large, multifaceted problems, much material is available for therapy and training outside of the formal group sessions. Many aspects of problems identified in the group become the basis for individual counseling and therapy and as targets for the token economy that exists on the residential treatment unit. Thus, this group not only provides a forum for learning problem-solving skills, it also identifies material for long-term treatment using other therapeutic modalities. This has been particularly useful with the chronic patient who tends to be withdrawn and noncommunicative in individual therapy. Often such clients have difficulty focusing on topics for treatment, and the problem situations identified in their homework provide a guide for the individual sessions.

Example of Problem Solving II

An example of one of the Problem Solving II groups will serve to illustrate this model of psychoeducational treatment. For the purpose of illustration, the group focusing on intimate and marital relationships will be presented. As mentioned before, this group consists of a didactic presentation, a case example, and an application to an individual personal problem. A didactic lecture begins the group.

> We are going to apply the problem-solving model to problems in dating and marital relations. Some of the problems that are specific to these relationships are jealousy, infidelity, financial incompatibility, household chore disagreements, in-law problems, step-family adjustments, sexual problems, disagreements regarding recreational activities, value differences, family planning issues, etc. What are some dating and marital problems you have experienced? [*Group brainstorming and discussion follow. The board is used to list the problems generated through discussion. The list is left on the board with space on the right to later list feelings and solutions.*]
>
> We all experience ongoing, long-term problems in intimate relations. What are some examples you have experienced? [*List on the board. Select one of these general long-term problems and break down into workable units so alternative solutions can be generated.*]
>
> Breaking the link in a chain of behaviors by solving one single instance of a long-term problem gives us control over our long-term problems and a reasonable way to solve them. If we can change our behavior and feelings in one instance of a problem [*give example by referring to the long-term problem with which you just dealt as a group*], then we make some real movement toward solving problems that continue day after day, over a long period of time. In order to deal with long-term, ongoing problems, we have to be able to make them specific, concrete, and behavioral, so that we can act on them.
>
> When dealing with a specific problem, such as dividing up household chores, discussions can become heated. For example, if my spouse eats and leaves his plate on the table, never offering to do the dishes or taking his plate to the kitchen after I have cooked a meal, I may feel angry regarding his lack of cooperation or sad regarding his lack of appreciation for my efforts. What are some of the feelings that these problems you have listed on the board have generated for you? [*Group discussion follows.*]
>
> When we have strong feelings about a situation, we often behave in ways that are

related to these feelings. For example, when I feel sad and angry about my husband not helping with the dishes, sometimes I may pout, get a headache, or refuse to make his favorite meals. What are some of your behaviors that happen when you have had the feelings listed on the board? [*Group discussion follows.*]

In forming a solution to the problem of my spouse leaving dishes, several alternatives are possible. What do you think could be done in this situation? [*List the alternatives on board.*] What alternative would you choose? Why? [*Group discussion follows.*]

In order to practice problem solution in the area of marital relations, let us choose one of these situations [*from board*] and list the feelings you might have and the behaviors that might accompany these feelings; then we will make a how-to statement. List at least five solutions and their consequences. Indicate which of the alternatives you would choose. [*Have group choose one situation. Apply problem-solving model to it.*]

In addition, dating and marital relations pose particular problems in communicating. For example, partners often find it difficult to shift from the communication style they adopt at work to a more intimate self-disclosing style in their personal relations. Often, one partner habitually assumes an aggressive or passive role, or we find ourselves being passive with regard to certain topics—in-laws, for example. What are some communication problems you have experienced? [*Group brainstorming discussion—write on chalkboard.*]

People often find themselves having more difficulty being assertive with dating or marriage partners for fear of hurting the other's feelings, of jeopardizing the relationship, or of increasing one's own vulnerability in exposing sensitive areas of concern through self-disclosure. Have you had some difficulty communicating with intimate persons? Write some examples. Examples: Last night, Amy's boyfriend was late to pick her up, but didn't say anything because she was afraid to make him angry; the girl John met at a party Friday said to call her for a date, but when John called today, she was busy and he was annoyed, but didn't say anything, etc.

In intimate relations, such as dating and marriage, we often become concerned with behaviors of the other person that ordinarily do not concern us. For example, it may become very important that our partner's politics, occupation, recreational interests, value system, etc. are similar to our own, whereas we are less concerned about these factors for friends, relatives, etc. What are some differences you have experienced in your concerns about intimate partners and other relationships? What problems have occurred in relation to these concerns? [*Group discussion*]

Often, our expectations are very important in defining intimate and marital relationships. What are some of your expectations regarding romantic partners, and how have these expectations been fulfilled? [*Group discussion follows.*]

After this presentation and discussion, the clients take a rest break and then take up the following case example

Example for Intimate and Marital Relationships

Arrange participants into dyads, preferably a male and a female in each pair. One partner will be assigned the role of *husband,* and one will be assigned the role of *wife.* Hand out role sheets to the appropriate partner.

Procedure

Clients are instructed to read the role sheet and then complete the Problem Solving Form for Problem Area 1 (managing money). Each partner tells the other the *how to's* without discussing their solutions with the partner. After completing Step 1, the dyad jointly completes one problem-solving form for Problem Area 1. During this time, they should tell each other how they are feeling about different aspects of the problem, basing some of the feelings and opinions on the role being played in the problem narrative. After completing this procedure for Problem Area 1 (managing money), Steps 1 and 2 are repeated for the two remaining problem areas listed on the role sheet.

After completing the entire task, the dyad takes a real problem in their own lives and completes a homework assignment sheet for this problem. The following are guidelines for the roles used in the case example.

Husband's Role

You have recently remarried after being a bachelor for about 3 years and have moved into a new home with your new wife and her two young school-age children from her previous marriage. You are employed as an auto mechanic at a busy local gas station nearby. You work Tuesday through Saturday from 9 A.M. until 6 P.M. Your wife has taken a job at a local department store, Monday through Friday, from 8 A.M. until 3 P.M. These hours are convenient because she is home when the children return from school

When you remarried, you felt that this was the beginning of a happier, more satisfying life for you, your new wife, and the kids. It was going to be nice to be part of a close, united family once again. However, after 3 months in this marriage you find yourself feeling very tired, depressed, and frustrated. This is not at all what you thought your new life would be like. You and your wife are not getting along well; you spend a lot of time arguing and complaining. Even though your wife says she is trying hard to make this marriage a good and happy one, you are realizing that you and she don't see eye to eye on some important issues of everyday living (for instance, you and she don't agree on what a wife's and a husband's roles and responsibilities should be in a marriage). You and your wife say you agree that a married couple has to share responsibilities, but you feel that you end up with the worst end of the deal. It seems to you that you are expected to give up and compromise more than is fair. You are tired of feeling taken advantage of and want complaints and problems between the two of you worked out more fairly.

Problem Areas

1. *Managing Money*. You have observed over time that your wife overspends whenever she goes shopping and you don't like seeing unexpected large bills coming in. You also feel that it is easier to manage a household's finances if just one person handles all cash and bills. So, you hold all the credit cards, the checking account, and most of the cash and give your wife all the money she needs for groceries, clothes, etc. That way, you know what money is going where. That's the way it was always done in your family, and it worked very well. Your wife doesn't like this arrangement and wants it changed.

2. *Meal Preparation.* After a long, physically exhausting day at work, you come home tired and really hungry. Since your wife is home by 3:30 it seems natural that she would cook you a good satisfying meal. A salad and fruit does not fill you. You would cook dinner except, one, you get home about 6:30, and the kids can't wait until 8 P.M. to eat; and, two, you don't know the first thing about cooking. You really don't feel that's too much to ask a wife to do for her husband and kids. You are tired of arguing about who is going to cook and what kind of meal to prepare.

3. *Outside Activities.* Since you married, you have really been going out of your way to be a good husband and father to your family. You always make sure that the family does at least one activity together per week. But, it's getting harder to plan something because your wife is out frequently at her club meetings. In addition, you feel like you're stuck home baby-sitting when you would like to have a night out with your men friends. Seems like now that you're married, you rarely get to go out for a couple of beers or go fishing or hunting with your buddies. You've asked your wife to go, but she's not interested in those kinds of activities.

After this exercise, as indicated in the directions, clients identify a problem in this area from their own lives and apply the problem-solving procedure to it. These individualized problems, as mentioned before, also become the basis for ongoing treatment on the residential unit.

As was discussed regarding the Problem Solving I module, Level II is also conducive to the daily addition of new members to the therapy group and the graduation or discharge of others. Again, consideration of a typical group will serve to illustrate the flexibility of the program in dealing with this problem. Each group session will have new members but also members who have been presented one or more of the topic areas. All members have completed Problem Solving I and have a good understanding of the model. Therfore, there is this basic foundation upon which all members of the group can build.

Those members who are participating in a session for the first time will experience the material as new. Those who are repeating Problem Solving II will be building on their previous learning and attempting to master the material. Once the program is "passed," the client will be presented the next problem area (for example, friendships and social support), and this will be new material.

Thus, this problem-solving program consists of two levels, awareness training and skills acquisition. The rotating format of each session has proven to be able to provide sequential training on an individual perspective while at the same time treating a group of clients with a constantly changing membership.

The material presented previously is only one of the many that comprise the set of lesson plans developed for use. The Problem Solving II example is one of six complete modules that comprise the groups presented. Each of the other five modules is similar in structure but deals with a different content area. All the modules for Problem Solving I and II were designed to be structured comprehensive guides for the practitioner. The specific material to be presented is contained in the lesson plan. These plans are helpful to the practitioner and essential to insuring a consistent quality of the program.

Evaluation of the Problem-Solving Program

The problem-solving program described in this chapter is part of a comprehensive treatment system comprised of many components, including several other skills training groups, a transitional program to approximate community living, psychiatric treatment, and individual therapy. Because of the compexity of the total treatment experience, a controlled study is necessary to identify treatment outcomes that are related exclusively to this problem-solving skills training program. Such a study has not yet been conducted, and current evaluation has been oriented to determining the type of client being given treatment and to the operational viability of the program. Therefore, only data related to these two issues will be presented at this time. The third type of evaluation is of a clinical-outcome nature, and two case studies will be presented to illustrate the clinical application of the program.

The present program was originally intended to serve the needs of the chronically mentally ill client. The target group of this treatment was to be those individuals who were identified for participation in a deinstitutionalization program designed to reduce state hospital census and provide treatment and long-term aftercare in the community. It was not anticipated that these clients would show a total rehabilitation after receiving this psychoeducationally oriented program and no longer need mental health care. Rather, it was expected that these clients would continue to be chronic users of mental health services and make a fragile adjustment to independent community living. It was expected, however, that this program would reduce clients' use of the professional health care system because of their increased social skills and competence.

The clients involved in this program were referred by community mental health agencies for residential, 7-day-a-week treatment. In some cases these clients were reentering the local community after being treated at a state hospital. For these clients, this program provided a transition from state hospital treatment to community mental health aftercare, usually in a supervised living situation. Other clients had recently experienced an acute episode of extreme disability and were referred to this program subsequent to acute care and stabilization. The third principal group of clients involved in this treatment were individuals who were involved in a long-term community aftercare program and had begun to evidence behaviors suggesting that their condition was deteriorating, but they were not in need of acute care.

Based on the first year of operation of the program, it is possible to describe the type of client receiving treatment according to several variables. Generally, the demographic information suggests that the client group may be described as the *new chronic*. Based on 153 participants, the program has addressed males (49.02%) and females (50.78%) equally, and there has been a slight underparticipation of black clients (Caucasion = 93.46%; Negro = 5.22%; other = 1.30%). The average age of the clients was 30.89 years with a range from 18.5 years to 59.6 years. The average client had 12.15 years of education, although the range was 6 to 18 years.

Also of importance are the descriptive data regarding the clients' diagnoses and psychiatric histories. Nearly all the clients were diagnosed as having either a schizophrenic disorder or an affective psychosis. Thus, most of the clients, as expected, were experiencing a major mental disorder and were severely handicapped. Consistent with the notion that these were chronic patients, the average number of hospitalizations for mental or emotional problems prior to admission to the present program was 4.34 with a range of 0 to 20 hospital admissions. Also, nearly every client treated had previously been admitted to a state-funded mental hospital at least once prior to being treated on this unit. The chronic disability of the group also was evidenced by the fact that the average client had experienced an average of 9.55 months of mental hospitalization (range 0–130 months) prior to being treated in this program.

Given this extensive and chronic history of mental disorder and treatment, is it possible to teach these clients "effective" behavior, or problem-solving skills? The answer is, of course, that the clients going through the program generally meet the criteria for completion of the various psychoeducational groups and the overall program. Thus, they seemed to learn the problem-solving model and how to apply it to a number of problem areas.

In this regard, it was of interest to evaluate how well the program, as described here, matched the learning abilities of this group of clients. That is, did everyone pass everything the first time it was presented or did it take a long, arduous time to finish? Or, did they seem to progress steadily in their learning? In the former case, it would be suggested that the program was too simple or superficial, and in the latter case, the program would perhaps be so difficult that these clients could not learn the concepts and behaviors. It was also of interest to determine whether the awareness training phase (Problem Solving I) was learned at the same or a different rate than the skills acquisition component (Problem Solving II).

In order to evaluate this issue, the records of 25 clients who completed the two phases of problem solving between November 1982 and May 1983 were reviewed. Each client's performance in the group was evaluated to determine the number of repetitions of each session required before performance reached criterion level. Figure 2 is a graphic representation of these data for Problem Solving I, and Figure 3 presents Problem Solving II.

As may be seen in these figures, the material was mastered in a reasonable time in both phases. The level of awareness training was mastered on the first presentation by about half of the clients (44%), and all 25 individuals mastered the material within five sessions. After the first session, approximately 10–20% of the clients reached criterion on each successive session. Because the Problem Solving I group is presented twice each week, everyone mastered the concepts within 2.5 weeks.

Similarly, the skills acquisition component (Problem Solving II) showed a progressive pattern of learning with about 10% of the clients reaching criterion after each successive session. As may be recalled, clients had to complete six problem areas before reaching the criteria for completion of Problem Solving II. It may be noted in Figure 3, that two (8%) of the clients met criterion in the minimum time. The skills acquisition Problem Solving II phase appeared to

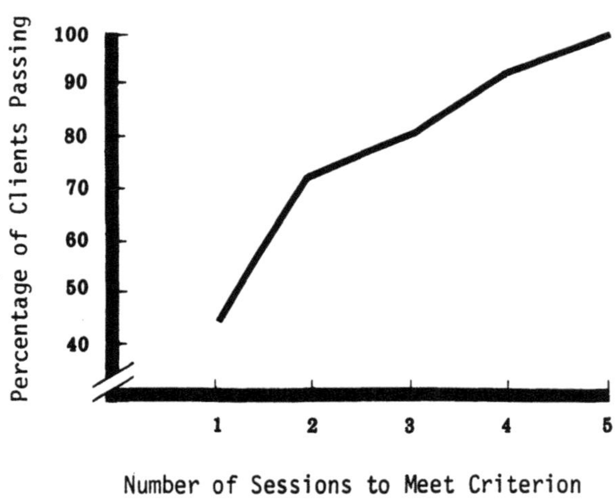

FIGURE 2. A graph illustrating the cumulative number of sessions required to meet criterion level in the Problem Solving I program.

represent more of a challenge to the clients because 44% of the clients passed Problem Solving I in the minimum possible time. Also, several clients took an extended number of sessions to complete the Problem Solving II program, considerably longer than most. This may be noted by the flattened characteristic of the curve shown after Session 16. This did not seem to occur in Problem Solving I. Also, it may be noted that the curve for Problem Solving I has a steeper slope

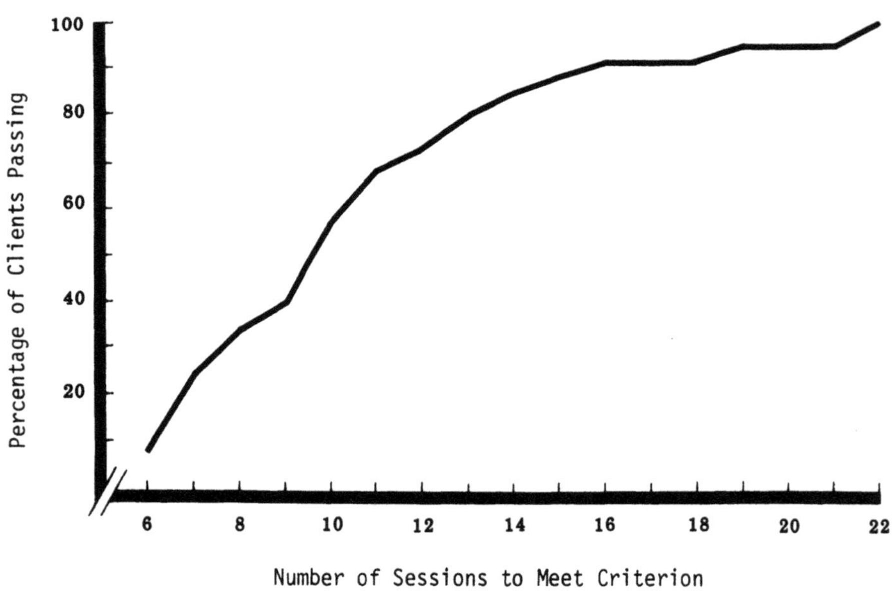

FIGURE 3. A graph illustrating the cumulative number of sessions required to meet criterion level in the Problem Solving II program.

than shown for Problem Solving II. This suggests more rapid learning in the first phase than in the second. This finding may suggest that awareness is acquired faster than is skills acquisition.

Thus, the program as developed matches the abilites of these chronic clients, and learning appears to be occurring. The speed of learning also seems to be in a reasonable range, with the slowest client completing the entire program in approximately 4 months.

Further research is in progress that will evaluate the recidivism of these clients after they leave this program. It is, of course, the durability of such learning that is important. Preliminary indications are that many of these clients have learned "effective" behavior and function at a higher level even outside the treatment setting than they did prior to receiving this training.

In order to illustrate the clinical application of the program, two case studies have been prepared to demonstrate the usefulness of this program with some "typical" clients.

Case Report 1

Background

A single, black, unemployed male, Tom, was admitted to the Intensive Residential Treatment Unit (IRT) at the age of 27; he had been transferred from a community-based crisis unit after experiencing periods of sleeplessness and agitated behavior. He was brought to the crisis unit by staff of the boarding home where he was residing, who reported he was staying out until 3 or 4 A.M. and returning with the smell of alcohol on his breath. The intake counselor at the crisis unit noted bizarre behaviors such as talking with the "walls and ceilings." Tom was given a diagnosis of schizophrenia, chronic undifferentiated type.

Tom was born and raised in a midsized Florida city and was the youngest of three siblings; he had a married brother 4 years older and a divorced sister 2 years older. His sister and her three children were living with his mother at the time of Tom's admission. There was no reported family history for psychiatric or emotional problems. Tom's mother, age 53, was a nurse's aide. His father, a chronic diabetic, died at age 61 in 1981.

Tom graduated from high school and reported an adequate school adjustment from elementary through high school. He reported making average to above average grades and being involved in a variety of extracurricular activities, such as football, high school choir, and a social club. Tom described himself as a "loner" outside school. He attended a junior college in his hometown for 2 years and pursued a liberal arts degree with a stated interest in prelaw, but Tom did not complete his A.A. degree.

Tom reported having worked as a bus driver for a year and as a stock and delivery man with a local department store for 11 months. He was in the Army for 7 months where he was training for the Signal Corps. Tom reports leaving the Army after 7 months because of a nervous breakdown. He reported working as a maintenance man for 1 year at a local nursing home in 1981; this was his last gainful employment.

Tom has no history of suicidal or homicidal behavior or intent. He has no history of alcohol or drug abuse, although he reported social drinking during adolescence. Tom reports having sold drugs when he was around 20 and having been picked up for an assault charge in connection with a dispute regarding payment for drugs. Charges were reportedly dropped, and Tom apparently has no police record.

Tom indicated that his emotional problems began in 1979 at the age of 23, when he was picked up by law enforcement officers while walking long distances. His family had notified police because they were unaware of his whereabouts. During this episode, he reported that his "inner voice went crazy." Tom was hospitalized at that time for 2 weeks.

Treatment

Tom's treatment plan focused on the identified problem areas of poor socialization skills, which were further defined as staying in his room, having superficial interactions with others, not self-disclosing feelings with others, not engaging in activities, and describing himself as a "loner." Short-term goals included increasing the amount of time out of his room, increasing activity with peers, and increasing self-disclosure of thoughts and feelings.

Tom adjusted well to the unit and participated in treatment groups. Initially, he did not interact with other clients during unstructured time. He expressed paranoid ideation and reported hearing voices during individual counseling sessions, but his demeanor was generally pleasant and appropriate. Tom's social behavior improved as a function of treatment, but he tended to isolate himself if not prompted by staff to interact.

Problem-Solving Group Performance

In Problem Solving I, Tom indicated as his personal problem a situation in which an acquaintance of his was involved in a fight. Although Tom had some insight into this situation, he did not pass the group criteria because he confused several problems into one and could not recognize the problem as his own.

After three additional sessions, Tom was able to focus on one problem at a time; he clearly identified his feelings regarding the situation, accepted responsibility for his part of the problem, and understood how he was blaming the problem on another person. Although his performance was consistent on the criteria of performance for the group, situations described were often superficial or concerned with the activities of others. Three more sessions were needed before Tom produced situations that were more personally significant, for example, a visit from his mother and its related conflicts. As Tom took the next step and started producing alternative solutions to his problem situations, his performance in areas where he had previously met criteria diminished. Several additional sessions were necessary to establish consistency in choosing relevant situations, describing them objectively, and generating reasonable alternatives.

Next, Tom proceded to Problem Solving II. At this point, he began verbalizing more delusional and fragmented material and writing what resembled hieroglyphic or symbolic writing on homework assignment sheets. This continued for several group sessions until Tom's homework assignment sheets returned to previous, adequate levels of performance. It was hypothesized that the additional difficulty of dealing with complex and highly important problems associated with Problem Solving II may have been overly stressful. In any event, Tom began working on meaningful problems such as, "I have trouble trying to quit smoking" (physical health topic area); "I get angry at peers when I shouldn't" (friendship and social support topic area); and "I can't find a love in my life" (intimate and marital relations topic area).

Tom eventually learned to take general, global problems and break them down into workable units. For example, in the intimate and marital relations group, his global problem was "I can't find a love in my life." Tom could not deal with such an overriding, global situation, and it seemed insurmountable to him. Using the problem-solving group, he began to solve this problem. First, he began to focus on current situations, rather than the past. For example, he began to look for and develop friendships on the unit. He learned to identify his tendency to blame his problems on others, (for example, ladies are not fair with him) and his internal process, (for example, his expectations that he should already have met a friend). In identifying his goal, or *how to,* Tom was able to specify his wish to meet and make better friends and to deal with his feelings of sadness. He generated alternatives and chose to work on better communicating his feelings to peers. It was interesting that Tom's choice of a problem area and solution were directly related to his identified problem area and treatment plan that involved improving his socialization skills.

Other significant treatment issues were also chosen by Tom for use as homework assignments including getting along with his family, postdischarge living arrangements, postdischarge employment and vocational training, and social issues such as prejudice and how to deal effectively with his feelings about prejudice when he encountered it.

Tom eventually began to perform well in his groups and to meet criteria for passing. He learned the problem-solving model and how to incorporate the model into relevant situations that would promote adjustment after discharge. He chose effectively from alternative solutions and consistently acted on decisions bringing his experiences back to the original situation to evaluate the effectiveness of the decision choice.

Discharge Plans

Tom was interested in returning to the boarding home where he resided prior to the last crisis hospitalization. The boarding home was willing to take him back, based partly on his progress in treatment. His family facilitated his discharge by aiding with weekend visits to his family's home, providing transportation for discharge and general emotional support. Tom was discharged to a local boarding home 2 months and 3 weeks after being admitted to the program.

Postdischarge Follow-Up

Follow-up at 6 months postdischarge indicated Tom only remained in the boarding home three nights before returning to his family's home. His family was agreeable to taking him in, and he left the boarding home on good terms. This change in residence was well thought out and may be considered effective behavior on Tom's part. He continues to maintain appropriate behavior in his family's home, continues his medication regimen, and is attending his follow-up aftercare appointments with his case manager. He is involved with vocational rehabilitation and is presently completing a work assessment, prior to entering vocational training.

Case Report 2

Background

Jane, a divorced 24-year-old female, was admitted to the Intensive Residential Treatment Unit from a crisis stabilization facility, exhibiting extreme depression, accompanied by physical immobility and reduced responsiveness to external stimuli. Jane had previously been diagnosed as schizophrenic, catatonic type, but the referring diagnosis for the present admission was hysterical neurosis, conversion type.

Jane was born in a midsized southern city and lived there all her life. She has one brother, 3 years her elder, and three half-sisters born to her father in his first marriage, all of whom are presently in their 40s.

Jane completed the seventh grade, but her psychiatric difficulties began in the eighth grade and her schooling was interrupted at that time. She completed the G.E.D. in 1982 while an inpatient at a state mental hospital. She has worked as a waitress for a total of 6 months, holding no other type of employment since maturity.

Jane was married twice, the first time at age 18 and again at age 23. Jane's first marriage lasted 18 months, and although her second marriage ended in divorce after a similar period, she only lived with her second husband for a short time.

Jane's psychiatric difficulties began at age 14, and her first hospitalization occurred after she was found to be "high on acid and LSD in class." Jane admits to frequent use of LSD, PCP, and cocaine between the ages of 14 through 17. Her first hospital admission for emergency treatment was followed by two private psychiatric hospital admissions and then a 6-month stay at a state mental hospital at age 15. This hospital stay was followed by three subsequent admissions to the same state facility between the ages of 15 and 18. At 23, she had two admissions to a second state mental hospital; the first admission lasted 7 weeks, the second admission lasted 9 months. Jane has had intermittent, ongoing contact with outpatient mental health facilities since 1976 and admits to two suicidal gestures, one at age 15 with a razor and one at age 23 with pills. Jane made a third suicide attempt while in treatment in the present program, attempting to cut her wrists the day after Thanksgiving in 1982. Jand had, in the past, been treated with a wide range of psychotropic medications, including Haldol, Thorazine, Mellaril, Elavil, and Stelazine.

Treatment

Jane's treatment plan identified problem areas of self-injurious behavior, social withdrawal, verbalizations that others do not like her, holding conversations with herself in the presence of others, unrealistic expectations of herself, and difficulty utilizing assertive communication and relaxtion skills.

Initial short-term goals for treatment focused on increasing time out of her bedroom and the frequency of self-disclosing communication. Subsequent short-term goals included increasing the following: positive self-statements and thoughts, assertive communication, use of relaxation skills when fearful or anxious, and statements of self-awareness.

Jane's initial behavior on the unit was attention seeking and charaterized by excessive verbalizations and intellectualization. She attempted to engage various staff into prolonged discussions of her "diagnosis" and the authenticity of her motivation for help. Her initial onunit behavior was contradictory in that she repeatedly sought attention of treatment staff while also seeking to be discharged from the unit. She attended groups and participated with peers. Fifteen days after admission, Jane cut the insides of both wrists with a safety razor. She was treated in an emergency room and returned to the unit for observation and evaluation. This was considered to be a serious suicide attempt, and the treatment staff took extra care to work with Jane both to prevent a recurrence and also to help her learn insight into the reasons for this behavior.

After working through this setback, Jane advanced in her groups and the unit level system. As she progressed in the program, she reduced her expressions of labile emotions, increased insightful comments, and increased independence in dealing with feelings of fear and impulses of self-harm. Although she expressed suicidal ideations several more times during her stay, she was able to discuss her feelings with staff and seemed to gain insight and behavioral control through individual treatment. Jane improved socializations, reduced suicidal statements, increased self-responsibility, and improved positive self-statements throughout the course of treatment.

Problem-Solving Group Performance

Jane initially had difficulty at all levels of problem solving. For example, when describing a situation, she always included judgments and blaming statements in her description such as, "I was very patient and I did not get the chance to ask because he left." Although Jane showed a relatively sophisticated ability to verbalize a situation and generate alternatives, her defined "cause" tended to be self-effacing and martyred, such as "I understand others are more important to help." Her solution alternatives were characterized by passivity and withdrawal, such as "Go to my room," "Walk away," "Go take a shower," "Cry alone," and the like.

As Jane began attending the problem-solving group, she quickly improved in making clear, objective statements describing the problem situation. She learned to keep judgments out of her written statements. Clinical contact with Jane indicated that although her written performance on group criteria indicated she understood the didactic material and performed in a competent manner, her verbal behavior continued to manifest judgmental statements in nongroup settings. Therefore, additional attention to this area was provided outside of the problem-solving group in individual counseling sessions.

Jane had more difficulty clarifying the "cause" statement and used issues that did not relate to the problem. By the seventh session, however, she was consistently stating the problem objectively, identifying her behavior and feelings in relation to the situation, and was able to specify the "excuse" or blaming statements and the "cause" or expectations of the situation consistently. In additional, Jane's solution alternatives became more assertive and direct in dealing with the situation concretely. At the same time, the use of alternatives that avoided dealing with the situation decreased in frequency.

In Problem Solving II, Jane dealt with issues like finding a satisfactory place to live, improving communication with her family, maintaining employment, improving thoughts and feelings about previous marriage difficulties, improving methods of getting emotional support, and increasing trust in others, and reducing her overweight condition and maintaining an exercise program. Jane dealt with significant global problems, was able to break these problems down into workable units, to prioritize those units according to criteria of emotional importance, ease of solution, concreteness, and the like, and to further specify the global problem through several short-term example situations from which to actually choose a solution and act on it.

Discharge Plans

Jane left residential treatment to return to her family. In order to prepare for her discharge placement, she took several extended leaves of absence, during which she applied socialization and problem-solving skills that she was learning on the unit to her family and community contacts. Her home visitations were congenial, and Jane reported improved relations with her family.

Jane was referred to vocational rehabilitation, and plans were made to enroll her in a vocational training program at a technical school. She was referred to a local mental health center for outpatient aftercare.

Postdischarge Follow-Up

After discharge, Jane adjusted well to her family and began vocational school. She kept outpatient appointments, maintained her medication regimen, initiated social contact with friends, and continued to stay active, avoiding her previous pattern of withdrawal. About 5 months after discharge, Jane moved into a supervised apartment and stopped living with her family. According to her case manager, this was a well-planned move that was designed to help her gain some independence from her family. Her adjustment remains good at the last follow-up, some 6 months postdischarge.

Summary and Conclusions

This chapter has presented a problem-solving skills training program, developed and used with the chronically, mentally handicapped. The major conceptual underpinnings of the program have been presented as well as a detailed presentation of a sample of the program materials. Ths use of the psychoeducational model to organize this treatment program was also illustrated. Although some evaluative data were presented, additional research is required to determine the efficacy of the problem-solving group *per se,* apart from other treatments and the durability of the behavioral changes shown as a function of this training program. Based on clinical and nonsystematic follow-up data, clients receiving this program often progress more than they have previously in any of the many mental health programs with which they have been involved.

Other issues of cost containment, the use of interdisciplinary treatment teams, and the utilization of junior-level mental health professionals have not been raised in detail in this chapter. These issues are, however, important and seem to be facilitated by the program described. In fact, the structured and objective nature of the treatment program that develops as a function of using the procedures described in this chapter seems to be a major factor in the effective treatment of these difficult chronic clients. As more emphasis is placed on deinstitutionalization, programs that are effective with this group of clients are needed. Traditional services do not seem to be overly successful (e.g., Caton, 1981; Pepper, Kirshner, & Ryglewicz, 1981). Innovative approaches are called for, and the program described here is, we hope, an example of one type of effective approach to the treatment of the chronically mentally handicapped.

References

American Psychological Association. *Standards for educational and psychological tests and manuals.* Washington, D.C.: Author, 1966.

Bedell, J. R., & Weathers, L. R. A psychoeducational model of skill training: Therapist-facilitated and game-facilitated applications. In D. Upper & S. M. Ross (Eds.), *Behavioral group therapy, 1979: An anual review,* Champaign, Ill.: Research Press, 1979.

Bedell, J. R., Archer, R. P., & Marlowe, H. A., Jr. A description and evaluation of a problem solving skills training program. In D. Upper & S. M. Ross (Eds.), *Behavioral group therapy, 1980: An annual review.* Champaign, Ill.: Research Press, 1980.

Caton, L. M. The new chronic patient and the system of community care. *Hospital and Community Psychiatry,* 1981, *32,* 475–478.

Doll, E. A. *Measurement of soical competence.* Minneapolis: Educational Testing Bureau, 1953.
D'Zurilla, T., & Goldfried, M. Problem solving and behavior modification. *Journal of Abnormal Psychology,* 1971, *78,* 107–126.
Foote, N. N., & Cottrell, L. S. *Identity and personal competence, a new direction in family research.* Chicago: University of Chicago Press, 1955.
Goldfried, M., & D'Zurilla, T. A behavioral-analytic model for assessing competence. In C. D. Spielberg (Ed.), *Current topics in clinical and community psychology.* New York: Academic Press, 1969.
Heppner, P. P. A review of the problem-solving literature and its relationship to the counseling process. *Journal of Counseling Psychology,* 1978, *25,* 366–375.
Heppner, P. P. The effects of client perceived need and counselor role on clients' behaviors. *Dissertation Abstracts International,* 1979, *39,* 5950A–5951A.
Heppner, P. P., & Petersen, C. H. The development and implications of a personal problem-solving inventory. *Journal of Counseling Psychology,* 1982, *29,* 66–75.
Horan, J. J. *Counseling for effective decision making: A cognitive-behavioral perspective.* North Scituate, Mass.: Duxbury Press, 1979.
Kanfer, F. H., & Saslow, C. Behavioral analysis: An alternative to diagnostic classification. *Archives of General Psychiatry,* 1965, *12,* 529–538.
Pepper, B., & Ryglewicz, H. Profile of the new chronic patient. *Roche report: Frontiers of psychiatry,* January 1, 1982, pp. 6, 11.
Pepper, B., Kirshner, M. C., & Ryglewicz, H. The young adult chronic patient: Overview of a population. *Hospital and Community Psychiatry,* 1981, *32,* 463–469.
Phillips, L., & Cowitz, B. Social attainment and reactions to stress. *Journal of Personality,* 1953, *22,* 270–283.
Platt, J. J. & Spivack, G. Real-life problem-solving thinking in neuropsychiatric patients and controls. Paper presented at the meeting of the Eastern Psychological Association, Atlantic City, April 1970.
Platt, J. J., & Spivack, G. Problem solving thinking of psychiatric patients. *Journal of Consulting and Clinical Psychology,* 1972, *39,* 148–151. (a)
Platt, J. J., & Spivack, G. Social competence and effective problem solving thinking in psychiatric patients. *Journal of Clinical Psychology,* 1972, *28,* 3–5. (b)
Platt, J. J., Spivack, G., Altman, N., Altman, D. S., & Peizer, S. B. Adolescent problem solving thinking. *Journal of Consulting and Clinical Psychology,* 1974, *42,* 787–793.
Richards, J. M., Jr., Holland, J. L., & Lutz, S. W. *The assessment of student accomplishment in college* (ACT Research Report, No. 11, March 1966). Iowa City: Research and Development Division, American College Testing Program.
Rotter, J. B. Generalized expectancies for internal versus external control of reinforcement. *Psychological Monographs,* 1966, *80*(1, Whole No. 609).
Shure, M. B., & Spivack, G. *Problem-solving capacity, social class and adjustment among nursery school children.* Paper presented at the meeting of the Eastern Psychological Association, Atlantic City, April 1970.
Shure, M. B., & Spivack, G. Means–ends thinking, adjustment and social class among elementary school-aged children. *Journal of Consulting and Clinical Psychology,* 1972, *38,* 348–353.
Spivack, G., & Levine, M. Self-regulation in acting-out and normal adolescents (Report M-4531). Washington, D.C.: National Institute of Health, 1963.
Stern, G. G., Stein, M. I., & Bloom, B. S. *Methods in personality assessment.* Glencoe, Ill.: Free Press, 1956.
Watson, J. B., & Rayner, R. Conditioned emotional reactions. *Journal of Experimental Psychology,* 1920, *3,* 1–14.

5

Long-Term Behavioral Group Psychotherapy

An Integrative Model

PERRY L. BELFER AND PHILIP LEVENDUSKY

This chapter proposes a new integrative model of long-term process-oriented behavioral group psychotherapy. This new model integrates clinical insights from interpersonal process-oriented group psychotherapy (Yalom, 1975) with previously delineated behavioral group therapy (Rose, 1977; Upper & Ross, 1979). This model of treatment intervention is proposed for individuals with complex clinical syndromes (e.g., agoraphobia), entrenched chronic difficulties (e.g., chronic depression, morbid obesity, individuals with "characterological" interpersonal difficulties), or for those who are profoundly disabled (e.g., communication/interpersonal skills deficits of schizophrenics). This model is also relevant for individuals with less "profound" psychological or behavioral disability, although the individual's length of treatment might be expected to be briefer. Such open-ended groups accept new members as needed and available and graduate members as they accomplish therapeutic goals. Thus, the group takes on a life of its own, independent of the participation of any particular member(s) or even leader(s). The long-term open-ended nature of these groups, degree of disability of their members, and changing membership over time lead to an unfolding of group processes that may be understood and managed. In contrast with traditional (primarily operant, short-term, symptom-focused, less interpersonally based) behavioral group therapy, these processes may be utilized in the proposed model to maximize each individual's and the group's therapeutic gains.

In recent years, behavioral group therapy has been utilized increasingly for the treatment of diverse disorders, including agoraphobia (Belfer, Schachter, Dooley, & Levendusky, 1980); depression (Lewinsohn, Steinmetz, Antonuccio, & Terri, 1985); bulimia (White & Boskind-White, 1981), and sexual dysfunction

PERRY L. BELFER • Harvard Medical School, Boston, Massachusetts 02115. PHILIP LEVENDUSKY • Harvard Medical School, Boston, Massachusetts 02115.

(McGovern, 1985). Frequently these groups involve the administration of behavioral interventions/techniques in a group setting (Rose, 1977). Often, the group is conceptualized as a social reinforcement machine (Liberman, 1970). Generally, these behavioral groups are short term and symptom focused. A parallel innovation is the development of cognitive therapy groups (Hollon & Shaw, 1979). As with most behavioral groups, these cognitive therapy groups also involve the admistration of cognitive interventions in group setting (Rush & Watkins, 1981).

In this chapter, a new, long-term process-oriented behavioral model of group psychotherapy will be outlined. Instead of simply applying behavioral procedures in a group setting, this model attempts to integrate innovations in cognitive as well as behavioral therapies in groups with treatment procedures, interventions, and understandings gained from long-term process-oriented group psychotherapy (Bion, 1961; Foulkes, 1946, 1964; Semrad & Arseman, 1951; Yalom, 1975). The unfolding of process within the group, including the nature of relationships among the members (and leader), and stages of group development through time, as well as group dynamics are an important focus of therapeutic concern within this model. This integrative model will propose the utility of process-oriented behavioral group psychotherapy, as opposed to behavioral therapies *administered* in a group.

Long-Term Process-Oriented Groups

Nonbehavioral clinicians have utilized long-term process-oriented group psychotherapy for many years (Berne, 1966; Foulkes & Anthony, 1957; Whitaker & Leiberman, 1964), with several conceptual models of group process having been proposed. The earliest therapeutic groups used a psychoanalytic frame of reference, emphasizing psychosexual stages of development, unconscious motivation, and the analysis of transference and resistance (Ackerman, 1946; Foulkes, 1946; Freud, 1940; Schilder, 1936, 1938; Slavson, 1940, 1947, 1953; Wender, 1936). The foci of these groups were intrapsychic phenomena. These early psychoanalytic group approaches attempted to apply the principles of individual psychoanalysis to group therapy (Durkin, 1974). In a similar manner, many behavior therapy groups offer individual behavior therapy in a group setting (Flowers, 1982; Rose, 1977). The psychoanalytic principles upon which these early groups were based as well as the therapeutic interventions they utilized are not held in high repute by either personality researchers or behavioral clinicians (Eysenck, 1961; Mischel, 1968). Yet, the clinical experience of early psychodynamic group therapists may be quite instructive to behavioral group psychotherapists.

Concurrent with the development of psychoanalytic group therapy, psychodramatic groups began to be introduced (Moreno, 1937, 1966). These groups, which attempted to apply sociological and social psychological findings to group therapy, also emphasized affect generation and expression. Moreno (1937) described structural characteristics of therapy groups and noted the importance of group processes as well as patterns of relationships among members. Group cohesion was noted as of importance, and the nature of group leadership was highlighted. In addition, the notion of the group as the agent of psychotherapeutic change was introduced.

These psychodramatic innovations were followed by the work of Wilfred Bion (1961) and others who were influenced by the Tavistock school (Foulkes, 1946; Foulkes & Anthony, 1947; Semrad & Arseman, 1951). These clinicians conceptualized the psychotherapeutic group as an entity in itself, which functioned by way of group dynamics and group processes. Groups as whole phenomena were emphasized. The role and functions of the group leader, social roles within the group, group norms, group cohesion, and stages of group development were all emphasized and have since been studied extensively. Bion (1961) emphasizes that groups may be conceptualized as task focused and that various interpersonal processes (termed *basic assumptions*) might greatly influence the process by which tasks are carried out. Bion outlines three types of basic assumption groups: *the dependent groups, the fight–flight group,* and *the pairing group.* The dependent group, for example, sees the group leader as the fount of all knowledge and the source of all change. Bion's notion of therapy groups as task focused is of particular relevance to behavioral group psychotherapists. Treatment based on impacting a specific target symptom (motor behavior, cognition, or physiological response) or constellation of symptoms implies a very specific task for the group. This is especially so for homogeneous groups (e.g., Belfer *et al.*, 1980) where members may share a common symptom cluster, but it also holds for heterogeneous groups (Flowers, 1982) where diverse interventions are structured to impact target symptoms.

With the publication of several seminal texts, Yalom has made an enormous contribution to the field of group psychotherapy. This contribution has special relevance for behavioral group psychotherapists. Writing from the here-and-now perspective of existential psychotherapy, Yalom delineates several principles of group psychotherapy that apply to groups run within varied theoretical frameworks. Yalom writes about long-term process-oriented outpatient psychodynamic-existential psychotherapy groups (Lieberman, Yalom, & Miles, 1973) as well as inpatient therapy groups (Yalom, 1983). Yalom's focus is that interpersonal relationships are interpersonal processes. His principles, differentially applied to diverse groups, have wide applicability. Two foci of Yalom's concern are of particular note: the "curative" factors in group psychotherapy and the tasks of the group leader.

Yalom (1975) describes 11 curative factors in group psychotherapy. *Instillation of hope* becomes operative as new members experience the support of their fellow group members and observe others improving and growing. Expectancy of success appears to be a major factor in positive psychotherapeutic outcome (Goldstein, 1962); therefore, instillation of hope can be a powerful curative factor. *Universality* refers to the experience of group participants that they are not alone; others also have problems in living. *Imparting of information* is the direct instruction, advice, and suggestions that members may be offered. *Altruism* refers to the help that members provide to each other. This occurs by way of positive group interactions, as individuals step back from their own pain to offer support to their fellow members.

Recapitulation of the primary family group refers to resolution of transference phenomena based on problematic early interactions. Yalom draws heavily on Harry Stack Sullivan's interpersonal theory of psychopathology and psychotherapeutic change (1953). Sullivan holds that based on life experiences, not all of which are parental in nature, individuals may develop inaccurate cognitions and unhelpful affective responses with regard to interpersonal relationships (parataxic distortions). Yalom suggests that these inaccurate and unproductive ways of thinking and feeling about others often appear in long-term process-oriented groups. By the process of members' sharing their cognitive and affective responses to others within the group, individuals may get feedback and, thereby, resolve these parataxic distortions.

Development of socializing techniques occurs by way of processes quite familiar to behavior therapists. Group members may observe more functional social models, practice new social behaviors, and obtain coaching and feedback from the group. *Imitative behavior* may occur with regard to social interaction as well as other problems a group member may present with. *Interpersonal learning* is the very purpose of the group. Members learn from their fellows. *Catharsis* may be of some help as members are able to share their deepest emotional experiences and psychological pain. *Existential factors* refer to the realities of life that members share and may become aware of during the course of their group therapy experience.

Yalom (1975) sees *group cohesiveness* as the primary and most important curative factor, comparable to the therapeutic relationship in individual therapy. As he conceptualizes cohesiveness,

> the group therapy analogue of the patient–therapist relationship is a broader concept, encompassing the patient's relationship to his group therapist, to the other group members, and to the group as a whole. (Yalom, 1975, p. 46)

Group cohesiveness is a precondition for effective treatment. It is the attractiveness of a group for its members; that is what keeps them in the group. This group attractiveness enhances the group's reinforcing value; members may change attitudes and behaviors as well as learn to feel differently for the group. In addition, a safe, secure treatment environment provides a context in which members can share embarrassing aspects of symptoms experienced or factors that may have hindered prior growth, development, and symptom resolution. This safe, secure environment, provided that adequate norms have been developed, provides the individual member with a sense of acceptance. Often this sense of acceptance leads to a capacity to make, or even consider, life changes. Thus, group cohesiveness, a sense of what Yalom calls *groupness*, may be considered the most important curative factor.

Yalom also delineates the tasks of the group leader (therapist). The prime tasks are creation and maintenance of the group and establishing group norms. The group therapist is solely responsible for selection of members and bringing the group together. The process of member selection and events in early group meetings are critical in establishing the behavioral norms that will govern the group. Establishing a safe therapeutic environment, open and honest communication, member–member support and sharing as well as establishing the group as a place where members change and grow are tasks accomplished through interventions by the group leader in very early sessions. Group traditions begin early and are enormously difficult to change once established. As new members join and the group matures and develops, it falls upon the group leader as well as other group members to properly enculturate new members into protherapeutic norms (i.e., the ways of the group). The group therapist accomplishes this task through action as a technical expert and a model-setting participant. The leader then supports the group in their positive attempts to enculturate new members.

In the Yalom model one of the prime functions of the group therapist is gate keeping. This includes maintaining the stablility of group membership. This issue is of concern in any therapy group, as a nonstable membership aborts the development of curative factors. New members may unrealistically expect or fear instantaneous cure. In either case, this may lead to rapid termination and must be addressed.

In the early stages of a new group the therapist serves as the "primary unifying force" (Yalom, 1975, p. 106). Members relate to each other through the therapist. For the group to function effectively member–member communication must be facilitated from the very beginning. This may be established by utilizing the frame of the group as a supportive environment, where the prime source of support is each member's fellow group members. One of the prime tasks of the group therapist is to "deter forces which threaten group cohesiveness" (Yalom, 1975, p. 106). These include lateness, nonattendance, member–member attacks, and disruptive extragroup socializing. Many nonbehavioral group therapists seek to limit or clearly structure members' extragroup socializing (Yalom, 1975). By contrast, behavioral group therapists often encourage such socializing as a means of enhancing generalization (Rose, 1977). Whichever model is utilized, expectations need to be clear.

In our clinical experience, a particular danger in therapy groups is the perception that group leaders are the fount of all knowledge and expertise. Yalom notes two roles the leader plays to establish norms: the role as technical expert and the role as model-participant. It is the former role, as expert, that may undermine the strength of the group. Group therapy requires a high level of expertise of the therapist in conceptualization of psychopathology as well as in group-treatment interventions. This expertise may easily be seen by group members as disempowering the suggestions and strategies the group members themselves might offer. Thus, the leader is at risk of unintentionally dominating the group and undermining potential sources of group cohesion. Our clinical experience suggests that this is a notable risk in behavioral groups, particularly with inexperienced group leaders, and is of potential danger in long-term groups where early norms may reduce the group's effectiveness. Thus, the nature of leadership in therapy groups involves a constant balancing of the need for expertise-based interventions and the constrasting need to empower the group and enhance cohesion.

Treatment Variables among Theoretical Models

Several treatment variables are of importance in considering the similarities and differences among long-term process-oriented psychotherapy groups, behavioral (and/or cognitive) therapy groups, and groups conceptualized within the integrative model of long-term process-oriented behavioral group psychotherapy proposed in this chapter. These variables, and the manner in which they are utilized as therapy groups develop and unfold, describe the differences among group therapy models and determine the nature of therapeutic work and outcome. The variables of concern include (a) style and methods of group leadership; (b) the group contract; (c) group norms and curative factors emphasized; (d) methods of utilization of therapeutic "techniques"; and (e) the purpose of the group.

Group Leadership

The group leader is the individual who convenes the group, selects group members, and whose role as technical expert and model sets the tone, boundaries, and many of the norms of the group. The group leader (or therapist, herein used interchangeably) is the most powerful member of the group, either by explicit, purposeful interventions or implicit, nonpurposeful actions (or inaction). As the group leader cannot help but influence the group's formation and development, we would propose the utility of purposeful, planned leader behavior. That point stated, How shall the therapist lead?

Early psychoanalytic group leaders attempted to apply the principles and methods of individual psychoanalysis to group therapy (Durkin, 1974). This implied the therapist functioning as the analytic "blank screen" in order to enhance the emergence of transference reactions and unconscious affect. Interaction between group therapist and group members was kept to a minimum lest the real relationship interfere with the recapitulation of early, primarily parent–child, relationships. Interaction between leader and each individual member primarily consisted of clarification of affect and interpretation of unconscious or preconscious dynamics. The group as a whole was minimally utilized, and therapy often resembled serial individual psychotherapies.

Early psychodramatic group leaders (Moreno, 1937, 1966), although often psychodynamically informed, were more actively engaged with group members, in part in order to generate affect. They were powerful participant shapers of the group experience and actively utilized and stage-managed intermember interactions and relationships. The group as a whole was a focus of concern and was often utilized to further therapeutic ends.

Many more recent interpersonal process-oriented group therapists (Yalom, 1975) employ a more real-life, genuine approach to leadership. Depending on the situation and clinical needs, the therapist may express his or her real feelings and interact with either individual members or the group as a whole. Yet, the primary locus of communication is member–member rather than leader–member communication. Therapist interventions are often directed toward facilitating intermember interaction in order to empower the group as the agent of psychotherapeutic change. Thus, as noted previously, group cohesion is of primary importance, and the leader's interventions are often aimed at enhancing cohesion by elucidating interpersonal and group processes.

Ironically, behavioral group therapists often employ a style with many similarities to that utilized by early psychoanalytic group therapists. Not in the sense of a nondirective blank-screen approach but in terms of doing individual therapy in the group. The therapeutic role is often of technical expert/teacher/trainer. Therefore, expression of affect, not often seen in teaching settings, may be suppressed or discouraged, and the group may come to see the therapist as extremely powerful—massively more powerful than the members. This approach can be problematic on several grounds. Excessive empowerment of the group therapist (and thereby disempowering the individual members) makes the group leader's job more difficult. The leader must do all the work to help people change: Make assignments, suggest behavioral interventions, establish contracts, accomplish the initial and ongoing behavioral and cognitive assessments, confront maladaptive behavior in the group, reinforce positive steps toward growth, and the like. This is an inefficient use of the group therapy treatment modality where group members can come to perform all these tasks. Given that members, especially in homogeneous groups, may share similar types of distress and experience, an individual's fellow members are often more likely to be effective than the leader! For example, in our experience with highly task-oriented groups (e.g., smoking cessation) members identify group interaction and esprit de corps as being among the most important factors in achieving their goals.

Therapist-centered behavioral groups, where the therapist is seen as the all-powerful technical expert, may lead to suppression of the expression of affect. Openly sharing feelings is an important part of the group experience as it allows the group to understand how the members experience their lives and symptoms. These data are critical in assessment of problem areas and design of individualized interventions. In addition, open, honest expression of feelings often deepens the relationship among members, increasing cohesiveness and the group's reinforcing value. Thus, the ability of the group to influence the individual member is enhanced.

Leader-centered groups may discourage generalization of response. To the extent that new behaviors are primarily associated with one stimulus, these behaviors are less likely to appear in novel settings. Thus, behavioral flexibility, application of newly learned material, and generalization of response are impeded. Generalization is critical; therapy serves little purpose if new responses learned are not applied in extratherapeutic settings and at times other than the therapy hour. When the all-powerful therapist is seen as the agent of change, the individual member, especially the highly disabled member, may come to see himself or herself as unable to make changes or function effectively without external impetus. In our clincial experience, this is less likely to occur with a highly empowered group that has many members who are much like each other and like their nonsymptomatic (nonclient) brethren. When the varied group members are the stimuli to which new behaviors become associated, there is an initial powerful step toward generalization. A closely related advantage of the nonleader-centered group is the maintenance (or establishment) of each individual's responsibility for his or her own behavior. This is, of course, critical as development of the notion of other's responsibility for our behavior makes us helpless. We cannot change what we are not responsible for! A sense of helplessness destroys the effectiveness of the group.

In the integrative model of long-term process-oriented behavioral group psychotherapy herein proposed, the leader serves as the technical expert who trains and empowers the group. This is accomplished through facilitating member–member communication. The leader is seen as both an expert *and* as a real person. Group empowerment becomes a primary goal (in many instances more important than any specific behavioral intervention). Group empowerment implies that the group is seen by its own members as the primary, but not sole, source of interventions, and group suggestions are highly valued. Individual responsibility, instead of leader responsibility, is emphasized. Affect expression is supported and encouraged in order to value the individual's personal experience and enhance cohesion. Generalization of response beyond the leader and beyond the group is encouraged. Finally, the group leader/therapist lets the group do the work whenever possible. The previous goals are accomplished by both procedural and process interventions. Procedures include role playing and dyadic exercises; process interventions relate to the facilitation of group interaction.

The role of the group leader in the integrative model of behavioral group psychotherapy differs from that found in an exclusively interpersonal process model (Yalom, 1975). In the latter model, the group leader's role is primarily to facilitate and model effective interpersonal interactions. In the integrative model the group leader also provides technical interventions that may be educative and/or symptom focused. As such, the role of the group leader in the integrative model emphasizes the role as technical expert more extensively than in the interpersonal process model.

The role of the group leader in the integrative model of behavioral group psychotherapy also differs from that role in other behavioral groups. In this instance, the former role emphasizes interpersonal process and the primacy of facilitating member–member communication and relatedness.

The Group Contract

Establishment of the group contract is a critical consideration in beginning any psychotherapeutic group. The contract is the shared agreement that binds group members together; it embodies the rules thay all members agree to abide by. As such, it is more explicit than the informal norms that become established through the process of the group. The contract helps establish a boundary around the group (Rice & Rutan, 1981); the group includes only those who have agreed to the contract. The group boundary "marks the outer limits of . . . a group" (Rice & Rutan, 1981, p. 297); it defines who is in and out of the group and how members enter and leave. The contract thus becomes a basic component of group structure.

Group contracts may differ markedly among different group leaders and among therapists of differing theoretical orientations. Most contracts, regardless of the orientation of the leader, include clauses related to time and place of the group sessions as well as fee arrangements. Here commonalities end. Within purely psychoanalytic groups, the explicit contract may be minimal: members are expected to share their feelings, thoughts, and images with little, if any censorship (the "free association" rule). The contract may be stated in pregroup interviews and restated as a new member joins the group.

Rose (1977) proposes a very explicit, written contract for behavioral groups including expectations of both members and leaders. He proposes a contract including explicit contingencies for noncompliance by group members (e.g., forfeiture of money for nonattendance at group meetings or noncompliance with homework assignments). As such, his approach to the contract is primarily an operant-reinforcement model. Parenthetically, in this model, contingencies for group leaders are omitted.

The contingency-based approach to group structure has much to recommend it. Foremost, contingency management works. Group members and individual organisms of all kinds respond to explicit contingencies. Therefore, establishing explicit contingencies is a powerful method of shaping the behavior of the group. In addition, the explicit nature of the contingencies proposed by Rose (1977) means all group members are clearly aware of these contingencies prior to entering the group. Provision of explicit rules is respectful of group members and provides members with helpful information as consumers of mental health care.

There are, nonetheless, several marked disadvantages to the contingency-based approach. Given that the keeper of the contingencies is clearly the group leader, this type of group contract excessively empowers the group leader (and thereby disempowers the members). This excessively authoritative, if not authoritarian, approach to the group contract, and thereby group leadership, may paradoxically reduce group cohesion and thus the effectiveness of the group. In addition, such an approach, in the authors' experience, may tend to suppress affective sharing and trust. Finally, the awkwardness of structured, monetary contingnecies may reduce the interpersonal focus of the group and thereby further disempower this modality of treatment.

Yalom (1975) suggests that potential group members be carefully prepared for their group therapy experience. In essence, the enculturative process begins prior to an individual's entrance into the group. Explicit expectations of sharing feelings and reactions are clearly stated. The *contract* (although Yalom does not use this term) is primarily interpersonal; it is made between the group therapist and potential member and later made between the new member and veteran group members. Most of the clauses of the contract are interpersonal in nature, emphasizing the interpersonal process nature of Yalom's model of group treatment. This model emphasizes the interpersonal deficits that bring individuals into psychotherapy and advocates an interpersonal environment as being curative. The structure of the group (e.g., number of members, open vs. closed nature, specific committments requested) is outlined to the potential member prior to entering the group. Yalom suggests clear pregroup preparation (when the contract is presented) to enhance the desirability of the group. This issue is, of course, discussed in greater detail in Chapter 1 of this volume.

A combination of Rose's (1977) pregroup behavioral contract and Yalom's (1975) group preparation models may be of substantial utility in long-term behavioral psychotherapy groups. A sample contract, used for homogeneous groups of agoraphobics, is presented in Table 1. The group contract is best

TABLE 1. Sample Group Contract: Agoraphobia Group

1. The purpose of the group is to help members overcome the difficulties associated with agoraphobia. These include the discomfort of agoraphobic anxiety as well as the constriction in one's life associated with agoraphobic avoidance.
2. The group meets weekly on (day) at (time) A.M./P.M.
3. As one of the prime purposes of the group is to help members overcome avoidance associated with anxiety, attendance at group meetings is critical. Therefore, avoidance of the group (other than for vacations, illness, etc.) is very problematic.
4. One of the purposes of the group is to provide a safe, supportive environment in which members may grow. Therefore, members may expect to receive support *from* their fellow group members as well as to provide it *to* their fellow members.
5. Upon entering the group, members are asked to make a 4-week commitment to stay in the group. Starting in a new group can sometimes be anxiety provoking, and we want to provide an opportunity to begin to benefit from the group (which may take several weeks).
6. Upon leaving the group, members are asked to inform the group as a whole at least 4 weeks in advance. This facilitates postgroup planning for the member leaving and allows all members to deal with saying goodbye.
7. If you know you will be missing a group please announce it in advance (if possible). Otherwise, please call the leader(s) prior to the group so your absence can be announced. All group members become important to the group and are missed if they are not present.
8. Confidentiality is critical for the group to be a safe place for members to share their experiences and feelings. Your own "business" you can, of course, share with anyone you chose; information about other group members and what happens here needs to stay in the group.
9. Homework tasks will be negotiated each week between the individual member, leaders, and other group members. Completion of homework is critical to success in overcoming agoraphobia.
10. Openness, honesty, and respect for fellow group members are important for the group. Providing and receiving honest feedback is an important part of the group experience.
11. Members may wish to get together between sessions, for example, to work on tasks related to the group (e.g., *in vivo* exposure). As members meet each other within the context of the group, such extragroup socializing is considered group business and must be brought back to the group.
12. Finally, the group meets for 2½ hours weekly. The first hour is spent in reviewing how members are doing, going over completed homework tasks, coaching in coping skills, and planning the next hour's experience. The second hour is spent doing *in vivo* exposure, exposing oneself to the situations and feelings that cause anxiety. This may be done accompanied by a group leader, another group member or members, or alone—whatever is most useful. The last half hour of the group is spent reviewing the *in vivo* experience and negotiating new homework tasks.

presented to potential members at pregroup screening sessions where the process of group enculturation begins. If a member is felt by the therapist to be appropriate for the group, desires to join, and agrees to the contract the person is then brought into the group. Beware of potential members who agree only in part or vacillate with regard to the contract clauses! In the authors' experience such members may not fully agree to the structure of the group. They may interpret the group therapist's silence or inattention to their lack of agreement as not valuing the contract. Thus, they may not value the contract. Such individuals, when they become group members, are often disruptive and become treatment failures.

It is best to repeat the contract at the member's first meeting so that all members are aware that the same contract binds them all. This helps to create a boundary around the group. It is recommended that expected cognitive and behavioral interventions be generally mentioned in the contract as a way of emphasizing the task focus of the group to the new member and maintaining the task focus for veteran members. Rather than explicit, structured (e.g., monetary) contingencies for compliance or noncompliance, the authors would suggest that the social approval of a cohesive therapy group is a sufficiently powerful group contingency. The interpersonal focus of the contract and contingencies for contract maintenance serve to empower the group. Over time, what is often found, is that the group has as much or more investment in the contract than the leader.

For long-term behavioral psychotherapy groups, the contract itself should include the explicitly stated purpose of the group, meeting times, special rules necessitated by the nature of the group composition or treatment interventions (see Table 1, Clause 3) as well as clauses about confidentiality, honesty, and support. In addition, particular commitments asked of members around scheduling should be included as well as rules about socializing. Finally, one or more clauses emphasizing the task-focused nature of the group are highly recommended in order to clearly maintain this frame over time and changes in membership.

The contract establishes an interpersonal context for the group. In long-term behavioral psychotherapy groups the group contract, in addition to providing training to group members in carrying out and utilizing cognitive and behavioral interventions and coping strategies, serves to provide a structure for the group and to empower group members. Thus, members become "therapists" for each other and for themselves. This can best occur in a safe therapeutic environment provided by a skilled group psychotherapist and an effectively implemented group contract.

Group Norms

The *group norms* are the behavioral rules that guide the interaction of the group (Yalom, 1975). Norms are rules that may or may not be verbalized. These rules may be purposefully shaped by the group leader or may occur as a result of inadvertant interventions. In all instances, norms are also established by the ongoing interpersonal process of the group. This is particularly so for the process of early group therapy sessions, those occurring in the first several months (even the first several weeks) of an ongoing long-term group. Norms may also be created by particularly powerful events in the history of a group. Once established, group norms are *very* difficult to change, even with explicit intervention. Given that norms are often evolutionary, it is best for potential group leaders to plan appropriate norms and build them in.

A variety of norms follow from the explicitly stated clauses of the group contract. For example, a contract may state that members are expected to attend each session and arrive on time. A norm of the group might then be that members rarely miss group meetings and everyone is in their seat when the time for beginning the group arrives. If a member is late, other members comment upon this and apply presure on tardy members to comply with the rules. All of this may occur without explicit intervention by the therapist.

Many procedural norms around attendance, lateness, paying fees, even style of dress of members (and leaders), are often shared by groups of widely differing theoretical persuasion and clinical type. For example, chronic nonattendance at meetings will destroy *any* group. Therfore, powerful norms around attendance help maintain the group, and, as needed, leader interventions to bolster these norms are strongly indicated. On the other hand, norms having to do with therapeutic process, what members and leaders are actually expected to do and talk about within and between sessions, may differ radically among groups run within different theoretical orientations.

Explicit consideration, development, and establishment of protherapeutic norms are an important task of the group leader. The specific norms chosen by any group leader as those worthy of facilitation will depend on personal predilication, theoretical orientation, and purposes of the group. The particular norms chosen for facilitation should relate closely to the curative factors the group therapist wishes to emphasize. Thus, the group therapists' understanding of the clinical objectives of the group and knowledge of the processes that underlie behavior change (in its broadest sense: including affective as well as cognitive changes) will determine the norms to be chosen.

Traditional behavior therapy groups depend heavily on techniques and therapeutic interventions developed under the broad rubic of *behavior therapy* and cognitive therapy. These include procedures such as self-monitoring, systematic desensitization, implosion, behavior rehearsal, self-instructional training, modeling, coaching, contracting, extinction, cognitive restructuring, positive reinforcement, and response prevention. These techniques are aimed at changing specific target behaviors in (potentially) quantifiable ways. The emphasis on behavioral intervention and behavior change, in part, determines the nature of desirable group norms. For example, in a behavioral group, members are expected to carry out a variety of assignments, participate in behavioral interventions (e.g., *in vivo* exposure, role playing), and their target behaviors are expected to change from time to time. As these occur, a common group norm would be member-to-member support and praise.

Norms in traditional behavior therapy groups serve to empower the interventions utilized and enhance specific, reportable changes in behavior. Consistent self-monitoring to establish baseline data for potential target symptoms and to provide feedback as to the effectiveness of interventions becomes critical. Therefore, a powerful group norm in support of completion of daily self-monitoring charts and bringing the charts to the group is highly desirable. In a similar manner, powerful norms around homework completion and *in vivo* application of behavioral interventions and new skills learned are important in behavior therapy groups. The leader may establish these norms in a variety of ways. Simply stating the group norm and reasons for it is a natural initial intervention (with restatement of the norm as necessary). Verbal reinforcement for completion of charts and homework tasks and the expression of mild disapproval when tasks are not completed are also commonly used. Eliciting comments from the group serves to encourage pronormative behavior as long as the group explicitly supports the norm under consideration. Many behavioral therapists will use concrete reinforcers, including fee rebates for attendance or homework completion, monetary fines for noncompletion of assignments, or even denying a member access to the group if criteria are not met. This last intervention assumes that attending the group is highly reinforcing for the member and is so radical that it should only be used with severe conditions, for example, potentially life-threatening anorexia nervosa (Dooley, personal communication, 1983).

Several common norms in traditional behavior therapy groups may be problematic in long-term behavioral group psychotherapy. Traditional behavioral groups tend to be extremely task focused. As such, clinical material brought up by members that does not mesh with the chosen agenda (e.g., particular behavioral intervention) may be de-emphasized. The most common result of this process is to reduce the expression of affect, specifically, speaking about affectively laden topics and concerns. As outlined previously, our clinical experience suggests that this strategy tends to reduce group cohesion and the investment of individual members in the therapy group. This intense task focus may, in fact, be appropriate for short-term behavioral groups with nonclinical populations (e.g., smoking cessation, minor obesity, assertiveness training or stress-management groups in industry). However, we would propose that such a norm of primary (exclusive) task focus and affect suppression is not appropriate with clinical groups composed of individuals with serious or long-standing difficulties. A major consideration in working with moderately to severely psychologically disabled populations is the demoralization such individuals experience. This demoralization—a sense of hopelessness, helplessness, and lack of self-worth—is often a prime clinical consideration. It may lead to noncompliance with behavioral assignments and the failure to report significant clincal information. Therefore, treatment ought to value the individual's affective experience. This process of valuing may be more significant than any other intervention made.

Yalom (1975) proposes that a prime consideration for the group therapist in long-term process-oriented group psychotherapy is culture building, that is, the construction of a therapeutic social system. This includes the establishment of therapeutic norms. Yalom proposes that the leader works to establish the group as the agent of psychotherapeutic change through his or her role as model-setting participant and technical expert. Within this process-oriented model of group psychotherapy several norms are suggested. For the group to become the agent of psychotherapeutic change, the members of the group must begin to take responsibility for what happens in the group. Yalom refers to this as the norm of the *self-monitoring group*. The leader may ask the group to evaluate the effectiveness of the session and comment on what they find helpful. Another important group norm is *self-disclosure*. Of course, members need to set the pace of their own self-disclosure, but the ultimate value of disclosure is woven into the fabric of the group. An atmosphere of trust, safety, and, above all, security in the confidentiality rule must be created in order to provide a context for the norm of self-disclosure.

The members must value the group in order to benefit fully from it. Therfore, Yalom proposes that all interventions by members or leader that enhance the value of the group be emphasized. This may include such interventions as enforcing the group contract (or norm) around attendance. Encouraging members to attend, announcing absences in advance, or at the least, members calling the leader(s) so they may announce the member's absence are all important. Emphasizing that members are missed when they are unable to attend and that fellow members will wonder where a member is if they are not present helps the members to value the group. Reinforcing testimonials to the group and encouraging progroup connections between members will help the group to value itself. Members' connections with each other between groups can be quite valuable as long as such extragroup contact is reported back to the group. Members may come to see each other as resources in times of crisis, even between group sessions.

Finally, Yalom proposes a norm of establishing the group members as agents of help. The group members themselves need to feel empowered as a major source of input to their fellows, and each member needs to value this input. The therapist may establish this norm by specifically pointing out helpful comments, asking group members to specify which contributions from others have helped, and ask for member-to-member comments even when the therapist is asked for input. Behavior by any group member that undermines the norm of mutual aid must be challenged. In this way the leader protects the group and maintains this norm.

Norm building is a critical task in long-term process-oriented behavioral group psychotherapy. The model herein proposed involves a melding of norms found in traditional behavioral groups with those more commonly found in long-term process-oriented group psychotherapy. Proposed group norms include self-disclosure, affect expression, group empowerment, group responsibility as well as the task focus found in more traditional behavioral groups. Norms should also include those specifically tailored to the clinical population served by and the particular purposes of the group. For example, the norms in a long-term process-oriented behavioral psychotherapy group for individuals with an impulse control disorder (e.g., borderline personality, drug addiction, aggressive outbursts, or morbid obesity) might differ markedly from therapeutic norms in a group of phobic or generally anxious or socially anxious individuals (e.g., agoraphobia group or communications skills group for chronic psychiatric patients). The norms in the impulse-control group might emphasize group support for suppression of maladaptive behaviors, development of alternative responses, and use of coping strategies to mediate overwhelming affect that might otherwise lead to self-destructive or other destructive behaviors. Norms in a group of anxious individuals would focus on group support for building new behaviors, for seeking out anxiety-provoking situations, and developing a more extensive behavioral repertoire with which to function effectively and cope with these problematic situations. Thus, it is the task of the group leader, prior to beginning a long-term behavioral psychotherapy group, to broadly understand the clinical needs of the population or populations to be served and to clearly specify those group norms that will enable the group to aid members in overcoming their difficulties.

The task of melding together group norms around self-disclosure, affect expression, and task focus is a difficult one for the leader in a long-term behavioral psychotherapy group. Self-disclosure and affect expression within the interpersonal process of the group will enhance group cohesion and allow members to be emotionally honest with the group (Lott & Lott, 1961). Empowerment of the group members and enhancing member–member help giving and help seeking will make the group maximally powerful as a therapeutic modality (Flowers, 1978; Flowers, Booraem, & Seacat, 1974). Yet, the task focus is critically important as a variety of cognitive and behavioral interventions have been shown to be quite helpful and often curative for many psychopathological conditions and behavior disorders. On a moment-to-moment basis, the group leader must weigh the utility of one intervention or another (group empowerment vs. use of cognitive-behavioral clinical intervention) and must help the group to make effective choices in terms of which direction to go. The authors have seen numerous examples of groups deciding to forego further discussion of affect-laden topics in favor of a return to behavioral interventions (e.g., *in vivo* exposure for an agoraphobia group or role playing for a communication skills group). On the other hand, groups will often decide that discussion of a particularly important topic should take precedence over a planned cognitive or behavioral intervention. It depends on the skill of the behavioral group psychotherapist and the level of sophistication of the group in helping the group to decide in which direction to go. It is frequently found that the preexisting structure of the group is helpful in these deliberations. For example, in a heterogeneous group, with members with many differing clinical problems, time may be set aside each week to allow for individualized behavioral contracting. This contracting might focus in on the specific tasks each member will complete before the next group in order to move toward overcoming their difficulties.

Use of Therapeutic "Techniques"

Many of the clinical considerations related to the use of therapeutic techniques have been outlined in the preceding sections on group leadership, curative factors, norm building, and group contracts. A few further considerations will be presented here briefly.

The issue of integration of therapeutic techniques into group treatment is primarily a consideration for traditional behavioral group therapists and those working within the model of long-term process-oriented behavioral group psychotherapy. Therapeutic technique in nonbehavioral therapy primarily focuses on considerations in the therapeutic relationship or what among the clinical data presented by the client the therapist should attend to. Thus, in individual psychodynamic psychotherapy there are a variety of interventions a therapist may make (Bibring, 1954), ranging from suggestion, to clarification of affect, to interpretation of unconscious dynamics. In some psychodynamic groups these same interventions may be made. In terms of technical interventions, Yalom (1975) emphasizes the importance of the group psychotherapist's focus on the here-and-now interactions of the group members, the interpersonal process. Elucidating and clarifying these interactions as they occur is a prime task of the therapist within the ongoing group.

In behavioral groups, whether of the traditional variety or long-term process-oriented model proposed in this chapter, the integration of therapeutic "techniques" is a central issue. Behavioral and cognitive "technologies" have been developed for addressing a variety of disorders for which an individual may seek treatment. These range from *in vivo* exposure for agoraphobia (Emmelkamp, 1982; Marks, 1973, 1975, 1977) to cognitive therapy for depression (Beck, Rush, Shaw, & Emery, 1979) to self-monitoring, stimulus control, and contingency contracting for morbid obesity (Stuart & Davis, 1972). Each of these treatments may either be administered in a group or woven into the context of a long-term psychotherapeutic group. In traditional behavioral group therapy, technical interventions are frequently administered in a group. People are gathered together with common or diverse difficulties and exposed to the treatment intervention (or arrangements are made for this exposure). Relatively little use is made of the group itself as a therapeutic modality or of the interpersonal processes of the group. We would suggest that this is an inefficient use of the group treatment modality and does not well serve the clinical needs of individuals who request services for their psychological pain and difficulties (except in limited instances, e.g., group desensitization for focal phobias).

The current model of long-term process-oriented behavioral group psychotherapy is proposed as an alternative. Therapeutic techniques are one part of what occurs in the group. Empowerment of the group members to offer suggestions and support to their fellow members in an important task for the leader. Facilitation of self-disclosure and expression of affect are important in increasing group cohesion as well as enhancing both the extensiveness of personal data presented for cognitive-behavioral assessment and the degree of compliance with subsequent behavioral homework assignments.

Purposes of the Group

Understanding the purpose of the group is a necessary requisite for both the leader and potential members. When discussing group psychotherapy, the purpose can be considered from two perspectives. The most common perspective is what is the overall goal of the group; in other words, what are both the members and the group leader attempting to accomplish by participation in the group. The other perspective on purpose is considering the means by which the ultimate goal will be achieved. In process-oriented group therapy, the typical purpose is the development of insight and personal growth (Yalom, 1975). Usually, these goals are accomplished by attention being paid to the personal interaction among members, transferential issues related to the leader, and observation of interpersonal communication styles. For most behavior therapy groups, the purpose is that of symptom resolution (Rose, 1977). In these groups, a specific symptom is focused on with a variety of behavioral techniques being introduced that are designed to help participants improve their ability to cope with their symptom situation. Formats are often didactic, and usually little attention is paid to interpersonal issues among group members.

As with most behavioral groups, the "purpose" in the current model tends to be issue or symptom focused. Two examples offered later in this chapter demonstrate this. In the first, a group designed to treat agoraphobia is described, and in the second example, the Therapeutic Contract Group, a systematic problem-solving intervention is reviewed. However, not only are specific goals delineated, but also the means to these ends are discussed with group members prior to the group's initiation. It is important for members to be informed that each group attempts to integrate specific behavioral skill training relevant to the group's problem area with an opportunity for members to learn from the group process and interaction. In other words, we are speaking of taking purposes that are dealt with in process-oriented groups and weaving them into those most usually seen in behaviorally oriented groups. Given that a focus on personal interaction and process are somewhat more ambiguous ways of accomplishing therapeutic goals, it is extremely important for members to periodically be reminded of the overall purposes and goals of the group. Although the use of various leadership procedures and technical interventions, described later, facilitate this, it is equally important for both leader and members to clearly articulate their anticipated objectives for involvement in group therapy. In short, any time the question is raised—"why are we meeting?"—it should be seen as an indication that the "purpose" of the group needs to be reclarified.

Clinical Examples

Having presented the outlines of an integrative model of long-term process-oriented behavioral group psychotherapy, two clinical examples of this model in action will be delineated. Each of the groups to be described have been led by one of the authors for a minimum of 4 years. Groups are ongoing and open-ended. New members are accepted as old members graduate. One of the groups is composed of outpatients (although other such outpatient groups have been conducted by the authors and their associates using the same model), and one group is composed of relatively long-term inpatients, with postdischarge continuation of group treatment for many members.

Agoraphobia Group

A sample contract for the group appears in Table 1. The group meets on a weekly basis for 2½ hours. As agoraphobia is a complex clincial syndrome (Chambless & Goldstein, 1982), treatment involves several components, and behavioral group psychotherapy includes several phases. The theoretical model that guides the group is that proposed by Goldstein and Chambless (1978) with modifications based on the work of Belfer and Glass (1982) and Marks (1973, 1975, 1977, 1979). As such, it is an interpersonal, cognitive-behavioral treatment with heavy emphasis on *in vivo* exposure.

The group itself is structured to achieve several clinical goals. First, it is structured as a support group. Agoraphobia is a very discomforting and disabling psychopathological condition. As such, it is often quite demoralizing to agoraphobic individuals. The experience of chronic high levels of anxiety, subjectively unpredictable and subjectively incomprehensible panic attacks, in addition to the commonly described life constriction (inability to drive, take public transporation, be alone, enter public places, etc.), all contribute to this demoralization. The experience of support from other similarly afflicted individuals, within the context of a therapeutic, hope-generating group environment, can be quite powerful. Members share their experiences and successes as well as failures and help each other through rough times.

The primary behavioral intervention in the group is *in vivo* exposure. *In vivo* exposure within a cohesive group has been shown to be an effective treatment for agoraphobic avoidance (Emmelkamp, 1982; Hand, Lamontagne, & Marks, 1974). The treatment entails reexposure to both the situations that are feared as well as the feelings that are feared. The feared situations are generated by the individual prior to entering the group and listed in an extensive hierarchy. The feelings that are feared include the very experience of anxiety, called *fear of fear* by Goldstein and Chambless (1978). Exposure to these feelings occurs naturally during *in vivo* exposure to avoided situations. Exposure occurs gradually, by small steps, up the hierarchy. Members may be accompanied by one or more fellow members, a group leader, or they may go out alone for the exposure. In any event, the hierarchical step chosen for exposure needs to be small enough so that anxiety will abate (extinguish or habituate) within the group time allotted for the exposure.

A substantial amount of coaching also occurs during the group. Coaching primarily focuses on use of self-control coping skills including multiple methods of relaxation training, systematic rational restructuring of catastrophic thoughts (Goldfried, Decenteceo, & Weinberg, 1974), and self-instructional training (Meichenbaum, 1977). In the authors' experience relaxation training and rational restructuring appear to be most effective for anticipatory anxiety, whereas self-instructional training seems most useful for facilitating exposure itself as well as coping with severe panic attacks. Finally, group time is spent in individual contracting with each member for continued exposure during the intersession week.

The group, which is 2½ hours in duration, is broken down into several phases. The first hour is spent in the office, in general discussion. How members are doing, results of the past week's homework (exposure), successes, failures, traumatic events, or anything else of relevance are covered. In addition, planning occurs for the *in vivo* exposure. The second hour is spent out of the office accomplishing the exposure. Members may walk, drive cars, take public transportation, go into stores or large public places as needed. This may occur alone, in small groups, or with a group leader. The last half hour of the group is spent processing the exposure and contracting for continued exposure prior to the next group meeting.

Several issues have been discussed at length as the proposed long-term process-oriented model of behavioral group psychotherapy was outlined. These include methods and style of group leadership, the group contract, group norms, and integration of behavioral techniques. Each of these has particular relevance to the agoraphobia group being described.

As with other behavioral psychotherapy groups, the therapist for an agoraphobia group serves as gatekeeper and the individual who maintains the boundaries of the group. These boundaries include both who is in and out of the group as well as between different phases of each group session (free verbal time, *in vivo* exposure, homework contracting). Slightly different roles may be played in each section. In the initial free verbal time, the behavioral group psychotherapist serves as a facilitator of group process, the individual who empowers the group. During *in vivo* exposure, the therapist serves as technical expert and cognitive-behavioral trainer and coach. In the final portion of the group there is a melding of roles. Of course, in reality the behavioral group psychotherapist should and does shift flexibly from one role to the next during all phases of each session, with the consistent goal of empowering the group; ultimately the group is the agent of psychotherapeutic change.

A sample group contract for a long-term process-oriented agoraphobia group is presented in Table 1. As the contract speaks for itself, only a few words will be added here. The contract serves to frame the group, to establish its purpose, basic rules, and outlines curative factors to be emphasized (e.g., group interaction, support, *in vivo* exposure). It also may set certain rules necessitated by clinical interventions or characteristics of the population to be treated as well as establish the basis for group norms. An example of the former function of the contract is seen in Clause 3 of Table 2. Agoraphobia involves avoidance as a prime clinical feature. When an agoraphobic individual feels anxious he or she is less likely to engage in certain activities. As the agoraphobia group may well meet in a setting beyond the comfort range of the client, there is a natural tendency to avoid. This is clearly countertherapeutic and is addressed by Clause 3. This clause must then be enforced by the leader with the help of the group.

A norm that follows closely from the group contract is exposure. It is critical that agoraphobic individuals work to expose themselves to both the situations and feelings that are feared. Activities that facilitate exposure (within clinical reason) are helpful. Attempting exposure is better than avoidance; exposure with retreat (partial escape) is better than no exposure at all. Support from fellow group members for attempted and successful exposure is critical. Establishing a clear understanding that exposure often entails the experience of anxiety (which is seen as positive) can be quite helpful. Support from fellow group members through the experience of anxiety can be very powerful. Thus, counterphobic norms (although not suggesting the induction of panic) should be facilitated.

Technical interventions, including *in vivo* exposure as well as coaching in the use of relaxation training, cognitive restructuring, and self-instructional training are clinical components of behavioral treatment for agoraphobia. Although everything must be done to enhance the power of these interventions, it should not be at the expense of the group. Members share a dilemma in grappling with agoraphobia. Although war stories, exploration of parental dynamics, and symptom listing are not particularly helpful, discussion of the practical and existential difficulties of coping with a disabling psychopathological condition may be curative. Thus, the behavioral group psychotherapist constantly grapples with the alternative needs to emphasize proven behavioral interventions with the need to empower the curative factors of the psychotherapy group. In this dynamic tension, effective treatment occurs.

Therapeutic Contract Group (TCG)

By contrast to the previously presented agoraphobia group, the Therapeutic Contract Group is used in the treatment of a heterogenous inpatient population and represents the core clinical component in the Therapeutic Contract Program (Levendusky, Berglas, Dooley, & Landau, 1983). Patients treated in the TCG come from a broad range of diagnoses with the affective categories being the most frequently represented. All patients in the Therapeutic Contract Program are expected to attend the TCG, which meets on a biweekly basis for 90 minutes. The average patient membership in the group is 12; in addition, the group leader and two to three staff members are also in attendance. The length of involvement in these groups is determined by the patient's length of hospitalization, with patients being introduced to the groups shortly after admission and typically continuing for 3 to 4 weeks after discharge. As a result, most patients will attend at least 25 group meetings.

The primary purpose of the TCG is to provide patients with a forum where they can actively develop problem-solving strategies to cope with the wide variety of situations that have led to their hospitalization. In these public settings, they are assisted in defining a series of long-term goals for their treatment and then operationalizing a number of short-term goals that are designed to help accomplish their long-term objectives. As can be seen in the sample contract (Table 2), these goals focus on a wide range of conflict issues.

The biweekly schedule of group meetings allows members to present a series of potential objectives in the first weekly session, and then several days later to evaluate their success in accomplishing these objectives. Because the

TABLE 2. Sample Contract

The following revised contract was prepared by the members of the treatment team and the patient:

A. Long-term goal: follow program to decrease anxiety and compulsions
   Short-term goals:
   1. Continue to identify and deal with feelings during flooding procedure.
   2. Do flooding at home if arrangements are made by behavioral therapist.
   3. Make and document one "I-feel" statement each day.
   4. Use relaxation tapes daily.
   5. Utilize worry talks.
   6. Document anger on anger chart at least twice this week.
   7. Use 5-minute maximum worry talks.

B. Long-term goal: improve self-esteem and personal presentation
   Short-term goals:
   1. Document two positive self-sttements daily.
   2. Make and document one assertive statement daily.
   3. Speak into tape recorder minimum of 20 minutes this week, play back, or tape conversations and play back; ask for feedback.
   4. Be aware of nonverbals: holding hands rigid or wringing them; others cue.
   5. Be aware of negative thoughts of being dirty, restructure thoughts; ask patients or staff whether or not they think your hands are dirty and verify what "dirty" is.
   6. Begin to deal with feelings regarding discharge and realities of going home; talk with patients and staff regarding feelings.
   7. Terminate with roommate before she is discharged this week.
   8. Give at least two patients feedback in Friday contract review meeting.
   9. Be more assertive with staff, especially when following program.
   10. Be aware of anxiety situations outside of hospital and document; discuss with staff member upon return.

C. Long-term goal: clarify family issues
   Short-term goals:
   1. Discuss with husband in depth his fears about my coming home and my difficulties with obsessive behavior.
   2. Meet with social worker Wednesday and talk extensively about husband's fears.
   3. Be aware of negative assumptions with husband; ask him to cue me.
   4. Meet with social worker to determine importance of second meeting with my sisters.
   5. Maintain correspondence with stepmother.

D. Long-term goal: continue vocational issues
   Short-term goals:
   1. Get resume typed, copied, and distributed to at least three companies this week.
   2. Set up at least two interviews and go to them this week.
   3. Make list of positive features of my secretarial background and working qualities and discuss with coordinator in staff talk.
   4. Work at craft studio Tuesday and Wednesday nights; extend Wednesday time to $1\frac{1}{2}$ hours.
   5. Meet with rehabilitation counselor Wednesday.
   6. Attend job group.

purpose of the two meetings is somewhat different, the format also varies. In the first session, members are expected to present their proposed objectives for the week and are encouraged to give and receive feedback in regard to the most effective means for accomplishing these. In addition, there is an overriding effort made by the leaders to facilitate each member's making an overt commitment to the accomplishment of their various goals in this highly visible social forum. To this end, each member actually produces a treatment contract (Table 2) that becomes the focus of their weekly treatment activity.

In the second session, which occurs at the end of the week, members review the contracts and publicly identify what has and has not been accomplished. As a result, the focus of the group is on each member's accountability to his or her commitments made in the previous session. It is felt that this biwekkly format provides an opportunity for both public declaration of goals, and then later an equally public "recounting" of accountability greatly facilitates each member's accomplishment of his or her therapeutic objectives.

As discussed in this chapter, the various treatment variables emphasized in the long-term process-oriented group therapy model are especially relevant to the therapeutic contract groups. In addition to the usual gatekeeping tasks, the goal of the group leader in the TCG is that of facilitating interaction among the members and modeling the type of constructive, supportive, or critical feedback that is necessary to help participants actively engage in the presentation and review of their problem-solving strategies. Rather than presenting each member with a prepackaged set of objectives, the leader tries to foster both the individual's ability to creatively develop goals and also to help other members to contribute to this process. In short, the leader's attention is toward operationalizing an active social learning therapeutic milieu.

Describing the group contract may be somewhat confusing when discussing the Therapeutic Contract Group, but, in this context, we are referring to the group treatment variable referred to as the *contract*. Consistent with the long-term model being described in this chapter, the TCG contract is of central importance. Each member is informed of it prior to entry, and, given the frequently shifting membership of the group, it is necessary to frequently review this contract. Simply stated, all members are expected to attend all scheduled meetings on time, all are expected to have their proposed or completed contract drafts, and they are also expected to actively participate. In addition, each member is instructed in how to give direct feedback to other members and to continue discussion of unresolved group issues in forums offered in the general therapeutic milieu. Experience leads us to report that this group contact is followed very closely with attendance close to 100%; all members have contracts; and the frequency of verbal interaction is high. This inpatient therapeutic milieu is composed of a diagnostically heterogeneous patient population with some preponderance of individuals with affective diagnoses (e.g., depression). The age range is from 19 to 50 years old.

The group norms and curative factors are particularly interesting in these groups. In ratings given by patients at the time of discharge, over 90% indicate that the contract groups are the most important component of their hospitalization. They further indicate that the opportunity to be open about their treatment objectives and to be able to give and receive feedback in regard to these helps foster an increased sense of "being in control" of the conflicts that resulted in hospitalization. In a systematic evaluation of the several process components of these groups (Berglas & Levendusky, in press), the import of the public declaration and problem-solving strategies appears to be confirmed. The correlations between accomplishment of treatment goals and the willingness to participate actively in the group is very high. Conversely, patients unable to reach their therapeutic objectives were much slower to involve themselves in the mainstream of group interaction.

Although a number of specific behavioral techniques have been used in the TCG, most take the form of operationalizing short-term goals on a patient's treatment contract (e.g., use relaxation 3 times/day, document assertive behavior twice this week, etc.), whereas the actual ingroup focus is on the facilitation of member interaction through the use of leader modeling and fostering interaction among members to more openly and publicly declare their treatment accomplishments or lack therof.

In summary, the therapeutic contract groups attempt to provide patients with skills to develop their own strategies with a functional analysis of problematic behavior (Zifferblatt & Hendricks, 1974). This goal is accomplished through a combination of members' learning to identify problem areas, applying relevant behavioral intervention, and increasing the probability of compliance to these interventions by fostering a group process that then holds each member accountable.

Summary and Conclusions

In this chapter, a new integrative model of long-term process-oriented behavioral group psychotherapy has been proposed. This model involves a melding of long-term process-oriented group psychotherapy (Yalom, 1975) with a model of behavioral therapy in groups (Rose, 1977). As such, this chapter may be considered part of the ongoing process of integration between behavior therapy and other schools of psychotherapeutic thought (Goldfried, 1982; Kendall, 1982; Wachtel, 1977).

Several variables have been emphasized as being of particular importance in this integration process, as it relates to group psychotherapy. These variables include the nature and style of group leadership, the group contract, choice and development of group norms as well as the use of therapeutic "techniques." Each of these variables is of critical importance and requires substantial attention by potential long-term behavioral group psychotherapists.

The model of long-term process-oriented behavioral group psychotherapy can be utilized in both homogeneous groups as well as heterogeneous groups. In homogeneous groups, all members may present with similar clinical difficulties. In heterogeneous groups, diverse problems in living may be represented in the group.

The type of group proposed here may be relevant for a variety of clients. The model was developed for use with clients who were notably disabled by their symptoms or who had complicated or treatment-resistant psychopathological conditions (e.g., agoraphobics, schizophrenics, the chronically depressed, the morbidly obese). Yet these individuals and those with similarly complicated problems in living represent a substantial part of the population seeking therapeutic assistance. Therefore, the model has wide applicability.

References

Ackerman, N. W. Some general principles in the use of group psychotherapy. In B. Glueck (Ed.), *Current therapies of personality disorders*. New York: Grune & Stratton, 1946.

Beck, A., Rush, A., Shaw, B., & Emery, G. *Cognitive therapy of depression*. New York: Guilford Press, 1979.

Belfer, P., & Glass, C. *Agoraphobic anxiety and fear of fear: A cognitive attentional model*. Poster presentation at the 16th Annual Convention of the Association for Advancement of Behavior Therapy. Los Angeles, 1982.

Belfer, P., Schachter, J., Dooley, C., & Levendusky, P. *Agoraphobia treatment manual: A group psychotherapeutic approach*. Unpublished manuscript, 1980.

Berglas, S., & Levendusky, P. The Therapeutic Contract Program: An individual-oriented psychological treatment community. *Journal of Psychotherapy: Theory, Research, and Practice*, in press.

Berne, E. *Principles of group treatment*. New York: Oxford University Press, 1966.

Bibring, E. Psychoanalysis and the dynamic psychotherapies. *Journal of the American Psychoanalytic Association*, 1954, *2*, 745–770.

Bion, W. R. *Experiences in groups*. London: Tavistock Publications, 1961.

Chambless, D., & Goldstein, A. (Eds.). *Agoraphobia: Multiple perspectives on theory and treatment*. New York: Wiley, 1982.

Durkin, H. E. Current problems of group therapy in historical context. In L. Wolberg & M. Aronson (Eds.), *Group therapy: 1974*. New York: Grune & Stratton, 1974.

Emmelkamp, P. *In vivo* treatment of agoraphobia. In D. Chambless & A. Goldstein (Eds.), *Agoraphobia: Multiple perspectives on theory and treatment*. New York: Wiley, 1982.

Eysenck, H. The effects of psychotherapy. In H. Eysenck (Ed.), *Handbook of abnormal psychology*. New York: Basic Books, 1961.

Flowers, J. The effect of therapist support and encounter on the percentage of client–client interactions in group therapy. *Journal of Community Psychology*, 1978, *6*, 69–73.

Flowers, J. *Behavioral group therapy with heterogeneous clients*. Paper presented at the 16th Annual Convention of the Association for Advancement of Behavior Therapy. Los Angeles, 1982.

Flowers, J., Booraem, C., & Seacat, G. The effect of positive and negative feedback on members' sensitivity to other members in group therapy. *Psychotherapy: Theory, Research and Practice*, 1974, *11*, 346–350.

Foulkes, S. H. Principle and practice of group therapy. *Bulletin Menninger Clinic*, 1946, *70*, 85–89.

Foulkes, S. H. *Group analytic psychotherapy*. New York: International Universities Press, 1964.

Foulkes, S. H., & Anthony, E. J. *Group psychotherapy: The psychoanalytic approach*. Baltimore: Penguin Books, 1957.

Freud, S. *Group psychology and analysis of the ego*. London: Hogarth, 1940.

Goldfried, M. On the history of therapeutic integration. *Behavior Therapy*, 1982, *13*, 572–593.

Goldfried, M., Decenteceo, E., & Weinberg, L. Systematic rational restructuring as a self-control technique. *Behavior Therapy*, 1974, *5*, 247–254.

Goldstein, A. *Therapist–patient expectancies in psychotherapy*. New York: Pergamon, 1962.

Goldstein, A., & Chambless, D. A reanalysis of agoraphobia. *Behavior Therapy*, 1978, *9*, 47–59.

Hand, I., Lamontagne, Y., & Marks, I. Group exposure (flooding) *in vivo* for agoraphobics. *British Journal of Psychiatry*, 1974, *124*, 588–602.

Hollon, S., & Shaw, B. Group cognitive therapy for depressed patients. In A. Beck, J. Rush, B. Shaw, & G. Emery (Eds.), *Cognitive therapy of depression*. New York: Guilford Press, 1979.

Kendall, P. Integration: Behavior therapy and other schools of thought. *Behavior Therapy*, 1982, *13*, 559–571.

Levendusky, P., Berglas, S., Dooley, C., & Landau, R. Therapeutic Contract Program: Preliminary report on a behavioral alternative to the token economy. *Behaviour Research and Therapy*, 1983, *21*, 137–42.

Lewinsohn, P., Steinmetz, J., Antonuccio, D., & Teri, L. A behavioral group therapy approach to the treatment of depression. In D. Upper & S. Ross (Eds.), *Handbook of behavioral group therapy*. New York: Plenum Press, 1985.

Liberman, R. A behavioral approach to group dynamics. *Behavior Therapy*, 1970, *1*, 141–175.

Lieberman, M., Yalom, I., & Miles, M. *Encounter groups: First facts*. New York: Basic Books, 1973.

Lott, A., & Lott, B. Group cohesiveness, communication level, and conformity. *Journal of Abnormal and Social Psychology*, 1961,. *62*, 408–412.

McGovern, K. Modifying sexual dysfunction: An analysis of behavioral group treatment programs. In D. Upper & S. Ross (Eds.), *Handbook of behavioral group therapy*. New York: Plenum Press, 1985.

Marks, I. The reduction of fear: Towards a unifying theory. *Canadian Psychiatric Association Journal*, 1973, *18*, 9–12.

Marks, I. Behavioral treatment of phobic and obsessive-compulsive disorders. In R. Eisler & P. Miller (Eds.), *Progress in behavior modification*. New York: Academic Press, 1975.

Marks, I. Phobias and obsessions: Clinical phenomena in search of a laboratory model. In J. Maser & M. Seligman (Eds.), *Psychopathology: Experimental models*. San Francisco: Freeman, 1977.

Marks, I. Cure and care of neurosis. *Psychological Medicine*, 1979, *9*, 629–660.

Meichenbaum, D. *Cognitive-behavior modification: An integrative approach*. New York: Plenum Press, 1977.

Mischel, W. *Personality and assessment*. New York: Wiley, 1968.

Moreno, J. Interpersonal therapy and the psychopathology of interpersonal relations. *Sociometry*, 1937, *1*, Nos. 1–2.

Moreno, J. (Ed.). *The international handbook of group psychotherapy*. New York: Philosophical Library, 1966.

Rice, C., & Rutan, J. S. Boundary maintenance in inpatient therapy groups. *International Journal of Group Psychotherpay*, 1981, *31*, 297–309.

Rose, S. *Group therapy: A behavioral approach*. Englewood Cliffs, N.J.: Prentice-Hall, 1977.

Rush, A., & Watkins, J. Group vs. individual cognitive therapy: A pilot study. *Cognitive Research and Therapy*, 1981, *5*, 95–103.

Schilder, P. Introductory remarks on groups. *Social Psychology*, 1936, *12*, 85–100.

Schilder, P. *Psychotherapy*. New York: Norton, 1938.

Semrad, E., & Arseman, J. The use of group process group dynamics. *American Journal of Psychiatry*, 1951, *108*, 358–363.

Slavson, S. Group therapy. *Mental Hygiene*, 1940, *28*, 414–422.

Slavson, S. (Ed.). *The practice of group therapy*. New York: International Universities Press, 1947.

Slavson, S. Common sources of error and confusion in group psychotherapy. *International Journal of Group Psychotherapy*, 1953, *3*, 3–28.

Stuart, R., & Davis, B. *Slim chance in a fat world: Behavioral control of obesity*. Champaign, Ill.: Research Press, 1972.

Sullivan, H. *The interpersonal theory of psychiatry*. New York: Norton, 1953.

Upper, D., & Ross, S. *Behavioral group therapy, 1979*. Champaign, Ill.: Research Press, 1979.

Wachtel, P. *Psychoanalysis and behavior therapy*. New York: Basic Books, 1977.

Wender, L. Dynamics of group psychotherapy and its applications. *Journal of Nervous and Mental Disorder*, 1936, *84*, 54–60.

Whitaker, D. S., & Lieberman, M. A. *Psychotherapy through the group process.* New York: Atherton, 1964.

White, W., & Boskind-White, M. An experiential-behavioral approach to the treatment of bulimarexia. *Psychotherapy: Theory, Research, and Practice,* 1981, *18,* 501–507.

Yalom, I. *The theory and practice of group psychotherapy* (2d ed.). New York: Basic Books, 1975.

Yalom, I. *Inpatient group psychotherapy.* New York: Basic Books, 1983.

Zifferblatt, S., & Hendricks, G. Applied behavioral analysis of societal problems. *American Psychologist,* 1974, *29,* 750–761.

6

Behavioral Group Therapy with Heterogeneous Clients

JOHN V. FLOWERS AND BERNARD SCHWARTZ

Previous reviews of the status of behavioral group therapy (Flowers, 1979a; Upper & Ross, 1977) concentrated in part on the distinction between behavior therapy done *in* a group, such as massed desensitization (Paul, 1966) or massed assertion training (Booraem & Flowers, 1977) and behavior therapy done *by* a group, in which the group interaction is a crucial part of the therapeutic process (Flowers, 1979a). Subsequent work in the field of behavioral group therapy (Upper & Ross, 1979, 1980, 1981) has clearly demonstrated that there are in fact four types of behavioral group therapy in present use. These groups can be differentiated by two variables: (a) the variety of behavioral techniques employed (singular vs. multiple); and (b) the degree to which the members share similar problems (homogeneity vs. heterogeneity). Although heterogeneity in this context has been primarily defined in terms of the presenting problem, the term *heterogeneity* in this chapter also means variance in terms of such associated variables as sex, socioeconomic status, previous experience in therapy, and the like.

The earliest entry of behavior therapy into the group therapy field was with homogeneous clients treated with a singular technique in groups such as those described by Paul (1966) and by Meichenbaum, Gilmore, and Fedoravicus (1971) who employed desensitization with phobics in groups or by Booraem and Flowers (1972) who employed assertion training with socially unskilled inpatients.

The second category of behavioral group therapy contains members with a set of relatively homogeneous problems who are treated with an assortment of behavioral techniques. These groups to date have focused on problems such as sexual difficulties (Lobitz & Baker, 1979; McGovern, 1979), obesity (Coche, Levitz, & Jordan, 1979; Heckerman & Zitter, 1981; Knauss & Jeffrey, 1981), depression both in the elderly (Gallagher, 1981) and in college students (Hodgson, 1981),

JOHN V. FLOWERS • Chapman College, Orange, California 92666. BERNARD SCHWARTZ • Santa Ana College, Santa Ana, California 92706.

male abusiveness toward women (Watts & Courtois, 1981), mentally disordered sex offenders (Wieand, Flowers, & Hartman, 1981), marital problems (Blau, 1980), and delinquency (DeLange, Lanham, & Barton, 1981; Hazel, Schumaker, Sherman, & Sheldon-Wildgen, 1981). These problems have been described and evaluated.

A third approach entails forming groups of a more heterogeneous nature that emphasize a particular behavioral technique. In addition to social skills training (Curran & Monti, 1982), groups with more heterogeneous clients have emphasized cognitive change (Lange, 1979; Shapiro, Shaffer, Sank, & Coghlan, 1981), problem solving (Edelstein, Couture, Cray, Dickens, & Lusebrink, 1980), and self-reinforcement (Cohn, Mann, Flowers, & Booraem, 1980). In each case the group members were experiencing a wide range of psychological problems including anxiety, depression, interpersonal difficulties, and the like.

The fourth type of behavioral group therapy employs a varied set of behavioral techniques for clients with heterogeneous problems and heterogeneous backgrounds (Flowers, 1979a; Goldstein & Wolpe, 1971; Lazarus, 1976; Sarri, 1974; Walker, Hedberg, Clement, & Wright, 1981). Although such a group is both more difficult to conceptualize behaviorally and assess, in the nonbehavioral realm it is the most common form of outpatient group therapy presently being practiced.

This chapter presents a behavioral theory and methodology for this latter form of group treatment, which in spite of its popularity, has no uniform model as a basis from which to operate. The proposed model follows the basic format of any behavioral therapy: test, operate, test, exit (TOTE) (Miller, Galanter, & Pribram, 1960). As Flowers (1979a) has pointed out, in behavioral group therapy this translates into processes of (a) disclosure; (b) assessment; (c) narrowing (focusing); (d) intervention; and (e) feedback.

Given the original disclosure, the assessment is the first "test"; the narrowing and the intervention are the "operation"; and the feedback is the second "test" of the TOTE model. If the original problem is sufficiently remediated by this process, the problem is considered resolved, and if the client has no further need of problem resolution, he or she exits from the group. In practice, this process is neither absolutely linear nor is it perfectly sequential.

Disclosure

There are four types of disclosure that occur in group therapy.

Voluntary Disclosure

In voluntary disclosure in therapy groups, the client voluntarily tells of a problem that he or she is having. Flowers (1979a) has found that this voluntary form of disclosure is influenced by a number of factors. First, there is more of this type of disclosure if the client perceives that the group is cohesive; hence this type of disclosure increases as a group becomes more cohesive and, in fact, can be used as a measure of cohesion. Secondly, if the norm of the group is to disclose, more clients will do so. Starting a group with an explication of this norm increases subsequent disclosure. Clients also disclose more if they are given homework assignments to write down and specify in depth the disclosures they might make in the session. This effect is further increased if the client is instructed to bring two written disclosures to group with the alternative of disclosing either, both, or neither, depending on the client's feelings that session. Each voluntary disclosure can also be clearly acknowledged and verbally reinforced by the therapists. This also increases the rate of subsequent disclosure. Thus, disclosure does not have to be left to chance but can be influenced behaviorally.

Indirect Disclosure

A second type of disclosure involves a change in the nonverbal behavior of a group member while another member's problem is being explored. Thus, a member who appears bored, restless, or preoccupied may be indicating that he or she has a difficulty that is being cued by the present discussion. One key to recognizing this type of disclosure is sensitivity by the group therapists to the nonverbal cues that abound in a group session.

As Flowers and Booraem (1975) point out, the specific nonverbal cues that are most often associated with emotional change are (1) eye contact with the speaker; (2) posture; (3) body movement; (4) arm and hand movement; (5) head movement; (6) facial expression; (7) vocal volume; (8) vocal tone and affect; (9) vocal speed; and (10) vocal latency.

Each group member has his or her own baseline of these behaviors that are common to his or her group participation. The key to understanding when these behaviors may be an indication of an emotional reaction is to notice when they change markedly from the client's own norm. At such times, at the appropriate opportunity, the client should be asked if the prior discussion has produced awareness of material that he or she would like to share with the group. Our present research indicates that disclosures of this type are as common as voluntary disclosures when therapists know when to ask for them, and are rated as more intense by both the discloser and the other group members.

Demonstrated Disclosure

In demonstrated disclosure the client demonstrates a problem by virtue of his or her inappropriate interaction with other members of the group. Common problems demonstrated are in the communication area, including (1) lack of clarity; (2) communications that are too long; (3) lack of appropriate affect; (4) excess of affect; (5) self-deprecation; (6) too little communication; (7) inappropriate nonverbals; and (8) communication difficulty with same or opposite sex member.

Again, in order to note such demonstrated difficulties, the group therapists must continually monitor the ongoing verbal and nonverbal processes. It is important that the therapists not comment on every communication or other difficulty observed, but that they select for discussion only those issues that seem connected to problem areas in the client's life. For example, if a client puts himself or herself down in front of the group and the client's problem is already known or strongly suspected to be one of low self-esteem, this demonstration would probably be chosen for discussion. This type of demonstrated disclosure can be one of the most important in group therapy because it not only demonstrates *what* is wrong, but, additionally, *how* the client behaves in a maladaptive fashion as well.

Previous Disclosure

The fourth type of disclosure material is prior information possessed by the therapist either because of individual therapy sessions or referral information. Because of client confidentiality, this is the most difficult source with which to deal if the client does not voluntarily share or demonstrate the problem. Although group therapists cannot share this information for the client or insist that it be shared, they can, prior to a member's first group session, establish the norm that important individual therapy material is always shared with the group.

General Issues

Disclosure is obviously an ongoing process. Clients disclose different facets of their problem and even different conceptualizations of their problem in session after session. The amount and intensity (Flowers, 1979a) of disclosure of all types is affected by, and affects, group cohesion. The disclosure process in behavioral group therapy differs from more traditional group therapy *only* to the extent that the behaviorist brings more specific tools to bear that can directly influence this process. In Flowers's research (1979a), the range and nature of problems disclosed in behavioral and nonbehavioral groups are very similar, but the behaviorally trained leader elicits nearly 1.75 times as many disclosures as nonbehavioral leaders with the same clientele.

Assessment

The assessment process differentiates the behavioral group from the nonbehavioral group even more definitively than does the disclosure process. Assessment usually begins right after a problem disclosure and continues intermittently throughout the problem's life in the group. Other group members and the therapists ask questions in a struggle to understand the discloser and the problem. Such assessment begins slowly and awkwardly in newly formed groups because the members do not have a model of what form of assessment elicits the most useful information.

The following assessment model, developed from the work of many others (Barlow, 1981; Cone & Hawkins, 1977; Kanfer & Saslow, 1965; Lazarus, 1976; Mash & Terdal, 1976; Roberts & LaGreca, 1981) has been found relatively easy for behavioral group therapy trainees to understand and employ. According to Lazarus (1976), all problems can be thought of as potentially having the following components: (a) *b*ehavior; (b) *a*ffect; (c) *s*ensation; (d) *i*magination; and (e) *c*ognition.

As readers of Lazarus will be aware, this is a shortened version of his BASIC ID that leaves out specific mention of the variables of *I*, interpersonal relationships, and *D*, drugs. In terms of teaching this model to group therapy trainees, it is easier to subsume the I and D variables under BASIC rather than present an even more complex model than the one here given.

With the exception of demonstrated disclosures that always involve behavior, the client's initial disclosure may involve one or more of these aspects; however, initial disclosures usually involve only the aspect of the problem that is troubling the client most. Thus a client might phrase a disclosure in terms of a behavior such as procrastination, an affect such as anxiety, a sensation such as numbness, an imagination such as a picture of a person in the closet ready to stab him or her or a cognition such as self-punishing ideas. The group's task is to fill out the assessment until all aspects of the problem are understood.

Behavior

In the process of assessing the *behavior* component one attempts to discover specifically what the client is doing or not doing that may be related to the disclosed problem. Even when the disclosure is itself a behavior such as procrastination, more specific information about the problem needs to be ascertained.

When the client discloses a problem emphasizing other aspects of BASIC, for example, when a client complains of depression, the group will ask what the client is doing when he or she gets depressed and what previously reinforcing behaviors have been given up. Is the client complaining to others, is there a change in exercise behavior, in sleeping or eating patterns, and so forth? When crucial behaviors are identified, the group often attempts to get as exact a measure of frequency or duration as possible to complete and even verify this aspect of the picture.

Affect

The assessment of *affect* involves ascertaining the client's various emotions and emotional changes when experiencing the problem. This is the most common category of initial disclosure in that many clients conceptualize their problems in terms of how bad they feel. Unlike behavior that tends to be assessed as a frequency function, the assessment of affect usually involves intensity, an assessment that can be aided by adapting a Wolpe-type subjective intensity scale (1969). Thus clients rate the intensity of emotions involved in the problem, for example, anxiety, discomfort, anger, excitement, and the like on a subjective 10-point scale. A record of behavior frequency or emotional intensity each gives a baseline from which to plan treatment and a measure against which to check progress.

Sensation

The assessment of *sensation* involves determining whether there are any sensation changes that accompany the problem. In some cases such as hunger, bodily pain, or dizziness, the sensation is reported quite clearly as the problem and does not require that the client concentrate to become aware of sensation changes that may have previously been unacknowledged. On the other hand, in this assessment model, depression is considered as a problem of too little sensation rather than as a problem of affect. This separates depression from its common consequent emotions such as anxiety and sadness and also helps the therapists to separate the treatment of the depression response from the treatment of the associated problems caused by the depression.

Imagination

The assessment of *imagination* involves consideration of whether there are any images (mental pictures) that accompany and might be implicated in the problem. For example, in a sexual-lack-of-desire problem, the client may be fantasizing someone other than his or her partner at all times when aroused. Although behaviorists are well versed in the use of imagination in treatment, whether it is for desensitization (Paul, 1966) or covert sensitization (Cautella, 1967), this area of problem assessment is often inappropriately overlooked or minimized.

Cognition

The assessment of *cognition* involves analyzing whether there are maladaptive thoughts that cause or maintain the problem. A common example is a shy and lonely person who, immediately before any social contact thinks, "I am going to make a fool of myself." This is a difficult area of behavioral assessment because of the frequency and variability of thoughts. Assessment of attitudes or generalized thought patterns does not answer the cognitive response question. Attitudes, expectations, values, and other generalized cognitions are actually antecedent stimuli that are brought by the client to the problem situation. In the present method of assessment, *cognitions* are defined as actual thoughts the client has when experiencing the problem. Because of this distinction of cognitions and attitudes, the assessment of cognitions almost invariably involves training the clients to sample and record their thoughts at crucial times.

Other Issues

The assessment process begins in the group and explores the *what's*, *when's*, *where's*, *who's*, *how's*, and *how often's* of the particular problem. If necessary, homework assignments are made to help with the assessment. For instance, a client with a troubled marriage might be asked to record the frequency and approximate duration of all communications with his or her mate, briefly record the content of each, and rate each for satisfaction. Each part of this homework assignment would correspond to an aspect of the problem wherein the therapists or group members felt they needed more information to get an accurate picture of the problem. At first, this system seems unwieldy and overwhelming to the group therapy leader-trainee, but it is quickly learned and employed.

Antecedents

After getting a sense of the problem response according to the BASIC analysis, the assessment is broadened into a standard antecedent–response–consequence chain.

A *potential antecedent* is that event that is found to frequently precede the troublesome response and therefore might cue it.

Two different types of antecedents are usually assessed: *internal antecedents* (AI) and *external antecedents* (AE). Common immediate internal antecedents involve temporary change in the person due to drugs, fatigue, recent prior experiences, and so forth as well as any aspect of BASIC that regularly occurs prior to the problem. A less immediate internal antecedent is a relatively permanent deviation of the person from an adaptive norm due to either learning history, genetic, or traumatic biological factors. In group therapy, attitudes are probably the most common of this class of antecedents. In assessing these long-term antecedent conditions, one must note that attitudes, though usually conceived of as cognitions, are really long-term internal antecedents (Johnson, 1980). Attitudes and general thoughts are seldom the cognitions that occur during the actual problem situation. This behavioral assessment separation of cognition and attitudes is crucial because the interventions for attitude change and cognitive change differ.

The assessment of external antecedents involves uncovering any commonality of environment that seems to cue the problem. The most common of these are time, place, or person. External antecedent assessment is usually easier than internal because the data are public and because the regularities usually show up quite clearly when the right questions are asked.

Consequences

The final part of this assessment strategy involves answering the questions of what happens after the response. As with antecedents, the group therapists should divide consequences into four categories: *short-term internal consequences* (SCI), *short-term external consequences* (SCE), *long-term internal consequences* (LCI), and *long-term external consequences* (LCE). Short-term consequences refer to what happens soon after a change in response, for example, How do significant others react (SCE) when the client displays anger, depression, and the like? How does the client feel (SCI) after eating, gambling, and so forth. As opposed to antecedents, which address the issue of cause, this assessment addresses the issue of how problems might be maintained.

Assessment of long-term consequences, like the assessment of historical internal antecedents, is less direct and less certain. The primary purpose of this assessment is to determine if the conflict the client feels is due to the relatively common condition of a difference in the reinforcement level between the short- and long-term consequences of the problem response. The short-term reinforcement of a party (SCE) can easily interfere with the long-term goal of getting into graduate school (LCE) just as the short-term aversion of exercise (SCI) can inhibit the long-term gains of stress relief and self-esteem that can come from being in shape (LCE) and can affect the client's general sense of self-esteem (LCI).

The Total Model

On any disclosure of a problem, the form that the group therapists should be able to fill in over time looks like:

AE ______	B ______	SCE ______
	A ______	SCI ______
	S ______	
	I ______	LCE ______
AI ______	C ______	LCI ______

As specified, this is a "bad times" assessment, that is, an assessment of the client when he or she is experiencing the problem. The group therapists also try to get a "good times" assessment, that is, an assessment of BASIC, antecedents and consequences, when the client is coping well. In order to have the assessment provide the data for adequate intervention, it is important that the client's strengths as well as weaknesses are assessed.

The assessment in behavioral group therapy is not as systematic as presented here, nor does it occur in a lock-step fashion. Assessment proceeds session after session, providing an ever more complete picture of the client as a functioning person in the environment and providing an ever clearer picture of what is happening when the client is functioning poorly. Because the questions are asked by all the group members as well as by the therapists, the process is both less systematic but potentially more complete than the same type of assessment done in individual therapy. As behavioral group therapy proceeds, the clients come to learn and employ the therapists' model. In order to shape the group's assessment methods, the behavioral group therapist will praise good questions and ignore or lightly confront poor ones. However, even after this shaping has occurred, the group members usually ask more varied questions than the group therapists would. Although this can be technically inefficient, it can also provide a more complete picture of the client and his or her problems, and even when the assessment runs into a "dead end" the assessment failure gives clues to the next step.

Induction Reduction

Often during the assessment phase, another process begins that can either help or impede subsequent intervention. Recent research (Flowers & Tapper, 1982; Flowers, Tapper, & Schwartz, 1983) has shown that as the client is remembering the problem situations, he or she often gets upset. This process is called *emotional induction.* Such induction is partly under the control of group variables and tends to go to higher levels if

1. one of the leaders is charismatic (has scored higher on the Affective Communication Test; Friedman, Prince, Riggio, & DiMatteo, 1980);
2. the group is more cohesive (especially as measured by eye contact with the speaker); and
3. the questions asked are more specific about consequences and subsequent affect responses.

The research has also clearly demonstrated that a client's resolution of a problem is significantly better the greater the difference between the induction during the assessment process and the subsequent emotional reduction prior to attempts at intervention. *Emotional reduction* occurs when the group shifts the focus from what is wrong to the client's strengths, alternatives, and to the narrowing of the problem to manageable size. Emotional reduction is also aided by touch, testimonial, and pure encouragement. In open-ended questionaires we regularly administer after therapy groups, the clients' own conception of this process is that the induction gives them the motivation to attempt change, whereas the reduction gives them the clarity to accomplish it.

Narrowing the Problem (Focusing)

Although this process could be included within the assessment section, we teach this as a separate process to insure that the behavioral group therapists attend to it clearly. Because the assessment process elicits more information than can be used in any single intervention, the therapists and group members must engage the client in a decision (D'Zurilla & Goldfried, 1971) to act on one of the 11 elements in the preceding chart (AE, AI, B, A, S, I, C, SCI, SCE, LCI, LCE). To determine which factor to address first, each must be assessed for its significance and for the ease with which it can be modified. For example, for one depressed client the narrowing might indicate that the best first intervention is to try to change his or her low level of behavior when depressed, that is, get out and do almost anything when feeling down, whereas another depressed client might narrow to attempting to change his or her attitude that anything not perfect is terrible.

This focusing often requires that the client try something in the world (intervention) and then return to the group and report the results for further focusing or refocusing. In the first example given, the client would report how his or her thoughts interfered with any action when feeling down. Following this, cognition rather than behavior might be focused on.

Another important part of this focusing process is to determine what approaches the client has already tried. It is very easy to be misled at this point. Clients often state that they have already tried to relax, to be assertive, limit their food cues, and so forth, but after inspecting the exact means by which they tried to change, the reasons for prior failures become evident.

The problem as presented is often overwhelming to the client, and it is the consequent hopelessness that is the client's worst enemy of change. The focusing process narrows the task and inspects resources for, and barriers to, change. Of course, the client wants the whole problem cured at once, but the group therapists and later the group members resist this agenda and try at first to select something that can be accomplished somewhat quickly, easily, and with maximum impact.

In a very real sense, this phase of treatment is the first intervention. Group pressure is being brought to bear to change the client's attitude about how to deal with his or her problems. Because this process is crucial, difficult, and often overlooked, it is separated in training from either assessment or intervention and made a separate entity in the conceptualization of behavioral group therapy.

Obviously in a therapy group the assessment does not end at one moment after which the narrowing or intervention immediately begins. Assessment, narrowing, and intervention in a client's problem can alternate over the course of a session. In addition, frequently one group member is still trying to assess while another is trying to focus, and still a third is trying to intervene. Although this process is less structured than individual therapy, it is potentially more powerful and complete.

Intervention

In the TOTE (test, operate, test, exit) model, intervention is the *O*. It follows and may precede assessment. Occasionally, intervention occurs because a client wants solely to disclose the problem without pursuing the matter further. Telling others is enough, and the client is satisfied, usually because of a consequent emotional relief. When such seems to be the case, the therapists should respect the client's wishes and try to insure that other group members do the same. If it subsequently becomes clear that this mere disclosure did not provide the necessary relief, the therapists and group can return to the problem for a fuller analysis.

Even more frequently, the assessment phase serves as an intervention. Sometimes the client reconceptualizes the problem during assessment and redefines it as either a nonproblem or places it lower on their hierarchy of concerns. In other cases, especially when homework recording assignments are given, the client finds that the problem is infrequent and sometimes even nonexistent. Problems that go away when they are assessed must be viewed with caution in that the solution of the problem can merely be a function of recording; thus the problem reoccurs as soon as the recording ceases.

Still more frequently, the focusing process provides intervention. Here, what usually happens is that the problem-solving aspect of the focusing procedure (D'Zurilla & Goldfried, 1971) gives the client a clear idea of how to intervene on his or her own without the group's having to help. The problem does not go away; it is intervened with effectively by the client before the group has a chance to provide any more assistance.

Each of these forms of change occur in individual as well as in group therapy; however, these forms of serendipitous intervention seem more common in group therapy. Disclosure as intervention in group therapy is a sharing of previously hidden material not just to a "purchased friend" (Scofield, 1964) but to peers as well. The other group members' lack of rejection is probably more important than the therapists' in this type of problem relief. Intervention through assessment is probably more common in group therapy than in individual because the reconceptualization of the problem that a client experiences is based on questions from the entire group and is, therefore, subject to the group's ability to change attitudes (Lieberman, Lakin, & Whitaker, 1968). The changes that occur because of the focusing are more powerful in a group because of the group's ability to change attitudes; in this case the attitude that a problem should be cut down to a manageable size before solution is attempted. When focusing resolves a client's problem without further intervention, what has usually happened is that the solution becomes obvious to the client without further group help.

The Range of Intervention

In behavioral groups where problems are disclosed ad lib, the range of necessary interventions is considerably greater than in groups where the clients are homogeneous with relation to the problems disclosed. The following list (Table 1) separates standard behavioral interventions into those most commonly and specifically used in behavioral group therapy, those used less often or informally, and those behavioral interventions seldom employed in behavioral group therapy as represented here.

As the following section will show, the list of these techniques is not meant to be either totally exclusive or exhaustive. For example, elements of role play and behavioral contracts are part of attitude change, and elements of desensitization are involved in behavioral rehearsal. The labels are really a utilitarian device for specifying common sequences of behavioral principles that are commonly employed with clients for certain ends.

The following section is devoted to the use of these techniques in behavioral group therapy. For more complete instruction in any specific technique, the

TABLE 1. Behavioral Techniques Employed in Group Therapy

Often employed	Sometimes employed	Seldom employed
Attitude change techniques	Modeling	Covert reinforcement
Homework assignments	Simulation games	Extinction
Instruction	Intermittent reinforcement	Flooding
Information giving	Relaxation techniques	Guided imagery
Differential feedback	Systematic desensitization	Paradoxical intention
Role playing	Self-instruction	Hypnosis
Behavioral rehearsal	Aversive conditioning	Programmed reading
Self-reinforcement	Cognitive restructuring	Satiation
Operant reinforcement	Token economy	Self-punishment
Problem-solving skill training	Reciprocal exchange contract	Thought stopping
Stimulus control techniques		Time-out
Shaping techniques		Covert sensitization
Incompatible response reinforcement		
Self-monitoring		
Behavioral contracts		
Self-control techniques		

reader may wish to peruse one of the many behavior modification texts available.

SPECIFIC INTERVENTIONS

Attitude Change

It may seem strange to some behavioral therapists to see *attitude change* differentiated from cognitive change, but such a distinction is crucial for behavioral group therapy. Obviously an attitude *is* cognition in the technical sense of the word. However, in terms of therapy technique, a useful and even essential distinction needs to be made. *Attitude* is here defined as a cognition with an accompanying value that defines the cognition as essentially true and unchangeable. A *cognition* here is defined as what the client actually thinks in the problem situation. Thus, a client about to go to a party to meet new people might actually think, "I am scared and will make a fool of myself." This is a cognition that actually occurs in the problem situation but is not necessarily an attitude (Johnson, 1980). In therapy, the attitude expressed might be, "I am not a worthwhile person." The crucial difference is that mere cognitions can be modified by therapeutic instruction, thought substitution, and distraction, whereas attitudes require considerably more therapeutic power (Johnson, 1980) and care to modify.

Attitude change is a common process in every form of group therapy. Technically, an attitude is an internal antecedent that is brought to the problem situation. An attitude has both cognitive and emotional components and is resistant to mere persuasional change techniques because it is not neutral; it is valued even when it is maladaptive (Johnson, 1980). An attitude can effect any or all of the elements of BASIC but most often effects B, A or C. An attitude can specify, "I should do *x*, I expect *y* and will be upset if I don't get it," or "I should be able to do *z* and am no good if I can't."

Once a maladaptive attitude's effects are assessed, the group intervention involves attempting to change this attitude to a more adaptive one. The most commonly employed method in almost all forms of group therapy is simple persuasion, which is usually accomplished by confronting the maladaptive attitude and supplying another presumably more adaptive one. Although such a process occurs in behavioral group therapy as well, and is sometimes effective, the behavior therapist has other more effective tools to bring to bear on this difficult and common problem.

In addition to employing the reinforcement and punishment power of the group more systematically than might occur in most traditional therapy groups, the behavioral group therapist leader reinforces the other group members for the use of direct persuasion in hierarchical fashion, that is, attempting to challenge and change weaker attitudes or parts of attitudes before attempting to change complex or strongly held attitudes. Thus, if a client was afraid of expressing her anger for fear of "destroying" someone perceived as weak, the group members would be reinforced for gradually encouraging the client to perceive the other as stronger and gradually supporting ever-increasing expressions of feeling. Group members would be confronted for attempting to persuade that client that the other person's problem of "falling apart" was not the client's concern and that the client should only think of honestly expressing herself regardless of the consequences. As in any change process, success at a easier level helps set the stage for success at a more difficult level.

The behavioral group leader can also bring the dissonance (Festinger, 1962) model to bear in a systematic manner and engage the client in role playing or behavioral contracts that weaken the attitude because the client is forced to behave in ways that are subtly different than what he or she believes. The client's attitude is also weakened if he or she is engaged in attempting to persuade another client to change a similar attitude. Research (Flowers & Booraem, 1980b) indicates that attitude change is more likely if the clients are encouraged to behave in more varied ways (more flexibly) from group session to group session. Thus, a client who shifts from listening to questioning, from challenger to supporter, from discloser to helper over a period of weeks is more amenable to attitude change than the client who adopts a more fixed pattern of group behavior.

Although attitude change has not been thought of as primarily a behavioral technique and is certainly not solely the province of behavior therapy, behavioral group therapy leaders can bring the entire spectrum of behavioral techniques to bear on this issue with powerful results.

Instruction

The purpose of *instruction* (Flowers, 1979b; Lazarus, 1966) is to show and/or tell the client how to do something that he or she needs to know how to accomplish. This technique is often included as a part of other techniques such as when instruction in nonverbal presentation of strength is coupled with behavioral rehearsal in assertion training.

In behavioral group therapy, instruction in how to communicate effectively is extremely common. Instruction tends to be more effective if what is instructed can then be practiced right in the group for immediate feedback and shaping. Most of the time, instruction as an intervention involves emotional reduction and is often employed, in part, to calm an emotionally induced client prior to any other intervention. There is, however, one notable exception when instruction is deliberately used to increase emotional induction.

Being in touch with one's emotions is a commonly heard mental health phrase that is vague yet persistent in the group therapy field. The vagueness occurs in part because the presumed problem is ill defined. When a client is not perceived as being emotional, it is first necessary to determine if this is, in fact, a problem rather than presuming on psychometaphysical grounds that emotional induction and expression is good *per se*. If this lack of perceived emotionality is in fact an integral part of the client's problem, it is next necessary to determine if the problem is primarily in the B or the A domain of BASIC. Some clients do not express emotions that they feel, whereas others do not feel emotions appropriate to the situation. Instruction is a common intervention in either case, but the instructions differ considerably, depending on the problem assessed. Instruction for emotional expression involves another technique—role playing—with an emphasis on the nonverbal elements of the communication. Instruction for emotional induction involves focusing the client's attention on any body changes, followed by having the client exaggerate the desired response. It is precisely this type of specificity that can be brought to bear by employing behavioral assessment and a variety of behavioral techniques in group therapy.

Information Giving

Information giving is a common occurrence in behavioral group therapy. It is clear that the impact of this technique depends on the quality and quantity of information possessed by the members of the group. Information is given for two primary purposes. The first is simply because the information is something that the client needs to know to cope with his or her problem. Such information can vary from where to apply for a type of financial aid to how the body works during sex. Group members and therapists possess a variety of experience and knowledge available for informational purposes. A second reason to share information is to relieve anxiety. Knowing that a panic attack is not a heart attack or that impotency after ingesting alcohol is common can help the emotional reduction process so necessary for subsequent intervention. Before sharing or encouraging sharing, a group therapist should always be able to answer the question: "What is my purpose in sharing this information?" in terms of what it does for the client. Information for information's sake is to be avoided.

Differential Feedback

Differential feedback, which is a term that includes both differential reinforcement and differential punishment when given from one group member to another, is a crucial intervention that is common in all group therapy. It can be defined as giving a positive response to adaptive behavior and a negative response to maladaptive behavior. Although it is easy to state that a group member's positive behavior should be supported and negative or self-defeating behavior should be confronted, getting this to occur requires considerable work. First, the therapists must clearly define for themselves the actions to be reinforced or punished. Both by modeling and by their reinforcement of others, the group members will soon participate in the same differential feedback system. Second, the therapists have to be sure that what is intended as praise or censure actually is received by the client as such. Although this process is usually highly informal, there is a process (Flowers, 1979a) wherein every intended positive feedback is accompanied by a blue token and every intended negative feedback is accompanied by a red token handed to the member for whom the feedback is intended. This procedure allows a clear statement of intent and allows quantification of the amount of member-to-member positive and negative feedback. Even if this procedure is not employed, the behavioral group therapist should be aware that this technique is one of the most powerful of group therapy and should always be able to specify what differential feedback he or she is attempting to elicit from the group and the purpose of such feedback for the individual client.

Role Playing

Role playing in group therapy (Booraem & Flowers, 1980) is usually employed for the purpose of improvement of communication skills and anxiety reduction. Occasionally, as specified before, it is for the purpose of emotional induction when the problem is one of lack of appropriate affect. Most role playing in behavioral groups involves becoming socially skillful in one of seven situations: (a) making a difficult request; (b) making a difficult refusal; (c) expressing a criticism; (d) receiving a criticism; (e) expressing a compliment; (f) receiving a compliment; and (g) negotiating a compromise.

Such changes in communication ability often involve anxiety reduction and attitude change as well as skill development. Thus, such role playing is often done in a hierarchy of perceived threat and in small steps of value change. The skills taught involve both verbal and nonverbal elements of communication. After performing the new behaviors, the group gives the client multiple sources of feedback that is compelling both in the reinforcement provided and in the fact that the client learns that other people respond in varied manners to that which he or she thought all people viewed similarly.

Other Aspects of Behavioral Rehearsal

Role playing is obviously a subset of the broader category of *behavioral rehearsal* (Flowers & Booraem, 1980a), and the role-playing distinction is simply made to separate the commonly occurring social communication categories mentioned previously from less common rehearsals that can also be helpful for a client. The rehearsals practiced in group include practicing deep breathing before responding in an anxiety-producing situation; talking more to threatening group members (such as members of the opposite sex); shortening or lengthening what he or she says; appearing deliberately silly or serious; and practicing self-reinforcement or self-instruction. It is clear that not everything can be rehearsed in group, but the behavior therapist should always be aware of ways in which the desired response or part of it can be practiced there. A member can, in fact, take a test during a group session in which he or she is being alternately ignored, intimidated, or praised. A member can perform a song for the group before he or she tries it at an audition. A client can have the group give her a mock job interview before she tries the real thing. The only limits of this technique involve the creativity of the therapists and the time available for such rehearsal.

Self-Reinforcement Techniques

Although all group therapy deals in the general area of self-esteem, few groups actually systematically employ *self-reinforcement* (Goldiamond, 1976; Kanfer & Marston, 1963) as a technique. Informally, a client is often challenged for being self-critical, but this is usually the extent of the assessment or intervention employed. Self-reinforcement and self-punishment are clearly *C* aspects of BASIC. Both in and out of group these covert operants can have an enormous impact on the client's life. The behavioral group therapist assesses self-reinforcement and self-punishment both in a client's problem situation and in the group sessions as well. At minimum, this involves specific questions aimed at eliciting, not the client's general attitude about self, but what thoughts are actually occurring in specific situations. A technique to make this ongoing process more public has been developed (Cohn *et al.*, 1980) and involves the clients' self-administering a blue token for a self-approval response and a red token for a self-disapproval response during the group session. This information about member self-reinforcement and self-punishment then becomes a primary issue for change. The type of change the group attempts to elicit depends on the pattern seen. Clients who reinforce themselves infrequently are encouraged by differential feedback to do so more often. A client who is too hard on himself or herself is a candidate for attitude change involving the definition of what should be reinforced, and so forth.

Operant Reinforcement

Operant reinforcement is a subset of the differential feedback section mentioned previously. It is included here as a separate category to emphasize the fact that there should be more reinforcement than punishment in behavioral group therapy. Differential reinforcement could mean a 1:1 ratio of positive and negative feedback. Human beings in general and groups in particular do not thrive under such a ratio. We have found (Flowers, 1979) that groups are maximally cohesive when the ratio of positive to negative feedback is between 4:1 and 5:1. Clients indicate that when the group is too negative they do not feel safe and therefore limit their disclosures, whereas when the group is too positive they do not trust the feedback as being valid.

Problem-Solving Skills Training

As opposed to problem solving, which is a common part of the narrowing or focusing procedure described previously, *problem-solving skills training* involves not merely helping clients solve their problem but teaching them the skills of problem solving in a more general sense (Mahoney & Thoresen, 1974). The assessment here should have demonstrated that the client is not merely having trouble with the problem disclosed but is having a problem becuase he or she does not solve problems well in general. When this technique is employed, instead of trying to solve the client's most pressing problem, the group therapists deliberately begin by concentrating on simpler and less emotionally charged problems. With the group's help the client is taught to

1. clearly define the problem and separate it, at least conceptually, from other problems;
2. generate all possible alternatives without any evaluation of consequences;
3. evaluate the most possible (not the most catastrophic) consequences for each alternative;
4. specify what information is necessary and how and when that information is to be gained if such an evaluation is not presently possible;
5. choose the first alternative to be attempted and commit to no rechoosing unless new *external* information is gathered that makes another choice superior;
6. inspect the resources the client possesses that could be employed to help make the attempt a success; and
7. eliminate or reduce barriers to achieving success with the chosen alternative.

There are, it is clear, some crucial points in this process that involve attitude change as well as skills development. Most poor problem solvers are also poor problem definers and separators. In many cases, it is the vagueness and complexity of the problem's definition that causes the client to feel overwhelmed and prevents him or her from any action. The group not only insists on a clear definition, it also insists that all possible solutions be created irrespective of their merit or prior failure. The client is led to the attitude of choosing the *best* alternative, not choosing a *good* alternative. Second, the client is offered a choice from among many alternatives, not a choice or whether to do *A* or *B*. If the client, as so many poor problem solvers do, says he or she cannot evaluate the choices, the task is shifted to how to get the best evaluation possible in a reasonable time. The attitude that the client must know the future and be sure that this alternative will work is always challenged. An alternative, once chosen, requires full commitment, but this is not the last word. Should the client gain information while trying the alternative that would indicate the need for a change, such change is possible. However, the group always attempts to get the client to stick by the decision in the face of insecurities or worry. The problem has been thought over many times, and more thought will not generate a better solution. A solution can only be changed, and even then only to a specifically defined alternative, if information from the environment indicates such a change is indicated. Finally, the reader should note that although the consequences are inspected prior to the choice, the barriers are inspected only after the commitment has been made. This is done because the inspection of barriers too early in the sequence tends to abort the commitment. The client's resources are inspected along with potential barriers so that the negative aspect of barriers is mediated by the resources available.

Adequate problem solving involves the skills to generate solutions and the attitudes that allow these solutions to be put into action. One of the themes of this type of group work is that it is usually better to take action in some direction, as long as it is not totally impulsive, than be frozen. Another theme is that in most situations the client can recoup from a wrong choice and even learn to make a correct choice because of it but that there is no recouping or learning from inaction.

Stimulus Control Techniques

The employment of *stimulus control techniques* depends greatly on the adequacy of the behavioral assessment (Karoly, 1980). These techniques are usually used in a behavioral group when the antecedents of the problem situation are clear and can be controlled. Thus, if most fights are elicited in conversations that occur within 30 minutes of getting home from work, a number of possible interventions could be suggested and tried in order to change this stimulus complex. Stimulus control can also be used to strengthen a desired response as well as to weaken an undesired one as in the example given previously. A poor student can be advised to set aside a certain place in the home to be used solely for studying in order to reduce the distraction cues and create a set of cues for productive study. Such techniques are often used in conjunction with other techniques. The limits of these techniques are determined by the assessment and the creativity of the behavioral group.

Shaping Techniques

Shaping, or putting tasks in a hierarchy of anxiety, difficulty, or any other important variable is common to almost all aspects of behavioral group therapy. Shaping should always be employed when the problem seems to exist within a hierarchy in which the client is more likely to fail as the situation becomes more difficult. This is commonly required in attitude change, role playing, behavioral rehearsal, problem solving, stimulus control, behavioral contracts, homework, self-monitoring, and self-control procedures.

Reinforcement of Incompatible Responses

In a very real sense, *the reinforcement of incompatible responses* is a special case of differential reinforcement. The major assessment issue involved in this technique is the identification of an incompatible response to the problematic response. Commonly in group therapy, relaxation is reinforced where prior anxiety existed, assertion is reinforced where prior passivity existed, talk is reinforced where prior silence existed, and emotional expression is reinforced where prior flatness of expressed affect existed. The group can also support the report of the incompatible response that has occurred outside the group. Examples might include the initiation of sexual activity; walking away rather than engaging in an argument; and asking what a person is thinking rather than reading his or her mind. All of these situations depend on the client's report and cannot be done *in vivo* by the group. Such incompatible actions are obviously events where self-reinforcement can be taught as an immediate support when the actions will not be quickly reinforced externally.

Self-Monitoring

Self-monitoring (Barlow, 1981) is often employed in the assessment phase of any problem solution, and, as stated before, can also serve as an intervention when the problem is redefined or reexperienced as a function of the monitoring (Ciminero, Calhoun, & Adams, 1977). Self-monitoring is also a method by which "insight" is generated in a behavioral group. The term *insight* is a difficult one to define in that it has multiple connotations and denotations in the therapy field. Despite charges to the contrary, the behaviorist and specifically the behavioral group therapist is not insensitive to the possible effects of insight. Insight into reasons for present undesired behavior can serve as motivation to change. If the problematic responses have clear and powerful alternatives that the client can emit, this insight alone can sometimes cause the change. What is true is that insight into the historical causes of a present behavior does not seem to be a particularly efficient assessment or intervention for the behavior therapist. On the other hand, insight into the pattern of one's behavior and the impact of that behavior on self and others can be extremely valuable both in terms of anxiety reduction and in terms of motivation to change. When self-monitoring is employed as an intervention technique, the behavioral therapists or group members should have assessed that the member needs to have a more accurate picture of his or her own behavior. Such self-assessment for intervention purposes can involve any of the 11 elements of the assessment package. When employed as an assessment, the behavioral group therapist should be relatively certain that the client's insight into this aspect of his or her behavior could cause a significant change in the problem. Self-monitoring should not be used for curiosity when the therapists cannot think of something else to do or because insight is presumed to be a metaphysical good, irrespective of the nature of the problem and the client.

Behavioral Contracts and Homework

Perhaps one of the most common interventions in behavioral group therapy is a *contract* (DeRisi & Butz, 1975; Homme, 1973) with the group, sometimes formal but more often informal, where the client commits to try to accomplish something outside the group. Such contracts can involve any of the 11 elements of the assessment package and always involve the client's changing at least one element of the problem. This is different than traditional group therapy in which the clients either do not make such commitments or make them in a much less structured way. In behavioral group therapy the commitment is made extremely clear as is the fact that the client will report back to the group the successes and problems encountered when attempting the contract. Such contracts can literally involve any aspect of a client's life and can be as simple as making a phone call to a friend and can be as complex as a full stress-management program. *Homework* can also be assigned for the purposes of assessment, focusing, and intervention. When homework and contracts are a specific intervention, they usually involve an attempt to change 1 or more of the 11 elements discovered in the assessment process. The presumption is that generalization from the group to anywhere else must be engineered and cannot be left to chance. The group is a place to learn skills for use in the outside world. Behavioral group therapy is not an end; it is a means. Although this may seem obvious, group therapy and even individual therapy have all too often become ends in themselves. The therapy group is not a community; it is a training ground for the community. A group without homework is essentially either implying that transfer of learning is an easy task, or it is implying that the group is the home. Either belief is unfounded and potentially dangerous for the client.

Self-Control Techniques

Self-control techniques (Kanfer, 1980; Watson & Tharp, 1972) are placed last in this section because they are fundamentally related to everything that has been stated up to this point. Self-control techniques *per se* are employed with problems of impulse control; however self-control techniques are an essential part of every client's therapy in that any transfer of what is learned in group to the world will usually involve self-control. Usually, whatever changes that are taught or planned are usually performed in the environment haltingly and with great effort by the client. Self-control requires that the clients understand the techniques so that it is more likely that they will actually attempt that to which they have committed. In a behavioral group, the variables of self-control are made explicit and are often made part of the contract or homework assignment in order to enhance both the possibility of success and teach the process of self-control. Long after the group's termination, the client will have to cope with new problems. The skills gained in group should be those that help with this task. The aim of therapy is to put itself out of business by training clients to deal with their own problems. Self-control in behavioral group therapy is made more likely if

1. The alternative to be attempted is specific, publically known, and accountable. If the alternative is difficult or complex, it has been broken down into steps for completion.
2. The time by which the attempt is to be made is public and specific.
3. The group is more cohesive, which in part means that the power of group reinforcement and punishment is increased.
4. Emotional induction and reduction with a maximum difference between the two have preceded the self-control attempt.
5. The client possesses the skills and resources to succeed and has reduced the barriers to success as far as possible.

Because many interventions do not immediately affect the problem as disclosed, such as exercise for depression, relaxation training for anxiety, or self-reinforcement for low self-esteem, such self-control is essential if the treatment is to ultimately effect the problem as the client experiences it. When the intervention immediately solves the problem as the client perceives it, self-control is not essential. However, this fortunate case wherein the problem is solved quickly is seldom a fact. Thus, self-control is usually essential for maintaining treatment until the results become self-perpetuating.

Feedback

The feedback part of the behavioral group therapy model corresponds to the second test of the basic TOTE model of behavioral psychotherapy. In voluntary disclosures, because the client initially identifies the problem, it is tempting to let him or her determine when the problem is solved or remediated enough for it to cease being of concern to the group. There are clearly two potential errors with depending solely on client feedback. The first is the often-acknowledged fact that there are factors within individual and group therapy that cause clients to either deceive the group to avoid further anxiety-laden situations or to deceive themselves (Fingarette, 1969) in order to please or accede to the implicit demands of the therapists and the group members to get better.

There is also a problem that, although the client did, in fact, disclose the problem, he or she did not assess it. Whatever element of BASIC that the client found most troublesome is precisely what he or she will depend upon to assess whether he or she has been helped. Thus, a client who initially reports anxiety as the major difficulty will usually assess his or her progress on how he or she feels and will not assess on how well the entire pattern of the 11 assessment factors have been changed to help immediate anxiety and protect against anxiety in the future.

The therapists are both better and worse judges of improvement. Well-trained therapists will not make the mistake of focusing too narrowly on the part of the difficulty that is most salient to the clients but have the disadvantage of a very biased view of clients, namely their behavior in the therapy group. Furthermore, the therapists often have an even greater vested interest in seeing improvement than the client and can be biased by their desires to be effective.

The risk of inaccurate therapist and client assessment of improvement is even worse when the disclosure was indicated by client nonverbal behavior. The indicated disclosure is often not clearly in the client's awareness until it is asked for, and our present research indicates that these disclosures are not only rated as more intense than voluntary disclosures on the average, but they are rated as more anxiety producing; hence, they are more subject to avoidance.

The demonstrated disclosure is actually the most accurately assessable by the therapists and even by the clients if the group have helped the client become self-aware of his or her own behavior. Because the maladaptive behavior occurs in group, therapists, other members, and the client can assess change over time. Here the potential assessment problem is one of transfer of learning. Without further assessment, the group has no feedback, other than the client's, as to whether the new skill is used or successful in the rest of the client's world.

To resolve this issue, one must go outside the group for feedback. Although researchers tell clinicians this all the time, it is clear that this will not usually occur unless it can be easily built into the therapy system. We (Flowers, 1979a; Flowers & Booraem, 1980b; Flowers, Booraem, & Hartman, 1981) have employed an easily implemented system wherein clients first list the problems they have disclosed and worked on in group and problems they have not yet (or may never) disclosed. Second, clients indicate a person they know outside the group who could reasonably rate their improvement or deterioriation on that problem. Depending on the group's length, goals, and so forth, these external raters can be contacted at set intervals to give simple external data for the therapists and clients to analyze.

The reason for giving raters problems that have and have not been disclosed is to be able to identify any rater's positive or negative bias. In our present ongoing research projects, employing these external ratings as the criterion, the difficulties with in-group assessment become clear.

In the case of voluntary disclosures, the other group members have the best match to the external raters; the clients themselves are next, and the therapist is worst. No match is particularly good.

In the case of indicated disclosures, the group members are again best, the therapists are next best, and the client is worst. This form of disclosure shows the worst match to external raters overall.

In the case of demonstrated disclosures, the therapists have the best match; the other group members are next best, and the clients are worst. This form of disclosure shows the best match of all ratings to the external raters assessment. However, this category also has a small subset where the client and the external raters indicate no improvement or exacerbation of the problem and the therapists and other group members rate substantial improvement. These cases seem to elicit an almost total lack of generalization from group to the environment.

In terms of the model presented here, the issue is clear. Unless the final test of the TOTE model is accurate, the therapy group does not know when to exit the problem, and ultimately the member does not know when to exit the group.

Employing the method described or any other method for collecting external data on client improvement is preferable to trusting the group or any part of it to make the feedback assessment.

When external data are not collected, the other members are generally the best assessors, albeit substantially less accurate than might be hoped. Specifically, the other members are best at assessing voluntary disclosures. The other members are also best at assessing indicated disclosures, but even they are so poor that the group should make every attempt to make this disclosure into another type—namely demonstrated.

Generally, when no external assessment is done, the best thing to do is to attempt to make the disclosure or some part of it into a demonstrated one wherein the entire group has greater assessment strength. This is generally accomplished in two ways. First, the aspects of the behavior change that can be role played in group should be. Second, outside indications of progress such as letters, evaluations, paid bills, tickets, marked newspapers, photos, obtained books, weight charts, exercise charts, and the like should be brought and shared with the group.

Accurate feedback is the essential step wherein the group decides whether to assess more, change or lengthen intervention, narrow differently, or change the outcome criterion. Without this feedback, both the client and the group are ungoverned. Although behavioral therapy and theory have much to offer group therapy, this issue of clear (or clearer) feedback governing the group system is the most important systematic change that a behaviorist has to make in traditional group therapy in order to make it truly behavioral.

References

Barlow, D. H. *Behavioral assessment of adult disorders.* New York: Guilford Press, 1981.

Blau, J. S. Changes in awareness and marital satisfaction after participation in an assertiveness training group. In D. Upper & S. M. Ross (Eds.), *Behavioral group therapy, 1980: An annual review.* Champaign, Ill.: Research Press, 1980.

Booraem, C. D., & Flowers, J. V. The reduction of anxiety and personal space as a function of assertion training with severely disturbed neuropsychiatric patients. *Psychological Reports,* 1972, *90,* 63–68.

Booraem, C. D., and & Flowers, J. V. A procedural model for the training of assertive behavior. In J. M. Whiteley & J. V. Flowers (Eds.), *Approaches to assertion training.* Monterey, Calif.: Brooks/Cole, 1977.

Booraem, C. D., & Flowers, J. V. The reduction of anxiety and personal space as a function of assertion training with severely disturbed neuropsychiatric inpatients. *Psychological Reports,* 1980, *30,* 923–929.

Cautella, J. R. Covert sensitization. *Psychological Reports,* 1967, *20,* 459–468.

Ciminero, A. R., Calhoun, K. S., & Adams, H. E. (Eds.), *Handbook of behavioral assessment.* New York: Wiley, 1977.

Coche, J., Levitz, L. S., & Jordan, H. A. Behavioral group psychotherapy for overweight children and adolescents. In D. Upper & S. M. Ross (Eds.), *Behavioral group therapy, 1979: An annual review.* Champaign, Ill.: Research Press, 1979.

Cohn, N. B., Mann, R. J., Flowers, J. V., & Booraem, C. D. Methods of increasing self-reinforcement in group therapy and the effects on therapy outcome. In D. Upper & S. M. Ross (Eds.), *Behavioral group therapy, 1980: An annual review*. Champaign, Ill.: Research Press, 1980.

Cone, J. D., & Hawkins, R. P. *Behavioral assessment*. New York: Brunner/Mazel, 1977.

Curran, J. P., & Monti, P. M. *Social skills training*. New York: Guilford Press, 1982.

D'Zurilla, T. J., & Goldfried, M. R. Problem solving and behavior modification. *Journal of Abnormal Psychology*, 1971, *78*, 197–226.

DeLange, J. M., Lanham, S. L., & Barton, J. A. Social skills training for juvenile delinquents: Behavioral skills training and cognitive techniques. In D. Upper & S. M. Ross (Eds.), *Behavioral group therapy, 1979: An annual review*. Champaign, Ill.: Research Press, 1981.

DeRisi, W. J., & Butz, G. *Writing behavioral contracts: A case simulation practice manual*. Champaign, Ill.: Research Press, 1975.

Edelstein, B. A., Couture, E., Cray, M., Dickens, P., & Lusebrink, N. Group training of problem solving with psychiatric patients. In D. Upper & S. M. Ross (Eds.), *Behavioral group therapy, 1980: An annual review*. Champaign, Ill.: Research Press, 1980.

Festinger, L. *A theory of cognitive dissonance*. Evanston, Ill.: Row, Peterson, 1962.

Fingarette, H. *Self-deception*. London: Routledge & Kegan Paul, 1969.

Flowers, J. V. A behavioral analysis of group therapy and a model for behavioral group therapy. In D. Upper & S. M. Ross (Eds.), *Behavioral group therapy, 1979: An annual review*. Champaign, Ill.: Research Press, 1979. (a)

Flowers, J. V. The differential outcome effects of simple advice, alternatives and instructions in group psychotherapy. *International Journal of Group Psychotherapy*, 1979, *29*, 303–316. (b)

Flowers, J. V., & Booraem, C. D. Assertion training: The training of trainers. *The Counseling Psychologist*, 1975, *5*, 29–36.

Flowers, J. V., & Booraem, C. D. Role playing and simulation II. In F. H. Kanfer & A. J. Goldstein (Eds.), *Helping people change: Materials and methods* (2d ed.), New York: Pergamon Press, 1980. (a)

Flowers, J. V., & Booraem, C. D. Three studies toward a fuller understanding of behavioral group therapy: Cohesion, client flexibility and outcome generalization. In D. Upper & S. M. Ross (Eds.), *Behavioral group therapy, 1980: An annual review*. Champaign, Ill.: Research Press, 1980. (b)

Flowers, J. V., & Tapper, B. *The use of the Affective Expression Test to predict group therapist's effectiveness, individually and in pairs*. Paper presented to the Western Psychological Association, Sacramento, April 1982.

Flowers, J. V., Booraem, C. D., & Hartman, K. A. Clients' improvement on higher and lower intensity problems as a function of group cohesiveness. *Psychotherapy: Theory, Research and Practice*, 1981, *18*, 246–251.

Flowers, J. V., Tapper, B., & Schwartz, B. *Group therapy cotherapists: differences in therapy group behavior based on cotherapist variables*. Paper presented to the Western Psychological Association, San Francisco, April 1983.

Friedman, H. S., Prince, L. M., Riggio, R. E., & DiMatteo, M. R. Understanding and assessing nonverbal expressiveness: The Affective Communication Test. *Journal of Personality and Social Psychology*, 1980, *39*, 333–351.

Goldiamond, I. Self-reinforcement. *Journal of Applied Behavioral Analysis*, 1976, *9*, 509–514.

Goldstein, A., & Wolpe, J. Behavior therapy in groups. In H. I. Kaplan & B. J. Saddock (Eds.), *Comprehensive group therapy*. Baltimore: Williams & Wilkins, 1971.

Hazel, J. S., Schumaker, J. B., Sherman, J. A., & Sheldon-Wildgen, J. The development and evaluation of a group skills training program for court-adjudicated youths. In D. Upper & S. M. Ross (Eds.), *Behavioral group therapy, 1981: An annual review*. Champaign, Ill.: Research Press, 1981.

Heckerman, C. L., & Zitter, R. E. Long-term follow-up of couples treatment of obesity. In D. Upper & S. M. Ross (Eds.), *Behavioral group therapy, 1981: An annual review*. Champaign, Ill.: Research Press, 1981.

Hodgson, J. W. Cognitive versus behavioral-interpersonal approaches to the group treatment of depressed college students. *Journal of Counseling Psychology*, 1981, *28*, 243–249.

Homme, L. *How to use contingency contracting in the classroom*. Champaign, Ill.: Research Press, 1973.

Johnson, D. W. Attitude modification methods. In F. H. Kanfer & A. J. Goldstein (Eds.), *Helping people change: A textbook of methods*. New York: Pergamon Press, 1980.

Kanfer, F. H. Self management methods. In F. H. Kanfer & A. J. Goldstein (Eds.), *Helping people change: A textbook of methods*. New York: Pergamon Press, 1980.

Kanfer, F. H., & Marston, A. R. Conditioning self-reinforcing responses: An analogue to self-confidence training. *Psychological Reports*, 1963, *13*, 63–90.

Kanfer, F. H., & Saslow, G. Behavioral analysis: An alternative to diagnostic classification. *Archives of General Psychiatry*, 1965, *12*, 529–538.

Karoly, P. Operant methods. In F. H. Kanfer & A. J. Goldstein (Eds.), *Helping people change: A textbook of methods*. New York: Pergamon Press, 1980.

Knauss, M. R., & Jeffrey, D. B. Group behavior therapy for the treatment of obesity. In D. Upper & S. M. Ross (Eds.), *Behavioral group therapy, 1981: An annual review*. Champaign, Ill.: Research Press, 1981.

Lange, A. J. Cognitive-behavioral group therapy and assertion training. In D. Upper & S. M. Ross (Eds.), *Behavioral group therapy, 1979: An annual review*. Champaign, Ill.: Research Press, 1979.

Lazarus, A. A. *Multimodal behavior therapy*. New York: Springer, 1976.

Lieberman, M. A., Lakin, M., & Whitaker, D. S. The group as a unique context for therapy. *Psychotherapy: Theory, Research and Practice*, 1968, *5*, 29–36.

Lobitz, W. C., & Baker, E. L. Group treatment of sexual dysfunction: Coping skill training for single males. In D. Upper & S. M. Ross (Eds.), *Behavioral group therapy, 1979: An annual review*. Champaign, Ill.: Research Press, 1979.

Mahoney, M. J., & Thoresen, C. E. *Self-control: Power to the person*. Monterey, Calif.: Brooks/Cole, 1974.

Mash, E. J., & Terdal, L. G. *Behavior therapy assessment*. New York: Springer, 1976.

McGovern, K. B. An analysis of behavioral group treatment programs designed to modify sexual dysfunction. In D. Upper & S. M. Ross (Eds.), *Behavioral group therapy, 1979: An annual review*. Champaign, Ill.: Research Press, 1979.

Meichenbaum, D., Gilmore, J., & Fedoravicus, A. Group insight versus group desensitization in treating speech anxiety. *Journal of Clinical and Consulting Psychology*, 1971, *36*, 410–421.

Miller, G. A., Galanter, E., & Pribram, K. H. *Plans and the structure of behavior*. New York: Holt, Rinehart & Winston, 1960.

Paul, G. L. *Insight vs. desensitization in psychotherapy*. Stanford, Calif.: Stanford University Press, 1966.

Roberts, M. C., & LaGreca, A. M. Behavioral assessment. In C. E. Walker (Ed.), *Clinical practice of psychology*. New York: Pergamon Press, 1981.

Sarri, R. C. Behavioral theory and group work. In P. Glasser, R. Sarri, & R. Vintner (Eds.), *Individual change through small groups*. New York: The Free Press, 1974.

Scofield, W. *Psychotherapy: The purchase of friendship*. Englewood Cliffs, N.J.: Prentice-Hall, 1964.

Shapiro, J. R., Shaffer, C. S., Sank, L. I., & Coghlan, D. J. Cognitive behavioral therapy groups: Methods and comparative research. In D. Upper & S. M. Ross (Eds.), *Behavioral group therapy, 1981: An annual review*. Champaign, Ill.: Research Press, 1981.

Upper, D., & Ross, S. M. Behavioral group therapy: I. Emotional avoidance and social skills problems of adults. In M. Hersen, R. M. Eisler, & P. M. Miller (Eds.), *Progress in behavior modification* (Vol. 5). New York: Academic Press, 1977.

Upper, D., & Rosa, S. M. *Behavioral group therapy, 1979: An annual review*. Champaign, Ill.: Research Press, 1979.

Upper, D., & Ross, S. M. *Behavioral group therapy, 1980: An annual review*. Champaign, Ill.: Research Press, 1980.

Upper, D., & Ross, S. M. *Behavioral group therapy, 1981: An annual review*. Champaign, Ill.: Research Press, 1981.

Walker, C. E., Hedberg, A., Clement, P. W., & Wright, L. *Clinical procedures for behavior therapy*. Englewood Cliffs, N.J.: Prentice-Hall, 1981.

Watson, D. L., & Tharp, R. G. *Self-directed behavior: Self-modification for personal adjustment*. Monterey, Calif.: Brooks/Cole, 1972.

Watts, D. L., & Courtois, C. A. Trends in the treatment of men who commit violence against women. *Personnel and Guidance Journal*, 1981, *60*, 245–249.

Wieand, L. A., Flowers, J. V., & Hartman, K. A. Training paraprofessionals to do assertion training with mentally disordered sex offenders. In D. Upper & S. M. Ross (Eds.), *Behavioral group therapy, 1981: An annual review*. Champaign, Ill.: Research Press, 1981.

Wolpe, J. *The practice of behavior therapy*. New York: Pergamon Press, 1969.

II

Clinical Applications with Specific Populations

The four chapters in Part II focus on the special procedures and problems associated with specific clinical populations.

Rose and LeCroy in Chapter 7 address the problem of improving social competence in children and describe a group treatment model that integrates cognitive-behavioral techniques with small-group approaches. Of special relevance for clinicians working with children are the description of how social skills training, problem-solving training, and cognitive restructuring can be integrated into a comprehensive treatment package and the authors' specific guidelines for establishing and maintaining children's groups in various settings.

In Chapter 8, Hazel, Sherman, Schumaker, and Sheldon review what they feel are the most important issues related to the development and more widespread use of social skills training groups with adolescents. Among these are the choice of skills to be taught and specific components of each, the procedures or combinations of training procedures employed, and the techniques used for evaluating treatment effectiveness. The authors' comprehensive critiques of the work to date on each of these issues should prove useful to clinicians, trainers, and researchers alike.

Kantor, in Chapter 9, discusses the clinical utility and cost-effectiveness of employing a broad range of time-limited, intensive, psychoeducational treatment approaches with a behavioral medicine population, and he uses a behavioral group therapy program aimed at modifying the Type A behavior pattern as a detailed example of such approaches. Many nuts-and-bolts details of the group program, from assessment through follow-up, are provided, and unresolved problems and directions for future work are discussed.

In Chapter 10, Steinmetz, Thompson, Breckenridge, and Gallagher address relevant issues and recent research on the use of behavioral group therapy with the elderly. The special problems associated with using a psychoeducational approach with this population (e.g., possible problems with memory, vision or hearing, chronic pain) are considered, and specific suggestions for enhancing the effectiveness of the therapeutic/educational process are offered.

7

Improving Children's Social Competence

A Multimodal Behavioral Group Approach

SHELDON D. ROSE AND CRAIG W. LECROY

INTRODUCTION

A child's social competence continues to receive extensive attention from researchers, developmentalists, and social practitioners (e.g., Edelson & Rose, 1981; LaGreca & Santogrossi, 1980; LeCroy, 1983; Swetnam, Peterson, & Clark, 1983). By *social competence* we are referring to the ability to produce desired effects on others in specific social situations. Research is revealing how important social interactions can be in the healthy development of children. This focus on social interaction can be facilitated through the use of small groups. Models for small-group treatment have lagged behind the development of new knowledge on helping children obtain a greater degree of social competence. In fact, many programs designed to help children develop better social skills have not even utilized the natural format of small groups for teaching children these skills. Many practitioners have continued to work individually with children ignoring the benefits the small group can provide.

The purpose of this chapter is to describe a model of group treatment that integrates cognitive-behavioral techniques with small-group approaches as a multimodal approach to improving social competence in children. It attempts to provide an overview, broad in nature, but of practical utility. The primary focus is not a review of research but a selection of empirically based methods and inclusion of research relevant to these procedures as well as a guide to the use of children's groups. We begin with a discussion of the purposes for conducting children's groups. Following this, a review of the major strategies used while working with children in groups is provided. These strategies include social skills, problem solving, cognitive restructuring, reinforcement, and small group. We then turn to an examination of the mechanics of leadership such as the size, number of leaders, themes, composition, and techniques for putting a group

SHELDON D. ROSE • University of Wisconsin, Madison, Wisconsin 53706. CRAIG W. LECROY • Arizona State University, Tempe, Arizona 85287.

together. The chapter concludes with a review of the research support for the various methods being advocated in the group treatment of children.

Purposes

The major purposes of the multimodal behavioral group approach are (a) to promote effective social skills; (b) to improve problem-solving skills, especially the development of consequential thinking; and (c) to increase the child's repertoire of cognitive coping skills primarily through the replacement of self-defeating cognitions with self-enhancing or coping cognitions.

Promote Social Skills

Social skills are critical for healthy development in children. Recognition of the importance of peer relations has been increasingly documented in research studies (Asher, 1978; Hartup, 1980; see Swetnam *et al.*, 1983, for a review). An emphasis on teaching social skills to children has grown in recent years because of the demonstrated importance of socially effective behavior on subsequent development. Research has shown a linkage between a lack of skills and future adjustment problems (see Conger & Keane, 1981; Hartup, 1979, for a review of this research).

Hartup (1980) in an article on peer relations and the growth of social competence suggests several reasons why peer relations are important: (a) lack of sociability in both boys and girls is associated with discomfort, anxiety, and a general unwillingness to engage the environment; (b) children master their aggressive impulses within the context of peer relations; (c) sexual socialization probably cannot take place in the absence of peer interaction; (d) peer relations are related to a child's ability for role taking, which in turn is related to social competency; and (e) children rejected by their peers have higher delinquency rates (Roff, 1961), are more likely to drop out of school (Ullman, 1957), and are at risk for emotional and behavioral difficulties (Cowen, Pederson, Babigian, Izzo, & Trost, 1973; Kohn & Clausen, 1955; Roff, Sells, & Golden, 1972).

Social skills have been defined as "those responses which, within a given situation, prove effective or, in other words, maximize the probablity of producing, maintaining or enhancing positive effects for the interactor" (Foster & Ritchey, 1979, p. 626). This definition is not without problems (see Conger & Keane, 1981, for a discussion on defining social skills), but it does stress a situational and interactional emphasis. Because interaction is the basis of group process, a peer group approach as opposed to an individual adult–child approach should be the most appropriate context for teaching social skills.

The group format is a natural context in which to help children learn more adaptive social skills. It gives children the opportunity to learn and practice many behaviors as they respond to the constantly changing group demands. Through reinforcement, modeling, and role-play practice, children learn many social skills that help them interact more effectively with peers. These skills may include communication and socialization skills such as starting conversations, sharing, coping with conflict, and expressing feelings. For adolescents, more advanced skills, such as carrying on an extended conversation or a job interview, dating or negotiating with parents, can be taught in the same way.

As a result of increased social skills development, a child's social status may change. The group leader can structure opportunities for group members to play roles quite different from those assigned to them by their peers. For example, the group leader may assist a child to assume a leadership role that allows the child to demonstrate a wider range of skills than previously observed by his or her age-mates. These kinds of experiences produce increased feelings of mastery, which may strengthen the child's sense of self-efficacy (Bandura, 1977).

Develop Problem-Solving Skills

Problem solving as a set of abilities in its own right has been given increasing attention in its application to problems of children. This has been spearheaded by Spivack and Shure's work on the assessment and teaching of interpersonal cognitive problem-solving skills (ICPS) to children (Spivack, Platt, & Shure, 1976; Spivack & Shure, 1974). Their research revealed consistent findings that showed that subjects with ICPS abilities were better adjusted (Spivack *et al.*, 1976). This led to their attempting to teach ICPS abilities to young children. The results of several studies (see Spivack *et al.*, 1976) found young children learned the cognitive abilities, that these gains were related to adjustment, and that the results were maintained over time.

Problem solving is a key competency that can maximize a child's adjustment and interpersonal effectiveness. The components that have been identified as primary skills include (a) alternative thinking, which is the ability to generate multiple alternative solutions to interpersonal problem situations; (b) consequential thinking, which involves the ability to anticipate short- and long-term consequences of a particular alternative and then to utilize this in decision making; and (c) means–end thinking, which refers to the ability to plan a series of specific means or actions necessary to carry out the solution to an interpersonal problem. This includes the recognition of obstacles that need to be overcome and implies that a realistic time framework is important in achieving a goal.

In group treatment, children are helped to explore different choices and to act out the consequences of each of their choices. In this way, they begin to learn the process of consequential thinking. Through role playing, children can experience various solutions and learn why one solution is a better course of action than another. Group members suggest to each other possible consequences as an interpersonal difficulty is discussed or roleplayed. The exposure to these various consequences teaches the children to think more consequentially about their behavior.

Increase Cognitive Coping Skills

Cognitions refer to thoughts, images, thinking patterns, self-statements, or private or covert events that may be inferred from verbal or other overt behavior.

Cognitive coping skills are those cognitions that facilitate coping with internal and social phenomena. Examples of such skills are analysis of one's cognitions, covert rehearsal, identification and elimination of self-defeating statements, self-instructions, and self-reinforcement. Though important skills in their own right, cognitive coping skills also mediate the attainment of the more observable social skills, as defined previously.

This goal of increasing cognitive coping skills is important as a means of correcting anxiety-inducing and behavior-inhibiting cognitions (Meichenbaum, 1977). Self-statements, such as "Everyone thinks I'm weird," not only produce anxiety, they promote inaction. Changing such a statement to something like "Sure, I'm different than other kids in many ways, some of which I like and some I'll change" may reflect a more accurate appraisal, may suggest avenues of change, is more self-respecting, and may even reduce anxiety. The group can be instrumental in identifying self-defeating statements, helping members to acknowledge them as self-defeating, and assisting them to find more effective and more accurate ways of describing themselves and their actions.

All of these preceding purposes, if achieved, serve to improve the assessment an individual has of him- or herself. Learning to perform more effectively with others, learning new, positively recognized social roles, learning to solve problems systematically, and finally learning to praise oneself rather than to put oneself down should result in an individual with much higher self-esteem and higher level of social competence.

The Function of the Group in Group Treatment

In the previous section we pointed out that the group is a natural format for peer-to-peer interaction with the added potential for guidance and protection by the adult. The group more nearly simulates the real world of most clients than does the situation consisting solely of a high-status therapist and a low-status child. As such, the group provides the child an intermediate step between performing a newly learned behavior in a therapy setting and transferring that performance to the community. Several other reasons for using the group can be delineated.

In the group, the child must learn to deal with the idiosyncrasies of other individuals. He or she must learn to offer other children feedback and advice and, as a result, can develop important skills for leadership. By helping others, the child usually learns to help him- or herself more effectively than when he or she is the sole recipient of therapy.

In group interaction, powerful norms arise that serve to control the behavior of individual members. If these norms (informal agreements among members as to preferred modes of action and interaction in the group) are introduced and effectively maintained by the leader, they serve as efficient therapeutic tools. The group pressures deviant members to conform to such norms as attending regularly, reinforcing peers who do well, analyzing problems systematically, and assisting peers to find solutions to their problems. Of course, if the group leader is not watchful, antitherapeutic norms also can be generated. Some group norms, indicated by such behaviors as erratic attendance, noncompletion of agreed-upon assignments, and constant criticism of therapists may work against the attainment of therapeutic goals.

To guard against such problems, the leader can call upon a vast body of experimentally derived knowledge about norms and other group phenomena in which individual behavior both influences and is influenced by the various attributes of the group (see Cartwright & Zander, 1968, for an extensive summary). In addition to modifying the norms of the group, the leader can facilitate the attainment of both individual and group treatment goals by such procedures as modifying the cohesiveness of the group, the status pattern, or the communication structure in the group. Much of the power of group treatment is lost if negative group attributes remain unbridled.

Another characteristic of behavioral group therapy is the varied opportunity for peer reinforcement. Each person is given the chance to learn or to improve his or her ability to mediate rewards for others in social interactive situations (with acquaintances, friends, family members, fellow group members, teachers, or employers). The leader can construct a situation in which each person has frequent opportunities, instructions, and rewards for reinforcing others in the group. Reinforcement is a highly valued skill in our society; there is good reason to believe that as a person learns to reinforce others, he or she is reciprocally reinforced by others and mutual liking also increases (see Lott & Lott, 1961).

More accurate assessment can be another major contribution of behavioral group therapy. The group provides the child with a major source of feedback about what in his or her behavior is annoying to others, which cognitions appear to others to be self-defeating, and what he or she does that makes him or her attractive. This is helpful especially when children cannot pinpoint their own problems or inappropriate cognitions. A very important fringe benefit is that the group provides a natural laboratory for learning discussion skills that are essential to good social relationships.

In addition to facilitating assessment, the group allows the leader to use an abundance of therapeutic procedures that are either unavailable or less efficacious in the therapeutic dyad. Among these procedures is the use of group reinforcement, which for many children is more powerful than individual reinforcement (see Wodarski, Hamblin, Buckholdt, & Perritor, 1973). The group provides an abundance of models, role players for behavioral rehearsal, manpower for monitoring, and partners for use in a "buddy system." Finally, the group also appears to be as effective and more efficient in terms of therapist cost than dyadic treatment methods (see, e.g., Kendall & Zupan, cited in Urbain & Kendall, 1980, who are among the few who compare, experimentally, children treated in groups versus children treated individually).

Major Strategies

Several major strategies are used in behavioral group treatment with children. Most prominent are social skills training, problem-solving training, cognitive restructuring, reinforcement, and group procedures. The incorporation of each strategy into group treatment is discussed in the following section.

Social Skills Training

The most common group approach to teaching social skills is based upon a social learning conceptualization (Ladd & Mize, 1983). A first step in this process is to select specific social skills to be taught. The skills selected depend upon the specific assessment of the children referred to the group and the overall goals for the group. For example, if the children are shy or withdrawn, the focus would be on increasing peer interaction by teaching conversational skills (e.g., Whitehall, Hersen, & Bellack, 1980) and/or approach responses. Such skills might include how to greet others, keeping interactions going, and being cooperative. Children identified as overly aggressive when not getting their way would need to learn alternative ways of dealing with such situations (e.g., Elder, Edelstein, & Narick, 1979).

Children need not be identified as having problems to benefit from social skills training. Many programs have been developed for normal children to strengthen their socialization skills (Clark, Wood, & Northrup, 1980; LeCroy, 1983; Oden & Asher, 1977; Swetnam *et al.*, 1983).

Once skills are selected, they are broken into their component parts for teaching purposes. A comprehensive social skills curriculum has been developed by Stevens (1978) that demonstrates how each social skill can be divided into smaller tasks. Under the major category of "interpersonal behaviors" (other categories are "self-related and task-related behaviors"), Stephens lists 10 subcategories. An example of a subcategory is "coping with conflict," which includes six subskills. For example, two of the skills for coping with conflict are (1) to walk away from peers when angry to avoid hitting; and (2) to respond to teasing or name calling by ignoring, changing the subject, or using some other constructive means.

LaGreca and Mesibov (1979) identified nine areas that they thought were important in teaching social skills to learning-disabled children. They include smiling and laughing, greeting, joining, extending invitations, conversation skills, sharing and cooperation, complimenting, play skills, and physical appearance and grooming. These skills are then further broken down into observable steps. For example, the joining sequence includes the following: smile, look at the person, use his or her name, stand nearby, greet him or her, ask to join nicely, ask a question to enter the conversation. Ideas for developing social skills curricula for elementary-school children can be found in Cartledge and Milburn (1980), and for adolescents, see Goldstein, Martens, Van Belle, Schaaf, Wiersma, & Goedhart, (1973) and Hazel, Schumaker, Sherman, & Sheldon-Wildgen (1981). Where most of the component steps are already familiar to the children, many of steps may be omitted and the more complex social skill may be handled as whole, early in the treatment program.

The teaching process involves all the familiar procedures of social learning theory. In some research, modeling alone has proven effective (Evers & Schwarz, 1973; Gottman, 1977; Keller & Carlson, 1974; O'Connor, 1969, 1972). However, this does not make sufficient use of the group to refine, reinforce, and promote outside use of the skills. Most programs supplement modeling with instructions, rehearsal, feedback (Bornstein, Bellack, & Hersen, 1977; Ladd, 1981), and coaching (LaGreca & Santogrossi, 1980; Oden & Asher, 1977). Coaching involves more emphasis on instruction as to how and when the skills are to be used and overlaps with the more complex procedures of instructions, modeling, rehearsal, and feedback. A relatively standard procedure for teaching social skills can be summarized as follows:

1. The leader explains the skill to the group, who discuss its utility.
2. The leader gives instructions on how to use the skill (reviews the steps in successfully performing the skill).
3. The leader or an experienced group member models the skill. The leader emphasizes the important aspects of how to perform the skill.
4. The members, one at a time, behaviorally rehearse the skill. For some children, coaching or prompting may be used. For more proficient children this may not be required.
5. After each rehearsal, the other members and leader provide feedback, including reinforcement for approximations of skill mastery, and provide critical suggestions for improvement.
6. Usually, a rerehearsal follows in which the feedback is incorporated.
7. Finally, homework to perform the skill in the real world may be designed with the group, and the children are instructed to carry it out. Contingencies with younger children (e.g., points awarded and exchanged for a field trip at the end of the group) are often associated with completion of the homework (see Rose & Roessle, 1980, for a more detailed example).

Although the teaching of social skills *per se* is not always difficult, the most effective leader will keep the group attentive, structured, participating, and enjoyable through sociorecreational activities.

In more sophisticated and experienced groups, breaking down each skill into its component parts is not required. The group can discuss a specific problem situation and come up with appropriate goals and a general set of guidelines for achieving those goals. The situation might then be modeled and rehearsed and feedback provided the target child as to his or her success in meeting the previously mentioned guidelines. In this variation, rather than using common situations, children are encouraged to bring in their own unique situations to work on.

In the following excerpt we see an example of how the group carries out the social skills training process.

LARRY: I have trouble asking my teacher for help, too. Yesterday, the teacher gave us a math problem I didn't understand. Then on the test later on in the day I flunked the test. I know I should have asked her. I just didn't know what to say.

TONY [*the leader*]: We discussed a number of ideas of what one can do and say when asking for help at the beginning of the meeting. Why don't we have someone who feels comfortable with asking for help show you what they would do.

LARRY: I'd like that. Maybe even a couple of guys could do it. How about you, Quint? You seem to have a lot of good ideas.

QUINTIN: OK, but who'll be the teacher?

TONY: How about me? I'd make a great teacher. [*Group members agree, laughing.*]

TONY: OK, here's a new math problem in which we reverse the A with the B. We know the value of A but we don't know the value of B. The first thing you do is to . . .

QUINTIN: Just a minute, Mr., ah, Jones, I've lost you. Could you explain that first part again, please?

TONY: [*in his role as leader*] Good! Anyone else want to demonstrate what he would say?

AL: How about, "You've lost me, Mr. Jones. I really need some help"?

TOM: I prefer, "I'm confused. I don't understand at all."

TONY: OK, Larry, notice how the model got the teachers attention and then kept the eye contact. Notice too how each person spoke in loud clear voice. And everyone asked for help. Now, why don't you try it? I'll still be the teacher. [*in role as teacher*] OK, here's a new math problem. The antisepsis and countersepsis are calculated by dividing then multiplying by two unknowns.

LARRY: Ah, eh, ah, Mr. Jones, ah, I'm lost. That's really confusing. I wonder if you could explain it to me once again, slowly.

TONY: Great, what did he do well, guys?

TOM: Well, he did what he said he wanted to do. He asked for help.

AL: And he did it in a loud clear voice.

ROGER: With good eye contact, so he would get his attention.

LARRY: Would anybody have done anything differently?

QUINTIN: Well, when he said that it was confusing. It might be better to say, he was confused, not the teacher. I guess it's better not to blame the teacher.

LARRY: Yeah that's a good idea. I'll remember that.

The leader would then have Larry try it again until he felt comfortable. Larry's homework assignment for the following week would probably be to try out asking for help from the teacher or another adult.

Closely integrated with social skills training is problem solving. In fact, as the reader will note in the following section many of the steps are similar or exactly the same. One might even regard social skills training as preparation for carrying out solutions to problems that are interactive in nature. Of course not all problems are interactive; yet the general problem-solving model is equally applicable as we shall see next.

Problem-Solving Training

Several different programs amenable to group training have been developed to teach children problem-solving abilities. They all have in common the basic problem-solving steps: (a) define the problem; (b) generate alternatives for solving the problem; (c) evaluate the alternatives; (d) make a decision; and (e) implement the solution.

In children's groups, each child is asked to describe a problematic situation, or the leader provides the group with a problem relevant to most of the group members, for example, being able to tell friends "no" when the adolescent is pressured to take a drink, or budgeting his or her time more effectively. Teaching children the criteria for identifying situations that call for problem solving is the first step. The leader models several problems that meet the criteria, and the members discuss in which way the criteria are met. Later, the children are asked to bring in their own problems that the group evaluates in terms of the criteria.

Also, in Step 1, each group member is prompted to identify the concrete aspects of the problem being presented. They usually ask questions about who is involved in the problem or how these people in the problem are affected by the situation. Questions are asked about what happened and/or what needs to be decided. The leader encourages all the group members to examine how the people involved in the problem might feel. Once the problem is clearly defined, solutions to that problem are generated.

In generating solutions, the leader encourages everyone to come up with at least one alternative. Children (with at least a third-grade writing skill level) are instructed simply to write down every idea that comes to their minds and not to be concerned whether or not the alternative is effective. When conducted enthusiastically, this part of the session can be the most fun and most productive. Care, however, must be taken not to evaluate in this phase, until all possible solutions have been identified; otherwise the evaluation ("Oh, that will never work," or "What a good idea!") may inhibit the members' further generation of other alternatives.

While evaluating the alternatives, the group members are exposed to various ways of reasoning about social problems. They begin to think more specifically in terms of consequences and learn to think ahead. The leader encourages the group in evaluating negative as well as positive alternatives. This way children can get exposure to many of the possible consequences of alternatives they may have proposed.

In decision making, the children are asked about which alternative or combination of alternatives is best and why, in terms of the long-term interests of the child. The comparative risk of each alternative is also examined. If the group is working with a specific child's problem, he or she is asked to decide upon an alternative to encourage implementation; the social skills training sequence is at this point often integrated into the approach. The solutions generated through brainstorming, if the solution is interactive, are modeled, and the child rehearses behaviorally the modeled behavior with or without coaching. Feedback and rehearsal follow. Following the social skills sequence preparation, additions and/or deletions to the solution can be made. There decisions are made by the child and group leader as they obtain feedback from the group members.

Last, the leader structures how the child will implement the decision outside of the group by asking such questions as, "When will you perform the solution? Where will it be performed? Who will be present when the actions involved in the decision are performed?" These types of questions are designed to increase the clarity of the decision and in so doing increase the likelihood that the decision will be carried out. The children are also asked to commit themselves publically to the group as to the details of the action they plan to take. Progress is reported back to the group for celebration and reinforcement.

In the following example, the leader assists the group to go through the initial steps of the problem-solving process.

PATRICIA [*group leader*]: Angie, could you tell us a little more about what happened when the other girls call you wierd?

ANGIE: Well, yesterday, I was walking down the halls and Licia looks at me and says, "you sure are wierd." It made me feel awful. She does it all the time and so does her friend, Annamarie.

PAT: Any questions about the situation?

BILLIE JEAN: What were you doing?

ANGIE: Nothing, just walking down the hall by myself. She just doesn't like me I guess. And she's so stuck up.

EILEEN: You don't sound wierd to me. I think she's just mean. She's mean to a lot of kids in class.

JANEY: What did you do?

ANGIE: Nothing, I just turned away. Maybe I stared at her a second, then I looked away in a huff. I guess she could see I was mad.

PAT: [*After a moment's pause*] Well, what else could she do? Why don't each of you write down as many ideas as you can. The important thing is to get a lot of ideas. You can write down ideas, too, Angie. [*After a few minutes*] What did you write?

JANEY: You could kick her and say, "I'll show you who's wierd."

ANGIE: Oh, I don't . . .

PAT: [*Interrupting*] Let's wait before we say whether an idea is any good or not. Let's hear all the ideas, first. Why don't you jot the ideas as they are described, Angie? [*All the members suggest about 10 different ideas.*]

PAT: OK, Angie, which of these ideas do you like best? And tell us, why.

ANGIE: Well, I think I should walk away and tell the teacher she's been teasing me.

PAT: Is there any risk in doing that?

EILEEN: Well, Licia and Annmarie might not like you any more.

ANGIE: They don't like me anyway, that doesn't bother me a bit. But other kids might think I'm a snitch.

HELEN: It's better than fighting, and you won't get a detention.

ANGIE: Yeah, I like telling the teacher best. That's what I'm going to do if it happens again.

Problem solving is basically a cognitive intervention strategy. Through this kind of training one learns a cognitive set and how to apply it to a wide range of problems. However, there are other cognitive change strategies that have been used with children. Among these is cognitive restructuring.

COGNITIVE RESTRUCTURING

Cognitive restructuring procedures are those that change self-defeating or illogical patterns of thinking that interfere with social functioning to self-enhancing or logical ones. It is assumed that, in a given set of circumstances, cognitions mediate overt behavioral responses. These cognitions include how one values oneself and one's actions and how one specifically thinks or responds covertly in a given situation. The child is taught first to identify, then to replace, self-defeating statements uttered to oneself in the face of stress with new more functional self-statements. This process consists of step-by-step verbalizations concerning the problem definition ("What's wrong with the way I'm thinking about this?"), problem focus ("What can I do about it?"), focusing of attention ("I should think about how that will get me in trouble"), coping statements ("If I keep relaxing I won't blow it!"), and self-reinforcement ("Wow! I did it! See, I can do it"). These components are discussed by Meichenbaum (1977) and Bash & Camp (1980) in more detail.

The procedures usually followed in this approach are described next. With the addition of covert rehearsal and a fading technique, cognitions are taught in much the same way as overt behavioral skills in social skills training.

First, each child chooses a stressful situation to be discussed at a given meeting. The situations are similar to or the same as those used in the social skills training strategy. After the child describes the situation to the group, the other members interview the client as to what his or her cognitions might be.

These thoughts are discussed by the group in terms of the effectiveness of such cognitions in facilitating achievement of client goals. For example, "I can't do it!" or "I'll never learn that!" are regarded as self-defeating statements because they render the child inactive and often anxious. These thoughts are targeted for replacement. In some cases, children are not able to verbalize their cognitions, but they are also not clearly saying anything to mobilize productive action. In both cases the leader and, in later sessions, the group members suggest alternative statements that the child evaluates and selects to help him or her cope better with the situation. These cognitions are then modeled aloud by the leader or one of the other members. At the same time the leader performs the desired overt behavior in the situation while the child and other group members observe. The targeted child then performs the task, instructing himself or herself out loud (the model will coach the child). The leader and a member model task performance while whispering the self-instructional statements. In later sessions other children do the whispering; this is followed by the target child's performing the task and whispering the self-instructional statements to himself or herself. The leader or child model performs the task using covert self-instructions with pauses and behavioral signs of thinking (e.g., scratching head, stroking chin, raising eyes toward the ceiling). This reminds the child to follow the self-instructional sequence. The target child performs the task using covert self-instructions; homework assignments are discussed by group; and the target child evaluates them and chooses an assignment to practice in the natural environment. Throughout this process, the group members provide feedback on how well each target child is doing and what might be done differently. Several of the steps are demonstrated in the following excerpt from a group of 11-year-old girls.

MARIELLEN: I guess I do get too mad whenever my Mom asks me to do something. I just can't control it.

WINNIE: Didn't we learn that "can't" is often a self-defeating statement? I'll bet you can control it if you give yourself a chance. You sure get in a lot of trouble, they way things are now, and you're always fighting with your mom.

MARIELLEN: I know, but what can I tell myself when my mom bosses me around?
JUANITA: For one thing you can say, "cool it" or "relax" like we learned in the group.
WINNIE: Yeah, and you could say, "She is my mom, she can tell me some things."
MARIELLEN: I suppose I could say to myself, "Hey, the room was a mess. Don't ruin everything. I don't want a fight." What do you think, Cynthia [*group leader*]?
CYNTHIA: You guys are doing fine without me. Would you like me to put a few of those things together in a role play?
MARIELLEN: Yeah, would you?
CYNTHIA: Ok, I'm imagining I just got home. My Mom asks me to clean up my room I left a mess this morning. I feel a pounding of anger rising up inside of me. Ok, cool it, take a deep breath, now relax, that's it. The room was a mess. No sense getting into a fight over it. I'll just go ahead and clean it [*pause*]. How did I do?
MARIELLEN: That was great. I wish I could do it like that.
CYNTHIA: You can do it. In fact why don't you try it now. I'll paint the picture for you.

The leader goes on to describe the scene, and she has Mariellen rehearse what she says to herself several times. In subsequent performances "Mom" is not quite as gentle as she was in the first rehearsal.

CYNTHIA: How did Mariellen do, oops, I mean, what did she do well? [*Group laughs.*]

The members go on to evaluate what Mariellen did. After the evaluation, she repeats the scene several times, first whispering, then going through the thinking part completely silent.

In both social skills training and cognitive restructuring much reinforcement is used by peers as well as the leader. These are not the only uses of reinforcement as we see in the following section.

REINFORCEMENT STRATEGIES

One of the major advantages of the group as the context of treatment is the opportunity to provide the members with the large number of reinforcing activities usually unavailable to the isolated child in treatment. Even such individualized activities as the making of airplane models appear to be more reinforcing when others are present. Except for the highly withdrawn or autistic child, who is not usually treated in groups, most clients value interactive over isolated activities. As a result, social interactive activities or group tasks comprise one of the major opportunities for reinforcement in group treatment.

For most children, contingently applied social reinforcement is sufficient to maintain desirable behaviors and teach new ones. However, for those children whose maladaptive behaviors are well learned, whose reinforcement repertoires are limited, and for whom the usual social reinforcement is ineffective, more concrete reinforcement, as we describe later is required. Many children in treatment fall into one or more of these categories.

Social reinforcement, either verbal or nonverbal, is seldom isolated from material reinforcement. Because many clients come from either socially or materially deprived backgrounds or both, material goods are powerful reinforcers, especially early in treatment. Praise and various nonverbal indications of interest or affection often represent ambiguous cues at best, and at worst are indications that someone is going to deprive them of something. For such children, material rewards such as nuts, raisins, small candies, and cut-up pieces of fruit are dispensed initially but are paired with praise and nonverbal encouragement in order to establish the latter as social reinforcement. One of the problems of material reinforcement is that highly valued objects may be too large to administer every time a person performs a desirable act, and it is for this reason that tokens are often used. Tokens have a small value and can be used, when a sufficient number have been accumulated, to purchase desirable material goods or social activities. "Tokens" may be poker chips, painted blocks, play money, clicks on a counter, tally marks on a tabulation sheet, pennies, or any other visible indicator of achievement. The tokens are later paired (by a system of exchange) with desirable objects or with activities such as a trip to the zoo or the right to be first in line to go to lunch.

Tokens are highly manipulable. They can be given with great frequency that increases their effectiveness as a teaching tool. Their value can be varied, and they are concrete and observable; children always know that they and their peers are getting something when they receive a token, which is not always the case with praise. Early in treatment, tokens are given immediately following conformity to group rules, completion of individual behavioral assignments, and performance of any spontaneous behaviors whose frequency the therapist wishes to increase. They also may be given following a predetermined time period when at least one or more desirable acts is performed or when a stated number of undesirable acts are not performed. In later sessions, the reinforcement schedule is usually thinned; (i.e., tokens are usually given on an increasingly infrequent basis).

In order to make use of the reinforcement value that peers have for each other in group treatment, contingencies are often designed for the entire group (Wodarski *et al.*, 1973). An example of how a group contingency is delivered is the following. Children often received points or tokens for completion of homework assignments or for predetermined in-group behavior. The value of these points is put on a large thermometer that, when filled, earns the group the right to a trip, attendance at a baseball game, a visit from an athlete, one dance lesson, a meal at McDonalds, or some other highly valued activity that the group members have determined in advance from a menu of possible group activities. Group contingencies engender much pressure on each member to perform what is expected of him or her in order that everyone obtains the reward. If the group is valued by the individual, the pressure is a highly effective device for behavioral change. However, if the individual has more attractive alternatives, the pressure may be ignored, or the child may even leave the group. The leader must therefore weigh whether he or she wishes to risk using the group contingency or whether to downplay the saliency of the reinforcers being used. One method to do this is to permit the children to use their individual tokens or points for both individual rewards as well as group contingencies.

Group Intervention

Adjunctive to the particular strategies mentioned before are some concrete group ingredients that appear to be active in helping children toward change. It may be the effective use of these procedures that is more important than the particular strategy of practice being utilized. These include group discussion, role playing, sociorecreational activities, and other group procedures such as the buddy system, each of which will be discussed next.

Group Discussion

Group discussion refers to child-to-child verbal interactions as well as child-to-leader ones. It is the essential stuff by which problems are laid out and considered, solutions are shared and evaluated, decisions are formulated and affirmed, values are examined, and friendships are made. Of course, it is a useful treatment vehicle only if everyone in the group has ready access to it. Dominance by the leader or a few members diminishes its usefulness to those who will not or cannot participate as much. For this reason, in group treatment maximum attention is given to the broadest possible distribution of participation.

Through group discussion the children build on the ideas of others. They try out new concepts and receive feedback from their peers. Through this exchange of ideas, members share values and are confronted with the values of others. Often they are forced to defend their ideas and sometimes, in discussion, to alter them.

By talking with each other in the protected setting of the treatment group, children gain confidence in their ability to speak reasonably. They gradually are able to transfer their speaking to other settings where speaking in groups is required.

Group discussion is fostered in children's groups in a number of ways. First, in early sessions, the group worker may shape participation through the distribution of tokens whenever anyone participates. If some dominate the discussion while others rarely speak, the leader may reinforce with a token until five tokens are received and then one token is deducted. The object of this "game" is to see how close the members can get to all receiving five tokens. The children have named this the *five token game.*

Another strategy is to provide children who participate too little in the group with cue cards. Whenever the leader asks a question for which they have been prepared in advance, they answer it with the help of the cue card. Later the card is faded. The child also receives token reinforcement that is also later faded.

A third strategy is to have the second leader or a highly active member coach the quieter children. A related approach is to use an inner circle of people who are permitted to participate while an outer circle of persons either serves as onlookers or coaches one member each.

A number of games can be used in which each person in turn is asked to explain something or describe an event. In this way children with slow response latency get a highly structured and protected opportunity to speak. For example, in a board game it is possible to insert the preceding instructions in one of the squares. When the person's piece lands on the square, he or she is required to help the group carry out a discussion on the given topic.

Group discussion is the cornerstone of all of the other strategies. Without adequate peer-to-peer discussion, little learning can take place. One particular form of group discussion occurs in and about role playing.

Role Playing

Role playing has repeatedly been an effective procedure for encouraging planned change. All of the strategies for working with children presented in this chapter could incorporate role-playing techniques to accommodate their various perspectives. In its most elementary form, *role playing* can be defined as the practice of roles in simulated conditions. The leader, by acting as a guide and structuring the role playing, influences the process and outcome of the role playing. If the leader is clear about the purposes of role playing, even through focused use, this technique can prove highly beneficial in promoting change. In social skills training, role playing is used both to demonstrate specific skills and to practice them. Demonstration is regarded as one form of modeling. Practice in a simulated setting is referred to as *behavioral rehearsal*. The steps of the modeling–rehearsal process have been discussed earlier.

A problem situation that is interactive may also be roleplayed to get a better understanding of the nature and details of the difficulty. Role playing will often reveal problem affect or problem behavior that mere description overlooks. Following brainstorming in the problem-solving process, it is helpful to roleplay the solutions, both good and bad. In contrast to role playing in social skills, where the leader directs the rehearsal, the focus here is on spontaneous role plays. The children are encouraged to play out in detail some of the possible alternatives. The leader directs the teaching process by following the role plays with discussions about feelings and consequences, including potential risks. The purpose is to guide the children to consequential thinking and a better understanding of the complexities of the problem.

Sociorecreational Activities

Sociorecreational activities involve the use of active games, board games, and dramatics that can be used to facilitate the achievement of therapeutic goals. Whittaker (1976) notes that,

> despite the popularity of group treatment as a mode of helping troubled children, many clinicians underestimate the potential of program activities as a medium for growth and change in groups. (p. 459)

Ross and Bernstein (1976, p. 127) state that "games and activities offer children and adolescents a workshop for discovering and developing new ways to manage obstacles."

Sociorecreational activities provide a highly satisfying set of stimulus conditions in which concrete skills can be informally practiced and reinforced. Sociorecreational activities form the initial basis for broad participation and increased group attraction. Furthermore, such activities provide the context for practicing social skills in a way that is more realistic and more entertaining than role playing.

Some commonly used examples for latency-aged children have been charades (to prepare for role playing), a detective game (to improve observational skills), competitive sports (to create the context for dealing with good winning and losing behaviors), board games (designed specifically to practice social skills), and puppet making (to increase motor skills, cooperative behavior, and create opportunity for public performance). It should be noted that in most cases activities are selected that have specific behavioral goals. The children may choose them themselves from an available list or from their own experience, but decisions are usually justified in terms of what one can learn.

In every group session, at least one such activity is incorporated into the program for all age groups. In the later phases of treatment with adolescents, they may choose to drop these activities. Failure to incorporate such activities into groups often results in dull group meetings and poorly motivated children.

In a group of 9- to 10-year-old boys, the following activities were incorporated into each of the sessions. The instructions were typed out and distributed to the children in advance so that they could teach the games to each other.

1. *Charades variation.* A child is chosen, and a card is attached to his or her back. This card identifies the child as a (a) bully; (b) best friend; (c) shy person; or (d) new person in the class. The others in the group act toward this child as if she or he was the character on the card. The "it" child then tries to guess which card is on his or her back. Repeat three more times.

2. *Making a group sign.* With a blank piece of poster board and colored markers, children are given time to help each other make a group sign identifying their group (or club).

3. *Eye spy.* Divide the group into two teams of two. Put out a tray with about 20 items and allow all to look at the tray for 2 to 3 minutes. Remove the tray and ask each team to write down as many of the things on the tray that they can remember. The team that remembers the most is the winner. Repeat one more time with new teams.

4. *Detective.* One child is chosen to be "it." The other children then "look over" this child. The "it" child then leaves the room and changes something about his or her appearance. When this child reenters the room, the other children try to guess what is changed. The first one to guess is the winner.

5. *Playing card basketball.* Divide the children into two teams. Divide a deck of cards into reds and blacks. Give one team reds and the other blacks. Then divide the colors among the children on the team. Put a bucket in the middle of a circle of all the children with each child facing a teammate. Set a timer or use a watch for 30-seconds. The teams must try to get all of their own color cards into the bucket before the time runs out (children should be just far enough from the

bucket to have to toss the cards). The team with the most in wins. Repeat several times.

6. *Wink! You're out.* Sit in a circle. Turn down the lights if you can. Pass out slips of paper to everyone; only one says, "You're it". The person who is "it" tries to wink at people without others seeing him or her. The person who is winked at waits a few seconds and then drops to the floor without telling who is "it." Others can guess who is "it," but if they are wrong they are out. The "it" child wins if she or he can wink all but the last person out.

7. *Miniature Olympics.* This consists of a Javelin throw with a straw, a shot-put with a balloon, and a low jump in "limbo" form under string held by two others (cannot touch the string). Let each child try each event.

Other Group Procedures

A number of group procedures are used other than those already mentioned. These include subgrouping, the buddy system, leadership delegation, and group exercises. These group procedures are unique to the group situation in that they are tasks that require the cooperation or effort of two or more persons.

Subgrouping is a simple procedure of working in subgroups of two to three persons in the group session as a means of getting broad participation. It also momentarily frees some of the children from the surveillance of the group leader and reduces, for some, the social pressure. It also provides some variety in the program as do the other group procedures.

> Terry, the leader, divided the girls into three groups of two, two, and three. She gave each subgroup the assignment of coming up with one suggestion within 3 minutes for a game that could be played next week and a homework assignment that each thought was important. She also noted that the game could not last longer than ten minutes.

The *buddy system* (Rose, 1972) is a subgroup of two or three members who meet outside the group either to carry out a homework assignment together, practice a role play, or encourage each other to carry out assignments. The buddy system, as with subgrouping, provides an opportunity for a semistructured, unsupervised interactive situation. Both forms of subgrouping also provide all parties with increased opportunities for leadership. This provides each child with an opportunity to participate in a high-status role. These leadership skills are usually valued in the classroom and represent an opportunity for each child to gain recognition outside the group for their accomplishments in the group. Another technique for training members in leadership skills is permitting the children themselves to serve as discussion leaders in the later phase of treatment.

Training is carried out first by evaluating what the group leader did when he or she led the sequence. The leader role is then rotated among all the members. With younger children, a cue card is given to the discussion leader. The cue card contains leader tips and the agenda. After each person plays the role, he or she receives feedback from the group.

Group exercises are as extensive as the imagination of the group leader permits. Discussion of case studies, sensitivity group exercises, and the "friendly seat" are all examples of exercises that fall outside the normal pattern of behavioral group therapy.

In the "friendly seat," all the children sit in a circle except the person who is "it" who sits in the middle. The children in the outside circle are numbered and then required to write down as many things as they can think of that the "it" person does well. As "it" calls the number of an outside person, that person responds with his or her praise statement. The exercise continues until all persons have given all their praise statements. Then another person is "it." The purpose of the exercise is to provide practice in the giving and receiving of praise. It also, like other exercises, serves to increase the attraction of the group.

Modifying Group Attributes

Group and individual procedures are often used together to modify group attributes that include the level of group cohesion, the distribution of group participation, the agreement to certain group norms or rules, the status of various children in the group, and the domination of a given member over others in the group. It is this concern for influencing group phenomena to mediate the modification of individual behavior that most dramatically distinguishes group from individual therapy. Most often when group data reveal a group problem (e.g., low satisfaction, low-homework-completion rate, group problem solving is used.

Modification of group process such as the communication pattern among adolescents was illustrated in a group of six children in which data revealed that two children spoke almost 60% of the time, and one less than 5% of the time. After we presented the data to the group, they agreed participation was a problem and developed a plan to implement at that meeting. The more active children agreed to reformulate the previous speaker's position before making a point of their own ("recapitulation"), and the less active children agreed to write down any thoughts they had relevant to the subject if they were disinclined to speak up. The leader agreed to call upon them to review their notes. The group practiced the complex plan for the following 5 minutes and decided to use it only twice a meeting for 20 minutes because it was somewhat disruptive. They also agreed to end it once the distribution of participation was somewhat more even. Thus, the plan utilized problem solving, recapitulation, cuing by the leader, and rehearsal.

In another group, teasing or "put downs" about in-group problems was reported by a child as having occurred between sessions. This infringement of an important group norm was immediately discussed as a group problem. The leader asked the members the consequences of the teasing to the both the tease and the person being teased. The group then developed a plan together to prevent its reoccurrance; this included confronting the tease assertively with what he or she was doing. The members roleplayed the confrontation in the group.

Another way of modifying group attributes is through the use of group rules. Several rules are explicitly established early in treatment. The first is that no one needs to agree to any specific homework suggestion, but once a child agrees to do it, he or she is expected at least to try to perform it. This rule is included in the group contract.

A second rule is that the therapist should be contacted if someone misses a meeting. In this way some of the new information as well as concerns about the meetings themselves can be handled over the phone.

A third rule involves each child's right to terminate criticism while receiving feedback if it is making him or her too uncomfortable. Although seldom invoked, this rule provides psychological protection to the child when his or her recent actions are being evaluated. A related rule is also designed to protect the child. No criticism can be presented to a child about his or her performance in a given situation until that same child has received positive evaluation over the same performance.

Of particular concern is the rule that personal information revealed in the group is not mentioned or discussed outside of the group. Jokes about behavior patterns are not acceptable inside or outside of the group. This is discussed at length in the first session.

Rules are sometimes made about personal aggression or other highly disruptive or damaging behaviors. These behaviors are dealt with as they occur either by the therapist or group so that clients can immediately experience the social consequences of such behavior. Even without rules, it becomes clear to the child that such behaviors will always be responded to immediately. The particular combination of the preceding procedures is selected only after a thorough assessment.

Assessment

Assessment is an integral part of all behavioral approaches. It refers to the strategies employed to collect information as a means of determining appropriate targets of change and of evaluating the ongoing effectiveness of therapy. In behavioral group treatment, assessment is also necessary for determining whether a person should be in a group, what kind of group that child should be in, the composition of groups, and the effect of ongoing group process. In general, the children discussed in this chapter are referred by the school or family member to the counselor or social worker who will be running the group. Occasionally, children refer themselves when they hear from acquaintances about the availability of a group. Recently, we have also been working with entire classrooms and in fact an entire grade (LeCroy, 1983) because of the school's interest in upgrading the social skills of all children in the given class. When children are referred, they are most often referred for friendship-making skills, social withdrawal, anger control, social problem-solving deficits, and other social deficits that parent, teacher, and/or child deem important. As we discuss in the section on group themes, not all groups are social skills or cognitive-behavioral skills training groups, although they rely heavily at some point on these procedures. For example, some children may be referred to a group consisting solely of children from recently divorced parents. A child is rarely excluded from a group once the referral process has been initiated. Only where the problem is so different from those in the group or where communication skills are extremely difficult because of age and/or socioemotional development would the child be referred elsewhere. This is discussed further in the section on group composition. Children are often seen simultaneously in group as well as individual treatment.

Assessment in groups often begins in a pregroup interview with the child and/or with significant others (e.g., parent, peers, teacher). The assessment process may involve the child and/or significant others. To a large extent, this depends upon the methodology used in assessment. To facilitate assessment, a number of procedures are used—a pregroup interview with the child and an interview with the adult who referred the child are particularly useful. Many leaders, particularly those concerned about using assessment for evaluation purposes, rely upon more objectively gathered information. For example, behavior checklists can be completed by parents or teachers who know the child (e.g., Miller, 1972; Quay & Peterson, 1967; Walker, 1970). For assessing social skills, a behavioral role-play test (Bornstein *et al.*, 1977; Edelson & Rose, 1978) can be used. This involves having children respond to a series of simulated situations as if they were in those situations. Sociometric testing (Gottman, 1977), where peers rate each other to determine a child's social status, is frequently used to assess the level of rejection by age-mates. Another assessment procedure is naturalistic observation of the child in the setting where problem behaviors occur (Rose, 1978). Last, self-report and self-monitoring procedures are often used, such as the Children's Action Tendency Scale (Deluty, 1979). These are easily administered and scored. An example of a self-monitoring procedure that is commonly used is a weekly diary in which the children keep track of problem situations and successful interpersonal exchanges. These descriptions of problem situations are used by the group leader more often than any other assessment procedure as a means of selecting specific treatment procedures to be used.

For purposes of assessing ongoing group process, observation of participation, estimating rate of homework completion, satisfaction as measured on a postsession questionnaire, and rates of attendance provide an empirical foundation for insight into how well the group is functioning (see Rose, 1984, for details).

Structure of Children's Groups

The *structure* of the group refers to the theme around which the group is organized, how the group is to be composed, the setting in which it takes place, the number of children in the group, the number and duration of each session, and the number of group leaders used.

Group Themes

There are many kinds of children's groups. The leader selects a theme based on the perceived needs of the population he or she expects to serve. If major focus is a simple social skills, for example, refusal responses when imposed on, a social skills group is the basic theme. Similar groups have been organized around themes of shyness or aggression.

If the potential clients are primarily deficient in problem-solving skills, this becomes the central theme of such a group. If the children are highly anxious, an anxiety-management or coping-with-stress theme is emphasized.

Some groups deal with children who are victims of abuse, unmarried teenage mothers, children of families in transition, siblings of the mentally ill, or adolescents in search of jobs. In these groups, the common theme shared by all is the social situation in which the children find themselves. In most of these groups, only a part of the program may be devoted to improving social competence. Other nondirective strategies may be used for dealing with grief, loss, and feelings of impotence. However, at some point many of these groups move toward improving or reinstating social competence with peers as an effective way of improving self-esteem and life satisfaction.

A theme is selected based on the needs of the population being served. In some cases, the referrals are so diverse that only a general treatment approach will be used in which diverse goals are pursued with diverse strategies. In long-term groups, this presents few problems. In short-term groups, the diversity often makes it difficult to provide sufficient relevant modeling and practice for every member in the time permitted. This is an issue of concern in the composition of groups.

Group Composition

Group composition refers to the way in which decisions are made as to the behavioral and population characteristics of children to be placed in a given group. At first consideration, group leaders may think about using a homogenous grouping. There would be practical advantages in this, for example, a group of all phobic children, would share common difficulties. But should groups be composed of children similar in such characteristics as age, sex, socioeconomic status, and emotional development? All of these attributes are considerations in group composition. In general, the more areas of similarity the greater the cohesion, but this is not always an advantage. For example, a group composed of all aggressive children of the same age and all male, although achieving a high level of cohesiveness, has on occasion led to antileader and antitherapeutic norms and a high frequency of in-group aggressive behavior. Based on our experience, a somewhat more complex basis for grouping than similar or dissimilar behavioral manifestations and population characteristics is suggested. We have used a system of ranking each of the group members' behavioral attributes as one methodology for grouping. The leader ranks the behavioral deficits or assets of each child on a scale from 1 to 10. The child is placed in a group in which at least one other member is near him on most of the continua. For each continuum, this may be a different person (see Rose, 1972, for examples). In this way every child has someone with whom he or she communicates (or whom the child feels understands his or her problem). There appears to be general consensus with regard to sex grouping. Most group experts suggest mixed-sex groups for young children but same-sex groups for elementary-school-aged children (Gazda, 1968). At the junior high level, mixed-sex groups are again recommended. When at least some of the problem is in relation to members of the opposite sex, mixed-sex composition is usually desirable. However, some adolescents are so disturbed by the presence of the opposite sex that in the early phases of treatment, same-sex groups for this particular complaint would be organized.

Similarity in age or social development seems also to be advisable. If the differences in age or social development are too great, the younger or less developed children tend to be excluded or lowered in status.

These are rough guidelines; there is no compelling research to suggest a particular grouping strategy. In fact, many of the groups we are involved with permit only a minimum of grouping decisions. This is frequently the case, where one only has a limited number of referrals or where the group is based on some form of self-selection.

Group Settings

Group settings are only limited by one's creative abilities in planning for groups. We have conducted young children's groups in nursery school and Head Start programs. Groups for older children have been organized in elementary, junior high, and senior high schools. Outpatient mental health centers and child guidance clinics have also made use of these behaviorally focused small groups. These types of groups can be an important adjunct in nonbehaviorally oriented settings. For example, in residential treatment centers, the use of short-term treatment groups has produced behavior changes that have ultimately affected the overall residential program (Elder *et al.*, 1979). This is particularly true when groups are oriented toward anger control, resisting peer pressure, and friendship skills.

The physical setting of the group does not seem to be a factor influencing outcome. Groups may end up in classrooms, homes, attics, storefronts, and even the back of stationwagons. The principles involved are twofold: simulate as nearly as possible the setting in which problems occur (Goldstein, Heller, & Sechrest, 1966) and find as attractive a setting as possible to increase group attractiveness.

Group Size

Group size is an important variable in group treatment with children insofar as it should allow for a high degree of interaction and participation among its members. Most experienced group workers limit their groups to three to eight members (Gazda, 1968). As size increases, the levels of participation, cohesiveness, and satisfaction are likely to decrease.

With adolescents, larger groups may be initially organized to encourage highly resistive adolescents to observe without getting involved. As the adolescents become interested in the program, intense subgrouping activities could be used to increase the therapeutic focus.

Frequency, Length, and Duration of Group Sessions

Although many group workers seek answers to questions regarding the frequency, length, and duration of groups, there is little research to provide guidelines. We assume that early in treatment the leader wants to increase group participation, build group cohesion, and provide ample reinforcement. Therefore, it may be beneficial to arrange a twice-a-week schedule to begin with, and then to fade the frequency of group meetings toward the end. A gradual fading of the group sessions helps in the maintenance of behaviors learned in the group once the group sessions have terminated (see the later discussion of this principle). In total, groups with children with a variety of behavior problems or severely troubled children should last between 10 to 16 sessions to maximize opportunities for behavior change. Groups with very defined and limited goals usually require fewer sessions to produce stable change.

The duration of group sessions, like almost everything else, tends to vary. Our groups have lasted from 30 minutes to much longer marathon sessions, although most last from 40 minutes to an hour. The younger the child, usually the shorter the duration of the group. Group leaders should consider the capacity of the group members to respond attentively if they are to learn effectively from the group experience. Practical considerations alone often play the determining roles in the decision as to the length of sessions. For example, in schools we are often restricted to the duration of lunch, recess, or left-over time from other classes.

Number of Leaders

In most groups, the number of leaders is one. Only when the leader or coleaders are in training have we added a second leader. Although having two leaders increases the richness of program ideas, it also tends to increase the amount of participation of the leader role. Furthermore, it can double the cost of treatment. However, in groups with severely acting-out children or large groups (nine or more), we do recommend more than one leader in order to have sufficient control over the group members and to monitor participation. An additional reason for having two leaders would be to provide male and female models in mixed-sex groups.

Phases of Group Treatment

One can identify at least four major, albeit overlapping, phases of group treatment: pregroup, orientation, treatment, and termination.

Pregroup Phase

During the pregroup phase the leader usually interviews the child, and depending on the referral source, the parent, teacher, supervisor, parole officer, or other significant persons in the child's life. The purpose of these interviews is to make three basic decisions: Is treatment necessary? Is group treatment appropriate? What kind of group would work for the potential child, and how should it be composed? The leader attempts to ferret out from each individual involved with the child at least some of the behavioral attributes of the child and to focus on specific incidents in which they are manifested. These interviews are usually brief, focused on precipitating events, and are geared toward the interactive pattern of the child and adult, and the interactive pattern of the child with other children.

In order to determine whether an individual should be treated at all, it is usually necessary to consider the ultimate consequences of his or her behavior were it to continue. In a given third grade, for example, the ultimate consequence would have been suspension from, or failure, in school for several boys involved in aggressive behavior. One also should not overlook the well-being of the teacher. There are also certain practical considerations in a recommendation for treatment. In the case of a teacher referral, Do the parents agree? Are adequate alternate resources available? Is there a danger that treatment will create only an additional handicap if the child, as a result, is labeled a "troublemaker" or "sick"?

As indicated previously, the group lends itself primarily to the treatment of interactive problems, and, as a rule of thumb, at least one of the child's major problems should be in the area of peer or sibling interaction. The reason for this rule is that the group provides an ideal laboratory for trying out new ways of interacting with peers. The leader can protect the child from the consequences of failure and can control the level of demand placed on each child as he or she is learning.

Orientation Phase

In the orientation phase, the leader introduces members to each other through group exercises. He or she attempts to build group cohesion through games and other social recreational activities.

It is helpful to establish some group rules early in the treatment. We have found that the children can usually voice all the necessary rules for being in a group that are conducive to making progress. The specific rules the leader needs to emphasize depend to some extent on the children in the group and the purpose of the group. In general, rules such as no fighting, no interrupting, and taking turns are of particular importance. The idea is to provide some general structure by sharing expectations about the group. Children quickly determine that the treatment group is much different than the classroom. For example, one does not need to raise his or her hand to talk; therefore, some initial group structure helps them understand what is expected of them.

It is also necessary to provide the children with a clear therapeutic contract. We let them know why they are being asked to be part of the group. We have found the following procedure for group orientation useful. Children were asked either in dyads or in the group, "What do you think this meeting is for?" The leader then discusses with the group the purposes of the group. Following this, it is helpful if the leader summarizes and adds the idea of normalization, for example, "All of us have problems doing something." Also, the leader usually stresses the interactional and treatment foci of the group and how the group is going to be oriented toward these.

Homework in this phase is usually a request for a description of situations in which the child has successfully and unsuccessfully coped with a stressful or problematic social situation. In this phase, most of the leadership functions are held by the group leader. The group session is usually highly structured, and there is a heavy use of concrete and verbal reinforcement.

Treatment Phase

In the treatment phase, problem situations are analyzed and solutions generated, modeled, repeatedly practiced, and evaluated. At first, common problem situations are worked on. Later, individual problem situations, which the child has recorded in his or her diary, are the focus of treatment. Homework to try out solutions to problem situations in the real world is designed, carried out between sessions, and subsequently monitored. Sociorecreational activities are continued but usually diminish in frequency. In this phase, preparation is already underway for transfer and maintenance of change. Responsibility for decision making is gradually shifted to the group and to individuals. The degree of structure begins to diminish, and reinforcement schedules are thinned.

Termination Phase

In this phase, the emphasis is on preparation for ending the group and generalization and maintenance of behavioral changes achieved in the group. Clients are prepared for termination by having them plan how they intend to apply what they learned in the group when the group finally ends. Possible self-referral sources are discussed, should the children feel they need it, such as the school counselor or a local clinic. The group leader identifies with each of the children the specific behavioral and cognitive cues for seeking outside help.

In order to help the group members end the relationship with the leader, the leader encourages members to establish relationships outside of the group and to become involved in extragroup activities, such as afterschool interests or sports groups, boy scouts, girl scouts, or YWCA groups. Furthermore, nongroup members whom they have befriended may be invited as guests to hear what they have achieved in the group. Assignments to carry out activities with these friends are encouraged. In this phase, material reinforcement is ended for homework completion and conformity to group rules. Homework, in fact, is less structured but more extensive. Preparation is largely in the hands of the child.

Monitoring is less strict. Social recreational and other cohesion-building activities are held to a minimum. Many of the leadership functions are performed by group members. Finally, as part of this phase, a follow-up could also include "booster" sessions 2 weeks to 2 months beyond termination. In the booster session the children have an opportunity to discuss their achievements and any new problems that may have arisen. If the group sessions end toward the end of the school year, it may be difficult to organize booster sessions in the fall as children go into other schools. Moreover, summer booster sessions are also difficult to arrange if the leaders are school personnel or if the children have diverse vacation plans. In private clinics or practice, practioners may arrange the booster sessions as part of the general package regardless of when the booster session occurs. School personnel are beginning to start their groups earlier so that booster sessions are possible in the spring.

Research Support

Thus far, a large number of assumptions and practice principles have been explicated. But what are the empirical foundations of the treatment package? There are a number of research studies that support components of this approach. Many of these have addressed, as we discussed, a given procedure. The direct social skills or assertion training approach has been demonstrated to be effective by Bornstein *et al.* (1977), Cooke and Apolloni (1976), Elder *et al.* (1979), Gottman, Gonzo, and Rasmussen (1975), and Minkin *et al.* (1976), using multiple baseline designs across behaviors. The target behaviors that changed as a result of treatment were conversational, socioemotional, and aggressive behaviors, with populations ranging from first-graders through adolescents. Kelly, Wildman, Urey, and Thurman (1979), Michelson and Wood (1980), O'Connor (1969, 1972), and Oden and Asher (1977) compared guided social skills training and/or coaching with control groups and found significant differences in favor of guided social skills training in various age groups. In our own studies with fifth- and sixth-graders, our results were less clear (Edelson & Rose, 1981), although the complex problem-solving, social skills training condition showed greater improvement on both the sociometric as well as role-play tests. The differences were not always significant.

The Oden and Asher (1977) study was the largest ($N = 99$) and methodologically the most elaborate and represents the best test to date of the largest component of the approach reported here. Using primarily coaching and a postcoaching review, Asher and Oden found that children in the experimental groups did better on a sociometric measure than groups of peers who merely played together or children who participated in isolated play. Ratings on a 1-year follow-up showed continued progress by the children in the experimental condition.

Michelson and Wood (1980) with two experimental and two control groups ($N = 80$) found that fourth-grade children receiving direct social skills training did better at follow-up and posttesting on self-report and teacher's ratings of their behavior than the controls. The authors also found that 16 hours of treatment were more effective than 8.

In summary, a broad base of empirical support exists for social skills training in groups for children and adolescents; however, many of those studies involved only small-sample designs. Where large-sample control group studies exist, the approach also is supported in almost all studies.

More modest support is found in the use of cognitive procedures with children. One of the few cognitive-behavioral studies using groups was the Kendal and Zupan (cited in Urbain & Kendall, 1980) study mentioned earlier. The authors compared a group and individual cognitive-behavioral approach with a nonspecific treatment control group. Thirty children, in the third to fifth grades, were randomally assigned to each of the conditions. Children in the individual and group conditions received self-instructional training with modeling and a response-cost contingency. There were 12 sessions of 45 to 55 minutes in length. Although all conditions showed improvement on impulsiveness as measured by the Matching Familiar Figures Test (MFFT) and on teacher ratings of hyperactivity, only the cognitive-behavioral conditions showed improvement on teacher ratings of self-control. No differences were noted between the group and individual cognitive-behavioral conditions.

Meichenbaum and Goodman (1971) in a controlled study trained impulsive children in individual sessions to talk to themselves as a successful means of developing self-control. McCullough, Huntsinger, and Nay (1977) and Strober and Bellack (1975) have reported case studies involving use of cognitive restructuring as one component in treatment programs that have reduced aggressive behavior. In addition, cognitive restructuring has shown some degree of success in group treatment programs with aggressive children and adolescents (Block, 1978; Camp, Blom, Herbert, & Van Doorninck, 1977; Goodwin & Mahoney, 1975; Robin, Schneider, & Dolnick, 1976). Spivack, Platt, and Shure (1976) report on various studies in which children have been effectively taught problem-solving skills, although the role of the group in these studies was not explicated.

As yet, the entire approach described in this chapter has not been tested, although several such studies are now in various stages of development. In our own study, where all of the intervention strategies were used, we found that social skills, problem-solving, and social-cognitive training did almost equally well in improving social competence, and all subjects did better than the subjects in an attention-placebo control group. A combined approach with seventh- and eighth-grade children seemed to be an improvement over the component approaches (LeCroy, 1983).

Summary

Research has supported the importance of children learning socially competent behaviors. As a result, practitioners have introduced treatment programs in a variety of settings to help troubled children become more socially adjusted.

We have presented a group model for enhancing social competence in children. This approach emphasizes empirically derived behavioral, cognitive-behavioral methods, and small-group approaches. It deals explicitly with the group context as the focus of treatment. Within that context the cognitive-behavioral strategies of social skills training, problem-solving training, and cognitive restructuring are introduced. The group model represents a comprehensive treatment package for group leaders and presents guidelines for establishing and maintaining children's groups within various settings.

This model presents a somewhat technical and structured group treatment approach. Although technical, we emphasize the importance of programming to make the group as attractive as possible without losing its treatment focus. As research continues in group approaches with children we foresee a practical group model with well-developed quidelines and interventive strategies. With procedures becoming more refined, we can look forward to a more scientific and effective approach to treatment aimed at improving the social competence of children.

References

Asher, S. R. Children's peer relations. In M. E. Lamb (Ed.), *Social and personality development*. New York: Holt, Rinehart & Winston, 1978.

Bandura, A. *Social learning theory*. Englewood Cliffs, N.J.: Prentice-Hall, 1977.

Bash, M. A. S., & Camp, B. W. Teaching training in the think aloud classroom program. In G. Cartledge & J. F. Milburn (Eds.), *Teaching social skills to children*. New York: Pergamon Press, 1980.

Block, J. B. Effects of a rational-emotive mental health program on poorly achieving, disruptive high school students. *Journal of Counseling Psychology*, 1978, *23*, 61–65.

Bornstein, M. R., Bellack, A. S., & Hersen, M. Social-skills training for unassertive children: A multiple baseline analysis. *Journal of Applied Behavior Analysis*, 1977, *10*, 183–195.

Camp, B. W., Blom, G. F., Herbert, F., & van Doorninck, W. J. "Think aloud": A program for developing self-control in young aggressive boys. *Journal of Abnormal Child Psychology*, 1977, *5*, 157–169.

Cartledge, G., & Milburn, J. F. *Teaching social skills to children*. New York: Pergamon Press, 1980.

Cartwright, D., & Zander, A. (Eds.). *Group dynamics: Research and theory* (3rd ed.). Evanston, Ill.: Row, Peterson, 1968.

Clark, H. R., Wood, R., & Northrop, J. The family and education: New directions for promoting healthy social interactions. In J. B. Jordan & R. C. Sarri (Eds.), *Disruptive youth in school*. Reston, Utah: Council for Exceptional Children, 1980.

Conger, J. C., & Keane, S. P. Social skills intervention in the treatment of isolated or withdrawn children. *Psychological Bulletin*, 1981, *90*, 478–495.

Cooke, T. P., & Apolloni, T. Developing positive social-emotional behaviors: A study of training and generalization effects. *Journal of Applied Behavior Analysis*, 1976, *9*, 65–78.

Cowen, E. L., Pederson, A., Babigian, H., Izzo, L. D., & Trost, M. A., Long-term follow-up of early detected vulnerable children. *Journal of Consulting and Clinical Psychology*, 1971, *41*, 438–446.

Deluty, R. H. A Children's Action Tendency Scale. Unpublished manuscript, 1979.

Edelson, J. L., & Rose, S. D. *A behavioral roleplay test for assessing children's social skills*. Paper presented at the Annual Convention of the Association for Advancement of Behavior Therapy, Chicago, 1978.

Edelson, J. L., & Rose, S. D. Investigation into the efficacy of short-term group skills training for socially isolated children. *Child Behavior Therapy*, 1981, *3*, 1–16.

Elder, J. P., Edelstein, B. A., & Narick, N. M. Adolescent psychiatric patients and modifying a juvenile behavior with social skills training. *Behavior Modification*, 1978, *3*, 161–178.

Evers, W., & Schwartz, J. Modifying social withdrawal in preschoolers: The effects of filmed modeling and teacher praise. *Journal of Abnormal Psychology*, 1973, *1*, 248–256.

Foster, S. L., & Ritchey, W. L. Issues in the assessment of social competence in children. *Journal of Applied Behavior Analysis*, 1979, *12*, 625–638.

Gazda, G. M. A functional approach to group counseling. In G. M. Gazda (Ed.), *Basic approaches to group psychotherapy and group counseling*. Springfield, Ill.: Charles C Thomas, 1968.

Goldstein, A. P., Heller, K., & Sechrest, L. B. *Psychotherapy and the psychology of behavior change*. New York: Wiley, 1966.

Goldstein, A. P., Martens, H. J., Van Belle, H. A., Schaaf, W., Wiersma, H., & Goedhart, A. The use of modeling to increase independent behavior. *Behaviour Research and Therapy*, 1973, *11*, 31–42.

Goodwin, S. E., & Mahoney, M. J. Modification of aggression through modeling: An experimental probe. *Journal of Behavior Therapy and Experimental Psychology*, 1975, *6*, 200–202.

Gottman, J. Toward a definition of social isolation in children. *Child Development*, 1977, *48*, 513–517.

Gottman, J., Gonso, J., & Rasmussen, B. Social interaction, social competence and friendship in children. *Child Development*, 1975, *46*, 709–718.

Hartup, W. W. Peer relations and the growth of social competence. In M. W. Kent & J. E. Rolf (Eds.), *Primary prevention of psychopathology* (Vol. 3): *Social competence in children*. Hanover, N.H.: University Press of New England, 1979.

Hartup, W. W. Peer relations and family relations: Two social worlds. In M. Rutter (Ed.), *Scientific foundations of developmental psychiatry*. London: Heineman Medical, 1980.

Hazel, J. S., Schumaker, J. B., Sherman, J. A., & Sheldon-Wildgen, J. *ASSET: A social skills program for adolescents*. Champaign, Ill.: Research Press, 1981.

Keller, M., & Carlson, P. The use of symbolic modeling to promote social skills in preschool children with low levels of responsiveness. *Child Development*, 1974, *45*, 912–919.

Kelly, J. A., Wildman, B. G., Urey, J. R., & Thurman, C. Group skills training to increase the conversational repertoire of retarded adolescents. *Child Behavior Therapy*, 1979, *1*, 323–336.

Kohn, M., & Clausen, J. Social isolation and schizophrenia. *American Sociological Review*, 1955, *20*, 265–273.

Ladd, G. W. Effectiveness of a social learning method for enhancing children's social interaction and peer acceptance. *Child Development*, 1981, *52*, 171–178.

LaGreca, A. M., & Mesibov, G. B. Social skills intervention with learning disabled children: Selecting skills and implementing training. *Journal of Clinical Child Psychology*, 1979, *8*, 234–241.

LaGreca, A. M., & Santogrossi, D. A. Social skills training with elementary school students: A behavioral group approach. *Journal of Consulting and Clinical Psychology*, 1980, *48*, 220–227.

LeCroy, C. W. *Promoting social competence in early adolescents: An experimental investigation*. Unpublished doctoral dissertation, University of Wisconsin-Madison, 1983.

Lott, B. E., & Lott, A. J. The formation of positive attitudes toward group members *Journal of Abnormal and Child Psychology*, 1961, *61*, 297–300.

McCullough, J. P., Huntsinger, G. M., & Nay, W. R. Self-control treatment of aggression in a 16-year-old male. *Journal of Consulting and Clinical Psychology*, 1977, *45*, 322–331.

Meichenbaum, D. H. *Cognitive behavior modification*. New York: Plenum Press, 1977.

Meichenbaum, D. H., & Goodman, J. Training impulsive children to talk to themselves: A means of developing self control. *Journal of Abnormal Psychology*, 1971, *77*, 115–126.

Michelson, L., & Wood, R. A group assertive training program for elementary school-children. *Child Behavior Therapy*, 1980, *2*, 1–9.

Miller, L. C. School Behavior Checklist: An inventory of deviant behavior for elementary school children. *Journal of Consulting and Clinical Psychology*, 1972, *38*, 134–144.

Minkin, N., Braukmann, C. J., Minkin, B. L., Timbers, G. D., Timbers, B. J., Fixsen, D. L., Phillips, E. L., & Wolf, M. M. The social validation and training of conversational skills. *Journal of Applied Behavior Analysis*, 1976, *9*, 127–139.

O'Connor, R. D. Modification of social withdrawal through symbolic modeling. *Journal of Applied Behavior Analysis*, 1969, *2*, 15–22.

O'Connor, R. D. Relative efficacy of modeling, shaping and the combined procedures for modification of social withdrawal. *Journal of Abnormal Psychology*, 1972, *79*, 327–334.

Oden, S., & Asher, S. R. Coaching children in social skills for friendship making. *Child Development*, 1977, *48*, 495–506.

Quay, H. C., & Peterson, D. R. *Manual for the Behavior Problem Checklist*. Champaign, Ill.: Children's Research Center, University of Illinois, 1967.

Robin, A., Schneider, M., & Dolnick, M. The turtle technique: An extended case study of self-control in the classroom. *Psychology in the Schools*, 1976, *12*, 120–128.

Roff, M. Childhood social interaction and young adults' bad conduct. *Journal of Abnormal Social Psychology*, 1961, *63*, 333–337.

Roff, M., Sells, S. B., & Golden, M. M. *Social adjustment and personality development in children*. Minneapolis: University of Minnesota Press, 1972.

Rose, S. D. *Treating children in groups*. San Francisco: Jossey-Bass, 1972.

Rose, S. D. *Observation system for the classroom*. Unpublished manuscript, University of Wisconsin-Madison, 1978.

Rose, S. D. Fun and games in children treatment groups. *Behavior Group Therapy*, 1983, *5*(1), 2–9.

Rose, S. D. The use of data in resolving group problems, *Social Work with Groups*, 1984, *7*(2), 23–36.

Ross, A. L., & Bernstein, N. B. A framework for the therapeutic use of group activities. *Child Welfare*, 1976, *56*, 776–786.

Spivack, G., & Shure, M. B. *Social adjustment of young children: A cognitive approach to solving real life problems*. San Francisco: Jossey-Bass, 1974.

Spivack, G., Platt, J. J., & Shure, M. B. The problem-solving approach to adjustment. San Francisco: Jossey-Bass, 1976.

Stevens, T. M. *Social skills in the classroom* Columbus, Ohio: Cedar Press, 1978.

Strober, M., & Bellack, A. S. Multiple component behavioral treatment for a child with behavior problems. *Journal of Behavior Therapy and Experimental Psychiatry*, 1975, *6*, 250–252.

Swetnam, L., Peterson, C. R., & Clark, H. B. In C. S. LeCroy, (Ed.), *Social skills training for children and youth*. New York: Haworth Press, 1983.

Urbain, E., & Kendall, P. Review of social-cognitive problem-solving interventions with children. *Psychological Bulletin*, 1980, *88*, 109–143.

Walker, H. *Problem Behavior Identification Checklist*. Los Angeles: Western Psychological Services, 1970.

Whitehall, M. B., Hersen, M., & Bellack, A. S. Conversation skills training for socially isolated children. *Behaviour Research and Therapy*, 1980, *18*, 217–225.

Whittaker, J. K. Differential use of program activities in child treatment groups. *Child Welfare*, 1976, *55*, 459–468.

Wodarski, J. S., Hamblin, R. J., Buckholdt, D. R., & Perritor, D. E. Individual contingencies versus different shared consequences contingent on the performance of low achieving group members. *Journal of Applied Social Psychology*, 1973, *3*, 276–290.

8

Group Social Skills Training with Adolescents

A Critical Review

J. STEPHEN HAZEL, JAMES A. SHERMAN, JEAN BRAGG SCHUMAKER, AND JAN SHELDON

INTRODUCTION

Over the past decade, social skills training in groups has become a popular method of therapy for adolescents. This treatment approach has evolved from work in several fields: research in applied behavior analysis focusing on social skills training with court-adjudicated adolescents (e.g., Phillips, Phillips, Fixsen, & Wolf, 1972); research by social psychologists (e.g., Argyle, 1972); work by clinical psychologists (e.g., Goldstein, 1973); and group work with children, adolescents, and adults (e.g., Rose, 1972; 1977). Group therapy programs have most often been implemented with "problem adolescents," those who are usually labeled as "acting out" and who frequently exhibit severe social skills deficiencies. Because group therapy is often considered an economical form of treatment, particularly when a large number of adolescents need the same type of therapy, it has been conducted in schools, group homes, and institutions.

On the one hand, a number of advantages have been ascribed to conducting therapy in groups. Upper and Ross (1977) and Trower, Bryant, and Argyle (1978) discuss the advantages in terms of efficiency with regard to the therapist's time, greater opportunities for behavioral rehearsal with a variety of people, greater generalization because practice can occur in the social context of a group of people, and because of the variety of stimuli provided by the participants, more effective feedback on performance, greater experience with a larger number of problem situations, more support for problem solutions, less intimidation for the youths because they are with people having similar problems,

J. STEPHEN HAZEL, JAMES A. SHERMAN, JEAN BRAGG SCHUMAKER, and JAN SHELDON • University of Kansas, Lawrence, Kansas 66045.

and greater social reinforcement. Sansbury (1979) proposed several hypotheses concerning the potential benefits of conducting therapy in groups. As applied to social skills training, the most relevant hypotheses include saving the therapist's time, the availability of multiple models, the enhancement of discrimination learning, and greater generalization of new coping behaviors to a wider range of situations.

On the other hand, Lieberman (1975) points out a number of potential disadvantages for behavioral group therapy. He argues that, in a group, the leader may not be able to remain in control of the situation. For example, whether the group reinforces appropriate behavior or not may be more a function of group norms than group leader input. Thus, the group therapy session, according to Lieberman, is an imprecise setting in which to conduct therapy because the leader may not be able to implement the procedure that he or she desires. Another problem with group therapy was raised by Kelly (1982) who stated that skills training in groups may be difficult with individuals who exhibit varying rates of skills acquisition. A pace for slow learners may bore the quicker learners, whereas a faster pace may frustrate slow learners. Trower *et al.* (1978) specified two possible disadvantages of group social skills training: (a) the poor or inappropriate modeling that might be exhibited by group members; and (b) loss of flexibility in dealing with individual problems.

Thus, a number of advantages and disadvantages have been discussed with regard to behavioral group therapy in general. It is not clear which of these factors plays a significant role in group social skills training with adolescents. A number of articles on group social skills training with adolescents emphasize that problem behaviors can occur in group settings (De Lange, Lanham, & Barton, 1981; Hazel, Schumaker, Sherman, & Sheldon-Wildgen, 1981b; Rotheram, 1980). Typical problem behaviors discussed by these authors include inattentiveness, disruptiveness, nonresponsiveness, inappropriately delivered criticism, peer pressure to behave inappropriately, and high dropout rates. Whether these problems negate the advantages of group training is unclear. These same authors offer possible solutions to many of the problems. In fact, a few studies have been conducted to specifically examine procedures to modify these problem behaviors. For example, Hauserman, Zweback, & Plotkin (1972) showed that token reinforcement could increase the rate of verbal initiations in an adolescent group in which the group members had a low rate of verbal statements. Therefore, specific problems that occur within the group therapy session with adolescents may be amenable to change through the use of behavioral contingencies and other appropriate procedures.

Although there may be problems associated with conducting group social skills training with adolescents, this type of training has been used extensively as a treatment of choice for problem adolescents. In addition to the advantages of group therapy described previously, the basic logic for the social skills training of adolescents in groups is that (a) social skills are behaviors that are learned; (b) large numbers of adolescents fail to learn these behaviors for a variety of reasons; and (c) without these skills, adolescents will encounter a variety of problems in their everyday lives because social interactions occupy a large amount of their time and appropriate social skills are important for obtaining desired rewards. A number of authors have used these rationales to focus attention on teaching social skills to groups of adolescents, particularly those adolescents who are experiencing problems in getting along with others at home, in school, or in the community. It has been hypothesized that, through training in social skills, these adolescents can learn more appropriate, alternative ways of behaving, can incorporate these new skills into their repertoires, and can use them as the need arises (Hazel *et al.*, 1981b).

Alternative hypotheses to the social skills deficiency hypothesis have been advanced with regard to deficits in social skills performance. For example, some theorists postulate that most individuals have learned how to perform a social skill, but some are inhibited, typically by anxiety, from performing the skill (Arkowitz, 1981). This type of analysis would shift the focus of social skills training away from the training of actual social skills to the training of techniques, such as relaxation techniques, that could be used in an effort to counter the anxiety experienced in social interactions. Although performance inhibition may be a significant problem in certain social performance areas (e.g., dating) (Arkowitz, Lichtenstein, McGovern, & Hines, 1975), little work has focused on alleviating it in problem adolescents. Thus, this review will focus on the literature concerned with the training of actual social skills to groups of adolescents and issues related to the training of social skills in group therapy sessions.

Because social skills training with adolescents is concerned with teaching those skills to adolescents that are necessary for successful social interactions, success of this training is dependent upon the determination of the necessary content for social skills training and the use of effective procedures to teach social skills to adolescents in groups. Because a number of problems continue to exist in specifying the appropriate content (i.e., social skills) and training procedures for adolescent social skills groups, neither of these determinations has been made.

In the following sections, the problems associated with the content of group social skills training programs and the teaching methods to be employed in group social skills training will be addressed in view of the goal of the development of an "ideal" group social skills training program for adolescents. A review of the methods that have been used to select social skills for training programs will be followed by a discussion of critical issues that must be considered with regard to the selection of skills to be trained. Next, a review of the methods used to select social skills components to be trained will precede a critical discussion of these and additional methods that might be used. Then the social skills that actually have been trained and the ways they have been defined and measured will be described. Next, the training procedures that have been commonly used in empirically based research studies focusing on the group training of social skills to adolescents will be reviewed. Finally, the outcomes of empirically based group social skills training studies will be evaluated, and recommendations for future research will be made.

The Content of Group Social Skills Training Programs for Adolescents

One of the most important decisions that must be made in developing a group social skills training program for adolescents is the determination of the skills to be trained. Only by correctly identifying the areas of social skills deficiency and choosing appropriate skills to remediate these deficiencies can developers of a program ensure that the program is functional for adolescent trainees. After the skills have been chosen, the next task is to determine the behaviors that comprise each skill.

Although the determination of the content for a social skills program is very important, it is difficult to make this determination because of the lack of an adequate definition of social skills. When we refer to a person as being socially competent or socially skilled, it indicates that the person has displayed a repertoire of behaviors in interacting with others that are judged to be appropriate and successful. Thus, although the term refers to a repertoire or set of behaviors of a person, it is based on the judgments or opinions of other people. If one refers to another person as "socially skilled," it is roughly equivalent to saying, "I have observed this person interacting with others, and this person behaves in ways that seem appropriate to me and that are likely to produce positive outcomes for the person with regard to getting along with others." The statement, of course, is deceptively simple. If the label *socially skilled* as a summary statement about the person's past performances is to have predictive utility about how the person's behavior will be judged by others in the future, it seems necessary that, at a minimum, the one providing the label must have observed the person's behavior in past situations that are similar to those that will occur in the future, must share with future observers common criteria for appropriateness and common expectations for what kinds of behavior will produce what kinds of consequences, and must respond to the situations as future observers would about what the person's purposes or goals are with regard to the interaction.

Further, the judgments about the person's social skills within a particular instance of social interaction must be sifted or passed through a series of filters that affect the judgment. These filters include the circumstances that surround the interaction and the characteristics of the people involved. For example, a particular set of behaviors that occur in the supermarket, such as those involved in starting a casual conversation, may be judged as appropriate in the supermarket but perhaps would not be judged appropriate on the job during busy working hours. The kinds of behaviors judged appropriate for a teenager in a particular interaction may be very different than those judged appropriate for a middle-aged person. The kinds of adolescent interactions judged likely to be successful with peers are somewhat different than those judged likely to be successful with an employer or teacher. Judgements about the purpose or desired outcomes of a casual conversation with friends will probably be different than those about the purpose or desired outcome of a negotiation of a problem between a brother and sister. The kinds of behaviors judged appropriate between two people who know each other well will vary from those judged appropriate between two people who have just met, and so on. Thus, the summary term *socially skilled* used about a person not only encompasses the behavior of the person and some commonly held notions about appropriateness, purposes, and probable success but also includes an extremely complex set of circumstances that surround a particular interaction and the characteristics of the participants.

In spite of the tremendous complexity involved in making a judgment about the general social skills of another person or even about making such a judgment with regard to a more specific skill such as maintaining a conversation, common experience suggests that these judgements can be made with some reliability. There are some people who are judged with a fair degree of reliability as being "socially skilled" in general; there are others who are consistently judged to be "not socially skilled." Even though it may be possible to make judgments about what is meant by socially skilled, unfortunately there are no agreed-upon methods for determining what social skills should be taught for particular social problems, how those social skills are to be grouped and defined, and for establishing the component behaviors of these skills. In this section, the methods that have been reported in the literature for selecting, grouping, and defining social skills and the behavioral components of these skills for group social skills training programs for adolescents will be reviewed. Additionally, alternative methods for selecting and grouping skills and their components will be discussed.

Selection Methods for Social Skills

A Review of Methods Used to Select Skills

A number of different procedures have been used to identify the social skills to be taught in adolescent group training programs. One procedure that has been used involves a review of research literature. For example, Hendrix and Heckel (1982) identified skills to be taught based on the research literature on social reinforcement and reciprocity. Minkin, Minkin, Goldstein, Taylor, Braukmann, Kirigin, and Wolf (1981) used a review of previous research with delinquent youths to identify peer criticism as an important skill. Spence and Marzillier (1979) chose skills that had been identified as important by other researchers. Similarly, a number of researchers focusing on assertion training (e.g., Lee, Hallberg, & Hassard, 1979; Ollendick & Hersen, 1979; Pentz, 1980; Pentz & Kazdin, 1982) relied on the research literature indicating the importance of assertion training for a variety of populations.

Another approach that has been used to identify skills to be taught relies on the clinical and professional experience of the program developers. For instance, Golden, Twentyman, Jensen, Karan, and Kloss (1980) based the skills to be taught in their program on their own previous experience and observation of skills deficits of juvenile offenders. In a similar fashion, Gross, Brigham, Hopper, and Bologna (1980) determined the skills to be trained based on their professional experience.

A third approach that has been used to identify social skills to be taught to groups of adolescents involves interviewing and/or surveying (through the use of questionnaires) the actual program participants, a representative sample of potential participants, or significant others in the youths' lives to determine common problem areas. De Lange *et al.* (1981), for example, interviewed 60 adolescents who identified common problem situations that were then grouped into skills categories. Sarason and Ganzer (1973) taught skills based on problem situations frequently mentioned by youths in a pilot study as being particularly difficult. Elder, Edelstein, and Narick (1979), in addition to interviewing the adolescent trainees, asked staff members at a psychiatric institution to describe behavioral excesses and deficits of the target population. Sarason and Sarason (1981) conducted interviews with a sample of students, former students, teachers, counselors, and employers about the common problems of students at a high school serving a student population with high rates of delinquency.

A fourth method that has been used to determine the social skills to be taught to groups of adolescents involves the observation of adolescent trainees in social interactions. From the resultant observational data, specific deficits are identified, and skills are targeted for training. This procedure relies on the judgments of the program developers to decide (a) what behaviors are to be observed; (b) what constitutes a deficit; (c) for the deficits identified, which social skills are related to ameliorating those deficits; and (d) which skills have the highest priority for training. Heimberg, Cunningham, Stanley, and Blankenberg (1982), in determining the necessary skills for job interviews, conducted a series of role-play job interviews with the participants. The participants' performances were evaluated to determine their skills deficits in this area.

Still other program developers have used combinations of the approaches described previously. By way of illustration, Hazel *et al.* (1981b) initially identified a list of skills to be taught to youths on probation by asking their probation officers to identify problem areas, by reviewing the research literature, and by selecting skills based on the developers' clinical experience. The identified skills were then validated by comparing the list to problem reports of parents and youths as well as by having parents and professionals rate the importance of the skills.

Thus, a variety of methods have been utilized to select particular social skills to be taught to groups of adolescents. Social skills selection has been based on literature reviews, the experience of the people developing the skills training program, interviews with and questionnaires completed by potential learners of the skills and people who are familiar with potential learners, observation of role-play performances, and combinations of these approaches.

Comments on the Methods Used to Select Social Skills

As indicated before, the selection of social skills to be taught in a training program is extremely important if the program is to achieve desired outcomes. Clearly, the popular methods for the selection of skills are heavily based on the opinions of people, as evidenced by the reliance on literature reviews, clinical and professional judgments of program developers, interviews with, and questionnaire surveys of, potential learners and people familiar with them, and observational methods. Are these reasonable methods for selecting the social skills to be taught?

A partial answer to the question lies in the success with which these methods have resulted in the teaching of social skills that have had clearly beneficial effects on the lives of participating youths and those around them. For example, assume that the goals of a program are to teach the skills of instruction following and accepting negative feedback so that adolescents are more likely to obtain and keep their jobs. If these skills are taught and participating adolescents are more likely to obtain and keep a job than initially similar adolescents who were not taught the skills, then most of us would agree that the social skills taught were (and are) important ones.

As will be discussed in more detail later in this chapter, the developers of a number of social skills programs have attempted to measure the effects of social skills training on the lives of the participating adolescents. Some of the effects have been determined through the use of questionnaires. For example, there have been questionnaires completed by the participating adolescents (e.g., concerning their self-concept, their anxiety level, their attitudes), and there have been questionnaires given to significant others in the learners' lives (e.g., concerning the changes they have perceived in the learner) before and after the training experience. Other developers have determined whether there were more objective or overt changes in the lives of the learners (e.g., by measuring changes in juvenile court contacts). Many of the studies conducted by these developers have suggested that beneficial changes in the lives of the learners resulted from the social skills training. These results would suggest that the use of peoples' opinions to select social skills to be taught is a reasonably good method.

Nevertheless, several qualifications need to be noted. First, few of the researchers in the area have attempted to provide an evaluation of the *direct* effects of group social skills training on learners' lives. Second, many individuals who have attempted an evaluation have not always employed an experimental design that allows the conclusion that the observed changes were specifically a result of social skills training. Third, there seem to be differences in the quality or importance of the measures that have been used to document changes in the learners' lives. For example, use of a self-report questionnaire may suggest some possible beneficial changes in a person's life; however, without some corroborating objective evidence of changes in the person's life, a self-report measure seems less socially significant than, say, measures of employment obtained, measures of school performance, and measures of juvenile court contacts. Thus, at issue here is what kinds of evidence are judged to be more important or more socially significant than others. Even if the types of appropriate evidence could be agreed upon, there appear to be important practical limitations on what can be done in evaluating the effects of social skills training on events in adolescents' lives. Often it is not clear when the actual outcomes or consequences of training will become evident and under what circumstances they will become apparent.

Thus, it is unclear when or where to look for the actual outcomes in the natural environment. Many times, researchers may need to rely on questionnaires or interviews with learners and significant others in the learners' lives to judge the success of social skills training programs. The fourth problem with relying on peoples' judgments is that validation of the importance of a social skill must then come after the fact. That is, developers must invest much time and effort in training a skill and measuring the effects of the training before they can be sure they chose the correct skill(s).

The validity of these qualifications probably could be evaluated through an increased emphasis on determining the effects of social skills training on the real-life behavior of the participating youths and the use of experimental designs that more clearly establish that the changes in real-life behavior are a result of the social skills training. Although these would be difficult tasks, they appear to be within current research capabilities.

Thus, as long as several qualifications are noted, selection methods that rely on peoples' judgments appear to be reasonably successful. At the present time, alternatives that do not rely on peoples' judgments do not seem apparent. One variant of the typically used skills selection procedures might offer more precision. This alternative procedure for selecting social skills to be included in group training programs for adolescents would involve the observation of people who are judged to be unsuccessful at a particular task and the comparison of their performances to the performances of people who are judged to be successful at that task. For example, one might observe the social skills of people who are judged to be successful at a particular job, or in obtaining dates, or in conversing with others, or in making friends, or in staying out of juvenile court (assuming that these are all judged to be socially important outcomes) and similarly observe the social skills of people who are judged to be not successful in these activities. Obvious differences in social skills displayed by successful and not-so-successful people would suggest the possible functional role of particular social skills. Clearly, this method relies on the judgments of people, but in this case it relies on judgments about who is successful and who is not, about what behaviors are to be observed, what constitutes a socially significant difference between the two groups, and what skills have higher priority than others for training. Nevertheless, the method allows one to examine and compare, in detail, particular behaviors displayed by people in representative life situations. Whether this approach will allow program developers to predict more accurately the social skills that are critical for successful functioning in real life remains to be seen.

Thus, for all practical purposes, it appears that the use of judgments of people will probably be a continuing characteristic in the selection of social skills to be taught, whether the judgments are used to select the skills directly or to select people judged as successful or unsuccessful at a particular activity and the behaviors to be observed in these people. Whether these judgments (of particular skills or of success) should be made by the developer of the social skills training program, the potential learners, significant others in the potential learners' lives, experienced professionals familiar with the potential population of learners, or some combination of all of these, is not known at the present time.

Additional research that specifies the relationship between the method of skills selection used and the outcomes of training programs is clearly needed.

Although it seems inevitable that the judgments of others will play a critical role in the selection of skills to be taught in programs or to be observed in successful and unsuccessful individuals, two additional cautions should be mentioned. First, developers should ensure that the skills that are selected for training include both "reactive" skills and "initiatory" skills. On the basis of our observations, there appear to be marked differences among various social situations in the extent to which a person is expected or obligated to respond. For example, if a teenager is told to do something by a teacher or employer, the teenager is expected to verbally acknowledge the instruction, ask for clarification, and perhaps explain why the instruction cannot be followed. Usually, he or she is expected to follow the instruction. Similarly, if someone approaches a youth and asks a question, rules of appropriate social conduct require an answer, an indication that the youth does not know the answer, or a suggestion of another person to ask. In contrast, few situations so strongly require someone to initiate a conversation, ask a question, or give criticism. Many situations may make these behaviors permissible or appropriate, but few make them obligatory.

It seems possible that relying on the judgments of people to select social skills to be taught or observed could result in a heavy emphasis on those behaviors that are obligatory or reactive to situations rather than those that are permissible or self-initiated, primarily because the failure to engage in those expected or obligatory behaviors is more obvious and viewed as more damaging than the absence of behaviors that are more permissible or self-initiated. On the one hand, this may be reasonable because a teenager's failure to respond in situations in which some kind of behavior is required is highly likely to result in the judgment that the teenager is not socially skilled. On the other hand, if all or a heavy preponderance of the social skills selected for a training program are of the obligatory or reactive type, the training program will not teach the kinds of social skills (e.g., initiating and maintaining conversations, making new friends, and dating skills) that have a high likelihood of enhancing the adolescent's own satisfaction with life. Thus, when one is determining the skills to be covered in a training program, a representative sample of the youths who are going to be trained should be asked for their input with regard to the initiatory skills they feel are missing in their repertoires. Others who are asked for judgments should be specifically prompted to suggest skills that are self-initiated. When observational methods are to be used, developers should take care to observe opportunities for initiatory skills and whether initiatory skills are used following these opportunities.

A second caution related to the use of judgments of people to select skills to be taught is that care should be taken to identify the specific kinds of situations to which the skills should be related in training. Typically, such judgments fail to indicate precisely the kinds of situations in which the skills need to be taught. For example, a teenager may be regarded as deficient in response to situations in which he or she is criticized. Nevertheless, the teenager may not respond appropriately when criticized by a teacher in school, yet he or she may well respond appropriately when criticized by an employer about a job performance. Alternatively, the teenager may respond appropriately to criticism from others when it is combined with some praise for appropriate behavior and given in a normal conversational voice tone, but he or she may respond inappropriately when criticism is given in a harsh or sarcastic voice tone and not accompanied by any praise. Furthermore, the teenager's response to criticism could depend on whether it is given in front of peers or privately. The existence of a problem in accepting criticism from teachers and not employers probably could be revealed by having judgments about the teenager from people in both categories; however, the existence of a problem with accepting criticism that is given in a certain way and not in other ways probably would not be revealed by soliciting judgments from a variety of people. In fact, the issue might only be confused if a teacher consistently gave criticism in a harsh voice tone, without any accompanying praise, and in front of peers, and the employer provided criticism in a normal conversational tone, preceded the criticism by some positive comments, and talked to the teenager privately. Based on the different judgments of the teenager's skill in accepting criticism from a teacher and an employer, one might assume that the person who gave it was the critical factor, whereas it might be the manner in which it was given that was the critical factor.

Because the judgments of people will not necessarily reveal details about the types of situations in which social skills deficits are evident or the specific kinds of stimuli that will occasion inappropriate or appropriate behaviors, it seems prudent to employ additional methods. One method that could be utilized entails observations of role-play performances in which various stimuli, such as the way in which criticism is delivered, are varied. Unfortunately, although this might be a convenient method, it may lack the necessary reality to produce behavior that is similar to what occurs in real life. Another method that seems preferable (but is more difficult to achieve) is to observe teenagers exhibiting "problems" in naturally occurring situations. Given that a general problem in accepting criticism is already identified for a group of teenagers through the judgments of others, it might be possible to observe various situations in which criticism is delivered and begin to pinpoint the various stimuli that occasion appropriate and inappropriate behaviors. Thus, in order to correctly identify the range of skills required by any group, it may be necessary to include both judgments of the teenagers themselves and other persons as well as observation of the teenagers. The observation task alone appears to present a significant challenge.

Two additional problems concerning the selection of skills to be taught need to be discussed. First, although the selection of social skills to be taught rests, in part, on the opinions of people, the organization of the skills into particular "units" for training seems to rest entirely on the intuitive judgment of the developer of the program. These units represent the "best guess" of the developer, and, although they may be based on some theoretical perspective, they rarely are based on empirical data. The task of organizing or grouping social skills is a taxonomic one. In what types of situations, under what surrounding circumstances, and with what personal characteristics are what variety of behaviors judged to be appropriate and probably successful? Again, the question is deceptively simple; there are a number of problems that immediately arise when one tries to proceed in making a taxonomy. For example, should one group general situations in which a teenager might display "assertive" behavior, or have more specific groupings such as a cluster of situations, that is, those that involve initiating a conversation with a peer or asking for a date? Does one similarly classify all situations in which a person is criticized, or should there be different groupings depending on whether the criticism is from a friend, an employer, or a teacher? What are the responses or behavioral units that might be classified together? Should a unit be called *making friends, maintaining a conversation,* or *asking questions of another person?* Do we group together several responses into a complex behavior, such as showing interest in what another says, or concentrate on simpler response groups such as headnods and eye contact?

In other words, to arrive at a taxonomy of social skills, one must make a very large number of decisions about the groupings of situations, of behaviors, of person characteristics, and of circumstances surrounding the situation; however, it is by no means clear how these decisions are to be made. Presumably, one could base some of the decisions on theoretical grounds as has been suggested elsewhere (e.g., McFall, 1982). Alternatively, decisions about the taxonomy might be based on the utility of the classification for teaching various skills to people who are regarded as socially deficient. Of course, one would be able to compare the utility of different classification methods only after the classification decisions had been made and the skills had been tuaght. Nevertheless, the criterion of teaching utility might allow program developers to choose between existing taxonomies that classify skills in different ways.

Another problem facing a developer of a group social skills training program concerns the identification of *common* problems for the target population. In deciding upon the skills to be taught, the developer of a group program that is to be widely used for adolescents cannot determine all of the skills deficiencies of each and every youth who might eventually participate in the training program. Instead, such a developer should determine the *common* skills deficiencies of a *representative* sample of the population to be served. For example, if one is developing a program for juvenile delinquents on probation, one might determine the social skills deficiencies exhibited by the majority of a sample of juvenile delinquents on probation and develop the content of the group program based on this information. Methods already discussed in this section including comparative observations between juvenile delinquents and youths with no history of court involvement could be used for this purpose.

Summary

The selection of the social skills to be taught is critical to the success of a group social skills training program for adolescents. It appears that the selection of skills has most often been based on the opinions of individuals who interact with adolescents. This approach appears to be successful as evidenced by the positive outcomes of several group social skills training programs; however, a number of cautions concerning the effectiveness of the programs need to be noted. These include the lack of appropriate measures of the direct effects on learners' lives, the use of inadequate experimental designs, and the failure to objectively measure changes. Another skills selection method was described here that also utilizes the opinions of others but may offer more precise judgments. This method involves comparisons between socially skilled and unskilled adolescents to determine necessary skills.

Given that the judgments of people will be used to select the social skills to be taught, two additional cautions were discussed. The first caution concerns the possibility of overemphasis on "reactive" with less emphasis on "self-initiatory" skills. A second caution concerns the importance of specifying the situational variables that can interact with social skills deficits and targeted social skills.

Finally, two additional problems concerning the identification of the content of a social skills training program were discussed. One problem concerns the organization of skills into "units" for training, and the second concerns the identification of skills that are common problems for the target population. All of these issues are important to consider in order to insure that the social skills selected are necessary and important skills for the target population.

Selection of Skills Components

A Review of Methods Used to Identify Skills Components

Once particular social skills have been selected and grouped together as units, the specific behavioral components of these skills need to be identified so that they may be taught. For example, the skill of asking a question contains a number of specific skills components such as eye contact, voice tone and volume, the type of question asked, and the like. In addition, the developer of a social skills training program must identify not only the components of the skills, but the *sequence* of these components. For example, an appropriate sequence for interrupting correctly would be to wait for a break in the conversation, say "excuse me," and then start talking rather than the reverse.

In a majority of studies that have focused on group social skills training with adolescents, there was no explicit description of how the component behaviors were identified and sequenced. Presumably, the developers of most of the social skills training programs identified and sequenced the component behaviors to be taught on the basis of their professional and clinical experience. Of the studies that did include a description of the methods used to identify component behaviors, several closely related approaches were employed.

A number of program developers have utilized professionals to identify the components of the skills. De Lange *et al.* (1981) asked four assertiveness trainers to identify what should and what should not be included as appropriate responses to each problem situation. Hazel *et al.* (1981b) first determined the specific behaviors of each skill based on the researchers' judgment. Then, these skills components were modified based on input from adolescent trainees and validated through ratings of the importance of the components by knowledgeable people and by judges' ratings of their satisfaction with skills performances before and after training. Heimburg, Cunningham, Stanley, and Blankenberg (1982) asked potential employers to describe possible responses to problem situations and to indicate which of these responses would be preferred. The identified components were later validated through ratings by employers of actual job interview performances. Golden *et al.* (1980) used a variation of this procedure by having project staff roleplay the situations requiring the skill, and, from these role-play performances, the specific response components were identified.

A second procedure that has been used to identify skills components involves asking the adolescents themselves to identify the specific behaviors necessary to improve their skills. Minkin *et al.* (1981) used this procedure to identify the components of peer criticism skills. In their study, the adolescent trainees met as a group and, in a series of meetings, discussed behaviors they thought would improve their peer criticism skills. The identified components were then validated by having judges rate the conversations prior to and after training.

In none of the studies reviewed was the issue of the sequence of the component behaviors to be taught directly addressed. Most developers probably relied upon their own judgment to determine the sequence of the skills components within a skill.

Comments on Methods Used to Identify Skills Components

The primary methods currently used to identify behavioral components of social skills have been very similar. Basically, they have involved asking people (directly or in role-play settings) to indicate the kinds of specific behaviors one should display in performing a general social skill. The people asked for these judgments have included teenagers (the potential learners), their employers, and others who work with the teenagers.

Although asking others to specify the component behaviors of skills has been useful and productive, other methods also offer considerable promise. One alternative method relies on direct observation in combination with judges' ratings. In using such a procedure, various behaviors of youths could be recorded as they participated in a standard social interaction. Measures of the various specific behaviors could then be correlated with judges' ratings of the youths' performances on several dimensions related to the successful nature of the interaction (e.g., Spence, 1981). Those components and sequences of components highly related to successful interaction could then be selected for training.

A variation of the direct observational approach involves the selection of youths who were previously rated as poor or very good on either general social skills or on a particular skill of interest and the observation of the two groups of youths in various relevant situations to attempt to determine exactly what behaviors distinguished the groups and, therefore, what might be taught as part of the skill. Observations of the youths rated as very good on the skill could also be used to help determine the criterion performances to be required of trainees by correlating judges' ratings of various aspects of behavior with quantitative measures involving frequency, duration, timing, variability, and the like of specific behaviors.

Another approach to determining the relevant behavioral components of particular social skills involves the direct manipulation of a suspected relevant component or the sequence of relevant components and the evaluation of whether changes in that component are accompanied by changed ratings of the performance of the skills by relevant judges. A variation of this approach involves teaching varying levels of frequency, duration, or variability of the suspected component behaviors and determining the effects of the varying levels on judges' ratings. This approach might result not only in the validation of the components as important to the skill but also in the identification of desired criterion performances for each component. This general approach seems to have considerable merit and deserves attention.

Summary

Social skills components have been identified either by program developers, by professionals in related fields, or by adolescents. How the sequence of skills components has been determined by program developers is unclear at this time. A number of approaches, all involving observation and judges' ratings, have been suggested for future developers' use to ensure that the skills components being taught are relevant for the population being trained.

Social Skills That Have Been Trained

Through the utilization of many of the methods discussed previously, several social skills have been identified and taught to groups of adolescents. This section includes a review of the skills that have been actually taught as well as a review of how those skills have been defined. In addition, suggestions are offered with regard to future endeavors in defining social skills.

A Review of Social Skills and Their Components

To provide a base for reviewing the various skills that have previously been taught, Table 1 lists a summary of a number of published studies that have focused on group social skills training with adolescents. Not all studies in the field are listed. For example, where the same authors have published several studies focusing on the same target behaviors and utilizing the same procedures, one study was selected as representative. In addition, other studies by the same authors that were not empirically based or that only indirectly focused on social skills were not included. Listed in the first column are the authors of the studies. The "social skills" column refers to the names of the skills taught by the authors, and the "skill definition" column refers to the way in which the skill was defined and, if appropriate, provides an example of the specific behaviors that comprised a social skill. As can be seen in the table, a variety of social skills have been taught to adolescents including negotiating, interrupting correctly,

TABLE 1. Types of Behaviors Taught to Adolescents in Groups

Author	Social skills	Skill definition
De Lange, Lanham, & Barton, 1981	Assertiveness	Assertive responses were specified for each situation by a set of criteria linked to a 5-point scale
Elder, Edelstein, & Narick, 1979	Interruption Requests for behavior change Responses to negative communication	Each behavior specified according to a 5-point rating scale with a criterion performance specified for each step on the scale
Filipczak, Archer, & Friedman, 1980	How to observe and report behaviors Verbal and nonverbal communication	Not specified
Golden, Twentyman, Jensen, Karan, & Kloss, 1980	Justifying actions Petitioning authority figures	Not specified
Gross, Brigham, Hopper, & Bologna, 1980	Discrimination Negotiation Contracting Others not specified (Specific social skills were embedded within each lesson, e.g., within discrimination, youths learned to accept criticism)	Not specified
Hazel, Schumaker, Sherman, & Sheldon-Wildgen, 1981b	Giving positive feedback Giving negative feedback Accepting negative feedback Resisting peer pressure Negotiation Following instructions Conversation Problem solving	Nonverbal behaviors, including facing the person, eye contact, facial expression, and posture; verbal behaviors, including voice tone and specific and sequenced verbal behaviors such as, "Ask if you can talk to the person," "Say something positive," "Tell how you feel," etc.
Heimberg, Cunningham, Stanley, & Blankenberg, 1982	Interactions between subject and receptionist Greeting the interviewer Breaking the ice Responding to interviewer questions Asking questions Gathering information	Verbal behaviors, including questions, self-statements, single word responses, and requests for future contact; paralinguistic behaviors, including voice-volume, affect, latency of response, and duration;

(*continued*)

TABLE 1 (*Continued*)

Author	Social skills	Skill definition
	Closing the interview	nonverbal behaviors, including gaze, frequency of smiles, frequency and appropriateness of gestures, and posture
Hendrix & Heckel, 1982	Offering praise Offering physical affection Offering verbal affection Sharing (nonobject) Cooperation Compliance Sharing (objects) Offering help Initiating social contacts Offering physical or verbal protection	Not specified
Hollin & Henderson, 1981	Posture Nonverbal communication	Eye contact, facial expression, personal space, and gestures
	Listening and talking Conversational skills	"Ice breaking" and use of appropriate topics
	Job interview Interactions with others Confrontations Conversation with opposite sex Handling aggressive encounters	
Lee, Hallberg, & Hassard, 1979	Assertion	Specified by a general definition
Minkin, Minkin, Goldstein, Taylor, Braukmann, Kirigin, & Wolf, 1981	Giving criticism to a peer	Praise statement, a statement of understanding, and a request for acknowledgment
Ollendick & Hersen, 1979	Assertion	Not specified
Pentz, 1980	Assertion	Attention to body feelings, identification of causal events, consideration of alternative responses, and assertion of rights or feelings

(*continued*)

TABLE 1 (*Continued*)

Author	Social skills	Skill definition
Pentz & Kazdin, 1982	Assertion	Recognition of dissatisfaction, identification of the cause, consideration of alternative responses, and assertion of rights or feelings
Sarason & Ganzer, 1973	Applying for a job Resisting peer pressure Taking problems to a teacher Passing up immediate gratification	Not specified
Sarason & Sarason, 1981	Job interview Resisting peer pressure Asking for help in school Asking questions in class Getting along with boss Dealing with frustration on the job Refusing to cut class Asking for help at work Getting along with parents	Not specified
Spence & Marzillier, 1979	Eye contact Refraining from fiddling Appropriate head movement Acknowledgment Question-type feedback	Specified by duration and/or frequency of each specific behavior
Spence & Spence, 1980	Eye contact Posture Dealing with teasing Dealing with bullying Accepting criticism	Not specified
Thompson & Hudson, 1982	Problem solving	Not specified

greeting, praising, resisting peer pressure, assertiveness, eye contact, and posture, to name a few. The skills that have been taught to groups of adolescents range from very specific skills such as eye contact to very broad skills such as assertion. A number of common skills were taught in several of the studies. The most commonly taught skills include assertiveness, resisting peer pressure, job interview skills, eye contact, and appropriate posture. Other skills that were taught in more than one study include praise, negotiation, accepting criticism, conversation, and problem-solving skills. The emphasis on these skills indicates that program developers believe that the target population has a wide range of deficits in interactions with others.

The studies shown in Table 1 also represent a range of ways in which the skills have been defined. Some studies did not specifically and objectively define the skills that were taught. In these studies, either the authors did not state any definition for the skills, or the skills were defined by general descriptive statements. For example, Lee *et al.* (1979) using a general descriptive statement, defined assertion as "the ability to refuse unreasonable requests and to stand up for one's own rights" (p. 459). Other authors have named components of the skill to be performed. Some of the components that have been specified are more objective and behavioral than others. For instance, Pentz (1980) used general statements to name four components of assertion skills:

> (a) attention to body feelings signaling dissatisfaction. . . ; (b) identification of the causal event; (c) consideration of alternative behavioral responses; and (d) assertion of rights or feelings in a direct and reasonable manner. (p. 79)

Others have specified the behavioral responses that should be performed in sequence to comprise a skill. For example, Elder *et al.* (1979) defined the interruption skill as comprised of three behavioral components: "saying 'excuse me,' interrupting, and saying 'thank you'" (p. 166).

Still other authors have defined the skills targeted for training in their studies using quantitative methods. For instance, some authors have measured the frequency or duration of specific behaviors or have used quantitative rating scales to score the quality of the performance of a given behavioral component. Spence and Marzillier (1979), for example, defined eye contact as "the total average amount of time in seconds that the subject looked directly at the trainer per minute during general conversation" (p. 10).

Finally, some authors have used all three methods of defining the skills. Hazel *et al.* (1981b) gave a general definition for a skill, named specific behavioral components of a skill, and had a 3-point rating scale for the performance of each component. By way of illustration, giving negative feedback was generally described as giving criticism to another person when the other person has upset or hurt one in some way. Giving negative feedback was further defined by 17 specific components beginning with "face the person," "keep eye contact," through "tell the person how you feel or what you think he/she did wrong" to "thank the person for listening and change the subject" (p. 121). Although not described in detail in the study, Hazel *et al.* paired definitions of the quality of the response with a numerical rating for each of the components. For eye contact, the youth had to look into the other person's eyes during 75% or more of the interaction to receive a 2 rating and during 50 to 75% of the interaction to receive a *1* rating. He or she received a *0* rating when he or she looked into the other person's eyes during less than 50% of the interaction.

Thus, the studies reviewed here involved the teaching of a broad range of skills. Also represented are a variety of ways of defining the targeted skills and their components. The definitional methods ranged from broad descriptions of the skills to specific and quantitative methods for measuring either the occurance or quality of a single behavioral response.

Comments on the Social Skills and Skills Components as Represented by the Reviewed Studies

Analyzing and comparing the social skills that have been taught to groups of adolescents present some problems. Frequently, enough information about the skills is not provided to enable such analysis or comparison. The skills may be named or generally defined, but the specific components of the skills are not specified. For example, the skill of apologizing to others may have been taught in two different studies, but, because the apologizing skill is not specifically defined in the studies, it is not clear that the same behaviors were taught. The converse can also occur; different names can be given to the same set of behaviors thus making it appear that different behaviors were taught when in fact the same behaviors were taught.

Another problem that precludes detailed comparisons from being made between studies is that the social skills taught in various studies differ considerably in terms of their complexity or inclusiveness. For example, a skill such as assertiveness presumably encompasses a broad range of behaviors whereas skills like appropriate eye contact or posture encompass much narrower ranges of behaviors. Eye contact and appropriate posture are skills that might be included in assertiveness, but many of the studies do not make these kinds of relationships clear. Thus, it is difficult to relate the targeted skills in one study to those targeted in other studies in the field.

These large differences in the range of behaviors included in the targeted skills, when combined with considerable differences in defining the behaviors involved in the skills, interact to affect the kinds of measurement systems employed in the literature. Studies in which a generally defined skill is taught and in which the component behaviors have not been specified typically have employed ratings by judges on general characteristics such as pleasantness, appropriateness, or potential employability as measures. Studies that have included descriptions of the component behaviors of a skill have often used checklists for scoring the presence or absence of specific behaviors in addition to ratings by judges based on general impressions. Studies that report the teaching of very specific behaviors often have used relatively precise measures involving frequency and/or duration of the particular behaviors.

The differences in the types of measurement systems used across various studies make it difficult to determine possible similarities and differences among studies with respect to the skills taught. The differences in the measurement systems may have other effects as well. The use of general definitions and general ratings by judges relates most closely to the concept that "socially skilled" is a function of whether relevant people judge a person to be performing appropriately in a given situation. Unfortunately, these general definitions and ratings do not provide much guidance for individuals who wish to replicate studies that have involved the use of these techniques. If a reader does not know exactly what behaviors were taught and the criterion levels of the behaviors required or achieved in a study, it is extremely difficult to try to replicate the effects of the study. Logically, the use of more precise definitions or measures of behaviors, such as component checklists or frequency and duration measures, would help to facilitate replication; yet the relevance of these more precise definitions and measures to the general construct of *socially skilled* may be ambiguous.

Summary

A variety of social skills have been taught to adolescents in groups. The skills taught range from very specific skills such as eye contact and appropriate head movements to very broad skills such as accepting criticism and assertion. These skills have been defined by general descriptive statements, by the behavioral components of the skills, or by quantitative methods. A variety of measurement systems including judges' ratings, checklists, and frequency counts have been used to assess the use of the skills. Because of the different types of definitions used to define the skills and the different types of measurement systems used, it is difficult to compare the skills taught across studies, and it would be difficult to try to replicate many of the training programs described in the studies.

Summary of Content Issues

The successful development of group social skills training programs for adolescents depends upon the identification and specification of the social skills necessary for particular subgroups of the adolescent population. This task is complicated by the lack of an adequate definition of *socially skilled;* however, some procedures are available to help determine the social skills needed by particular subgroups. These procedures include asking significant others to identify needed social skills, observing representative samples of socially unsuccessful youths in role-play performances requiring various skills, and comparing their performances to the performances of socially successful youths, and asking representative samples of the teenagers themselves.

After the identification of the target skills, the specific components of each skill must be identified. Similar procedures to those used to identify the social skills to be taught may be used to determine the components of the skills. One procedure involves asking others or the teenagers themselves to identify the components. Other procedures include identification of the components based on clinical judgment validated by ratings of importance by others. Additional methods include direct observation of persons performing the skills or manipulation of specific behaviors to determine whether changes in the performance of these behaviors affect judges' ratings.

In reviewing the social skills taught to adolescents in groups, a wide range of skills have been targeted. The skills range in use from those to be used with peers, such as resisting peer pressure, to those to be used with authority figures, such as job interview skills. The social skills that have been trained were defined in a number of ways with very little commonality across studies. Therefore, at this point in the development of the field, it seems appropriate to recommend that authors employ both general definitions and ratings that relate closely to what seems to be meant by *socially skilled,* as well as more precise specifications and measurement of behavioral components to facilitate replication by others. The use of overlapping types of definitional and measurement systems may also help future reviewers to see more clearly the similarities and differences across studies appearing in the literature in the future.

Training Procedures

Besides determining the appropriate content for a group social skills training program for adolescents, the developer of any program should also incorporate the use of effective instructional procedures for teaching that content. This section includes a review of the instructional procedures that have been used in empirically based studies in the area. Additionally, recommendations are made with regard to future research in the area.

A Review of Commonly Used Training Procedures

Most group social skills training programs for adolescents have been based on the assumption that the targeted social skills are not in the youths' repertoires. Thus, the instructional procedures selected for training programs have been designed to aid the acquisition of new skills. Through a review of the studies presented in Table 1, a number of apparently similar procedures have been identified that have been used to successfully teach social skills to groups of adolescents in empirically based research studies. These training procedures can be conveniently grouped into four categories of procedures: descriptive, modeling, practice, and application procedures.

Descriptive procedures include those primarily verbal procedures used by the trainer to explain what a skill is, why it is important to learn the skill, where the skill should be performed, and the specific steps in a skill (e.g., Hazel *et al.*, 1981b). These descriptive procedures are typically used within a discussion format to involve the adolescents in the group in the training process as much as possible. The explanation or definition of the skill usually includes a verbal description of it. For example, the definition of the skill, *resisting peer pressure,* might be, "Resisting peer pressure is the skill of saying 'No' to your friends when they are trying to talk you into doing something that might get you into trouble." This type of explanation presumably helps the youths understand what skill they will be learning.

Another descriptive step can be used to explain why it is important to use the skill. This step typically involves a discussion of rationales that describe the causal relationship between the adolescent's use of the skill and the specific environmental consequences that typically follow the use of the skill. For example, a rationale for resisting peer pressure might be, "If you are able to say 'No' to your friends in a nice way, you will be more likely to keep your friends and less likely to get into trouble with authorities." The use of rationales is an attempt to "motivate" the learner to learn and use the skill.

A third descriptive step that has been utilized is a discussion of the general characteristics of situations in which the skill can be used as well as examples of specific situations. The general characteristics of situations in which the skill of resisting peer pressure could be used would be situations in which other people try to talk the youth into doing something that is illegal, against the rules, dangerous to someone, that the youth prefers not to do, or that has a high likelihood of hurting someone's feelings. In a discussion about these characteristics, the social skill being trained is typically related to specific situations to enable the learners to discriminate when it is and is not appropriate to use a skill. For example, it seems appropriate for a teenager to use the skill of resisting peer pressure when her or his peers are trying to talk her or him into skipping school. It probably would not be appropriate to use the skill when her or his parents are trying to talk her or him into doing her or his homework. Thus, specific example situations that would be discussed within the context of the resisting-peer-pressure skill would include situations when friends try to talk a youth into skipping school, staying out past the family curfew, going to a movie he or she prefers not to see, using drugs, or playing a dirty trick on someone.

Another descriptive step that appears to be crucial is a discussion of the specific steps or components that should be used in performing the social skill, the reasons for performing each skill component, and the specific requirements for mastering each skill component. Skill components or steps that are typically discussed include both the nonverbal (e.g., facial expression, posture, eye contact) and the verbal (e.g., voice tone, duration of speaking, specific types of statements) components that comprise the skill. The specific statements for resisting peer pressure might include saying something positive, making a statement that you will not do something, giving a personal reason for not doing it, suggesting something else to do, repeating that you will not do it, and, if the suggestion is not accepted, leaving the situation (Hazel, Schumaker, Sherman, & Sheldon-Wildgen, 1981a). To describe the requirements for each skill component, the trainer might tell the youths what they must do to receive a perfect score on each component as the components are discussed.

The use of these four descriptive procedures is an attempt to help the learner understand the basic requirements for successful skill performance. A group setting seems particularly appropriate for these descriptive procedures because the contribution of several participants in a group discussion can increase the variety of rationales, examples, and ideas that are experienced by the trainee. As a result, all of the participants will be more likely to be interested in learning the required information. In addition, through a group discussion, the group leader can determine that each person understands the information.

The second teaching procedure commonly employed with groups of adolescents is *modeling*. Because of the complexity of many social skills, a simple verbal explanation of a skill may not be sufficient to allow the youths to perform it themselves. Modeling consists of some type of simulated presentation of the skill. Through modeling presentations, the trainer shows a simulation of the use of the component behaviors that comprise the social skill in their appropriate sequence. A variety of types of modeling procedures have been used in social skills training with adolescents. Some modeling presentations have included both good and poor models (e.g., Heimberg *et al.*, 1982), whereas others have included only appropriate examples of the skill (e.g., Ollendick & Hersen, 1979). The models have been presented live (e.g., Sarason & Ganzer, 1973), through audio (e.g., Golden *et al.*, 1980) or videotape presentation (e.g., Thelen, Fry, Dollinger, & Paul, 1976), through imagery (Pentz & Kazdin, 1982), or through a combination of these techniques (e.g., Pentz, 1980).

Modeling in adolescent groups can have a particularly powerful effect. Individuals are more likely to imitate models who are similar to them (Bandura, Ross, & Ross, 1963) and who are reinforced for correct performance (Bandura, 1965). Both of these conditions can exist in adolescent groups if the models and their performances are properly arranged. For example, Hazel *et al.* (1981a) developed videotaped modeling scenes showing adolescents using social skills when they encounter typical problems. Those youths who perform the skills well are shown receiving positive consequences on the videotapes, whereas those who fail to use the skills are shown receiving negative consequences. If such videotapes are not available, a group training session still allows an adolescent to observe a large number of modeling demonstrations of the skills by peers as long as he or she can witness peers practicing the skills and peers being reinforced by the group leader or group members for correct performance. Such models by peers increase the likelihood of correct skills performance.

The third category of training procedures widely used is *behavioral rehearsal of the skills*. Behavioral rehearsal usually consists of practice of the skills by the group members in simulated situations in which the group members each attempt to perform the skills in front of the group (e.g., Goldstein, 1981). The function of rehearsal is to give the adolescents an opportunity to use the skills in simulated situations prior to actual skills performance in naturally occurring situations. A group training session provides a unique opportunity for adolescents to rehearse the skills with a variety of other individuals across a large number of simulated situations. The content and outcome of these situations can, to some extent, be controlled by the group leader. This increases the chance that the individual will be reinforced for correct skills performance.

A critical component of the behavioral rehearsal procedure is the feedback that is given the individual regarding his or her role-play performance. Feedback typically focuses both on those aspects of the adolescent's performance that were appropriate and those that were inappropriate. Feedback has been given by group leaders (e.g., Elder *et al.*, 1979) or by group leaders and members (e.g., De Lange *et al.*, 1981). It has also been provided through discussion of audiotaped (e.g., Golden *et al.*, 1980) or videotaped (e.g., Spence & Marzillier, 1979) replay of the performance. In social skills training, the importance of positive feedback for correct performance is critical. Positive feedback for correct performance is assumed to provide substantial social reinforcement for the performance of the skills. Because in a group training session the number of individuals who provide feedback can be larger than in individual therapy, the likelihood of finding someone whose feedback is reinforcing to each individual is increased. This may be particularly important in an adolescent group in which peer feedback may be more important than adult feedback.

Another important component of behavioral rehearsal is the use of a mastery criterion to signal the successful completion of training (Hazel *et al.*, 1981b). The use of a mastery criterion requires that each person in the group must meet some specified level of skills performance before he or she is considered to have learned the skill. This insures that each group member can at least perform the skill to a certain performance level in simulated situations. In a group, a mastery criterion may be easier to implement than in individual therapy because group members can observe that the criterion can be met by other group members and therefore is realistic.

The final category of training procedures consists of techniques, which will hereafter be called *application procedures,* that are designed to increase the likelihood that the adolescent will use the skills outside of the training setting and maintain this use over time. This training step is critically important because the adolescents' use of trained skills outside of the training setting should be the primary goal of most social skills training programs. A variety of procedures have been used to promote generalization of the skills. Pentz (1980) implemented between-session practice with teachers to enhance generalization. Ollendick and Hersen (1979) instructed the adolescents to use the skills outside of the training setting. Hazel *et al.* (1981b) used homework assignments and home notes that required the adolescents to use the trained skills, to record situations in which they used the skills, and to record their performance of the skills. These home notes and problems encountered in performing a skill were reviewed at the beginning of each group meeting.

In summary, a number of different instructional techniques have been used by the authors of the studies listed in Table 1 to teach social skills to groups of adolescents. These procedures can be classified into descriptive, modeling, rehearsal, and application procedures. Different combinations of the techniques reviewed here have been utilized and the emphases on specific techniques have varied. Although all of the techniques are rarely used in combination, it seems logical that programs incorporating all of the techniques would have a higher probability of success than others in terms of producing adolescents who can actually perform social skills outside of the training setting.

Comments on the Training Procedures Reported in the Studies

Similar to the problem that was encountered in reviewing the social skills that have been taught and the components that have comprised those skills, the review of training procedures also revealed a lack of specificity in the descriptions of the procedures used in studies targeting group social skills training for adolescents. For example, although a number of different authors reported that they have used "behavioral rehearsal," it is not clear that one person's definition of *behavioral rehearsal* is the same as another's. This lack of specificity makes it difficult to evaluate the actual similarities and differences between the procedures used in various studies.

A second difficulty encountered when reviewing the training procedures used in different studies relates to the way the training procedures have been combined into comprehensive training "packages." Because few component analyses with adolescent groups have been conducted to determine the contributions of each training procedure in the "package" (see Pentz, 1980, for an exception), it is very difficult to evaluate the relative importance of specific procedures. It may not be critical which procedures are most effective if the overall training program is effective and if individual techniques are not costly or time consuming, but it still remains difficult to evaluate and recommend whether certain techniques should be incorporated into a training program if component analyses have not been conducted.

Additionally, the importance of functions of the group has rarely been analyzed. For example, some studies may report that both the group leaders and the participants provided feedback on role-play performances. In others, just the group leader or just the participants have provided feedback. The relationship of this type of within-group procedural variation to the success of training has rarely been examined.

Finally, there is a general lack of emphasis on real-life, functional use of the skills across the reviewed studies. It may be contended that what is required within the training situation is an emphasis on "fluency" of use of a skill before a youth can be considered to have learned that skill. Analogous to speaking a foreign language, one becomes fluent when one can perform the skills immediately wthout hesitation, in the appropriate situations, without faltering and in a flowing manner, and with responsiveness and variability according to the time, place, and person with whom one is interacting. The question of primary importance then becomes, How does one teach a person to become fluent in the use of social skills?

Haring, Lovitt, Eaton, and Hansen (1978) hypothesize that learning occurs in four stages. First, there is the *acquisition* of the behavior or skill. This is when the person first learns the new response. After acquiring the new skill, the learner may move into the second stage, *proficiency,* by practicing the skill frequently and ensuring that all the steps in the skill flow together smoothly. The third stage, *generalization,* requires the learner to use the skill in new settings outside of the training situation and to maintain the use of the skill over time. Finally, there is the fourth stage of learning, *adaption,* where the learner, by using the skill frequently in a variety of situations and with a variety of people, learns to adapt the skill appropriately and to use it in combination with other skills depending on the stimulus conditions present at the time of skill use. When a person has mastered these four stages, one might say that the person can perform the skill fluently. These four stages and, where appropriate, ideas for promoting fluent use of social skills by adolescents within this four-stage framework are discussed in the next four subsections.

The Acquisition Stage

Most of the group social skills training studies thus far conducted have focused on the first stage of learning, the acquisition or initial mastery of the skills. This is obviously the point to begin because, without this step, it is impossible to move on to the subsequent stages; however, most social skills programs do not progress beyond this initial mastery stage. There are very valid reasons for concentrating one's efforts at this stage. Often, the participating youths have several deficits in the social skills area, and it is desirable to attempt to remediate these deficits as quickly as possible by teaching them the necessary skills. Thus, many people believe it is better to teach the initial mastery of several skills than to devote all of the training time to one skill. Group training offers an efficient and effective way to teach the initial mastery of several social skills. Additionally, social skills training is usually not part of a school curriculum, and, therefore, the youths are asked to devote extra time outside their regularly scheduled school day to the social skills training. The more quickly the training can be accomplished, the higher is the probability that the youths will complete the training. Thus, it appears logical that if training can only occur for short periods of time (e.g., 6 to 10 weeks), the training should concentrate on teaching fundamental elements of the social skills to ensure that the youths are cognizant of the appropriate skills and when they are to be used, and that the youths are able to perform them correctly in the training setting.

In spite of the strong reasons to concentrate training efforts on just the acquisition of the social skills, it is evident that much more is needed to allow a person to become truly fluent in the use of social skills outside the training setting. Although initial mastery of the skills is a necessary condition to becoming fluent in the use of social skills, it does not appear to be sufficient to accomplish this goal.

The Proficiency Stage

As mentioned before, a second stage in learning following the acquisition stage might be characterized as the proficiency stage. In this stage, one becomes quite adept at using the social skills. The youth becomes able to perform the skills correctly and with great facility. To become proficient at using the skills, one might need to develop abilities in three different areas.

The first of these areas is the ability to discriminate stimulus situations that require a particular skill. Most people who are characterized as having poor interpersonal or social skills typically do not respond appropriately in situations calling for social behavior. This may be due to a lack of a skill (e.g., not knowing how to accept criticism appropriately); however, the inappropriate behavior may alternatively be the result of an inability to recognize a situation as requiring a particular social skill. This lack of discriminative ability can contribute to a lack of generalization after training, even though the trainee has clearly demonstrated that he or she has acquired a skill and can perform it appropriately in cued situations.

For example, Schumaker and Ellis (1982) showed that youths trained in specific social skills, although able to perform those skills in role-play situations, did not consistently use those skills when presented with surprise situations in the natural environment. When the youths were subsequently questioned about their failure to use the skills, they often responded quizzically, stating that they did not realize that the situation called for the use of one of the skills. Once the situation was pointed out, they stated that they could understand that they should have used the appropriate skill, but it did not occur to them at the time.

The question arises as to why adolescents are able to respond appropriately in a novel role-play situation but not to a situation occurring in the natural environment. The answer may be in part due to the fact that a role-play situation sets the occasion for the youths to use one of their newly learned social skills. They know that they should be using one of their social skills; they only need to decide which skill would be appropriate for each particular role-play situation. In real-life situations, the cues that were available in role-play situations (e.g., a therapist/observer is present; the situation takes place in an experimental room at a time shortly following training; a tape recorder is in the room) are nonexistent. Thus, if the youth has not learned to recognize the stimulus conditions that set the occasion for the use of a skill and has not consistently practiced recognizing these cues in everyday situations, the youth may have difficulty in engaging in the appropriate skill at the appropriate time.

Recognizing the stimulus situation that requires the performance of a certain skill is a necessary, but not sufficient, condition for an adolescent to become proficient in using a skill. Another requirement for proficiency is that the youth, once he or she knows that a particular skill is required, be able to begin the skill immediately without faltering. Rather than taking several seconds to decide how to begin to use a skill or to begin an inappropriate response and then change to an appropriate one, the youth should be able to begin the initial response pattern immediately. Unfortunately, for many youths there may be strong competing inappropriate responses. These youths have developed fairly strong behavior patterns of responding inappropriately. Though they may recognize the need for the use of a particular social skill, they may find it difficult to use the skill because they are so accustomed to responding in a different way. For example, youths can be taught how to appropriately accept criticism. They may also be taught to recognize situations that require the use of that skill. They may, however, have a long history of responding inappropriately (e.g., by becoming angry or hostile) when they do, in fact, receive criticism. This long history makes the inappropriate behavior fairly engrained in the person's behavioral repertoire, and, thus, a behavioral chain may have been formed that is difficult to break. To become proficient at using the appropriate social skills, the youth must practice responding immediately with the appropriate skill required by the stimulus situation.

The third area to address in attempting to make a youth proficient in the use of newly taught social skills is the performance of the entire skill in such a manner that all of the steps flow naturally and smoothly together. This can present a problem for those youths who have been through programs where skills are taught consisting of several steps that are to be chained together. For example, Hazel *et al.* (1981b) taught the skill of "Giving Negative Feedback" that consisted of 17 specific steps. Adolescents who have learned these steps but who have not practiced them over and over again may periodically leave out one or more steps. Often, they will realize that they have left out a step and will pause to try and remember it, or, if the adolescents forget a step, they may begin performing the sequence of steps again in order to remember the step that has been forgotten. This may be necessary because the adolescents may only remember the steps as part of a chain, with each step acting as a discriminative stimulus or prompt for the next step. When a youth pauses or begins again, he or she obviously does not give the appearance of being socially skilled; instead, he or she appears to be unsure of him- or herself and unskilled. Thus, to become truly proficient at using social skills, one must know the skills and have practiced them so well that all of the steps flow together in a smooth, unfaltering sequence.

These requirements for training discrimination, immediacy of response, and natural flowing sequences of responses suggest that practice of a skill in a few cued role-playing situations may not be sufficient to promote proficient use of that skill. Thus, group training programs should probably include numerous opportunities for practice in cued as well as noncued situations. Noncued situations should be actively programmed into group training sessions by the trainers, and feedback should be given to group members about their responses to the situations. For example, criticism can be given to a youth who has just roleplayed a skill to determine the youth's proficiency in accepting criticism. Youths who have difficulty with these noncued situations can be cued in advance of their occurrence (e.g., "In 5 minutes, I'm going to give you an opportunity to use one of your skills"), and cues can be faded according to the youth's progress. Only by permeating the training situation with many opportunities for noncued practice can trainers hope to promote a high level of proficiency in the youth's use of skills.

The Generalization Stage

The third stage of learning, *generalization,* focuses on use of the skills in novel situations outside of the training setting and across time. Besides the application procedures that have been used in a few of the studies described before and those procedures described to enhance proficiency (e.g., the use of noncued practice situations), there are a number of other procedures that could be implemented to enhance the chances of generalization of skills to settings outside the training setting and across time. Stokes and Baer (1977) have described seven procedures that may increase the generalization of the skills from the training setting to the real world. Some of these procedures seem adaptable to group training with adolescents and could greatly enhance the effectiveness of training. One procedure advocated by Stokes and Baer is to teach skills that have a high likelihood of entering into a natural community of reinforcers. That is, social skills should be designed so that the adolescents will tend to be reinforced when they use the skills. For example, the skill of resisting peer pressure must be designed so that the adolescent is able to "save face" with his or her friends even while declining to participate in an activity. If skills are not designed such that it is likely that the person will be reinforced, it seems unlikely that the youths will use the skills. The adolescent group is a good setting in which to discuss and to demonstrate the most effective ways to procure reinforcement through use of the skills. Adolescents should be encouraged to give their opinions on what kinds of statements they would accept or reject and why. During rehearsal, if the youths observe individuals receiving reinforcement for skills performance and they themselves receive reinforcement, then they will be more likely to use the skills outside of the training setting. This peer reinforcement is particularly powerful in adolescent groups because of the importance of peer influence at this age.

An additional way to insure that the skill enters into a natural community of reinforcers is to specify the social rules that should be followed when using a particular skill. By following accepted social rules, the youth is more likely to receive reinforcement for skills usage. For example, an important social rule for conversations might be, "Do not interrupt the other person." If the youth follows this rule, it is more likely that he or she will have positive outcomes when engaging in conversations with others.

A second procedure proposed by Stokes and Baer involves the *utilization of multiple exemplars*. This procedure is based on the premise that the more examples that are used while a skill is being trained, the greater variety of stimuli to which the skill will generalize. An adolescent group is particularly well suited to this because of the great variety of models and situations to which the adolescents can be exposed during group training. By discussing, modeling, and implementing practice activities involving a large range of situations in which a skill can be applied, trainers can insure that the adolescents will be more likely to generalize to such a range of situations.

A third procedure recommended by Stokes and Baer is to *train loosely*. This procedure is an attempt to increase the variability during training to more closely resemble the real world. An adolescent group is again well suited to this. Adolescent group meetings themselves, although goal oriented, tend to be less formal settings than one-on-one training might be. The adolescents should be encouraged to be spontaneous and, in practicing with each other, to genuinely represent situations as they might occur elsewhere.

Expanding the limits of the training contingencies is a fourth training procedure specified by Stokes and Baer. This kind of procedure can be implemented by giving feedback to the youths on their use of a skill at all times after they have been trained on that skill. For example, informal discussion periods between the group leader and individual youths before and after group sessions, peer interactions before, during, and after group sessions, and interactions between the youths and their parents at the end of each group session are all opportunities for providing feedback on the youths' use of new skills and thereby expand the limits of the training contingencies.

Stokes and Baer also propose that trainers should *include stimuli in training settings that are likely to be present in the generalization setting*. The adolescents in the group can serve this function if they are present in both training and generalization settings. This is often the case with adolescent groups in that the youths often come from the same community and can interact with each other on a daily basis outside of group sessions.

Besides being concerned with generalization across settings, social skills trainers should also be concerned with generalization of the skills across time (skills maintenance). In general, the same procedures that enhance generalization to new settings will also enhance maintenance of the skills. For example, proper design of the skills, expanding the limits of training contingencies, and reinforcing generalized skills use outside the training setting can all increase the likelihood that skills usage will be maintained. One additional procedure, peer reinforcement for skills performance, is particularly appropriate to adolescent groups. A major determinant of maintenance of social skills is continued reinforcement for correct skills performance. Group members can serve this function by reinforcing correct skills usage after training is completed if they are taught how to reinforce appropriate skills use.

The Adaption Stage

The fourth stage in learning, after the adolescent has become proficient in and can generalize the use of the social skill, might be characterized as *the adaption stage.* In this stage, the skills become so much a part of the youth's repertoire that the youth can easily adjust the use of the skills depending on the requirements of new or different situations.

There are a variety of different ways in which the adolescent might learn to adapt previously learned social skills. If the adolescent has learned the skills by learning particular steps in a sequence, he or she needs to learn when to appropriately adapt those steps according to the stimulus situation. First, it may not always be necessary to use all of the steps, so the adolescent must be able to discriminate when it is appropriate to leave out certain steps. For example, in the "Giving Negative Feedback" skill taught by Hazel *et al.* (1981b), the first verbal step involves asking to talk to the other person. If a youth has been engaged in a conversation with another person and decides, in the middle of that conversation, to give the other person some negative feedback, it would be inappropriate to say, "May I talk with you for a moment?" Rather, the youth should adapt the skill step sequence by either leaving out that particular step or by changing it to something more appropriate for the situation like, "May I talk with you about something that has been bothering me?"

Second, the youth must learn to adapt the skill in order to be responsive to the person with whom the youth is interacting. Thus, one would behave differently depending on certain factors such as age, intimacy, and relationship with the other person. For example, in acceping negative feedback, a youth would probably use most of the steps in the skill whenever he or she uses the skill; however, depending on the age and status of the other person, the youth may choose to ultimately agree or disagree with the criticism. If the person giving the criticism is a friend of the youth, he or she may listen and discuss the criticism but eventually say, "I'm sorry; I still disagree with what you are saying." If the person giving the criticism is the youth's boss and the youth has tried to present his or her case, the youth might do best to accept the criticism even if he or she disagrees with it. Thus, the youth has learned to vary the skill, depending once again on stimulus conditions, as in this case, the person with whom he or she is interacting.

Third, a youth must learn the skill well enough and feel comfortable enough with it that he or she can vary the wording used for individual steps so that he or she does not sound like a tape recording when using the skill. For example, in many skills, a verbal step is to say something positive about the person. One phrase that youths frequently like to use is, "You are a really good friend." Although it may be appropriate to use this phrase periodically, it may not be appropriate to use this same phrase each time the youth interacts with a person. In order to use the skills convincingly, the specific content of each step should be varied with the goal of fulfilling the step while creatively adapting the content of the step to the situation at hand.

Fourth, when using a social skill, the youth must not only adapt the skill to different situations but also must adapt it to what the other person is saying. That is, the youth must tailor his or her responses to the feedback that he or she receives from the other person. This feedback can range from the very obvious, such as the person's saying that he or she does not have time to talk to the youth, to more subtle feedback, such as the voice tone and body posture of the other person. Regardless of the type of feedback, the youth must learn to respond appropriately to this feedback to insure the success of the interaction.

Finally, the trainee who can fluently use the social skills must be able to determine when a situation calls for combining two or more skills or beginning one and appropriately switching into another skill. For example, a teenager may start using the negotiation skill with his or her parents. After going through several steps of the skill, it may become apparent that the topic under discussion is nonnegotiable in the parents' view. Rather than attempting to continue to negotiate, it may be best for the youth to begin to use either the skill of "Accepting No" or "Following Instructions," depending on the situation. The trainees who are able to combine skills appropriately demonstrate that the skills are firmly engrained in their repertoires and that the skills are at their disposal whenever they need them.

In order to teach youths to adapt the skills to a variety of situations, trainers will need to emphasize adaption. After each skill is learned to mastery and proficiency levels, discussions and further practice regarding that skill should be focused on adaption of the skill. Each kind of adaption should be described to the youths, and group members should be encouraged to provide examples. Then, possibly in a game format, hypothetical situations can be posed by the trainer or group members varying the circumstances, the person(s) involved, the level of intimacy, what has happened previously, and so forth. Youths can take turns showing how they might adapt the skills to fit these situations. Individuals outside the training setting can be recruited to present noncued opportunities to each youth for adaptive use of the skills. Only by actively programming training for this stage of learning can trainers insure that the youths have fully integrated a skill within their repertoires.

Thus, a variety of methods can be used to increase the chances of generalization and maintenance of newly learned skills. These methods include procedures that focus on teaching the skills not only to acquisition or even to proficiency levels, but to a level at which the youth can generalize and adapt the skills to the changing requirements of various individuals and situations. The utilization of all of these techniques would enhance the chance of generalization of the social skills to new settings and the maintenance of skills usage across time.

Summary

The training procedures that have been used in empirical studies focusing on the group training of social skills in adolescents, although far from standardized, can be grouped into four categories: descriptive procedures, modeling procedures, rehearsal procedures, and application activities. Although several authors in the field report using these procedures in different combinations, it is unclear how they have been specifically used because of the general nature of the descriptions presented in their studies. Furthermore, few studies have involved component analyses to determine which of the teaching techniques are crucial for producing the achieved effects and to determine the nature of the roles of the group participants in the instructional process. Finally, there has been an emphasis on the use of methods to promote acquisition of social skills in the literature with little emphasis on methods for promoting fluent and proficient generalized use of skills. Further research is needed that combines careful description of instructional procedures with analyses of the need for those procedures. Although some methods for promoting proficient and generalized use of skills have been suggested here, research that focuses on the best methods for this promotion is required if programs are to insure actual and long-term use of skills outside of training settings.

Outcomes of Group Social Skills Training with Adolescents

Thus far, the social skills content and the training procedures that have been utilized in empirical studies focusing on group social skills training of adolescents have been reviewed. This section includes a discussion of the outcomes of those studies. First, four evaluation issues that must be considered when analyzing the outcomes of studies are addressed and are illustrated with examples from the literature. Next, an example is highlighted with regard to how the authors of one study addressed each of the issues. Finally, comments regarding future research needs are offered.

Four Evaluation Issues

In reviewing the outcomes of group social skills training programs for adolescents, a useful approach is to review the effects that have been demonstrated by specific training programs. In social skills training, four issues can be addressed in the evaluation of the outcomes of a study. These issues, although not mutually exclusive, do provide a useful method of describing and analyzing the studies. The first issue concerns whether an effect was demonstrated and whether this effect was the result of training. This focuses attention on whether there was a change in a youth's social skills performance as measured on some type of valid and reliable behavioral measure and on whether an appropriate experimental design was used to show that the change that occurred was caused by the treatment. The second issue concerns the significance of the change. Was the change judged to be socially significant by the youth and significant persons in the youth's environment? Preferably, this determination should be made in real-life settings rather than in simulated situations because research has shown that performances of skills in the two types of settings are not necessarily related (e.g., Schumaker & Ellis, 1982). The third issue concerns the generalization of the trained social skills to other settings. Was generalization of skills use across settings assessed, and was it achieved? The final issue concerns the maintenance of skills over time. Was maintenance of skills usage assessed, and were the trained skills maintained?

Measures and Designs

With regard to the first issue, whether an effect of social skills training was demonstrated, a variety of measures have been used to demonstrate the effects of group social skills training with adolescents. These measures range from questionnaires that address an adolescent's behavior to observation of skills use in naturally occurring situations. Questionnaires, although relatively easy to administer, have the disadvantage of being only indirect measures of social skills performance; however, a number of researchers have used questionnaires to assess changes in skills levels. These questionnaires require the youth, parents, teachers, or other significant persons either to rate the youths' performances of social skills or to indicate changes in some other aspect of the youths' lives. For example, Hollin and Henderson (1981) compared self-report measures of personal problems before, during, and after training and showed a reduction in problems following training. Pentz (1980) used a self-report measure of assertion that was situation specific to adolescents and found increases in assertion ratings following training. Sarason and Ganzer (1973) used a self-description inventory, a word-rating scale, a goal scale, an activity preference scale, an internalization–externalization scale, and behavior rating scales completed by cottage counselors to assess changes in skills levels. Significant improvements were found for the majority of these measures following training. Sarason and Sarason (1981) showed differences following training in social problem-solving skills on a problem-solving measure and on alternatives generation tests as compared to a control group. Spence and Marzillier (1979) showed a slight, though nonsignificant, improvement in the youths' social behaviors following training as rated on staff questionnaires.

A second type of assessment device, used in a variety of studies, involved the use of some type of behavioral role-play test. In this type of assessment, the subject is required to respond to a stimulus presentation, and then the subject's response is rated according to specified criteria. This type of measure yields a more direct assessment of the youth's social skills performance than do questionnaires. De Lange *et al.* (1981) used a behavioral role-play test that required the adolescent to respond to 10 videotaped vignettes covering different types of assertion situations. The subjects' responses were scored using specific response criteria on a 5-point rating scale. They found no significant changes following training in assertion. Elder *et al.* (1979) measured role-play performance during the group training session as one measure of the effects of training. Significant improvements were found for ratings of interruptions, requests for behavior change, and responses to negative communications following training. Golden *et al.* (1980) showed some change in the two trained skills of petitioning and justification as assessed through role-play tests presented through an audiotaped stimulus. Hazel *et al.* (1981b) used live presentation of situations in a role-play test to measure social skills performance and showed substantial changes in skills levels following training. Heimberg *et al.* (1982), using a simulated job interview to assess changes in skills performance, found significant improvements in several specific verbal (e.g., single- versus multiple-word responses) and paralinguistic (e.g., voice volume) behaviors following training but no differences in nonverbal behaviors. Minkin *et al.* (1981) showed substantial improvements following training in three components of peer criticism skills using videotaped role-play tests. Ollendick and Hersen (1979) used a role-play test involving both positive and negative situations to assess assertion. They found significant improvements on some of the measures such as eye contact, aggressive content, requests for new behavior, latency of response, and number of positive statements. Pentz and Kazdin (1982) used a behavioral role-play test in which the adolescents were presented with audiotaped situations requiring assertive responses. They found significant improvements from pre- to post-training on some of the test situations, particularly those involving interactions with teachers.

Finally, another method used in some studies to demonstrate the effects of training is observation of skills use in naturally occurring situations. This type of assessment is the most direct evaluation of the youths' performance of the skills. For example, Filipczak, Archer, and Friedman (1980) used observational data in social skills classes to assess changes in adolescents' performances following training. They showed significant improvement in a variety of social behaviors such as following directions and working well with others.

Of further concern is the type of experimental design that has been used in each of the group social skills training studies to determine whether changes in social skills performance of the youths resulted from the training procedures. The reviewed studies can be classified into three different groups with regard to the designs used: those using a control group or comparison group design, those using a multiple-baseline design, or those using a combination of these two designs.

A majority of the studies reviewed (e.g., Heimberg *et al.*, 1982; Lee *et al.*, 1979; Ollendick & Hersen, 1979; Pentz, 1980; Pentz & Kazdin, 1982; Sarason & Ganzer, 1973; Sarason & Sarason, 1981; Spence & Spence, 1980; Thompson & Hudson, 1982) used some type of control group design with random or quasi-random assignment to groups or used some type of comparison group design (De Lange *et al.*, 1981; Hollin & Henderson, 1981). In most of these studies, pre- and posttraining measures were collected for both groups of subjects. This type of design permits a comparison between the average performance of one group and the average performance of the second group. Hendrix and Heckel's (1982) study presents a straightforward example of this type of design. In their study, 30 male delinquents were randomly assigned to either the experimental or control group. All subjects were observed in free activity sessions prior to training. Social skills training was administered to the experimental group, whereas the control group received information in a nonrelevant area. All subjects were again observed during free activity periods after training with the result that the trained youths exhibited significantly more of the target social skills than the untrained youths.

The second type of design that has been used is a multiple-baseline design. In a multiple-baseline design, a series of assessments are made before, during, and after training. The onset of training occurs sequentially across different target behaviors or across individuals. This type of design allows a determination of the effects of training through a comparison of the performance of trained skills (or trained persons) and untrained skills (or untrained persons). The use of a multiple-baseline design was reported by Minkin *et al.* (1981) where baseline data were collected on three specific behaviors. Training was then implemented sequentially on each of these behaviors, and measurement was continued on all behaviors. As training was implemented on each behavior, substantial changes were noted in each behavior but only after training was implemented. Baselines remained stable on the untrained skills until they were trained. Other authors who used a multiple-baseline-across-skills design include Elder *et al.* (1979) and Spence and Marzillier (1979). Gross *et al.* (1980) conducted a multiple-baseline design across groups of subjects.

A study conducted by Hazel *et al.* (1981b) used a combination of these two designs. A multiple-baseline-across-skills design was used to assess changes in skills levels, and a comparison group design was used to compare differences in recidivism data. The authors generally found an increase in the use of each social skill as each skill was trained and a substantial difference in recidivism between the trained and untrained subjects. This combined approach is useful because each type of design may be most appropriate for evaluating the effects of training with different types of data.

In summary, the group social skills training studies that have been conducted with adolescents, although not always demonstrating significant changes in specific social skills performances following training, do as a group demonstrate that the social skills performances of adolescents can be measured in a variety of ways and that, generally, positive changes are found following training. The majority of reviewed studies used either questionnaires, observations of behavioral role-play performances, or combinations of these two procedures to assess the effects of social skills training. Only two studies used some type of observation procedure to measure the effects of training on social skills performance in natural settings. In terms of the type of designs employed, the majority of the reviewed studies used a multiple-baseline design, a control group design, or a comparison group design. In others, a combination of these designs was used. In some of the studies reviewed, however, the experimental designs or the procedures used were not adequate for assessing the effects of training.

Social Significance

The second issue that should be addressed in evaluating the group social skills training studies concerns the social significance of the obtained changes in the youths. Two methods were used in the studies reviewed to assess social significance: consumer satisfaction ratings and judges' ratings. Procedures to obtain consumer satisfaction ratings usually have included asking the youths and other significant persons in the youths' lives to rate their satisfaction with the goals, procedures, and effects of the program (Wolf, 1978). This type of evaluation gives a subjective impression of the respondents' reactions to the program. In one study that utilized this procedure, Gross *et al.* (1980) asked the youths, their parents, and representatives of the agencies who referred the youths if they were satisfied with the changes they had observed in the youths' behaviors. Generally, these respondents positively evaluated the program and the effects of the program. Hazel *et al.* (1981b), in a similar fashion, showed a high level of satisfaction with the goals, procedures, and effects of the program as assessed by the participating youths and their probation officers.

The second way to assess the significance of the obtained changes is to have independent judges rate the social skills performance of the youths. Usually, the procedure involves having judges either watch youths' live performances or watch and/or listen to taped performances and rate each performance on a number of dimensions. For example, Hazel *et al.* (1981b) audiotaped youths' performances during role-play interactions before and after training. Independent judges listened to these performances in a random order. They indicated a high level of dissatisfaction with the pretraining performances and a high level of satisfaction with the posttraining performances. Similarly, Minkin *et al.* (1981) had judges listen to audiotaped samples of situations in which criticism was delivered in actual family conferences. Their judges, including both adolescents and adults, gave significantly higher ratings to posttraining performances as compared to pretraining performances.

Thus, both consumer satisfaction and judges' ratings can be useful for determining the social significance of the changes in skills performance that resulted from training. The few studies in which the social significance of changes in the youths was assessed generally showed a high level of satisfaction with the training goals, procedures, and outcomes.

Generalization

The third evaluation issue concerns generalization of skills use from the training setting to real-life settings. A variety of measures have been used to assess generalization. One type of measure has involved the use of novel role-play situations to demonstrate that the youths can use the skills in situations they have never before experienced. This type of measure, although having the potential to show substantial increases following training, is limited because of two reasons: (a) the tests typically occur within the same setting as treatment; and (b) the youths know they are expected to perform social skills in these tests. Nevertheless, novel role-play situations have been used to demonstrate generalized use of social skills by researchers. For instance, Hazel *et al.* (1981b) showed that trained youths showed good performance of the skills steps in novel role-play situations after training to a 100% criterion. If this criterion was not enforced, the youths exhibited only minimal use of the skills in novel role-play situations. Thus, novel role-play situations can be useful in obtaining one measure of learning and the generalized use of social skills. Unfortunately, the relation of role-playing measures to measures of real-life use of social skills remains unclear. The results of one study (Schumaker & Ellis, 1982) have indicated that use of a social skill in a role-playing situation does not necessarily mean the youth will use the skill elsewhere. Thus, caution must be exercised when drawing conclusions from this type of measure.

Another procedure used to measure generalization of social skills usage involves direct observation of the skills outside of the training setting using behavioral observation systems. For example, Elder *et al.* (1979) observed participants' use of trained skills in the cafeteria and dayroom and showed generalized use of the skills. Hendrix and Heckel (1982) observed the adolescents' use of trained skills during periods of free-time activities within a juvenile institution. They found increased use of the skills following training. Minkin *et al.* (1981) assessed use of peer criticism skills during family conferences and found increased use of the skills following training. Pentz (1980), working in a school setting, observed youths' use of assertion skills in a novel but "real" situation involving a teacher. She found significantly better performance of the skills in these generalization tests for the trained, as compared to the untrained, subjects. Spence and Marzillier (1979), using a technique that approximates natural observation, assessed adolescents' use of social skills during a conversation with an unknown adult. Following training, the adolescents showed increased amounts of eye contact and decreased time spent fiddling but no significant changes in the number of appropriate head movements or in listening skills. Observation in natural settings appears to be the most useful way to assess generalization because, through direct observation, developers can get a true picture of how the youths behave when they have not been "cued" to use their skills.

A third measurement technique that has been used in studies to assess generalized use of social skills is the questionnaire. Through questionnaires, the adolescents or significant persons in the adolescents' environments are typically asked to rate the adolescents' performance on the skills or general changes in behaviors. By way of illustration, Gross *et al.* (1980) utilized behavior checklists and showed that parents and teachers rated the youths following training as exhibiting fewer problem behaviors in the home and school, respectively. Heimburg *et al.* (1982) showed substantial differences between trained and untrained subjects on a number of job interview variables as rated by employers following actual job interviews. Lee *et al.* (1979) showed no significant differences following training between treatment and control groups on peer ratings of aggression but did find a significant increase in participating youths' self-report ratings of assertion.

Other investigators have used attitudinal or cognitive questionnaires as measures of generalization. De Lange *et al.* (1981), although not showing any effects, used a number of attitude questionnaires designed for measuring such constructs as self-concept, locus of control, and self-expression to reflect changes in skills levels. Ollendick and Hersen (1979), using locus of control and anxiety scales, showed positive changes following training. Pentz and Kazdin (1982) generally showed positive, though nonsignificant, changes in self-reports of self-efficacy with regard to how youths felt they would perform in novel situations from pre- to posttraining for the various treatment groups. Spence and Spence (1980) administered locus of control scales and self-esteem questionnaires as measures of generalization and showed short-term, positive changes that were not maintained at a 6-month follow-up. These types of questionnaires, although not providing direct evidence of skills changes, can provide some indirect evidence concerning the effects of skills acquisition. Nevertheless, because they do not provide actual measures of generalized use of skills, questionnaires should probably not be relied upon as the only generalization measure.

A final way of assessing the generalization of social skills training that has been used is the measurement of the occurrence of other behaviors that might be affected by changes in social skills. For example, Elder *et al.* (1979) used measures derived from the token economy being used in an institution to determine the generalized effects of social skills training. They found a reduction in the number of token economy fines for inappropriate interruptions and inappropriate requests for behavior change but an increase in inappropriate responses to negative communications following training. They also found that seclusion orders decreased from baseline to posttraining measures. Filipczak *et al.* (1980) took global measures of school performance (e.g., school grades, discipline, and attendance) to show the generalization of skills usage. They found the students who had received training were significantly better in relation to comparison youths with regard to a majority of these measures following training. Gross *et al.* (1980) collected data on a variety of measures of school performance including number of suspensions, school and class attendance, and grades as well as police arrest data to demonstrate generalization. They found a decrease in school class absences during and following treatment, no suspensions during or following training, unclear results regarding grades, and a decrease in arrests during and following the program. Hazel *et al.* (1981b) used both a self-report delinquency scale and recidivism data from court records to measure the effects of their program and found a decrease in the number of delinquent acts reported and in the number of court contacts following training. Hollin and Henderson (1981) used institutional reports of problems to show generalization of skills use. They found a decrease in the number of institutional reports received by the social skills trainees following training as compared to before training. Ollendick and Hersen (1979) used points earned and number of instances of disruptions as measures of generalization. The trained youths showed a significant increase in the number of points earned as compared to the control youths, but no significant differences were found for disruptive behaviors. Sarason and Ganzer (1973) collected recidivism data from official records to assess the impact of social skills training on the court involvement of juvenile delinquents after training and showed a reduction in recidivism for youths who participated in the program as compared to untrained youths. Sarason and Sarason (1981) used tardiness, behavior referrals, and absences from school as measures of generalization. They found subjects in the two treatment groups to be significantly better than the control subjects following training on the first two measures, but only one of the treatment groups was significantly better than the control group on number of absences.

The results obtained with all four types of generalization measures indicate that following social skills training, the youths do, to some extent, generalize their use of the trained skills. Certainly, a clearer picture of youths' generalized use of trained skills can be obtained if as many of these measures as possible are used. It is critical that data from these types of measures be collected if developers are to determine whether their social skills training program has a meaningful impact on the participating youths' lives.

Maintenance

The final evaluation issue concerns the measurement of the use of trained skills over time. This becomes particularly important because Thompson and Hudson (1982) reported that some effects of group counseling did not appear until 15 weeks after group training had ended. It is also important because, if youths do not maintain their use of the skills over time, there may be a significant problem with the skills taught or the training procedures used. Unfortunately, few program developers have measured the effects of their training programs after considerable time has elapsed. Exceptions to this include Elder *et al.* (1979) who used discharged rate from the hospital and ability to remain in the community as measures of maintenance of effects. Sarason and Sarason (1981), as described previously, assessed the number of incidents of tardiness, behavioral referrals, and absences in the year following the program. Both of these studies, although using indirect measures of the effects of training, found positive changes in these measures following training. A number of studies have assessed maintenance of the skills through recidivism rates (Gross *et al.*, 1980; Hazel *et al.*, 1981b; Sarason & Ganzer, 1973) and showed a decrease in recidivism. Unfortunately, these types of measures offer only an indirect assessment of the youths' continued use of the skills. None of the reviewed studies directly assessed the social skills performance some time after the completion of group training. Hazel, Schumaker, Sherman, and Sheldon-Wildgen (1982) showed retention of social skills in role-play tests conducted 8 months after the completion of the group; however, no studies have shown maintained use of skills in natural environments.

Thus, although a number of methods for assessing maintenance of trained skills over time are available, they have rarely been used following group social skills training with adolescents. If the true usefulness of social skills training programs is to become understood, authors of future studies should endeavor to include maintenance measures among their measurement plans.

Summary

In summary, four evaluation issues need to be addressed in research studies if developers of group social skills programs for adolescents are to convince the public that their programs cause changes in the social competences of the participating youths, that these changes are socially significant, that the youths can and do use newly learned social skills outside of the training setting, and that the changes are maintained over time. Examples of how each of the four evaluation issues have been addressed in the past have been described. Unfortunately, the adequacy with which the issues have been addressed through the literature in the field is in question.

A Review of the Adequacy with Which the Four Issues Have Been Addressed

Although a number of examples were described previously to show how each of the four evaluation issues has been addressed in the literature, few studies have addressed all four issues adequately. Each of the studies represented in Table 1 addresses some of the issues better than others, but none of the studies presents an "ideal" example of how all four issues should be addressed. Nevertheless, one study that addressed most of the issues will be briefly reviewed here for illustration purposes.

Heimburg *et al.* (1982) trained the social skills necessary for job interviews. After a determination of the necessary social skills based on a series of interviews, these job interview skills were taught to unemployed teenagers in a group format. Subjects were assigned to treatment or control groups in a quasi-random fashion based on the time they entered the program. Before and after training, subjects participated in role-play job interviews that were videotaped and rated by individuals blind to the subjects' treatment condition. Each subject's performance was rated on a number of specific verbal, paralinguistic, and nonverbal measures. In addition, each subject's overall interview performance was rated. Also, self-ratings were collected concerning anxiety and performance. The final dependent measures consisted of performance measures collected during actual job interviews in which each subject's performance was judged by the interviewing employer. Heimburg *et al.* found significant improvements for a number of the specific measures as well as overall job interview performance as measured during role-play interviews. Thus, the assessment systems showed that there was an effect of training. Employers' ratings of performances during actual job interviews showed significant differences between treatment and control groups on a number of the measures. These results indicated that the outcome of the training was socially significant and that generalized use of the skill in natural settings was achieved. Finally, with regard to maintenance, role-play interviews were conducted 1 week after training, and actual interviews were conducted some time after training. These measures showed maintenance, albeit short term, of the skills. This study illustrates how the four evaluation criteria can be met in a study focusing on the effectiveness of a social skills group program.

With regard to the adequacy with which the other studies have addressed the four evaluation issues, the majority of group social skills training studies represented in Table 1 did show an effect using an adequate experimental design. A number of these studies can be criticized for the dependent measures selected particularly for their reliance on questionnaires and role-play assessments without observation of skills used in naturally occurring situations.

With regard to the social significance of the changes in the youths' behavior, only a few of the studies included assessments of this. Those that did include such assessments found a high level of satisfaction with the results of the training, but they rarely showed the long-term social impact of the training on the youths' lives.

The generalized use of the trained skills to novel settings was mainly assessed by roleplaying novel situations, questionnaires, attitude measures, and the measurement of other related behaviors that might be affected by training. It was rarely assessed through observation of skills use in settings other than the training setting; however, the results, though far from conclusive, are promising and indicate that generalized use of social skills by youths can occur.

In the studies reviewed, maintenance was assessed by measures of related variables such as recidivism or through role-play performances. No studies assessed maintenance in real-life settings. This issue needs to be addressed to determine if youths continue to use the newly learned skills over time.

Although, in aggregate, all of the evaluation issues have been addressed by the studies, few studies addressed all four issues. This limits the conclusions that one can draw with regard to group social skills training programs for adolescents. Nevertheless, the results are promising, and future researchers should utilize the broad base of sensitive measures and effective procedures used in the studies reviewed herein while insuring that they address the significant issues in social skills evaluation.

Conclusion

Social skills training with groups of adolescents has evolved into a common therapeutic approach in the past 10 years. A review of the literature in this field shows that although the results of a number of the studies are promising, problems continue to exist. These problems seem to center on the identification of the skills to be trained, the identification of the specific components of each skill, and the definition of selected skills and components. The teaching procedures that have been used tend to be less problematic. The majority of reviewed studies reported the successful use of a number of similar procedures. Unfortunately, because of poor descriptions of the techniques and a dearth of component analyses, it remains unclear which techniques or packages of techniques are the most efficient, effective, and practical. The studies that were reviewed in this chapter generally have shown positive results; however, these outcomes must be interpreted with caution because a number of the studies fail to fulfill some significant evaluation requirements. Nevertheless, taken as a whole, the studies in this field demonstrate that group social skills training holds promise as an effective approach for teaching social skills to adolescents. Important questions remain with regard to the effectiveness of this training for generalized use of the skills to new settings and situations across time. In the future, social skills training programs will need to focus not only on the initial acquisition of skills but on the teaching of skills to appropriate levels of proficiency and adaptation. Only by insuring that the youths are highly fluent in social skills, as well as that they demonstrate generalized use of those skills over time, can program developers be sure that their social skills training programs have reached their goal of producing socially competent individuals. Future researchers in this area are encouraged to take care in selecting and defining the skills of their programs, in selecting and describing the training procedures they use, in evaluating the usefulness of particular training procedures, and in evaluating the outcomes of their training programs.

References

Argyle, M. *The psychology of interpersonal behaviour* (2d ed.). Harmondsworth, England: Penguin, 1972.

Arkowitz, H. Assessment of social skills. In M. Hersen & A. S. Bellack (Eds.), *Behavioral assessment: A practical handbook.* New York: Pergamon Press, 1981.

Arkowitz, H., Lichtenstein, E., McGovern, K., & Hines, P. The behavioral assessment of social competence in males. *Behavior Therapy*, 1975, *6*, 3–13.

Bandura, A. Influence of model's reinforcement contingencies on the acquisition of imitative responses. *Journal of Personality and Social Psychology*, 1965, *1*, 589–595.

Bandura, A., Ross, D., & Ross, S. A. Imitation of film-mediated aggressive models. *Journal of Abnormal and Social Psychology*, 1963, *66*, 3–11.

De Lange, J. M., Lanham, S. L., & Barton, J. A. Social skills training for juvenile delinquents: Behavioral skill training and cognitive techniques. In D. Upper & S. Ross (Eds.), *Behavorial group therapy, 1981: An annual review.* Champaign, Ill.: Research Press, 1981.

Elder, J. P., Edelstein, B. A., & Narick, M. M. Adolescent psychiatric patients: Modifying aggressive behavior with social skills training. *Behavior Modification*, 1979, *3*, 161–178.

Filipczak, J., Archer, M., & Friedman, R. M. In-school social skills training: Use with disruptive adolescents. *Behavior Modification*, 1980, *4*, 243–263.

Golden, K., Twentyman, C. T., Jensen, M., Karan, J., & Kloss, J. D. Coping with authority: Social skills training for the complex offender. *Criminal Justice and Behavior*, 1980, *7*, 147–159.

Goldstein, A. P. *Structured learning therapy: Toward a psychotherapy for the poor.* New York: Academic Press, 1973.

Goldstein, A. P. *Psychological skill training: The structured learning technique.* New York: Pergamon Press, 1981.

Gross, A. M., Brigham, T. A., Hopper, C., & Bologna, N. C. Self-management and social skills training: A study with predelinquent and delinquent youths. *Criminal Justice and Behavior,* 1980, *7,* 161–184.

Haring, N. G., Lovitt, T. C., Eaton, M. C., & Hansen, C. L. *The fourth R: Research in the classroom.* Columbus, Ohio: Charles E. Merrill, 1978.

Hauserman, N., Zweback, S., & Plotkin, A. Use of concrete reinforcement to facilitate verbal initiations in adolescent group therapy. *Journal of Consulting and Clinical Psychology,* 1972, *38,* 90–96.

Hazel, J. S., Schumaker, J. B., Sherman, J. A., & Sheldon-Wildgen, J. *ASSET: A social skills program for adolescents.* Champaign, Ill.: Research Press, 1981. (a)

Hazel, J. S., Schumaker, J. B., Sherman, J. A., & Sheldon-Wildgen, J. The development and evaluation of a group skills training program for court-adjudicated youths. In D. Upper & S. Ross (Eds.), *Behavioral group therapy, 1981: An annual review.* Champaign, Ill.: Research Press, 1981. (b)

Hazel, J. S., Schumaker, J. B., Sherman, J. A., & Sheldon-Wildgen, J. Group training for social skills: A program for court-adjudicated, probationary youths. *Criminal Justice and Behavior,* 1982, *9,* 35–53.

Heimberg, R. G., Cunningham, J., Stanley, J., & Blankenberg, R. Preparing unemployed youth for job interviews: A controlled evaluation of social skills training. *Behavior Modification,* 1982, *6,* 299–322.

Hendrix, C. E., & Heckel, R. V. The effects of a behavioral approach on modifying social behavior in incarcerated male delinquents. *Journal of Clinical Psychology,* 1982, *38,* 77–79.

Hollin, C. R., & Henderson, M. The effects of social skills training on incarcerated delinquent adolescents. *International Journal of Behavioral Social Work and Abstracts,* 1981, *1,* 145–155.

Kelly, J. A. *Social-skills training: A practical guide for interventions.* New York: Springer, 1982.

Lee, D. Y., Hallberg, E. T., & Hassard, H. Effects of assertion training on aggressive behavior of adolescents. *Journal of Counseling Psychology,* 1979, *26,* 459–461.

Lieberman, M. A. In F. H. Kanfer & A. P. Goldstein (Eds.), *Helping people change.* New York: Pergamon Press, 1975.

McFall, R. M. A review and reformulation of the concept of social skills. *Behavioral Assessment,* 1982, *4,* 1–33.

Minkin, N., Minkin, B. L., Goldstein, R. S., Taylor, M. W., Braukmann, C. J., Kirigin, K. A., & Wolf, M. M. Analysis, validation, and training of peer-criticism skills with delinquent girls. In D. Upper & S. Ross (Eds.), *Behavioral group therapy, 1981: An annual review.* Champaign, Ill.: Research Press, 1981.

Ollendick, T. H., & Hersen, M. Social skills training for juvenile delinquents. *Behaviour Research and Therapy,* 1979, *17,* 547–554.

Pentz, M. A. W. Assertion training and trainer effects on unassertive and aggressive adolescents. *Journal of Counseling Psychology,* 1980, *27,* 76–83.

Pentz, M. A., & Kazdin, A. E. Assertion modeling and stimuli effects on assertive behavior and self-efficacy in adolescents. *Behaviour Research and Therapy,* 1982, *20,* 365–371.

Phillips, E. L., Phillips, E. A., Fixsen, D. L., & Wolf, M. M. *Teaching family handbook.* Lawrence: University of Kansas Printing Services, 1972.

Rose, S. D. *Treating children in groups.* San Francisco: Jossey-Bass, 1972.

Rose, S. D. *Group therapy: A behavioral approach.* Englewood Cliffs, N.J.: Prentice-Hall, 1977.

Rotheram, M. J. Social skills training programs in elementary and high school classrooms. In D. P. Rathjen & J. P. Foreyt (Eds.), *Social competence: Interventions for children and adults.* New York: Pergamon Press, 1980.

Sansbury, D. L. The role of the group in behavioral group therapy. In D. Upper & S. Ross (Eds.), *Behavioral group therapy, 1979: An annual review.* Champaign, Ill.: Research Press, 1979.

Sarason, I. G., & Ganzer, V. J. Modeling and group discussion in the rehabilitation of juvenile delinquents. *Journal of Counseling Psychology,* 1973, *20,* 442–449.

Sarason, I. G., & Sarason, B. R. Teaching cognitive and social skills to high school students. *Journal of Consulting and Clinical Psychology,* 1981, *49,* 908–918.

Schumaker, J. B., & Ellis, E. S. Social skills training of LD adolescents: A generalization study. *Learning Disability Quarterly,* 1982, *5,* 409–414.

Spence, A. J., & Spence, S. H. Cognitive changes associated with social skills training. *Behaviour Research and Therapy*, 1980, *18*, 265–272.
Spence, S. H. Validation of social skills of adolescent males in an interview conversation with a previously unknown adult. *Journal of Applied Behavior Analysis*, 1981, *14*, 159–168.
Spence, S. H., & Marzillier, J. S. Social skills training with adolescent male offenders: I. Short-term effects. *Behaviour Research and Therapy*, 1979, *17*, 7–16.
Stokes, T. F., & Baer, D. M. An implicit technology of generalization. *Journal of Applied Behavior Analysis*, 1977, *10*, 349–367.
Thelen, M. H., Fry, R. A., Dollinger, S. J., & Paul, S. C. Use of videotaped models to improve the interpesronal adjustment of delinquents. *Journal of Consulting and Clinical Psychology*, 1976, *44*, 492.
Thompson, D. G., & Hudson, G. R. Values clarification and behavioral group counseling with ninth-grade boys in a residential school. *Journal of Counseling Psychology*, 1982, *29*, 394–399.
Trower, P., Bryant, B., & Argyle, M. *Social skills and mental health*. Pittsburgh: University of Pittsburgh Press, 1978.
Upper, D., & Ross, S. M. Behavioral group therapy: I. Emotional, avoidance, and social skills problems of adults. In M. Hersen, R. M. Eisler, & P. M. Miller (Eds.), *Progress in behavior modification* (Vol. 5). New York: Academic Press, 1977.
Wolf, M. M. Social validity: The case for subjective measurement or how applied behavior analysis is finding its heart. *Journal of Applied Behavior Analysis*, 1978, *11*, 203–214.

9

Modifying the Type A Behavior Pattern

A Behavioral Group Approach in Behavioral Medicine

LYLE E. KANTOR

INTRODUCTION

During the first half of the 20th century the prevention and cure of infectious diseases occupied prominent medical attention. Since that time, however, there is growing recognition that health habits and chronic behavior patterns play an increasingly important role, along with infectious disease and genetic factors, in the determination of the onset and course of disease. This realization has led to the evolution of the field of behavioral medicine.

The discipline of behavioral medicine originated in the 1970s with the first formal definition appearing as an outgrowth of the Yale Conference on Behavioral Medicine. At that time, Schwartz and Weiss (1977) defined behavioral medicine as follows:

> Behavioral medicine is the field concerned with the development of behavioral science knowledge and techniques relevant to the understanding of physical health and illness and the application of this knowledge and these techniques to diagnosis, prevention, treatment, and rehabilitation. (p. 369)

Others (Blanchard, 1977; Pomerleau & Brady, 1979) have offered definitions assigning a more important role to behavioral assessment and intervention methods derived from experimental psychology. There is widespread agreement, however, that the field of behavioral medicine can be clearly distinguished from the related areas of liaison psychiatry and psychosomatic medicine by virtue of (a) its multidisciplinary nature with active collaboration between the basic and applied sciences; (b) its attention to important interactions among environmental, psychological, physiological, and biochemical processes; and (c) an empirical orientation emphasizing the demonstration of clinical and medical efficacy and replications.

LYLE E. KANTOR • Department of Behavioral Medicine and Psychiatry, Lahey Clinic Medical Center, Burlington, Massachusetts 01805.

As one might expect, clinical applications of behavioral medicine principles have been more readily accepted than traditional psychiatric approaches by the empirically oriented medical community. Patients who are not prepared to fully accept the possibility of a psychogenic component to their medical condition also find a behavioral medicine approach, with its emphasis on learning new habits and coping skills, a desirable alternative to long-term psychotherapy grounded in a psychopathology model.

There have been four major lines of development in the clinical aspects of behavioral medicine (Pomerleau, 1979): (a) interventions to improve patients' adherence to the treatment regimen (e.g., patient instruction, self-monitoring, building in family reinforcement, tailoring treatment to individual life-styles); (b) interventions to modify a specific behavior or response pattern that in itself is a health problem (e.g., chronic pain behavior, headaches, insomnia, hypertension); (c) interventions to modify the behavior of health care providers (e.g., providing feedback on laboratory tests ordered or referral patterns to specialists); and (d) preventive interventions to modify behaviors that constitute risk factors for disease development (e.g., smoking, dietary practices, Type A behavior).

This chapter will focus on the Type A behavior pattern to represent an application of a behavioral group treatment perspective to a problem within the field of behavioral medicine. After summarizing the existing intervention literature, I will address the conceptual issues and decisions that underlie a group intervention program for the Type A behavior pattern. The "nuts and bolts" of the group, from assessment through follow-up, will then be presented. Lastly, conclusions and unresolved problems will be addressed, and directions for future work outlined.

The group intervention program for Type A behavior patterns described in this chapter is conducted within the Department of Behavioral Medicine and Psychiatry at the Lahey Clinic Medical Center. Lahey is a private, nonprofit medical center comprised of a 200-bed hospital and a comprehensive network of ambulatory care clinics. When the Lahey Clinic moved from Boston to its new quarters in Burlington in 1980, the considerable increase in patient flow made it clear that cost- and time-efficient methods of assessing and treating patients needed to be implemented. The Lahey Clinic's Health Maintenance Organization (HMO) opened simultaneously, further contributing to the number of consultation requests to the department. We have therefore developed a broad set of time-limited, intensive, and psychoeducational approaches to treatment that have proved to be both clinically effective and cost-efficient. The group treatment program for individuals with Type A behavior patterns described later is among these.

The Type A behavior pattern (TABP) has been characterized as a constellation of behaviors with a "driven" quality: a great desire to achieve, a chronic sense of time urgency, competitive striving, unnecessarily rapid mental and physical functioning, underlying hostility, impatience with the speed of activities or interactions, and a pervasive difficulty in relaxing (Friedman & Rosenman, 1959; Rosenman, Brand, Jenkins, Friedman, Straus, & Wurm, 1975). As one might expect, not all Type A individuals display each and every one of the mentioned behaviors.

There are several important reasons for the interest within behavioral medicine that is being directed at understanding and modifying the TABP. What is most important is that there is growing evidence over the past 10 years identifying the TABP as a major independent risk factor for coronary heart disease (CHD), which is the number one cause of death in the United States. This evidence was recently reviewed by a panel of experts convened at the National Heart, Lung, and Blood Institute, with the conclusion being that the data revealed a significant association between TABP and CHD (Review Panel on Coronary-Prone Behavior and Coronary Artery Disease, 1981). The largest scale and most frequently cited prospective study investigating the TABP, the Western Collaborative Group Study (Rosenman *et al.*, 1975), classifed over 3,000 middle-aged men as Type A or Type B (Type B being the relative absence of Type A qualities). Follow-up of their cardiac status over an 8½-year period revealed that Type A men experienced twice the rate of new CHD as did the Type B men even when standard biological risk factors such as obesity, elevated blood pressure, cigarette smoking, elevated serum cholesterol levels, and lack of exercise were controlled for. In addition, those Type A men who experienced a first myocardial infarction within the study period had twice the risk of developing a subsequent one (Jenkins, Zyzanski, & Rosenman, 1976). This may well have been the first time that a psychosocial variable, in this instance a set of observable behaviors termed *Type A behavior*, was elevated to a level of medical attention comparable to that of the more traditional clinical symptoms and biological risk factors for CHD. It is not surprising, therefore, that health psychologists and other professionals working in the behavioral medicine field have seized upon this important opportunity to demonstrate the utility of a behavioral medicine approach to health risk reduction.

An additional reason for the attention to TABP within behavioral medicine circles is related to the burgeoning of general stress management programs. With recent estimates of the prevalence of Type A individuals in the work force approaching 50% (Rosenman, 1974), more attention is being directed to the stress-inducing nature of Type A behavior. In a sense, the very Type A behaviors relied upon by individuals as responses to environmental challenges and other stressors, in and of themselves (a) can be subtle stress triggers (e.g., hurrying); (b) can leave the individual overreactive to potential stressors (e.g., hypersensitive to time cues; imposing unreasonable deadlines); and (c) can promote a life-style that does not allow the individual sufficient access to stress-relieving mechanisms (e.g., relaxation methods, vacations). Therefore, general stress management programs are more frequently addressing the relationship between the TABP and stress.

Can We Alter the Type A Behavior Pattern?

Although early writings on the TABP were often pessimistic about the likelihood of its modification, several controlled studies within the past decade offered evidence of successful intervention. Suinn (1975) reported a cardiac stress management training procedure that was provided to Type A individuals with preexisting heart disease. The training included both anxiety management training (AMT, a procedure for learning and practicing muscle relaxation skills as a coping response to control a stressor), and visuomotor rehearsal (the imaginal practice of behaviors incompatible with Type A behavior prior to their *in vivo* application). Results revealed self-reports of behavior change and measured decreases in lipid levels. No standardized measures of Type A behavior were used. Suinn and Bloom (1978) modified this earlier intervention by comparing AMT by itself to a waiting list control procedure in a sample of Type A men without evidence of heart disease. Significant decreases in Type A behavior were demonstrated on two of the Jenkins Activity Survey (Jenkins, Zyzanski, & Rosenman, 1971) factors (Hard Driving/Competitive and Speed/Impatience) as well as on both the Trait and State scales of the State Trait Anxiety Inventory (Spielberger, Gorsuch, & Lushene, 1970). There were no significant changes in blood pressure, cholesterol, or triglyceride levels in either group.

Roskies, Spevack, Surkis, Cohen, and Gilman (1978) recruited a sample of men between the ages of 39 and 59 who were free from heart disease. These 27 subjects were randomly assigned to either a brief psychodynamically oriented psychotherapy group or to a behavior therapy group in which self-monitoring and muscle relaxation skills were taught. Although neither group showed significant changes in measured observable behaviors (e.g., work, recreation, and health habits), both groups experienced significant reductions in serum cholesterol levels and systolic blood pressures. Significant pre-post changes for both groups were also revealed on a general health, life satisfaction, and time pressure survey. Roskies, Kearney, Spevack, Surkis, Cohen, and Gilman (1979) extended the previously mentioned study by including an additional behavior therapy group composed of men with confirmed heart disease, and by extending the duration of their evaluation period to include a 6-month follow-up. The treatment benefits reported in the previous study were also experienced by the additional behavior therapy group. Examination of the 6-month follow-up data revealed that the sample as a whole showed good maintenance of gains, with a trend indicating that changes in the behavior therapy groups were more pronounced at 6-month follow-up than were those experienced by participants in the psychodynamic psychotherapy group.

A cognitive therapy approach to the modification of Type A behavior (based on concepts derived from Rational Emotive Therapy) was introduced by Jenni and Wollersheim (1979), and this treatment was compared to a combination of AMT and covert behavioral rehearsal similar to that developed by Suinn. Although both treatments emphasized the need to recognize early cues of tension, they taught very different methods of tension reduction. Cognitive therapy was more effective in reducing the Bortner scale (Bortner, 1969) Type A scores of the "high" Type A individuals than were the AMT and control groups. Both of the treatment groups reported successful reductions in anxiety levels, whereas neither of the groups demonstrated significant changes on physiological measures of cholesterol and blood pressure.

Levenkron, Cohen, Mueller, and Fisher (1983) investigated self-initiated self-control training as an intervention for disease-free Type A men. Three treatments offered in a group format were compared: brief information (a single lecture by a cardiologist and psychologist), group support (group discussion and support for behavior change), and comprehensive behavior therapy (self-initiated self-control training aimed at modifying both responses and stimulus events). Significant positive changes were reported by the comprehensive behavior therapy group on all measures of Type A behavior, and by the group support condition on two of the four standard scores derived from the Jenkins Activity Survey. Only one change measure, the Jenkins Activity Survey Job Involvement scale, reflected a significant positive change in the brief information group. The self-initiated self-control condition also demonstrated significant alterations on several physiological measures, including serum triglycerides and free fatty acid levels. Neither of the comparison groups evidenced significant physiological modifications.

Most recently, the ambitious Recurrent Coronary Prevention Program has been undertaken in the San Francisco area as a 5-year trial aimed at reducing morbidity and mortality among greater than 1,000 postmyocardial infarction men and women (Thoresen, Telch, & Eagleston, 1981). The treatment of interest is targeted at cognitive, behavioral, environmental, and physiological aspects of Type A behavior. Comparison groups include a more medically focused group conducted by a cardiologist, and a group of patients receiving routine medical follow-up care. Results at 3-year follow-up are promising, with the combined cardiology and behavioral Type A counselling group experiencing significantly lower rates of coronary recurrences and more marked reductions in Type A behavior (Friedman, Thoresen, Gill, *et al.*, 1984).

Comparisons across these intervention studies are difficult to make due to the variability of target populations, outcome measures, control groups used, and the frequently small sample sizes. Nonetheless, successful interventions are reported for both males and females as well as for individuals with and without the presence of CHD. In short, the outcome evidence thus far on short-term changes, although far from definitive, is promising, and suggests that aspects of the constellation of Type A behavior including related physiologic functions can be modified by brief interventions ranging from 6 to 14 sessions.

The Selection of Treatment Targets

Who to Change?

There are several target groups who may profit from intervention addressing the TABP. One target group would be those adolescents or adults who have yet to develop TABP. In this application of primary prevention, individuals would be seen with the goal of preventing the development of Type A behavior. As suggested by Roskies (1980), subsamples such as women about to reenter the work force would be particularly well suited for this form of timely preventive intervention. Perhaps the most obvious candidates for intervention are those individuals who by virtue of their well-developed Type A behavior are at a higher risk for the development of CHD. A secondary prevention intervention could be offered to a cross section of such Type A individuals or to a more circumscribed subgroup who are at a particularly vulnerable stage (e.g., preparing a group of tax accountants for the April 15th onslaught). Another target group is those Type A individuals who have recently experienced the onset of CHD. Here, tertiary prevention efforts could be aimed at assisting these individuals in behavioral changes to decrease the likelihood of further morbidity/mortality. One might expect this target group to have a particularly strong motivation for change.

Being situated within a general medical center community, we have focused intervention efforts on secondary and tertiary prevention work. We have also purposely composed treatment groups with a mix of males and females (although to date our program has been composed of 80% men), and a heterogeneous grouping of individuals with and without heart disease. A heterogeneous mix of patients can be helpful in broadening the participant reference groups, in providing exposure to a wider variety of coping models, and in gaining feedback from individuals with more diverse perspectives.

What Are the Appropriate Targets for Change?

There is considerable debate over the question of which aspect of the TABP to concentrate intervention efforts upon. We could focus on one or more aspects of the TABP, but what criteria should be used to select the target behavior? For example, we could address (a) the most obviously well-developed Type A behaviors for the particular individual; (b) the Type A behavior the individual is most highly motivated to change; or (c) the Type A behavior or behaviors that have been demonstrated in prior research to have the highest degree of association with CHD. Alternatively, we could attempt to modify all observable Type A behavior and to bolster such modifications with broader life-style changes as well. A case can also be made for changing environmentally based reinforcement for Type A behavior, because many Type A behaviors such as attention to deadlines, perfectionism, competitive striving, and an over-developed achievement orientation are frequently rewarded at a societal level.

Several assumptions and a review of existing data have guided our decision relative to the preceding questions on the issue of what to change. It is important to recognize that because TABP intervention is in its infancy, there is little research that can be relied upon as a definitive guide to the previously mentioned decision. As noted none of the Jenkins Activity Survey three-factor scores were found to be predictive of CHD in WCGS patients (Zyzanski & Jenkins, 1970). In contrast to this finding, Matthews, Glass, Rosenman, and Bortner (1977) found the factors of competitive drive and impatience derived from the structured interview to have the greatest degree of association with CHD onset. Subsumed within the factor of competitive drive is the high potential for hostility that Williams, Haney, Lee, Kong, Blumenthal, and Whalen (1980), Thoresen *et al.* (1981), and Matthews (1982) have also identified as the characteristic most highly associated with CHD onset. Thus, aspects of the TABP may be more "malignant" than others. In addition, certain Type A behaviors may be quite "benign," and all Type A behavior cannot be considered "coronary-prone" behavior. Although the initial evidence is pointing toward the hard-driving and potentially hostile behavior of Type A's as most malignant, until there is a firmer empirical base from which to proceed we believe it is prudent to moderate the spectrum of Type A behaviors, including potentially hostile behavior. Moreover, we do not view the Type A's potential for hostility as an entity unto itself. It is our contention that this hostility is intricately connected to the Type A's belief system, competitiveness, and time urgency, and will require a broadly based change strategy.

Research has yet to determine precisely the extent to which Type A behaviors need to be altered to meaningfully decrease CHD risk. Therefore, we have worked to assist Type A individuals in moderating the extremes of their Type A behaviors. If an individual is highly motivated to change a particular behavior, we certainly would recommend capitalizing on such motivation by using this behavioral target as a point of entry from which to build a positive collaboration and a base from which to generalize the application of behavior change methods. Although we strive to impact "life-style," we do so by successively focusing upon and altering clearly identified individual target behaviors. We strongly encourage efforts to modify the environmental reinforcers for Type A behavior. The work place in particular appears to be an appropriate site for intervention because it often provides praise, financial incentives, and promotions for sustained Type A behavior. In light of our medical center-based practice and general time constraints, however, we have limited our intervention efforts thus far to the Type A individuals themselves who present in the clinic.

Conceptual Model for the Lahey Clinic Intervention Program for TABP

The Type A individual is subjected to many of the same external circumstances and demands (potential stressors) as is his/her Type B counterpart. What appears to distinguish Type A individuals is (a) their tendency to interpret a broader range of potential stressors as being threats or challenges; and (b) their use of stress-coping mechanisms that create an increased number of self-generated stressors, such as self-imposed deadlines, hurrying, insufficient leisure/vacation time, and oversensitivity to time cues. These two factors are likely to contribute to the heightened emotional and physiological levels of arousal detected in Type A individuals.[1] For example, Glass (1977) and Friedman, Byers,

[1]The preceding represents our working conceptualization of Type A behavior. The reader is referred to Matthews's (1982) review of other conceptualizations that view Type A behavior as the outcome of person–situation interactions, and to Krantz & Durel's (1983) article describing Type A behavior as a response stimulated by underlying biological factors.

Diamant, and Rosenman (1975) have reported that Type A individuals experience a sharper rise in autonomic nervous system functions and neuroendocrine responses under perceived challenge, coupled with a slower rate of return to baseline. Alterations in the autonomic nervous system and a sense of feeling challenged/threatened may elicit a subjective state of anxiety/loss of control, and these feelings are repeatedly responded to with Type A behavior aimed at restoring control. The Type A behavior may possibly decrease the "press" of the challenging event (be it external or self-generated), but not without a price: increased fatigue, alienation of colleagues or family members, missed or hurried meals, and ultimately a progressively greater risk of developing CHD. This vicious cycle is depicted in Figure 1.

Given the cyclical nature of the TABP, there are multiple points in this chain of behavior at which to intervene. Prior intervention studies have not directly compared the outcomes of comprehensive behavioral approaches (e.g., the Recurrent Coronary Prevention Program) with those directed at a single target in the Type A behavior chain. Only Jenni and Wollersheim (1979) attempted to evaluate the differential effect of intervening at different points along the chain of Type A behavior. Their findings offer very limited direction, however, because the only measure of the several assessed that distinguished the two treatment groups (i.e., a cognitive group focusing on event interpretations and an AMT group focusing on applying a relaxation method) was the Bortner Type A

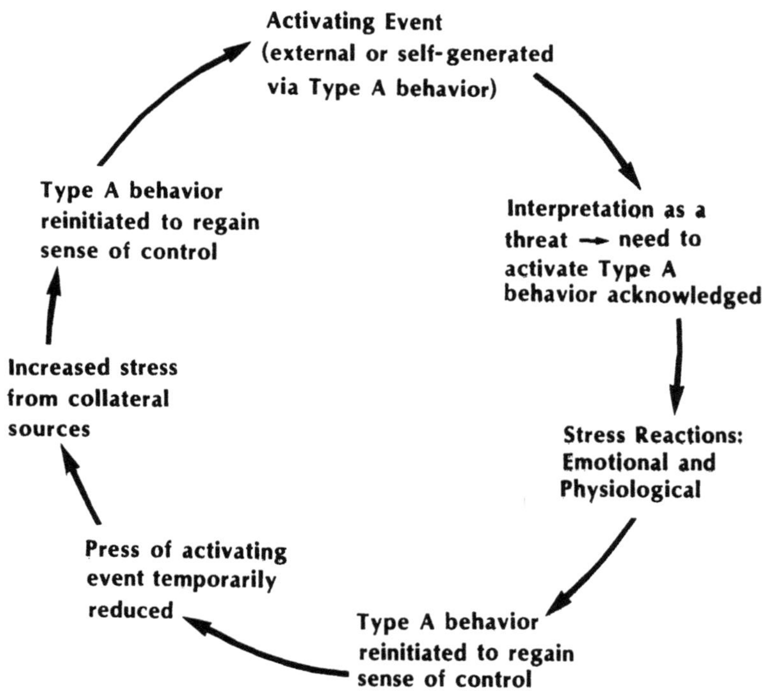

FIGURE 1. The Cycle of Type A Behavior.

Scale, on which scores of a subset of "high" Type A individuals were more improved by a cognitive approach. In light of the dearth of empirical direction, we have chosen to intervene in a comprehensive way, striving to alter both appraisals of stressors and the resulting Type A behavior itself. In our Type A behavior modification program several points on the cycle are targeted for change:

1. Activating events: Environmental sources of stress in the work and home settings are identified and targeted for change where appropriate. In addition, stressors imposed by Type A behavior itself are approached directly. Behaviors such as hurrying, the setting of unnecessarily stringent deadlines, and impatience can be altered through covert rehearsal, behavioral cuing (i.e., placing written reminders in key locations around the work or home environment), and *in vivo* practice.

2. Interpretations: Appraisals of threat and challenge to the individual's sense of personal control are addressed within a cognitive-behavior modification module focusing on underlying beliefs, expectations, and self-talk.

3. Stress reactions (emotional and physiological): Although learning a relaxation response in itself is not seen as a sufficient intervention, teaching a tension-reduction procedure within a self-control framework can be quite valuable. The relaxation response can be presented as being of general value and particularly useful in providing a means of controlling one's own internal responses, even when an external event is out of one's control. This strategy also offers Type A individuals the further benefit of fairly rapid and visible results.

4. Type A behavior initiated to regain control: Alternative modes of responding adaptively to stressors can be learned. A set of coping responses including relaxation methods, time management strategies, the delegation of responsibilities, and communications skills can offer additional tools to the Type A individual.

The Behavioral Group as an Intervention Approach for the TABP

Type A individuals are well suited for an intervention approach that emphasizes skill building and behavioral self-control. In contrast to focusing on psychodynamic conflicts or psychopathology, a behavioral self-control model poses far less of a threat to the Type A individual's sensitivity to loss of personal control. There are several reasons why we feel that a group format is preferable for the intervention: (a) problem-solving strategies and behavioral alternatives to the TABP can be modeled by various group participants; (b) the Type A individual working toward behavior change can profit from the availability of a reference group and support system; (c) as Roskies (1980) has noted, no self-respecting Type A individual will allow him- or herself to be any less motivated to benefit from the group than other participating Type A's; and (d) given the practical time constraints on psychological services, the group approach offers a time- and cost-efficient utilization of therapists' time.

Group leadership functions for the TABP group have been shared by a PhD-level health psychologist and a cardiology department nurse clinician. This collaboration has been found to be advantageous. Professionally, there is a mutual educative function served, whereby each discipline can benefit. Psychologists offer skills aimed at facilitating, among other things, self-control, compliance, generalization of behavior change, and the group's reinforcement value. Moreover, although most psychologists are quite comfortable delivering interventions in a group format, medical practitioners often are less accustomed to the group modality. The cardiology nurse clinician is well schooled in underlying medical conditions, heart disease, traditional biological risk factors, and physiological aspects of stress. It is clear that this collaboration broadens each professional's expertise. The TABP program participants themselves profit from multidisciplinary co-leadership as well. The credibility of efforts to increase attention to the medical/behavioral/life-style interface is heightened through multidisciplinary coordination and modeling strategies within the group. Furthermore, a broader range of areas of expertise can be offered.

Group Formation and Preparation

Referrals to a TABP group come from a number of sources. Medical practitioners, most commonly cardiologists and internists, are in the best positions within the medical center to identify at-risk Type A individuals. In order to solicit their referrals, however, (a) information on Type A behavior needs to be provided to medical practitioners to aid in the identification process; (b) criteria for appropriate group candidates need to be clearly specified; (c) physicians need to understand the nature and goals of the intervention program; and (d) outcome data substantiating the benefits of participation need to be presented. Even the physician sensitive to behavioral risk factor reduction work may need frequent reminders about the availability of the intervention program. Such reminders can be provided through brief written memos distributed to each referring physician announcing the start date for an upcoming TABP group, or by regularly providing written or verbal feedback to referring physicians on the progress of their patients. Demands of the acutely ill cardiac patient and a generally busy practice often overshadow interest in facilitating preventive health efforts, however.

Asymptomatic Type A individuals rarely request treatment of their own accord. Often, neither the patient nor significant others in his or her environment may see the Type A behavior as problematic. Moreover, even the prospective group participant who does recognize problematic aspects of TABP can present several barriers to active engagement in the program. There is general concern or threat posed by a new involvement under the direction of an outside authority. More specifically, individuals often demonstrate a fear that the intervention will have an adverse effect on their achievement and productivity (which are the Type A individual's "bread and butter"). There is also likely to be discomfort about altering immediately gratifying Type A behavior for a longer term promise of health benefits that may or may not be forthcoming.

Perhaps the best way to address the previously mentioned reservations is to step back and consider the reinforcements for the TABP. If we can strive to make behavioral alternatives equally or more reinforcing while offering a lowered health risk, then one might expect Type A individuals to have a greater willingness to participate. Among the positively reinforcing elements of the TABP are the following: (a) Type A behavior is presumed to preserve and restore a sense of personal control through productivity; (b) Type A behavior allows the individual access to multiple projects that provide an ongoing sense of personal challenge and the potential source of esteem-bolstering accomplishments; and (c) Type A behavior can reduce the press of the immediate activating event and is societally reinforced in the form of pay raises, promotions, and the like. The TABP is negatively reinforced as well because excessive commitments/activity allow the Type A individual to avoid the anxiety that can accompany unstructured, non-goal-directed time.

During the process of screening Type A group candidates, the group intervention is presented to prospective participants with these reinforcing elements in mind. Specifically, the reduction in personal control that the Type A individuals may fear through their group participation is addressed in several ways. First, a written, courselike outline for the psychoeducational group is provided. In this way, the individual is better informed about what to expect and can thereby minimize the sense of being out of control. A face-to-face individual screening session can also be useful in reducing skepticism about working with a psychologist. Here, an active, structured, and here-and-now interaction style (free of the stereotyped couch and early childhood focus), can serve a further rapport-building function.

The Type A individuals should be given the clear impression that the psychologist understands them and the TABP and is confident in assisting them in changing their behaviors. Fears related to reduced productivity and self-esteem can be addressed by describing ways in which the behavior change can actually *increase* personal efficiency. The positive effects of pacing activities, focusing the presently undifferentiated energies, and providing restorative relaxation can be described, with Type A functioning being likened to the inefficiency of an engine constantly idling at full throttle. The Type A individuals can also find it reassuring at this early stage of the intervention process to hear that they are not likely to be transformed into thoroughly "laid-back" Type B individuals. Rather, we present our aim as the moderation of counterproductive extremes of the behavior pattern, with the goal of "Type A− or B+ behavior." Finally, Type A individuals can be provided with the knowledge that the anxiety that now may accompany slowing down can be diminished as the skills of being more relaxed without compromising productivity are learned.

Assessment for Group Treatment

Although a comprehensive discussion of the assessment of Type A behavior is beyond the scope of this chapter, several points regarding assessment will be made on the basis of a review of the literature.

First, it seems clear that one or more standardized assessment measures with documented association with CHD outcome should be included in an assessment battery. The structured interview (Rosenman, 1978) has been shown to possess the greatest predictive power for this purpose. Its drawback is the necessity of a face-to-face method of administration and a scoring method that requires training and time to implement. The Jenkins Activity Survey (Jenkins *et al.*, 1974) and the Framingham Type A Questionnaire (Haynes, Feinlieb, & Kannel, 1980) are alternatives to the structured interview that offer the advantage of being self-administered questionnaires, but with a clear compromise of accuracy in predicting CHD.

Second, due to the partial independence of self-report, behavioral, and physiological measurements, it would appear to be valuable to assess multiple response systems. Thus, in addition to pencil-and-paper or interview measures of Type A behavior, physiological measures, self-ratings, and ratings from key significant others can be taken. Several studies have reported that Type A individuals respond with greater physiological reactivity to challenging, competitive tasks (Dembroski, McDougall, & Shields, 1977; Goldband, 1980). In light of this finding, laboratory-based stressors (e.g., serial subtraction with strict time limits; hand immersion in cold water with instructions highlighting the task difficulty and importance of doing well) can be applied while monitoring physiological measures such as serum cholesterol, triglycerides, and plasma-free fatty acid levels, and blood pressure concurrently. Self-ratings of variables that will be targeted for change can also be made on a pre-post basis. Such ratings could include number of total work hours, number of overtime hours, number of hours of work conducted at home, number of recreation hours, number of minutes per day at lunch, and vacation days per year. These data can be corroborated by the independent ratings on the same variables by significant others, such as work colleagues or family members. Adjunctive questionnaire measures to assess broader behavioral changes, such as the Anger Inventory (Novaco, 1975) and the State Trait Anxiety Inventory (Speilberger *et al.*, 1970) can be included as well.

Conducting the Type A Behavior Patterns Behavioral Group

There is expanding literature on the physiological underpinnings and behavioral manifestations of Type A behavior as well as on the outcome of intervention efforts. Although authors have speculated on the important elements to be included in a TABP intervention program, there is yet to appear in the literature a detailed "nuts-and-bolts" description of TABP modification written from a cognitive-behavioral group perspective. What follows is such a description, which is grounded in the TABP intervention program conducted at the Lahey Clinic. As was mentioned previously, the group is co-led by a health psychologist and cardiology nurse clinician. Its general philosophy is consistent with a behavioral self-control model. As you will see, a broad range of target behaviors and alternative coping skills are addressed, with an effort to assist group participants in individualizing approaches best suited to their particular needs and life-styles. The group sessions themselves are quite structured, and provide for a combination of didactic presentations and group participation. There is an agenda of material to be covered each week, and group participants are provided with written summaries of principles, articles of interest to the week's topic, and a concrete statement of homework to be accomplished between sessions.

The group is composed of 8 to 15 Type A individuals who meet once weekly for a 1½- to 2-hour session. There are a total of nine sessions, eight of which are delivered on consecutive weeks and with the ninth scheduled following a 4-week interim period. This 4-week interval can provide an opportunity for group participants to experience a consolidation of gains, to further practice applying newly learned skills in the natural environment, and to allow time for additional questions to surface. Thus far, the group has attracted significantly more men than women, with a typical distribution of 70–80% men in each group. The individuals have ranged in age from 21 to 69, and approximately 10% of these participants have had a diagnosable cardiac condition (including postmyocardial infarction, angina, and coronary artery disease). Screening criteria for group participation include the following:

1. A subset of Type A behaviors evident from at least two modes of assessment: subjective report during screening interview, observable behavior during the screening interview, and Jenkins Activity Survey Scores
2. No major psychiatric disorder that might interfere with the individual's ability to attend to and implement behavior change principles, or with the efficient conduct of the group
3. Subjective report of motivation to actively participate in the TABP Group

Course of the Group

Session 1

The goal of the initial group session is twofold: to impart a clear, credible, and shared rationale for the group's work and to actively engage the Type A individuals in beginning efforts aimed at understanding and identifying their sources of stress (stressors) and Type A coping modes. The characteristics of the TABP are identified and brought to life with specific illustrations. This commonly elicits participant involvement and the comment that "that's me to a T."

The question of why we are channeling our efforts to alter aspects of Type A behavior is then addressed. Although the reinforcing elements of Type A behavior are identified, we emphasize the counterproductive aspects of the TABP and discuss how this behavior, which is often implemented as a response to a stressor (e.g., hurrying, setting stringent deadlines, preoccupation with time cues, and overextending), is in itself stress inducing. We then distinguish between being responsible and adopting a pressured approach to responsibility. It is illustrated that, in the latter case, the work overload can lead to inefficiency, a neglect of other aspects of life concerns, insufficient time for the necessary rest and recreation, and a heightening of somatic problems such as fatigue and tension. The scientific evidence relating TABP to a higher incidence of CHD also is reported.

It is stressed that the alternative behavioral self-control skills that we will offer over the course of the group will not negatively impact achievement/productivity. On the contrary, we liken Type A behavior to the inefficiency of an engine idling continuously at high throttle and emphasize increased efficiency and decreased physiological strain as likely outcomes of the intervention. An outline of the course of the group is distributed, which describes the progression through modules addressing physiological, cognitive/self-generated, behavioral, and environmental sources of stress and their management. Responsibilities of group participants are also enumerated: to attend regularly and to participate actively. Taking an active role in order to maximize benefits includes, among other things, participating in group discussions, completing homework, and providing feedback, support, and suggestions to other group members. The Type A group participant is reminded that we view behavioral and self-control practices as something he or she can do, not something he or she is necessarily born with or without. The change process is discussed, making it clear that we see change as a gradual building process and not a sprint race.

The assignment of self-monitoring of stress cycles is presented. Stress logs calling for the date and time of the stress experience, situational events, automatic thoughts/self-talk, emotional/physical stress reactions and their duration, and coping actions are distributed with directions for their proper completion. A copy of the stress log is provided in Table 1.

Sessions 2/3

Sessions 2 and 3 comprise a module on the physiology of stress, the relaxation response, and physical health habits. Session 2 begins with a review of

TABLE 1. Stress Log

Date/time	Events	Automatic thoughts/self-talk	Emotional/physical reactions	Coping actions	How long does it last?

participants' experiences and findings on their self-monitoring work. An attempt is made to help participants identify temporal, environmental, and interpersonal patterns related to their stress reactions. These stress reactions are discussed with an eye to the range of possible responses that individuals can experience across behavioral, cognitive, affective, and physiological systems. Participants are encouraged to make particular note of their idiosyncratic early cues that signal the onset of tension and stress. By so doing, people can learn to apply relaxation methods at the most opportune point for intervention.

The cardiac nurse clinician directs the presentation on the physiology of stress. Here the activating response of the autonomic nervous system is described, and it is noted that Type A individuals have been reported to experience more frequent and heightened arousal to tasks/situations that pose a challenge. It is further explained that although our early ancestors could diminish autonomic nervous system arousal through fight-or-flight behavior, these two behavioral alternatives are rarely appropriate for us in today's more civilized world. We then introduce the notion of a relaxation exercise, a natural counteractive relaxation response that can be learned.

Type A individuals have been told time and again to relax, but this directive has never been translated easily to a successful course of action. We believe that in part this is due to the Type A individuals' personal belief system, and in part to their having never been provided with a structured, credible method for doing so. Progressive muscle relaxation is presented as a means of actively mastering control over our bodies. Progressive muscle relaxation, in particular, is selected as a relaxation method because it offers a concrete and active approach to the elicitation of the relaxation response and an excellent way for Type A individuals to learn to better discriminate their varying levels of tension.

Participants are led through the progressive muscle relaxation exercises within the session and directed to practice under relatively calm circumstances; however, we do inform participants that toward the latter weeks of the program they will be directed in integrating the use of their newly acquired relaxation skills into their day-to-day activities. Thus, we strive to encourage an approach to the practice of relaxation as a purposeful accomplishment rather than a waste of time. Recording sheets are provided (see Table 2) on which participants enter the date and time and duration of their daily practice, the muscle groups easily relaxed as well as those that are more difficult to relax, and subjective units of discomfort (SUDS) ratings of tension levels before and after the relaxation exercise. Each of the remaining six group sessions concludes with a brief practice of progressive muscle relaxation and/or related relaxation techniques.

Session 3 begins with a review of home-based relaxation practice. Primary focus for this session is on the physical health habits of diet and exercise. Although concerns about health habits are by no means unique to the Type A individuals, we believe that they deserve mention in a program aimed at promoting cardiovascular risk reduction and more successful methods of stress management. Moreover, recent research suggests that significant reductions in Type A behavior have been experienced by subjects exposed to a 7-week aerobic physical exercise program (Lobitz, Brammell, Stoll, & Niccoli, 1983). In an at-

TABLE 2. Log for Relaxation Practice

Date and hour of practice	Duration of practice	Body areas easily relaxed	Body areas with tension	Tension level before	(0–100)[a] After

[a]0–100: 0 = nonexistent tension; 100 = maximum tension.

tempt to relate this unit to our overall conceptual model, we present physical health practices as areas that the Type A individuals can control even when external events may be out of their personal control. In our presentation on dietary practices, we address the role of salt in fluid retention and elevations of blood pressure. Caffeine and other sympathomimetics (i.e., substances that can simulate sympathetic nervous system reactions) are also discussed, drawing attention to their tendency to stimulate what may be an already overstimulated physiological system. It is pointed out that caffeine ingestion can mirror the responses of the body to an acute stressor in that it can produce elevations in catecholamine levels, blood pressure, and heart rate. Products with large amounts of salt and caffeine are identified in handouts, as are acceptable alternatives.

Aerobic exercises that can condition the heart and lungs are identified and distinguished from isometric, muscle-toning exercises that can help improve coordination and muscle tone and offer tension reduction but that do not condition the heart and lungs nor burn off many calories. A sample exercise program is provided that emphasizes the need to incorporate a warm-up, brisk state, and cool-down period during each regular exercise period. Exercising at least three times per week and allowing for graduated increments in exercise intensity and duration are stressed. This session concludes by having each participant complete the Habit Change Planning Sheet, on which specific physical health-related behaviors are targeted for change. This sheet is presented in Table 3.

Sessions 4/5

The fourth and fifth sessions comprise a module that focuses on cognitive/self-generated stressors. After reviewing and reinforcing individuals for their efforts to alter dietary practices and levels of physical exercise, the topic of cognition is introduced. Individuals are informed about how self-talk, interpretations of events, and underlying beliefs can stimulate stress reactions.

This notion is derived from the conceptual model of Rational Emotive Therapy (RET) (Ellis & Harper, 1975). At this stage we also describe how ones personal belief system can influence a wide variety of ones behavior. For example, the competitive, time-urgent, impatient, and hostile behaviors of Type A individuals are depicted as logical outgrowths of the Type A belief in Type A individuals proving themselves through visible accomplishments. These interrelationships, which have been discussed in detail by Price (1984), are further highlighted in each remaining group session. Unreasonable beliefs that are especially common among Type A individuals are identified along with their corresponding stress-disposing elements. Among the beliefs addressed are the following:

- I must be thoroughly competent in all tasks that I attempt.
- I should take responsibility for the outcome of all problems that I am personally aware of around me.
- Most of my actions are so weighty that my self-esteem is always on the line (win-lose orientation).
- I am only worthy if I accomplish something tangible.
- If I slow down or set limits for myself, people will disapprove and view me less favorably.
- I must have things my way and not be inconvenienced when I do not care to be.
- If things move out of my control, even temporarily, something disastrous will result.

Moment-to-moment self-talk is also attended to, and participants are informed that the question is not whether they talk to themselves (because all of us do subvocally) but rather how well they do this. Examples of problematic self-talk are provided from participants' experiences during instances where they may be setting stringent deadlines, responding to provocations, or interacting with someone who they perceive is acting unfairly. A written handout is distributed that familiarizes participants with common, unreasonable beliefs and self-talk distortions (e.g., overgeneralization, exaggerated self-criticism, disregarding the positive). The way in which ones beliefs can shape self-talk is also

TABLE 3. Habit Change Planning Sheet

	Mon	Tues	Wed	Th	Fri	Sat	Sun	Mon	Tues	Wed
1. Old habit										
Change to (new habit)										
2. Old habit										
Change to (new habit)										

described to participants. They are further encouraged to use the appearance of any stress symptoms as a signal or reminder to pause to consider if they have imposed an unreasonable belief or expressed negative self-talk. To assist in recognizing stress-inducing cognitions, participants are required to self-monitor over the course of the upcoming week using the format presented in Table 4.

Session 5 is formulated around the premise that Type A individuals must be provided with a concrete method of disputing and restructuring the unreasonable beliefs and negative self-talk that may account for increases in felt stress and undue activation of Type A behavior. The steps involved in the cognitive restructuring process are taught using examples from one or two of the participants' daily monitoring forms. The group is engaged in the task of posing dispute questions to challenge the validity of the associated beliefs and self-talk, and then of constructing more reasonable cognitions by answering these dispute questions.

An example of this cognitive restructuring process that relies on fairly standard RET methodology is presented in Table 5.

In working with the Type A individual in particular, it is important to emphasize that the process of changing one's thinking habits is a gradual one and that it often incorporates the following elements: becoming more aware of one's thinking; challenging unreasonable beliefs and negative self-talk in what often feels like a mechanical way; challenging more fluidly, without the aid of structured forms; catching oneself in the act of beginning to think in a stress-inducing manner and becoming more able to shortcircuit this; and, finally, thinking more reasonably and constructively in response to everyday activating events.

TABLE 4. Daily Monitoring Form

Date: ______

A. Activating event
   (Briefly describe the situation or event that seemed to lead to your emotional/physical upset at C)

B. Beliefs or self-talk
   (List each of the things that you said to yourself about A.)
   1.
   2.
   3.
   4.
   5.
   (Now go back and place a checkmark beside each statement that is nonconstructive, an unreasonable expectation, or negative self-talk)

C. Emotional/physical consequences
   (Describe how you felt when A happened.)
   Emotionally, I felt: ______
   Physically, I felt: ______

TABLE 5. Cognitive Restructuring Form

(A) Activating event: I got passed up for a managerial promotion.

(B) Unreasonable beliefs/ negative self-talk	(D) Disputes (questions)	Reasonable beliefs/positive self-talk (replies)
1. I should have worked harder.	1 (a) What evidence do I have that I didn't work hard enough? (b) Is hard work the only criteria used to decide promotions?	1. I really have no evidence that I didn't work hard enough. There are definitely other criteria like who you know and what openings are coming up in the near future.
2. I obviously don't have a future in this company.	2 (a) Does the fact that I didn't get this promotion have to mean I can't get another? (b) Isn't there other evidence that the company values me?	2. I could be eligible for other promotions. This is only one of many positions. My strong reviews and salary increases suggest that I am valued here.
3. My associates will think less of me and it's going to be awful.	3 (a) How likely is this to happen? (b) If some colleagues think less of me, will this be tragic?	3. I doubt that my associates most familiar with me will think less of me. It may be uncomfortable for a while, but not awful or tragic.
(C) Emotionally, I felt: angry; disappointed in myself; like a failure Physically, I felt: more tense; had bowel problems		Additional reasonable beliefs and positive self-talk —I feel that I handled myself well during the interview process. —Maybe they're grooming me for a senior position.

Group participants are further encouraged to use their self-talk to their best advantage by praising their own change efforts when completing a restructuring form or noticing even slight changes in their self-expectations, self-talk, or resulting emotional or physical reactions. The assignment for the week is to routinely complete cognitive restructuring forms, using the appearance of stress reactions as a cue to make entries. The importance of recording as soon after the actual occurrence of the activating event and associated beliefs/self-talk is highlighted.

Sessions 6/7

The initial part of the sixth session is spent reviewing the group's cognitive restructuring forms and behavior change efforts. Following this, a general review of progress to date is conducted. An emphasis is placed on encouraging group social reinforcement and self-reward for sustained behavior change efforts. At this stage, we also conduct a verbal survey to identify any remaining outstanding needs of the participants, so that these can be integrated into our remaining sessions.

The sixth and seventh sessions address the Type A individual's sense of time urgency and the resulting behaviors of unnecessary hurrying, impatience, and frustration/anger. These behaviors and emotional responses are presented as logical extensions of the Type A individual's unreasonable self- and other-directed expectations. Hurrying can take several forms: in speech, while walking, driving, or eating, even when there is not an external time constraint to be concerned about. Another common behavioral manifestation of the Type A sense of time urgency is polyphasic activity (i.e., doing several things at once). We illustrate how each of these behavioral practices can serve as unnecessary stress triggers for both the Type A individual, and others around him or her, can be physically taxing, and can interfere with one's enjoyment of what one is doing.

Group participants are taught several strategies to modify undue hurrying. First, they are directed to attempt to catch themselves in the act of hurrying, using this identification as a cue to purposely slow the pace of their actions. Second, participants are encouraged to place visible cues for themselves around the environment that might prompt a slowing of behavior. These can take the form of adding environmental cues such as a sign on the dash of the car, or taking away an unnecessary cue such as leaving one's wristwatch at home during a pure leisure activity. Third, participants are trained in covert visuomotor rehearsal (Suinn, 1975). Here they practice experiencing in imagination all aspects of a situation associated with hurrying, and rehearse through imagery new, more adaptive ways of behaving in this situation. For example, they may imagine themselves engaging in more conversation at the dinner table in an attempt to pace their eating, or driving at a leisurely speed while being passed by another driver. After several repetitions of their imaginal modeling/practice, participants are encouraged to approach these situations *in vivo* to practice implementing the desired alternative behaviors.

Each of the preceding intervention strategies is also applied to the Type A's related difficulties with excessive impatience. Type A individuals often describe a jittery feeling associated with waiting in lines (e.g., store checkout counters, the bank, traffic jams), or in situations where other individuals are not moving or speaking rapidly enough. Irritation can frequently result when external circumstances or interactions are slow and can be perceived by Type A individuals as a barrier to their productive flow. This may be particularly troublesome for Type A individuals because they have assumed more and more responsibilities with accompanying time pressures and have never learned to be comfortable with slower paced activities or less active pursuits. Participants are taught that behavioral cueing and covert rehearsal also can be applied to counteract impatience. Although the preceding two strategies are preferable, certain individuals also may choose to reduce their discomfort in this area by avoiding triggering situations/interactions (e.g., avoiding the banks on Friday afternoon; the expressway at rush hour).

The goals of Session 7 are to recognize how the relentless drive toward greater productivity and time urgency and their behavioral derivatives of hurrying and impatience can leave one more subject to increased frustration, irritability, and anger. Type A individuals tend to view situational inconveniences or less than competent, fair, or agreeable people as barriers that were created expressly to foil them. In addition to recognizing the unreasonable beliefs that can perpetuate this aspect of the TABP, we discuss the general product orientation that many Type A individuals have evolved, from which they view getting things done in order to achieve rewards as the only mode of operation. Because of this orientation, the actual here-and-now activities and interactions lose their intrinsic reward value and pleasure. We also focus on communication skills in an effort to convert aggresive communications into more effective, assertive ones and to improve listening skills. Didactic presentations, modeling, behavior rehearsal, videotaped feedback, and feedback from other group members are all utilized to aid the communication skills training.

In addition to cognitive and skill-building approaches to anger management, we teach a series of brief applied relaxation techniques that can be used to interrupt a sequence of angry behavior. The skills of diaphragmatic breathing, applying pleasant imagery, progressive muscle relaxation without the tension phase, and differential relaxation are all presented. Examples of how such relaxation methods can be used in the natural environment to disrupt frustration and anger are provided, along with suggestions about how to generalize the use of these skills to a range of other stressful emotional and physical states. Homework during this unit involves the following: "planting" written cues in key places in the work and home environment aimed at prompting modifications in hurrying, impatience, and anger; practicing covert rehearsal of adaptive behaviors on a daily basis; actively trying out newly learned listening and assertion skills; and continuing to identify, challenge, and restructure cognitions that may underlie the excessive sense of time urgency and anger.

Session 8

The eighth and last weekly group session addresses environmental sources of stress and triggers for Type A behavior. At the outset of this session, participants' efforts to change behaviors related to irritation and anger are reviewed and reinforced. We then proceed to new material, opening with the notion that because our work and home environments are composed of several stressful unalterable fixtures, it becomes all the more important to employ prudent stress management strategies in areas of one's life where control can be exerted.

Effective management of environmental stressors begins with knowing the goals toward which one is headed. For Type A individuals, it is particularly important to structure this goal-setting task such that goals are set in personal and family/interpersonal areas, as well as in the career area. Participants are also encouraged to consider goals of "being" (e.g., personal qualities to be developed or furthered), as well as more performance-oriented goals. Following the setting of reasonable intermediate goals, these goals are prioritized, with a manageable number of actions to be taken targeted for immediate attention. We also address issues of time management: the avoidance of inappropriate, excessive commitments through delegation and assertion; and control over the obstacles of perfectionism and procrastination. Perhaps the greatest imbalance in the time distribution of Type A individuals is their tendency to carry work-related projects or worries into the home environment. We highlight the importance of separating the work from the home setting and recommend several strategies in this regard. These include leaving work at the office and establishing an end of the workday ritual to provide a clearer transition to a leisure mode. Finally, replenishing adaptive resources through relaxation breaks, exercise, and vacations (which Type A individuals often forego), and leaving oneself unscheduled time are presented as important means of buffering the unavoidable environmental stressors of day-to-day living.

Session 9

The ninth and final session is conducted 1 month after the last weekly session. This provides an opportunity for group participants to further practice applying newly learned skills in the natural environment, to experience a consolidation of gains, and to allow time for additional questions to surface. After reviewing and appropriately reinforcing the members' behavior patterns over this 1-month interval, a brief presentation is delivered on strategies aimed at promoting the maintenance and generalization of gains. Several points are highlighted.

1. The importance of continuing to set intermediate and attainable goals is emphasized, tying the attainment of these with predefined rewards (self-administered or provided by significant others).
2. The necessity of continuing to practice newly learned skills (e.g., relaxation, cognitive monitoring/self-talk, appropriate assertion, time management) is stressed. We also assert that further facility with the coping skills can be gained by teaching these skills to someone else, and we encourage participants to do so.
3. Participants are encouraged to vary the setting, timing, and situations under which these applications are occurring to enhance the likelihood of broader generalization.
4. The nature of progress is discussed so that participants will realize that it does not necessarily follow an upward climbing, linear course. Brief periods of "backsliding" are to be expected and not to be viewed as a total failure and reason to put aside what the participants have learned. Participants are also encouraged to develop a plan in advance for coping with situations that may carry with them a high risk of eliciting Type A behavior.

The final session concludes with discussions aimed at soliciting feedback from participants on the group's strengths and weaknesses, and by answering any remaining questions. Participants are then praised for their change efforts and asked to complete posttesting instruments.

Minimizing Noncompliance to the Treatment Regimen

Even the most effective medical or behavioral interventions are compromised if patients do not adhere to the recommended regimen. For example, recent surveys have shown that fewer than 30% of patients with hypertension benefit from treatment because of failure to comply with their treatment regimens despite convincing evidence that antihypertensive medication is effective in lowering blood pressure and associated health risks (Hypertension Detection and Follow Up Program Cooperative Group, 1979).

Several efforts are taken to minimize noncompliance within the TABP intervention program. As described previously, an initial screening/orientation interview is conducted, at which time the group intervention is described both verbally and in writing. The TABP group is presented in a manner that is consistent with the needs and alert to the resistances of the Type A individual. The intervention is described as a potential source of improvement to the Type A individuals' efficiency and productivity, and not one that will convert them to Type B's. Expectations regarding the nature of progress are also discussed at the outset, with attention to the peaks, plateaus, and valleys to be expected as part of the customary nonlinear course of progress. This latter strategy as well as providing individual contacts for participants who miss a group session can help to minimize dropouts.

During the course of the group, efforts are made to clearly detail information for participants in both verbal and written formats. Self-monitoring sheets are also provided for relaxation practice, cognitive monitoring and restructuring tasks, and habit change to add structure and accountability to these homework assignments. Wherever possible, directions on the application of coping strategies are individually tailored to increase the likelihood of initial compliance and long-term maintenance. Selection of ways to build exercise into an individual's activities of daily living or to choose a time, place, and type of exercise to pursue are examples of decisions that we assist the participant to make on an individual basis. Compliance is further bolstered by providing reinforcement from group leaders and other participants for behavior change efforts and improvements.

Outcome

Preliminary results of the preceding group intervention program have been clinically evaluated through the administration of the Jenkins Activity Survey (JAS) and the Trait Scale of the State Trait Anxiety Inventory (STAI) pre- and posttreatment. These data should be interpreted cautiously because complete data are reported on only 25 cases and are evaluated without the benefit of a controlled comparison group. The JAS data revealed statistically significant changes in the desired direction of the overall Type A score and in each of the three factor scores: (a) the overall Type A score ($t = 4.02$, $p < .001$); (b) the Speed and Impatience factor addressing time urgency, impatience with others, frank expression of irritation, and having a strong temper ($t = 5.06$, $p < .001$); (c) the Job Involvement factor reflecting dedication to occupational activities, a tendency to work overtime, and to work with frequent deadlines ($t = 1.73$, $p < .05$); and (d) the Hard-Driving and Competitive factor involving the perception of oneself as being more hard driving, competitive, and conscientious than other people ($t = 1.79$, $p < .05$). In addition, an adjunctive measure, the STAI, which is a brief self-administered instrument designed to measure more enduring aspects of anxiety, also revealed significant pre-post reductions in reported anxiety levels of group participants ($t = 2.99$, $p < .01$). Encouraging anecdotal reports of modifications in Type A behavior provided by group participants and their significant others adds further confidence to these preliminary outcome data. A better test of ourcome will come with time, as analyses including physiological monitoring during behavioral challenges, measures relating Type A behavior changes to coronary heart disease end points, and long-term follow-up of a larger number of program participants can be conducted.

Pitfalls and Directions for Future TABP Work

Program descriptions such as the one provided in this chapter can often leave the reader with the misconception that behavioral group intervention is a static process that runs like clockwork. In reality, we have encountered several pitfalls in our work with Type A individuals. I will summarize the most significant of these briefly, so that future efforts in this area can profit from our experience.

As one might expect, many Type A individuals erect an initial barrier to their group participation by claiming to be too busy to attend regular sessions. We have tried to use this concern as further justification for the appropriateness of the Type A group for these individuals. That is, we discuss how overextended these individuals must be to be unable to attend a brief series of meetings in the early evening. There are many individuals who are appropriate for the group who nonetheless choose not to participate for this reason. We respect their decision and place their name on our waiting list for a subsequent Type A group. In some cases, a further experience of stress symptoms, the onset of CHD, or added encouragement from a physician can increase an individual's motivation to participate at a later date. Reluctance to participate can also take on another common form, with the prospective participant commenting, "I've attended a lecture on stress management just last month." Here our approach is to highlight how our group intervention can be distinguished from a single lecture on the basis of its efficacy, focus on Type A behavior as it relates to stress, and more individualized attention.

Even after making a firm commitment to attend, many Type A individuals will ask for explicit assurances that the time they invest in the group will be productive. Although it is tempting to fall back on our empirical foundations and simply cite outcome data, we believe that this response is insufficient. It is also important to provide feedback to the Type A individual about what may be an unreasonable request for guarantees and how this may be representative of an unreasonable belief that *all* time can or must be spent constructively. Thus, group participation and the participants' willingness to allow the intervention to proceed without the assurance of a thoroughly productive expenditure of time is reframed for them as an initial step toward moderating Type A extremes. It is also important to be alert to group participants who may adopt a Type A approach to the change process: hurrying their efforts, being impatient at the pace of behavior change, taking on too many change projects at once, and chasing several ambiguous goals. We have found it best to predict such behavior at the outset of the group, and to repeatedly indicate how this course of action is counterproductive whenever it is reported by a group participant.

A final potential pitfall that we have encountered pertains to relaxation work with Type A individuals. Let me first say that we have found it beneficial to teach a relaxation method fairly early in the group. It offers fairly quick and visible results and can provide the Type A individual with a method for maintaining internal control even when external circumstances may be somewhat out of control. This rationale has been readily accepted. In general, we believe that it is desirable to begin the group by proposing the least threatening changes. Therefore, we have chosen to focus first on physical health habit modifications, of which relaxation training is a part.

After trial-and-error experimentation, we have decided upon tense-release progressive muscle relaxation as the relaxation method of choice for the majority of Type A individuals. Progressive muscle relaxation offers the Type A individual an active process and one in which a tensed and relaxed state can be most readily differentiated. Moreover, our experience in teaching Type A individuals to apply Benson's relaxation response was disappointing. It appeared that this more passive mode of eliciting the relaxation response failed to provide the Type A individuals with sufficient direction in overcoming their basic discomfort with being relaxed while sitting still.

Before suggesting directions for further Type A behavior modification work, I would like to mention a way in which interdisciplinary collaboration in behavioral medicine can serve as a basis for further expansion of behavioral medicine services. By demonstrating a range of interventions for Type A behavior that could be offered by a behavioral medicine staff person, the needs of other target groups within the cardiology department have now been identified. A psychoeducational group for individuals diagnosed with mitral valve prolapse (a minor heart defect that can trigger chest pain, palpitations, or shortness of breath) has been proposed, with the goal of providing information on mitral valve prolapse, minimizing patients' fearfulness, and decreasing the likelihood that newly diagnosed patients will develop any untoward life-style restrictions.

In regard to future directions for work on modifying the TABP, there are at least three pressing areas requiring further attention. The first of these involves the assessment of the TABP. This assessment has been closely tied to the prediction of CHD, and assessment instruments or interviews have been evaluated on the basis of their ability to predict disease end points. This has been advantageous from the standpoint of the global identification of individuals in need of health risk-reduction work. Assessment for the purpose of designing the optimal behavior change program, however, will require a more finely tuned, individualized behavioral analysis in the future. Behavioral observations in the natural environment would be of value in describing the characteristics of antecedent situations that may tend to elicit Type A behavior as well as providing a more specific identification of each individual's constellation of Type A behavior.

Second, during the past decade, great strides have been made in drawing attention to the importance of the TABP as a health-risk factor. Nonetheless, I believe that we have far to go before assessment and intervention work with Type A individuals is accepted into routine medical practice. My experience is that medical providers screening for coronary risk factors will usually identify a patient's traditional risk factors, and at times presentations of marked stress, but only infrequently refer for assessment/modification of the TABP. Repeated reminders about the availability and efficacy of the TABP group intervention must be provided to these medical practitioners. An additional obstacle to the "mainstreaming" of Type A intervention work is posed by current third party reimbursement policies. As is true for other health risk-reduction interventions (e.g., weight reduction, smoking cessation), individual patients are usually required to pick up the cost of treatment. I would hope that the credibility of behavioral medicine services for Type A individuals will be strengthened, and eligibility for third party payments approved, as the efficacy of Type A behavior intervention efforts continues to be demonstrated without the appearance of untoward side effects.

Third, the clinical evidence reported from our Lahey Clinic Program and the controlled outcome data summarized earlier provide initial evidence for the efficacy of brief behavioral interventions for the modification of TABP. Although these demonstrations of short-term changes are promising, long-term maintenance of reduced health risk remains elusive and deserves further attention in our behavioral medicine work. Perhaps the approach of the Recurrent Coronary Prevention Program can serve as a model for this. Their intervention will be maintained for a five-year period, with a gradual reduction of the frequency of group sessions over time. Future efforts to improve long-term maintainance of behavioral change with Type A individuals may profit by including significant others who can be important sources of reinforcement (e.g., spouses, parents, work colleagues) as active participants in the intervention process. Ultimately, the utility of TABP modification efforts will be decided on the basis of their ability to effect behavior change that generalizes across time and settings, and results in reduced cardiac morbidity and mortality.

References

Blanchard, E. B. Behavioral medicine: A perspective. In R. B. Williams, Jr., & W. D. Gentry (Eds.), *Behavioral approaches to medical treatment*. Cambridge, Mass.: Ballinger, 1977.

Bortner, R. W. A short rating scale as a potential measure of Pattern A behavior. *Journal of Chronic Diseases,* 1969, *22,* 87–91.

Dembroski, T. M., MacDougall, J. M., & Shields, J. L. Physiologic reactions to social challenge in persons evidencing the Type A coronary-prone behavior pattern. *Journal of Human Stress,* 1977, *3,* 2–9.

Ellis, A., & Harper, R. A. *A new guide to rational living.* North Hollywood, Calif.: Wilshire, 1975.

Friedman, M., & Rosenman, R. H. Association of specific overt behavior pattern with blood and cardiovascular findings. *Journal of the American Medical Association,* 1959, *169,* 1286–1296.

Friedman, M., Thoresen, C. E., Gill, J. J., *et al.* Alteration of Type A behavior and reduction in cardiac recurrences in postmyocardial infarction patients. *American Heart Journal,* 1984, *108*(2), 237–248.

Friedman, M., Byers, S. D., Diamant, J., & Rosenman, R. H. Plasma catecholamine response of coronary-prone subjects (Type A) to a specific challenge. *Metabolism,* 1975, *24,* 205–210.

Glass, D. *Behavior patterns, stress, and coronary disease.* Hillsdale, N.J.: Erlbaum, 1977.

Goldband, S. Stimulus specificity of physiological response to stress, and the Type A behavior pattern. *Journal of Personality and Social Psychology,* 1980, *39,* 670–679.

Haynes, S. G., Feinleib, M., & Kannel, W. B. The relationship of psychosocial factors to coronary heart disease in the Framingham Study: III. Eight-year incidence of coronary heart disease. *American Journal of Epidemiology,* 1980, *111,* 37–58

Hypertension Detection and Follow-up Program Cooperative Group. Five-year findings of the hypertension detection and follow-up program. I. Reduction in mortality of persons with high blood pressure, including mild hypertension. II. Mortality by race, sex and age. *Journal of the American Medical Association,* 1979, *242*(23), 2562–2577.

Jenkins, C. D., Rosenman, R. H., & Zyzanski, S. J. Prediction of clinical coronary heart disease by a test for the coronary-prone behavior pattern. *New England Journal of Medicine,* 1974, *290,* 1271–1275.

Jenkins, C. D., Zyzanski, S. J., & Rosenman, R. H. Progress toward validation of a computer-scored test for the Type A coronary-prone behavior pattern. *Psychosomatic Medicine,* 1971, *33,* 193–202.

Jenkins, C. D., Zyzanski, S. J., & Rosenman, R. H. Risk of new myocardial infarction in middle-aged men with manifest coronary heart disease. *Circulation,* 1976, *53,* 342–347.

Jenni, M. A., & Wollersheim, J. B. Cognitive therapy, stress management training, and the Type A behavior pattern. *Cognitive Therapy and Research,* 1979, *3,* 61–73.

Krantz, D. S., & Durel, L. A. Psychobiological substrates of the Type A behavior pattern. *Health Psychology,* 1983, *2*(4), 393–411.

Levenkron, J. C., Cohen, J. D., Mueller, H. S., & Fisher, E. B. Modifying the Type A coronary-prone behavior pattern. *Journal of Consulting and Clinical Psychology,* 1983, *51*(2), 192–204.

Lobitz, W. C., Brammell, H. L., Stoll, S., & Niccoli, A. Physical exercise and anxiety management training for cardiac stress management in a non-patient population. *Journal of Cardiac Rehabilitation,* 1983, *3,* 683–688.

Matthews, K. A. Psychological perspectives on the Type A Behavior Pattern. *Psychological Bulletin,* 1982, *91,* 293–323.

Matthews, K. A., Glass, D. C., Rosenman, R. H., & Bortner, R. W. Competitive drive, Pattern A, and coronary heart disease: A further analysis of some data from the Western Collaborative Group Study. *Journal of Chronic Diseases,* 1977, *30,* 489–498.

Novaco, R. W. *Anger control.* Lexington, Mass.: D. C. Heath, 1975.

Pomerleau, O. F. Behavioral medicine: The contribution of the experimental analysis of behavior to medical care. *American Psychologist,* 1979, *34,* 654–663.

Pomerleau, O. F., & Brady, J. P. The scope and promise of behavioral medicine. In O. F. Pomerleau & J. P. Brady (Eds.), *Behavioral medicine: theory and practice.* Baltimore: Williams & Wilkins, 1979.

Price, V. A. *Type A behavior pattern: A model for research and practice.* New York: Academic Press, 1982.

Review Panel on Coronary-Prone Behavior and Coronary Heart Disease. Coronary-prone behavior and coronary heart disease: A critical review. *Circulation,* 1981, *63,* 1199–1215.

Rosenman, R. H. The role of behavior patterns and neurogenic factors in the pathogenesis of coronary heart disease. In R. S. Eliot (Ed.), *Stress and the heart.* New York: Futura, 1974.

Rosenman, R. H. The interview method of assessment of the coronary-prone behavior pattern. In T. M. Dembroski, S. M. Weiss, J. L. Shields, S. G. Haynes, & M. Feinleib (Eds.), *Coronary-prone behavior.* New York: Springer-Verlag, 1978.

Rosenman, R. H., Brand, R. J., Jenkins, C. D., Friedman, M., Straus, R., & Wurm, M. Coronary heart disease in the Western Collaborative Group Study: Final follow-up experience of 8½ years. *Journal of the American Medical Association*, 1975, *233*, 872–877.

Roskies, E. Considerations in developing a treatment program for the coronary-prone (Type A) behavior pattern. In P. Davidson & S. Davidson (Eds.), *Behavioral medicine: Changing health lifestyles*. New York: Brunner/Mazel, 1980.

Roskies, E., Kearney, H., Spevack, M., Surkis, A., Cohen, C., & Gilman, S. Generalizability and durability of treatment effects in an intervention program for coronary-prone (Type A) managers. *Journal of Behavioral Medicine*, 1979, *2*, 195–207.

Roskies, E., Spevack, M., Surkis, A., Cohen, C., & Gilman, S. Changing the coronary-prone (Type A) behavior pattern in a nonclinical population. *Journal of Behavioral Medicine*, 1978, *1*, 201–216.

Schwartz, G. E., & Weiss, S. M. Proceedings of the Yale conference on behavioral medicine (U.S. Department of Health, Education, and Welfare Publication No. (NIH) 78-1424). Washington, D.C.: U.S. Government Printing Office, 1977.

Spielberger, C. D., Gorsuch, R. C., & Lushene, R. E. *Manual for the State-Trait Anxiety Inventory*. Palo Alto, Calif.: Consulting Psychologists Press, 1970.

Suinn, R. M. The cardiac stress management program for Type A patients. *Cardiac Rehabilitation*, 1975, *5*, 13–16.

Suinn, R. M., & Bloom, L. J. Anxiety management training for Pattern A behavior. *Journal of Behavioral Medicine*, 1978, *1*, 25–35.

Thoresen, C. E., Telch, M. J., & Eagleston, J. R. Approaches to altering the Type A Behavior Pattern. *Psychosomatics*, 1981, *22*(6), 472–480.

Williams, R. B., Haney, T. L., Lee, K. L., Kong, Y. H., Blumenthal, J. A., & Whalen, R. E. Type A behavior, hostility, and coronary atherosclerosis. *Psychosomatic Medicine*, 1980, *42*(6), 539–549.

Zyzanski, S. J., & Jenkins, C. D. Basic dimensions within the coronary-prone behavior pattern. *Journal of Chronic Disorders*, 1970, *22*, 781–795.

10

Behavioral Group Therapy with the Elderly

A Psychoeducational Approach

JULIA STEINMETZ BRECKENRIDGE, LARRY W. THOMPSON, JAMES N. BRECKENRIDGE, AND DOLORES E. GALLAGHER

INTRODUCTION

Older adults comprise a rapidly increasing proportion of the population in the United States. In 1980, 9.9% of the population was 65 or older; between the 1960 and 1970 censuses, the number of aged increased 21.1% (Brotman, 1973). Pfeiffer (1980) reports that 11% of our population is over age 65, and 25% of these persons are thought to have psychological difficulties warranting professional attention. Approximately 25% of all suicides in this country are committed by persons over age 65 (Butler & Lewis, 1977). There is a well-documented gap, however, between the mental health needs of the elderly and the provision of services to meet these needs (Zarit, 1980). At least two-thirds of all psychologists do not work clinically with elderly clients (VandenBos, Stapp, & Kilberg, 1981). Only 4 to 5% of the case load in outpatient mental health clinics consists of elderly clients (Redick & Taube, 1980), and an even smaller percentage of elders are thought to be treated by private practitioners (Gottfredson & Dyer, 1978).

Underutilization of services by the elderly has been partially attributed to a complementary relationship between older adults' reluctance to seek mental health services and professionals' resistance to use psychological interventions in treating elderly persons with apparent psychiatric problems. Regarding the hesitancy of elders to use psychological services, Zarit (1980) notes that the elderly may doubt that mental health personnel can be effective in helping them reduce their psychological discomfort. Given the history of medical difficulties and the regular use of medications typical of many elderly persons, it seems likely that those elders who do view their difficulties as psychological might

JULIA STEINMETZ BRECKENRIDGE, LARRY W. THOMPSON, JAMES N. BRECKENRIDGE, and DOLORES E. GALLAGHER • Veterans Administration Medical Center, Palo Alto, California 94304. This chapter was supported in part by grants R01-MH37196 and T01-MH17621 from the National Institute of Mental Health.

anticipate pharmaceutical remedies rather than behavioral treatment. They may also fear that consulting a mental health professional is tantamount to acknowledging severe pathology. Other elders may deem the admission of psychological difficulties to be a sign of personal weakness (Lawton, 1978) and feel that they should be able to handle their problems without professional assistance. Moreover, those elders who do seek professional assistance are often discouraged by shortages of low-cost, time-limited services—a difficulty encountered by most adults, but of particular concern for those living on limited retirement incomes.

Elders' judgments about the appropriateness of psychological help also may be influenced by incorrect or inadequate information regarding the course of "normal aging." The elderly are routinely confronted with the consequences of declining health and diminishing physical stamina and ability. Depressive signs such as insomnia, poor appetite, or fatigue may be construed primarily as age-congruent physical deterioration rather than as psychosocial in origin. Thus, many essentially psychological disturbances may be mistaken as "just a part of growing older" and not amenable to intervention. There is substantial evidence, moreover, that health practitioners may mistakenly attribute psychological symptoms to merely physical causes (Okimoto, Barnes, Veith, Raskind, Inui, & Carter, 1982). Kline (1976), for instance, cites several studies indicating that primary care physicians recognize clinical depression in only 10 to 33% of geriatric patients with depressive disorders.

Regarding the attitudes of professionals, Butler and Lewis (1977) suggest that clinicians may be reluctant to treat older persons because of negative views about the likelihood of beneficial outcome. Tacit beliefs that older persons are more rigid, less "psychologically minded," and more likely to have concomitant organic pathology underlie the conviction that the elderly are poor therapeutic candidates. Biases of this kind have been seriously challenged in the literature. For instance, elderly patients have been found to be faithful in attending therapy sessions, to engage thoroughly in the psychotherapy process, and to show therapeutic gains comparable to younger adults (e.g., Gallagher & Thompson, 1982; Mintz, Steuer, & Jarvik, 1981).

It is also possible that the training of many mental health service providers inadequately addresses the special concerns of older adults. In addition to the usual preparation for clinical responsibilities, work with aged populations demands knowledge of the behavioral correlates of prevalent physical disorders among the elderly as well as normative expectations for biological and cognitive function in later life. Few programs for mental health practitioners have offered extensive training in gerontology; Storandt (1976) reports fewer than 100 psychologists trained specifically in gerontology. Niederehe (1980) and Cohen and Cooley (1983) have recently documented the paucity of training currently available in this area.

Despite the substantial numbers of elderly who might benefit from psychological intervention and despite the well-documented deficiencies in service delivery, few outcome studies concerning psychotherapy of any orientation have employed older samples. Indeed, many exclude participants over age 60, and those studies that have included elders rarely report treatment effects broken down by age group. This state of affairs seems to be changing recently, however, as greater attention is directed to more thorough training of professionals in clinical gerontology, the development of specialized treatments for elders, and innovative outreach and education programs. The recent influx of state and federal monies to support research and training in aging has been instrumental in stimulating the development of such programs.

Behavioral group therapy, and particularly behavioral treatment offered in a psychoeducational framework, offers great promise for older populations. This chapter briefly reviews recent work in applying behavioral techniques to the problems of aging in a group format and presents the efforts of the authors to make behavioral techniques available to elders in a manner that is responsive both to their characteristic hesitancies regarding psychological treatment and to their physical, cognitive, and economic limitations.

Behavioral Group Therapy for Elders

The central, defining characteristics of the variety of approaches labeled as *behavior therapy* are well suited to the concerns of elder clients. Kazdin and Wilson (1978) identify two fundamental assumptions of behavioral approaches: a rejection of intra-psychic, quasi-disease models of mental illness and a commitment to scientific method in measurement and evaluation. Emphasizing primarily current, specific determinants of behavior, difficulties are construed as problems of living and subject to the same processes that influence normal behavior. This focus lessens the potential stigma associated with a stress on intrapsychic disease and enhances the potential for a collaborative approach to the elder client's complaints.

Clients who have misgivings about the nature and efficacy of therapy are frequently encouraged by the routine provision of a rationale for each procedure employed and the pragmatic format of behavioral approaches to treatment. Typically, clients record and monitor relevant activities, and treatment goals are broken down into a series of specific tasks. Interventions center on a single problem, or at least a restricted set of problems, shifting to other difficulties only with the achievement of objectives or the realization of new "data" concerning the target problem. This emphasis on the evaluation of progress and the concrete measurement and specification of problems is critical to work with older adults.

As the rationale for behavioral therapy procedures is developed in early sessions, differences in client and therapist expectations can be minimized. Such differences may be especially significant in the treatment of older adults, who are likely to have had little prior experience with psychotherapy of any kind (Zarit, 1980). Unlike their younger counterparts who have grown up in a culture where psychotherapy is a relatively common and accepted procedure, elder patients may see therapy as a mysterious and threatening process. The elaboration of client complaints in terms of specific behavioral objectives helps alleviate elders' uncertainties about the aims and appropriateness of intervention. In addition, behavioral treatment is usually brief and time limited, factors that are appealing to persons who are anxious to use their later years to best advantage. The active role assumed by the behavior therapist, together with the concentration on concrete issues, may be especially appropriate for elderly clients, a group who are said to benefit from higher levels of structure and support (Pfeiffer & Busse, 1973).

Further, the contingencies affecting elders in need of assistance often necessitate the development of new skills. Thus, the elderly frequently must learn skills to compensate for the many physical and emotional losses they encounter. An elderly widow, for example, may have to acquire new skills for managing financial resources and meeting needs for social interaction. Stroke, disease, or generally deteriorating health also entail the development of new behavioral skills to accomodate the loss of function. Behavioral approaches can provide effective training in the development of such skills.

The collaborative character of behavior therapy augments the client's sense of self-control over those behaviors that achieve and maintain positive change. Self-efficacy perceptions are enhanced by a growing appreciation of the factors influencing targeted problems—an understanding bolstered by self-evaluated monitoring of environmental/behavioral relationships. These are crucial assets for the treatment of distressed elderly because, as they witness the loss of abilities they once relied upon and sense others' lowering estimations of their capacities, elders' confidence in their capabilities may be attenuated. Few elders can depend upon extensive external support and assistance; therefore, treatments that strengthen personal control may be especially beneficial for older populations. The majority of behavioral interventions discussed in this chapter are aimed at increasing clients' self-control and facilitating more positive self-efficacy perceptions.

Finally, behavioral treatments have been specifically developed (although not always with the elderly in mind) for many of the physical and psychological symptoms commonly observed among older persons. Thus, procedures for the remediation of urinary incontinence (e.g., Atthowe, 1975), sexual dysfunction (e.g., Marks, 1976), chronic pain (e.g., Fordyce, 1976), sleep disturbance (e.g., Coates & Thoresen, 1981), alcohol addiction (e.g., Miller & Taylor, 1980), and eating disorders (e.g., Abrams, 1979) are readily available. In addition to these, behavioral approaches for increasing compliance with medical treatment regimes, enhancing social skills, developing assertive behavior, and reducing anxiety address significant needs of elderly patients.

A group treatment format offers further advantages over individual therapy for the elderly. Provision of services to groups of participants permits efficient dissemination of instructional material and can reduce costs, an appealing advantage to elderly with limited economic resources. Group formats enable participants to receive positive reinforcement from peers and provide increased opportunity to model both peer and leader behavior. The availability of several participants permits guided rehearsal and practice of certain social skills, and performance may be enhanced with feedback from multiple sources. Group members can also draw upon the example of others—they may observe peers attempting to cope with difficulties similar to their own as well as problems significantly different from their own, thus increasing their appreciation of the generalization of intervention principles. The interaction among group members is often quite enjoyable and serves to reinforce participants' commitment to the treatment. The social interaction itself may be especially salient for elders, a group for whom loneliness and isolation are common problems. Further, group treatment offers a "normalizing" function, permitting help-seeking elders to recognize that their problems are not unique but represent typical difficulties shared to a great extent by their peers. The participation of peers is particularly beneficial in work with older adults, when group leaders may be several decades younger than group participants.

Despite the promise of group behavioral therapy for elders, recent reviews have found very few reports of its use (Gallagher, 1981; Richards & Thorpe, 1978). Richards and Thorpe (1978) note that most published reports concern inpatient populations. The primary focus is often on the attenuation of negative behaviors that may be problematical to staff, such as incontinence or demandingness rather than on "clinically significant" behaviors such as depressive cognitions or social withdrawal. Richards and Thorpe's review thus encompasses the use of behavioral methods to modify institutional staff behavior and attitudes toward the elderly. These authors strongly advocate an increased emphasis on the use of behavioral methods for enhancement of skill, functioning, and satisfaction in elders (Richards & Thorpe, 1978).

A review of the most recent literature yields few additional published reports of behavioral group treatment with the elderly. The two most recent comprehensive annual reviews of group therapy literature provide a vivid illustration: of the 536 published reports of group therapy appearing in 1980 (reviewed by Silver, Lubin, Miller, & Dobson, 1981), *none* focused specifically on the elderly. Their review of the 1981 group therapy literature was slightly more encouraging: of 717 articles, four were concerned with the elderly (Silver, Miller, Lubin & Dobson, 1982). None of these four, however, was concerned with the use of behavioral group therapy.

A search of the major gerontological and psychological journals of the past 2 years yielded only a few published reports of group therapy with elders that is explicitly behavioral. An example of recent work is Evans and Jaureguy's (1981) description of a cognitive-behavioral group program for visually impaired elderly, utilizing telephone conference calls. Treatment goals include provision of social support and interaction, building of problem-solving skills, provision of information about resources, and enhancement of confidence. The authors report that program participants, in contrast to controls, exhibited significant reductions in loneliness, increases in outside social activity, and improved management of daily household routine. This approach is notable for its innovative outreach aspects; for example, telephone intervention made the group much more accessible to the participants and did not preclude social contact and support.

Patterson and Eberly (1983) describe a modular behavioral group treatment program to improve daily living and social skills in the elderly. This multicomponent program is designed to be administered to groups of patients in inpatient settings. Some components emphasize primarily traditional behavioral procedures (e.g., use of tokens to reinforce desired responses), whereas others are more educational in nature (e.g., training modules on self-care behaviors and social skills). This differentiation between the direct application of behavioral procedures in a therapeutic relationship or milieu and the teaching of behavioral skills and principles so that a client can use them independently is elaborated upon in the following section.

A Psychoeducational Model of Behavioral Group Treatment

In the last several decades, *behavior therapy* has denoted a broad array of interventions. Behavioral treatments have ranged from interventions relying primarily on classical and operant conditioning paradigms to those emphasizing the role of cognitive mediation in behavioral change (Kazdin & Wilson, 1978). Illustrations of treatments for the elderly using classical (Cautela, 1969) or operant (Hoyer, 1973) approaches are given elsewhere. What is here termed a *psychoeducational* approach to behavioral group treatment is most closely associated with the social learning conceptualization of behavior therapy (Bandura, 1977). Social learning theory emphasizes the role of vicarious, symbolic, and self-regulatory processes and accords individuals an active role in the modification of their own environment. Thus, the individual's capacity for self-control is accentuated. Whereas classical conditioning processes and external reinforcement systems are clearly important to psychoeducational approaches, interventions focus primarily on the active role of individuals in mediating environmental influences on the acquisition and maintenance of behaviors. Individual functioning is viewed as the result of continuous reciprocal interactions among environmental, behavioral, and cognitive processes. Psychoeducational procedures strongly emphasize attention to specific environmental events, their impact on behavior, and the manner in which they are perceived.

A psychoeducational approach makes relatively little effort to directly control the antecedents or contingencies of clients' behavior. In contrast to behavior modification procedures for increasing elders' activity levels (e.g., Libb & Clements, 1969) the psychoeducational treatments described here emphasize learning through instructional materials and guided exercises. Instructional materials are intended to modify clients' perspectives regarding target problems, and clients are encouraged to attend to cognitive, behavioral, and environmental antecedents and consequences of salient behaviors. Clients are *taught* the rationales of conditioning processes, and these relationships are demonstrated by a variety of "homework" activities (e.g., self-monitoring of mood/behavior relationships or personal contracting). Although guided exercises aim at immediate beneficial change, they also contribute to the maintenance of new perspectives and continued self-directed intervention in future difficulties.

Psychoeducational approaches fundamentally assume that target difficulties are the consequence of specific skills deficits, that is, that the distressed individual is unable to track and evaluate events in a manner that permits self-directed intervention. Such skills are taught through verbal instruction (supplemented with a series of reading materials), graduated practice with feedback, and opportunities to model peer and leader behavior. Assertive training and social skills training are familiar examples of psychoeducational interventions. Early psychoeducational programs in institutional settings are exemplified by the work of Bakker and Armstrong (1976). For the treatment of depression, McLean's (1976) skills training approach, Lewinsohn's social learning treatment (Lewinsohn, Sullivan, & Grosscup, 1980) and Rehm's (1981) self-control therapy are notable examples of psychoeducational interventions.

Psychoeducational interventions are frequently offered as "classes" or "workshops." It should be stressed, however, that the procedures employed constitute behavioral treatments whether they are presented as educational or therapeutic. Strictly educational formats are differentiated from the explicit provision of therapy by the commitment made by group leaders to participants, and, to a much lesser extent, by client characteristics. Under a therapeutic contract, the therapist commits to a much broader range of responsibilities than those required by the promise to teach the principles of self-change. The educational format is probably most appropriate for elders with mild disorders, but it may also be employed as a supplement to other forms of treatment or as a preventive intervention for persons at risk for future disorders.

As Levy, Derogatis, Gallagher, and Gatz (1980) have noted, there is a need for innovative interventions that have appeal for the elderly and in which older adults can engage without needing to identify themselves as patients. The educational format of psychoeducational behavioral interventions is particularly responsive to these concerns. The educational format precludes the labeling of participants as *patients* or *clients*, preferring the label *students*. Group leaders are called *instructors* rather than *therapists*. Such pedagogical titles may reduce the stigma that reluctant elders may attach to the use of mental health services. As is the case for other educational formats, the interventions are time limited, with goals, procedures, and requirements clearly defined at the outset. If class members are screened to assure that those requiring more intensive intervention than can be offered in a classroom setting are referred to other more appropriate resources, groups are relatively homogeneous, further reducing anxiety or stigmatization that might be experienced by group members.

When presented as a class for the elderly, the psychoeducational model carries with it the benefits of group behavioral therapy discussed previously. In addition, this approach provides a number of unique and attractive features. Perhaps what is most important is that courses can readily be made available in nonmental health settings. Senior centers, for instance, can schedule such classes among their regular offerings. This outreach capability is further strengthened by the fact that classes may be led or co-led by paraprofessionals, given appropriate background and training. Thus, the ability to provide mental health services to older adults is greatly expanded.

The remainder of this chapter is devoted to a description of our continuing work with psychoeducational behavioral groups for the elderly. Most of our research to date has been concerned with the treatment and prevention of depressive disorders in older adults. Applications to other problem areas common to older adults are being developed, and these are described as well.

The Coping with Depression Course

As noted earlier, depression is a common problem among the elderly. Approximately 5 to 7% of community-residing adults over 65 years of age are in a clinically significant episode of depression at any point in time (Blazer & Williams, 1980; Gurland, 1976; Vernon & Roberts, 1982). Lifetime rates in this age range, of course, are even higher. No reliable figures are available for the prevalence of subclinical depressions, but estimates have ranged from 15 to as high as 50% (Pfeiffer, 1980).

Two studies have recently demonstrated the effectiveness of behavioral group therapy for the treatment of depression in the elderly. Steuer, Mintz, Hammen, Hill, Jarvik, McCarley, Motoike, and Rosen (1983) compared psychodynamic and cognitive-behavioral group treatment for older adults diagnosed as having major depressive disorders. The cognitive-behavioral treatment followed methods proposed by Beck, Rush, Shaw, and Emery (1979), using weekly activity schedules, procedures for monitoring perceived mastery and pleasure of daily activities, and graded task assignments in addition to recording of negative cognitions and examination of cognitive distortions. The psychodynamic groups focused on development of group cohesion and of insight into patterns of socially maladaptive behavior. The two approaches had comparable results, each significantly reducing depression in their participants.

Gallagher (1981) also compared group supportive and behavioral therapies for treatment of depression in an outpatient sample of elders. Behavioral treatment followed the protocol of Lewinsohn *et al.* (1980) for improving social skills and increasing the frequency of engaging in pleasant activities. The supportive treatment was unstructured and nondirective, focusing on expression of feelings and development of group cohesion. Both groups of participants evidenced comparable and significant pre-post improvement in depression. Those who had been treated with behavioral therapy, however, were rated by observers as significantly more socially skillful. Compared to those in the nondirective groups, behavioral clients evidenced greater skill over time in giving and receiving positive feedback (rated by blind observers from behind a one-way mirror). There were also fewer instances of critical, negative interactions among behavioral group members by the 8th session of the 10-session protocol. In addition, behavioral clients were somewhat more improved at the 2 month follow-up compared to those treated with supportive group therapy.

The prevalence of depression among the elderly and the low utilization of mental health services by this group might indicate an appropriate situation for applying a psychoeducational behavioral treatment model. The "coping class" approach for the treatment of depression, designed by Lewinsohn and his associates at the University of Oregon (Lewinsohn, Antonuccio, Steinmetz, & Teri, 1984), seemed promising for application to older adults. Lewinsohn's "coping classes," based on his social learning model of depression (Lewinsohn, Biglan, & Zeiss, 1976), represent a reorganization of some of the traditional strategies used in the behavioral treatment of depression (Lewinsohn, Muñoz, Youngren, & Zeiss, 1978) into a course that can be offered to small groups in an educational format. This course consists of 12 meetings emphasizing self-control techniques relevant to thoughts, pleasant activities, relaxation, and interpersonal interaction (see Chapter 11 in this volume by Lewinsohn, Breckenridge, Antonuccio, and Teri for a more detailed description).

Thompson and his colleagues at the University of Southern California initially undertook an evaluation of the effectiveness of Lewinsohn *et al.*'s psychoeducational course with community elders (Thompson, 1981). The course was advertised as an educational experience directed toward acquiring skills to gain control over negative mood states ("the blues"). Because depression is frequently an episodic disorder, with periods of remission and exacerbation, the course was open both to older individuals who were self-described as depressed and to those who reported minimal difficulties. Preliminary data indicated that the pace of the course was too fast for many elderly participants. Although some individuals could undoubtedly stay abreast of proposed assignments, the majority fell behind. Many points had to be demonstrated repeatedly before individuals caught on. Homework assignments were frequently not completed because students had forgotten or become confused about the relevant material after leaving the class.

In response to this initial pilot course, the protocol was modified to allow more time for the presentation of each component skill. Fewer components were presented because simply slowing the pace of the original protocol to fit the needs of the elderly students would have made the course impractically long. The most basic skills, such as mood monitoring and the development of self-change programs to increase pleasant and decrease unpleasant events, were retained. More specialized skills, such as relaxation and assertion training, were removed from the basic course. These components may be presented in separate, brief "advanced" courses for which individuals may register according to need or preference.

This revised coping class for older adults was evaluated by Thompson and his colleagues at the University of Southern California (Thompson, Gallagher, Nies, & Epstein, 1983). Meetings were held once a week for 2 hours each over 6 weeks. Six to eight persons were enrolled in each class, to be taught by a team of two co-leaders. As in Lewinsohn and colleagues' course, *Control Your Depression* (Lewinsohn, Muñoz, Youngren, & Zeiss, 1978) was used as a text, and a participant workbook was also provided. Each class followed a similar format. Classes began with a general discussion of how things had gone for participants during the past week. An agenda was set, principles embedded in the current homework assignment were reviewed, and a "workshop" utilized the completed homework to illustrate the new principles taught in that session. A short break for socialization and refreshment was followed by a 10- to 15-minute minilecture on principles of the next week's homework and a short workshop to be sure that participants understood how to apply the new material.

In each class meeting, a single new behavioral skill was taught. In the first class the focus was on mood monitoring, that is, learning to be attentive to fluctuations in mood from day to day and to record a numerical mood rating each evening. The second class focused on identification of everyday pleasant events, teaching participants to record and monitor these on a daily basis. Participants also learned to graph the relationship between daily mood and frequency of occurrence of pleasant activities. In the third class, members learned to identify unpleasant events affecting their mood and again track and graph these on a daily basis. The lists of pleasant and unpleasant activities for tracking were specific to each student and were individually generated with the assistance of the co-leaders.

Participants typically had recognized a clear relationship between activity level and mood at this point and had begun to experience some control over mood through manipulation of activities. Reports of such progress were typically reinforced by other class members, and such supportive experiences appeared to enhance learning.

In the fourth class, a specific problem area amenable to change was identified for each person, a concrete goal for change was developed, and members were taught to reward themselves for steps representing progress toward that goal. Strategies for implementing a self-change plan were presented. Participants were encouraged to choose specific and attainable goals such as getting some physical exercise every day despite arthritic pain or selecting a new setting likely to encourage social interaction. Inappropriate goals, such as those centered on changing the behavior of others, or unrealistic goals, such as drastically improving one's financial status, were discouraged. In the fifth class, the self-change program was reviewed and expanded by the selection of a second reachable and meaningful behavioral goal. Finally, the sixth class focused on the maintenance of progress after the end of the course. All skills taught were reviewed, and the class discussed how to use these skills in anticipated future situations. Potential problems with motivation (e.g., continuing to do homework on one's own, rewarding oneself for progress toward goals, etc.) were also aired at this point to further reinforce the need for continued practice and utilization of behavioral methods for maintaining control over mood. Also, plans were made for a "reunion" meeting in 2 months that all class members were expected to attend. At that final session, problems that arose in the interim were discussed, and the main points of the course were again reviewed.

Pilot work during modification of the course indicated that elderly community volunteers were less depressed and reported greater satisfaction with their lives after taking the course, as indicated by self-report questionnaires such as the Beck Depression Inventory and Neugarten's Life Satisfaction Index (Thompson, Gallagher, Nies, Epstein, & Machon, 1981). A related study (Hedlund & Thompson, 1980) revealed that community elderly who were experiencing an episode of major depressive disorder also showed substantial improvement as a result of taking the course. A comparison with individuals who were receiving *individual* behavioral therapy indicated that the rate of improvement over the course of treatment was comparable for both approaches. It is clear that this psychoeducational course could have a positive effect on the level of distress experienced by community elderly in general as well as older individuals diagnosed as having a depressive disorder.

As noted before, one advantage of an educational model is that mental health services can be provided by specially trained paraprofessionals rather than therapists. A greater service effort can thus be implemented at considerably less expense, utilizing existing personnel in community settings serving the elderly. A secondary benefit of simplifying and reducing the length of the original coping course was to better facilitate the introduction of paraprofessionals as leaders or co-leaders of the course. Reducing the complexity of the material covered not only made it easier for participants to grasp the course material but also was intended to minimize problems in the presentation of more complex principles that might best be handled by more highly trained mental health professionals.

A trial application of this approach with paraprofessional leaders indicated that individuals who are interested in older persons and who have received appropriate specialty training can be effective in teaching this type of course, irrespective of varied levels of training in the mental health professions (Thompson *et al.*, 1983). If instructors are carefully selected and appropriately trained to present the course material clearly and to deal with commonly encountered problems, they can be quite effective teachers of the course. We have found that individuals who have successfully participated in the class as students and subsequently co-teach a class effectively with an experienced instructor are then able to function relatively independently as course instructors. Professional consultation is made available on an ongoing basis.

Despite the effectiveness of this version of the coping course, however, a systematic evaluation indicated a number of ways in which it could be improved to better serve elderly participants. First, some students still apparently had difficulty learning and using the range of skills and ideas presented in the course effectively. In particular, there had been only one session devoted to systematic self-change principles, a relatively complex topic. A more extensive treatment of steps and strategies for self-change appeared to be called for, allowing time for collecting and understanding baseline data in order to promote more informed selection of realistic goals for change. Second, a few participants and also a number of senior center staff members had remarked that "Coping with Depression" seemed to have a rather negative tone as a title for a class that taught such "positive" skills. It was suggested that a more upbeat title would attract a broader range of students and still accomplish the same purpose of teaching important coping and mood-maintenance skills. A title that emphasized a more preventive or mood-enhancement focus would also make it clear that the course was appropriate for older adults who were not currently depressed but who were interested in preventing future episodes of depression or simply improving their sense of control over the quality of their lives. Our current efforts to develop and evaluate the psychoeducational course along these lines are described in the next section.

The Life Satisfaction Course

Many older adults who would not describe themselves as depressed nevertheless report a low level of satisfaction with their lives (George & Bearon, 1980). Spencer (1980) states that the primary educational need of older adults is to maintain subjective well-being. Indeed, life satisfaction in the elderly has been the focus of much gerontological research (Larson, 1978). Research on life satisfaction has tended to identify two major components of experienced satisfaction: the presence of positive mood, associated with experienced pleasure in personally meaningful activities, and the absence of negative mood, associated with low stress and/or good problem-solving or coping abilities (Zautra, Kochanowicz, & Goodhart, 1982).

The Life Satisfaction Course is an adaptation of the Coping with Depression course of Thompson *et al.*, designed to address these broader concerns of the elderly. Similar to the earlier coping classes, this intervention teaches skills for monitoring mood, identifying potential sources of increased pleasure, and skills for developing a systematic "self-change plan" to increase the frequency and enjoyment of salient activities. Basic behavioral strategies for self-change are covered in greater detail in this course to provide participants with specific skills to be used in the future for effecting needed changes and coping with stressful life events. The presentation of step-by-step "self-change skills" proceeds at a much slower pace than in the earlier interventions. The more detailed treatment of this topic was intended to maximize the elderly participants' capacity to absorb the material and implement the techniques within their daily routines. Subsequent use of these strategies was expected to be more likely when the material was initially fully understood and applied.

The course has a parallel theme of managing time effectively so as to maximize positive outcomes and experiences. Lawton (1982) has found skillful time management to be directly related to life satisfaction in the elderly. Time management is not meant in the sense of being *efficient,* but rather in regard to arranging one's schedule to ensure that there is enough time for rewarding activity, to balance inevitable neutral and unpleasant tasks and events. Self-change plans are introduced in terms of first developing habits to assess one's daily routine and its effect on mood and then identifying specific activities that can be feasibly changed or added to daily routines in order to enhance positive mood and satisfaction.

The Life Satisfaction Course extends across a broader range of concerns than were emphasized in the Coping with Depression course. It is appropriate for elders who may be most interested in increasing their current satisfaction and sense of control over certain aspects of their lives, whether or not they feel depressed or are concerned about coping with future stressful events. For instance, participants may want to develop self-control skills for increasing exercise, improving organization and management of daily routine, or identifying more pleasurable and satisfying ways to use their postretirement time. This broader agenda allows participants who may be hesitant to enroll in a "mental health" course to learn skills and develop coping abilities that will be useful to them both at present and in the future. Regardless of each participant's current mental health and personal reasons for enrolling, the development of self-efficacy and behavioral skills for the prevention of pathological response to future stress is an important emphasis (Steinmetz, Zeiss, & Thompson, 1983).

The current intervention is designed for use with male and female community residents aged 60 and older. Participants are usually self-referred and learn of the course through senior centers, notices in senior newsletters, articles in general circulation newspapers, or by word of mouth. The course can be held at senior centers and senior residences and is offered as a regular class within each center's activity program. Applicants are given an individual "screening" appointment with one of the course instructors. The screening interview has three purposes: (a) to inform prospective participants about the nature of the class, making sure they understand its psychoeducational nature and that their expectations are appropriate; (b) to gather sufficient information to determine whether an applicant might better be referred to an alternative treatment (i.e., to assure absence of prohibitive organic or psychological impairment); and (c) to gather pretreatment data to provide a basis for evaluating the impact of the course.

Applicants diagnosable as having major depressive disorders or evidencing other serious psychopathology are referred elsewhere for more intensive treatment. Those meeting criteria for minor or intermittent depressions or more chronic conditions such as dysthymic disorder are invited to participate in the class along with those not reporting distress other than low life satisfaction. Persons not claiming any current adjustment problems but wishing to learn the skills are free to participate as well. Limiting class participation to those not suffering from severe depression serves two purposes. It allows the course to be taught by leaders lacking extensive mental health training and provides for a less "intimidating" group for elders experiencing some distress who nevertheless may be reluctant to seek "psychological treatment."

The Life Satisfaction Course emphasizes the acquisition of self-change skills in which most participants are deficient, but the leaders do not promise to provide a "healing experience." The course consists of nine 2-hour sessions in 9 weeks, plus "reunions" at 1 month and 6 months posttreatment. Each class has two leaders, and class size is limited to 6 to 10 participants. A seminar format is employed, with students and leaders seated around a table in a room with a blackboard.

Leaders follow a detailed outline for each session, and students are provided with a "participant workbook" for each meeting, including an agenda listing material to be covered, a synopsis of the main ideas presented during that session, and a homework assignment for the following week (Steinmetz, Zeiss, Hill, Parke, & Thompson, 1983). The workbook contains all of the forms that will be needed during the class session and during the subsequent week to complete the homework assignment. Students are also provided with a textbook (*Control Your Depression,* Lewinsohn *et al.*, 1978) to supplement these materials.

The first meeting of the class is an "orientation" session. Pretreatment assessment packets are collected and checked for completeness, and students are provided with a notebook containing the course materials. An important item on the agenda for the orientation session is a "getting acquainted exercise" to allow participants and leaders to introduce themselves and to foster a spirit of congeniality and collaboration in the class. A final task of the orientation session is to review the "ground rules" for the course, stressing the positive, problem-solving focus, consideration of others in the group, and confidentiality. Each ground rule is discussed, and members are explicitly asked for their agreement to follow each of them.

The eight remaining sessions following the orientation meeting share a consistent agenda. Homework is reviewed and discussed, leaders and participants reinforce progress and work together to solve any problems that have arisen in the homework assignment, new material is presented in a lecture by one of the leaders, there is a workshop to allow participants to begin to apply the new material with individual supervision from the leaders, and homework is assigned for the next week. Approximately halfway through each 2-hour session participants take a 10-minute break, usually accompanied by coffee and a snack brought by one of the students or leaders.

Session 1 begins with a presentation and discussion of the goals of the course. Students then hear a lecture on the topic of fluctuations in mood in response to environmental events and influences, and they are taught to monitor mood and life satisfaction on a daily basis. Session 2 focuses on the relationship between mood and key events, and students' daily mood data are perused for evidence and examples. Salient pleasant activities are identified using the Older Person's Pleasant Events Schedule (Hedlund, Gilewski, & Thompson, 1981), and a personalized list of 10 target pleasant events is developed for each student to keep track of daily. In Session 3, students learn to graph mood and activity data, and correlations are discussed. Leaders help students to discover specific relationships between daily events or activities and mood, relying on modeling and reinforcement by peers to further strengthen learning. Each individual's list of activities is then revised to reflect his or her growing understanding of the reciprocal relationship between events and mood. At this point in the class, many students realize the potential for personal influence on mood and satisfaction inherent in that relationship.

In Session 4, after 2 weeks of data collection, students are ready to identify personal problem areas, and leaders help them through a step-by-step process to pinpoint a behavior for change. In Sessions 5 and 6, further self-change skills are taught, and each student designs and implements a behavioral self-change plan, including the choice of appropriate rewards for meeting intermediate behavioral goals. Antecedents and consequences of target problems are identified, and strategies for overcoming "roadblocks to self-change" are developed. At this point, the leaders are able to focus on specific roadblocks frequently encountered by elders. A distinction is drawn between "internal" roadblocks (e.g., cognitions such as "I'm too old to change"), and "external" roadblocks (e.g., constraints in resources or physical abilities), many of which can be overcome or bypassed with creative thought and effort. The final two sessions focus on revision of self-change plans, generation of new plans to systematically increase positive and satisfying activity in salient areas, and generalization of skills to other problem areas. During the eighth session, plans for maintaining positive mood and anticipating and coping with future difficulties are discussed. The 1-month and 6-month reunions serve to review salient points, check on and reinforce student progress, and further discuss generalized application of self-control skills.

A number of professionals working with the elderly have requested training for administering this course in their own settings. Based on the experience of Thompson *et al.* (1983), we believe it to be feasible for nonpsychologist service providers to the elderly and for paraprofessionals to learn to administer the course. The structured nature of the class is important in this regard, and we agree with Christensen, Miller, and Muñoz (1978) that paraprofessional therapists should be employed only with well-specified treatment procedures. In addition to careful selection of such paraprofessionals and detailed training in the treatment protocol, instruction regarding selection of appropriate group participants and handling of commonly encountered problems is essential. Also, it is advisable that paraprofessional group leaders have ready access to an experienced professional for consultation on an "as needed" basis.

Coping with Care Giving Classes

Older adults who provide home care to frail or demented relatives are an additional group for whom psychoeducational group treatment may prove useful. Recent economic trends in this country have resulted in the greater burden of care giving being shifted away from institutions (such as nursing homes) back to the nuclear family. Often family members are ill prepared to provide the types of services needed by "frail elder" relatives—that is, those whose functional abilities have considerably declined, for instance, due to a severe stroke or Alzheimer's disease. The literature has long recognized that between 15 and 30% of those found within an institutional setting are functionally comparable to community-dwelling residents (Butler, 1978; Smyer, 1980). Conversely, there also is a sizable group of community elderly who are functionally comparable to the institutionalized (Brody, Poulshock, & Masciocchi, 1978; Shanas, Townsend, Wedderburn, Friis, Milhoj, & Stehouwer, 1968). This differential usage of services by impaired elders raises issues about the role of the family as both a buffer from institutionalization and a link to alternative services.

The consequences of prolonged care giving for family members have been comprehensively reviewed by Blumenthal (1980). Others have also commented upon the increased stress experienced by care givers who assume this role on a regular basis. Care givers themselves become vulnerable to development of physical and psychological symptoms (Archbold, 1979; Fengler & Goodrich, 1979; Klein, Dean, & Bogdonoff, 1967). Further discussion of the negative effects of prolonged care giving can be found in the literature on palliative treatment of Alzheimer's patients. For example, Blumenthal (1980), Zarit and colleagues (Zarit, Reever, & Bach-Peterson, 1980; Zarit & Zarit, 1982), Rabins, Mace, and Lucas (1982), and Lezak (1978) have described the impact of dementia on the family in terms of severe disruption of normal interaction patterns and development of depression, fatigue, and anger in the care givers. Although experiencing substantial burden on a daily basis, many care givers nevertheless choose not to institutionalize their family member. Thus, care givers comprise an important group of elders in need of services to strengthen their capacity to continue in their roles. Adult children and spouses who are burdened with the care of older family members, particularly family members with dementia, are likely to benefit from psychoeducational intervention.

The prevalence of dementia is 3 to 6% over age 65 and increases gradually to 20% over age 80 (Roth, 1978, 1980). As the population at large grows older, it is clear that the number of persons with dementia will increase. Thus, the problem of dementia and its treatment will probably become an even higher priority area in the health care delivery system. Similar increases can be expected in the number of elderly with other problems that result in a need for continual care, such as those with Parkinson's disease, severe strokes, or cancer. Multiple illnesses, independently less serious than these, can additively result in a reduced ability to care for oneself and an increased dependency on care givers.

At present, there are no satisfactory treatments for many of the illnesses experienced by this group, nor are there any likely breakthroughs on the horizon. Treatment typically is palliative/supportive and intended to optimize functioning and minimize stress in individuals who are experiencing a progressive degenerative process. This type of treatment is best offered by family members and/or interested community volunteers. The burden of care for these individuals is immense, and care givers frequently become discouraged and call for help from the health care system. At present the health care delivery system has few intermediate care options available, and the decision to institutionalize the patient is often made far sooner than necessary. The economic toll from institutional placement is exorbitant, to say nothing of the negative impact on other family members. Institutional placement could be delayed and in many instances avoided if intermediate programs were available that would assist care givers substantively and also help them feel less stressed by their burden. Courses designed to help individuals cope with stress and affective disorders could provide a practical and comparatively inexpensive alternative to immediate institutionalization.

A number of self-help programs and support groups are currently being utilized to assist care givers (e.g., Crossman, London, & Barry, 1981). In the support groups, the presumed mechanism of change is empathy and emotional support derived from sharing problems with others in similar situations. Behavioral treatment in a psychoeducational format can uniquely supplement this growing array of supportive interventions. It provides a more intensive focus on teaching skills for coping with the stresses of care giving, through instruction in systematic problem-solving and mood maintenance techniques. Support and encouragement by leaders and fellow students are not precluded and can be an important component of such groups.

Several efforts in this direction have been made by other research groups, within an individual rather than group format. For example, Levine, Dastoor, and Gendron (1983), working individually with a small sample of care givers of demented elders, found that use of a skills training program was helpful in improving problem-solving abilities, positive self-talk, and active use of beneficial coping strategies. The program is described as a multimodal approach consisting of motivational enhancement, social skills training, meditative relaxation, and training in problem-solving. Pinkston, Green, and Linsk (1981) report a program for teaching care givers procedures for social reinforcement, behavioral contracting, and scheduling of the frail elders' problematic behaviors (e.g., toileting at certain regular times during the day to reduce the likelihood of bladder and bowel accidents). They report that family members were eager to learn and were able to successfully carry out these procedures at home, leading to self-reported increased daily satisfaction and social contact.

The model currently being developed at our center to address these needs is a 10-session course entitled "Coping with Care Giving" (Gallagher & Rappaport, 1983). Each session lasts 2 hours and begins with a didactic presentation on a common care-giving problem (e.g., nighttime wandering behavior). After a break, a 60-minute workshop allows each participant to individually apply the material discussed to his or her particular situation. Finally, the group comes together again for discussion and mutual encouragement. At each session, individual homework assignments are reviewed, and completion of homework is encouraged and emphasized as a critical ingredient for success.

Participants first learn the usefulness of the problem-solving approach, and then are taught to implement the strategies and evaluate their efficacy expectations over time. For example, for some care givers, incontinence is a major issue; for others, nighttime wandering behavior is the most disturbing. Each of these problems is broken down into its component parts, and possible coping strategies are generated. Then care givers analyze the success and failure of their coping attempts, and that information is used to generate new plans of action. Relevant homework assignments are developed, and each class member plans to report back to the group about the usefulness of the new strategy. In addition to learning more effective ways of dealing with daily burdens, care givers also learn that they *can* tackle problems that seemed unsurmountable. According to Bandura (1982), this improvement in self-efficacy is likely to enable the care giver to feel more confident about coping with problems that may arise in the future. Indirectly, such a program could reduce the need for institutional placement. If care givers are less stressed and are able to obtain somewhat more satisfaction in their daily lives, they may be able to function effectively in that role for a longer period of time. The Coping with Care Giving class is currently being evaluated in regard to both short- and long-term effects.

Only those care givers who are attending some type of formal program to obtain relief or "respite" are eligible to participate in this research and service program. This is an important screening factor because some care givers find it difficult to admit the extent to which they are having problems—they may feel that caretaking is their "duty" and feel that seeking assistance constitutes unwarranted "complaining." Those who have already sought out a respite program, however, usually have come to terms with their limitations and seem more flexible and interested in learning ways to improve tbeir daily living situation. Because the model has an outreach orientation and can probably be used effectively by nonprofessionals after a training period, the program could conceivably be offered in a wide range of settings (such as respite programs, senior day health centers, and the like) without taxing the present health care delivery system.

As with the other courses described, enrollment is limited in order to encourage maximum individual participation. In the care-giver courses it has seemed impractical to have more than eight persons in a class. A small group of between six and eight members allows time for careful assessment of problem areas and thorough teaching and application of coping skills, with adequate attention given to each individual member.

Many of the care givers are themselves frail and in poor health, and so unavoidable absences are fairly common. Telephone contact or scheduling an individual time for "catching up" is appreciated in these instances. Many care givers are unable to attend any classes or individual makeup sessions unless provisions have been made for the care of their frail elder during that time. For some, this is not a major issue because they have engaged ongoing supportive services in the home (e.g., a visiting nurse or a family member to elder-sit for specific intervals); for others, however, it is a serious deterrent to their regular participation. This issue needs to be discussed in advance of class enrollment. Wherever possible, class leaders assist those care givers in making adequate arrangements. Scheduling classes while the frail elder is participating in a respite-type program obviates much of this difficulty because the care giver can feel free to attend classes that are concurrent with his or her relative's participation in a supervised program.

Coping with Bereavement Classes

Elders experiencing spousal bereavement are also appropriate candidates for psychoeducational classes. Prior intervention studies in the bereavement literature have generally focused on the usefulness of self-help approaches, such as the Widow-to-Widow programs (Silverman, 1970). These have developed as essentially leaderless (or peer-directed) support groups in several areas of the country. Although no controlled studies of their effectiveness have been reported, the sheer number of such groups suggests their ability to be of assistance to a wide range of widows and widowers. The present authors have found, however, that elders often do not feel comfortable seeking out such groups; reasons have included fear that talking about the death would result in greater discomfort and apprehension that the absence of a trained leader might result in more (rather than less) distress. For instance, a widow may fear that once problems have been revealed, peers going through the same experience might be unable to generate helpful solutions.

Professionally led counseling groups for the bereaved have been described by Gerber, Rusalem, Hannon, Arkin, and Battin (1975), Hiltz (1975), and Burnside (1978). These appear to have been focused primarily on sharing of feelings and on encouragement for attempting new roles and new activities as a single person. Gerber also reports the effective use of telephone counseling for the bereaved, indicating that the ease of availability made it particularly desirable for elders who then did not have to deal with transportation problems, scheduling of appointments, and so forth. In one of the rare empirical studies of the effectiveness of groups for the bereaved, Barrett (1978) found that several methods were effective in comparison to a waiting list control group, including a self-help condition, development of a specific confidant, and what she termed *consciousness raising* groups. Little work has focused specifically on the problems of bereaved *elders*, however, and little attention has been directed to the efficacy of a psychoeducational approach for working through the grief process and the adjustment problems that follow upon spousal loss.

Our efforts on this topic began with several pilot studies conducted at the University of Southern California by Gallagher and colleagues, using the basic model described earlier in this chapter. It soon became apparent that careful prescreening of members was essential, so that those suffering from clinical depression or other serious forms of psychopathology would be referred to appropriate resources. Combining bereaved who were clinically depressed, for example, with persons experiencing a relatively normal grief reaction (which was problematic for the individual but not of sufficient magnitude to be regarded as pathological) was counterproductive. The depressives tended to monopolize the sessions and demanded more attention from the leaders between sessions than did those persons experiencing normal grief reactions. In fact, after three or four such meetings, the "normal grievers" tended to drop out of the pilot program. They did not feel their needs were being adequately addressed. The Beck Depression Inventory (BDI; Beck, Ward, Mendelson, Mock, & Erbaugh, 1961) is a helpful screening instrument to assist the clinician in detecting this difference. The BDI is an easily completed, 21-item, self-administered scale. In general, elders experiencing normal grief can be distinguished from elder depressives on the basis of responses to items reflecting a negative cognitive set (e.g., perceived worthlessness, pessimism about the future, intense feelings of failure, etc.) that characterize depressives but not "normal grievers" (cf. Gallagher, Breckenridge, Thompson, Dessonville, & Amaral, 1982).

An additional concern that emerged in our pilotwork was the importance of attending to various phases of the grief process in choosing group participants. It is known that different problems emerge as one moves through the first 2 years of bereavement (Parkes, 1972). On a practical level, this suggests that grouping elders according to the time elapsed since the loss may prove to be a significant factor influencing success of the intervention. For example, concerns at 6 months after spousal loss often involved practical matters such as finances and housing, whereas by 12 to 18 months group members typically discussed ways to cope with loneliness and to construct new life-styles as single persons.

Bereaved participants in pilot groups reported that a highly structured psychoeducational program was unsatisfying; thus, the format was substantially modified (see DeBor, Gallagher, & Lesher, 1983). For example, the agenda of topics to be covered at each meeting was determined by consensus between leaders and participants at the start of each class. Then a short lecture was delivered by the co-leaders on that topic, and group members discussed their individual reactions, working to apply general principles of the problem-solving approach. Participants reported that this combination of new information, validation of thoughts and feelings and focused problem-solving, was effective in helping them recover from grief. Data collected from 20 elders (14 women and 6 men) completing this modified program indicated that they had gained a better understanding of the grief process and were better able to cope with the stresses of bereavement (DeBor *et al.*, 1983). Because no control group was used, however, it is not possible to attribute positive changes made to the intervention *per se*—it may have been that those who sought this kind of help were ready to take an active approach to dealing with their new status and so would have benefited from any one of a number of possible interventions. Nevertheless, the results are suggestive of the efficacy of a psychoeducational approach for coping with bereavement.

Future research is planned to evaluate this model more stringently. Traditional supportive group counseling will be compared with "Coping with Bereavement" classes to determine more precisely which critical ingredients promote positive adaptation. This research will be conducted within a prevention framework—that is, elders likely to be at risk for poor adaptation to spousal loss will be invited to participate in the research, and follow-up evaluation will assess the effectiveness of the interventions for prevention of subsequent clinical depression in women and mortality in men. Prior research has found that men and women respond differentially to spousal death: the risk of increased mortality is greater for men (Stroebe & Stroebe, 1983), whereas women who are adjusting poorly are more likely to report depression and/or increased somatic complaints (Clayton, 1982).

Summary and Conclusions

This chapter has reviewed issues and recent research in the use of behavioral group therapy with older adults. A psychoeducational model has been described, and the appropriateness of this approach to treatment for the elderly has been discussed. Finally, a series of applications of this approach to some specific problems common to the elderly have been presented. We would like to conclude with some observations and recommendations about the practice of group behavioral therapy with the elderly.

We have clearly found older adults to be enthusiastic participants in group behavioral therapy, particularly when it is presented in a psychoeducational model. Despite lore to the contrary, many elderly are quite able to learn and apply new skills and new ideas. The learning process seems to be facilitated by an appropriate and carefully monitored pace in presentation of ideas and skills, supplemental written material to reinforce learning, clearly defined homework assignments, and age-appropriate examples and illustrations. We also feel it is important that behavioral treatment be delivered in a warm, empathic, collaborative manner, with the group leader in the role of educator and consultant.

Although the preceding recommendations probably apply equally to *any* age group, some special considerations are necessary for the elderly. As we have noted, older adults seem to learn new material at a slower rate, and thus the pace of treatment should be expected to be slower. Many elders have physical or organic difficulties that require special consideration: memory problems require more extensive use of written material; patients with chronic pain or other disabilities may need special modifications in such procedures as systematic relaxation training; group participants with hearing or visual impairment will require special attention and compensation.

An additional concern is differences in age between therapist and client, as a therapist will often be one or even two generations removed from an elderly client. In behavioral therapy, with a strong emphasis on application of well-defined principles and teaching of specific skills, an acknowledgment of differences in life experience seems to be a sufficient response to client concerns about a "generation gap." The psychoeducational emphasis on teaching individuals how to improve and maintain their own mental health is especially appropriate when such an age difference exists, particularly because clients themselves gather data about situations and behaviors related to their difficulties. It is their knowledge and experience with their own lives in conjunction with the training and professional expertise of the therapist that determine the course of treatment. The collaborative approach is, thus, especially well suited to work between clients and therapists who may have many years' difference in age.

Based on our experience conducting group behavioral therapy and behaviorally oriented psychoeducational classes with the elderly, we join many others in strongly advocating the use of such approaches with older adults. Although it may require creativity and persistent effort to overcome the hesitancies of many elders to seek mental health services, we have found them to be a receptive and responsive population once services are begun. Despite the many losses and declines that are inevitable late in life, the elderly maintain a significant capacity for positive development and change. We have found the approaches described in this chapter to be effective both for interesting elders in such change and for providing them with tools to bring it about for themselves.

References

Abrams, D. B. Clinical developments in the behavioral treatment of obesity. *Clinical Behavior Therapy Review*, 1979, *1*, 1–14.

Archbold, P. An analysis of parent-caring by women. *Home Care Services Quarterly*, 1979, *3*, 5–26.

Atthowe, J. Controlling nocturnal enuresis in severely disabled and chronic patients. In R. C. Katz & S. Zlutnick (Eds.), *Behavioral therapy and health care: Principles and applications*. New York: Pergamon Press, 1975.

Bakker, C. B., & Armstrong, H. E., Jr. The adult development program: An educational approach to the delivery of mental health services. *Hospital and Community Psychiatry*, 1976, *27*, 330–334.
Bandura, A. Self-efficacy: Toward a unifying theory of behavior change. *Psychological Review*, 1977, *84*, 191–215.
Bandura, A. Self-efficacy mechanism in human agency. *American Psychologist*, 1982, *37*, 122–147.
Barrett, C. J. Effectiveness of widows' groups in facilitating change. *Journal of Consulting and Clinical Psychology*, 1978, *46*, 20–31.
Beck, A. T., Ward, C. H., Mendelson, M., Mock, J., & Erbaugh, J. An inventory for measuring depression. *Archives of General Psychiatry*, 1961, *4*, 561–571.
Beck, A. T., Rush, A. J., Shaw, B., & Emery, G. *Cognitive therapy of depression*. New York: Guilford Press, 1979.
Blazer, D., & Williams, C. D. Epidemiology of dysphoria and depression in various adult age groups. *American Journal of Psychiatry*, 1980, *137*, 439–444.
Blumenthal, M. D. *Mental deterioration and family burden: Some theoretical perspectives*. Paper presented at annual meeting of the Gerontological Society of America, San Diego, 1980.
Brody, S. J., Poulshock, S. W., & Masciocchi, C. F. The family caring unit: A major consideration in the long-term support system. *The Gerontologist*, 1978, *18*, 556–561.
Brotman, H. B. Who are the aging? In E. W. Busse & E. Pfeiffer (Eds.), *Mental illness in later life*. Washington, D.C.: American Psychological Association, 1973.
Burnside, I. M. *Working with the elderly: Group processes and techniques*. Belmont, Calif.: Wadsworth, 1978.
Butler, R. Alzheimer's disease—senile dementia and related disorders: The role of NIA. In R. Katzman, R. Terry, & K. Bick (Eds.), *Alzheimer's disease: Senile dementia and related disorders*. New York: Raven Press, 1978.
Butler, R., & Lewis, M. *Aging and mental health* (2d ed.). St. Louis: Mosby, 1977.
Cautela, J. R. A classical conditioning approach to the development and modification of behavior in the aged. *The Gerontologist*, 1969, *9*, 109–113.
Christensen, A., Miller, W. R., & Muñoz, R. F. Paraprofessionals, partners, peers, paraphernalia, and print: Expanding mental health service delivery. *Professional Psychology*, 1978, *33*, 249–270.
Clayton, P. J. Bereavement. In E. S. Paykel (Ed.), *Handbook of affective disorders*. New York: Guilford Press, 1982.
Coates, T. J., & Thoresen, C. E. Treating sleep disorders: Few answers, some suggestions, and many questions. In S. M. Turner, K. S. Calhoun, & H. E. Adams (Eds.), *Handbook of clinical behavior therapy*. New York: Wiley, 1981.
Cohen, L. D., & Cooley, S. G. Psychology training programs for direct services to the aging (Status report, 1980). *Professional Psychology*, 1983, *14*, 720–728.
Crossman, L., London, C., & Barry, C. Older women caring for disabled spouses: A model for supportive services. *The Gerontologist*, 1981, *21*, 464–470.
DeBor, L., Gallagher, D., & Lesher, E. Group counseling with bereaving elderly. *Clinical Gerontologist*, 1983, *1*, 81–90.
Evans, R. L., & Jaureguy, B. M. Group therapy by phone: A cognitive behavioral program for visually impaired elderly. *Social Work in Health Care*, 1981, *7*, 79–90.
Fengler, A. P., & Goodrich, N. Wives of elderly disabled men: The hidden patients. *The Gerontologist*, 1979, *19*, 175–183.
Fordyce, W. E. *Behavioral methods for chronic pain and illness*. St. Louis: Mosby, 1976.
Gallagher, D. Behavioral group therapy with elderly depressives: An experimental study. In D. Upper & S. Ross (Eds.), *Behavioral group therapy: An annual review*. Champaign, Ill.: Research Press, 1981.
Gallagher, D. E., and Rappaport, M. *Enhancing caregivers' capacity to care for frail elders*. NIH Grant Application AG04572-01, approved for funding by the National Institute on Aging, 1983.
Gallagher, D., & Thompson, L. W. Treatment of major depressive disorder in older adult outpatients with brief psychotherapies. *Psychotherapy: Theory, Research, and Practice*, 1982, *19*, 482–490.
Gallagher, D., Breckenridge, J., Thompson, L., Dessonville, C., & Amaral, P. Similarities and differences between normal grief and depression in older adults. *Essence*, 1982, *5*, 127–140.
George, L. K., & Bearon, L. B. *Quality of life in older persons*. New York: Human Sciences Press, 1980.

Gerber, I., Rusalem, R., Hannon, N., Arkin, A., & Battin, D. Anticipatory grief and aged widows and widowers. *Journal of Gerontology*, 1975, *30*, 225–229.
Gottfredson, G. D., & Dyer, S. E. Health service providers in psychology. *American Psychologist*, 1978, *33*, 314–338.
Gurland, B. The comparative frequency of depression in various adult age groups. *Journal of Gerontology*, 1976, *31*, 283–292.
Hedlund, B., & Thompson, L. W. *Teaching the elderly to control depression using an educational format*. Paper presented at annual meeting of the American Psychological Association, Montreal, September 1980.
Hedlund, B., Gilewski, M., & Thompson, L. The older person's pleasant events schedule. In D. Gallagher & L. Thompson, *Depression in the elderly: A behavioral treatment manual*. Los Angeles: University of Southern California Press, 1981.
Hiltz, S. R. Helping widows: Group discussions as a therapeutic technique. *The Family Coordinator*, 1975, *24*, 331–336.
Hoyer, W. J. Application of operant techniques to the modification of elderly behavior. *The Gerontologist*, 1973, *13*, 18–22.
Kazdin, A. E., & Wilson, G. T. *Evaluation of behavior therapy: Issues, evidence, and research strategies*. Lincoln,: University of Nebraska Press, 1978.
Klein, R., Dean, A., & Bogdonoff, M. The impact of illness upon the spouse. *Journal of Chronic Diseases*, 1967, *20*, 241–248.
Kline, N. S. Incidence, prevalence and recognition of depressive illness. *Diseases of the Nervous System*, 1976, *37*, 10–14.
Larson, R. Thirty years of research on the subjective well-being of older Americans. *Journal of Gerontology*, 1978, *33*, 109–125.
Lawton, N. P. *Clinical geropsychology: Problems and prospects*. Master lecture delivered at annual meeting of the American Psychological Association, Toronto, August 1978.
Lawton, N. P. *The varieties of wellbeing*. Distinguished contribution award address, Division 20, presented at annual meeting of the American Psychological Association, Washington, D.C., August 1982.
Levine, N. B., Dastoor, D. P., & Gendron, C. E. Coping with dementia: A pilot study. *Journal of American Geriatrics Society*, 1983, *31*, 12–18.
Levy, S., Derogatis, L., Gallagher, D., & Gatz, M. Intervention with older adults. In L. Poon (Ed.), *Aging in the 1980's: Psychological issues*. Washington, D.C.: American Psychological Association, 1980.
Lewinsohn, P. M., Biglan, T., & Zeiss, A. Behavioral treatment of depression. In P. Davidson (Ed.), *Behavioral management of anxiety, depression, and pain*. New York: Brunner/Mazel, 1976.
Lewinsohn, P. M., Muñoz, R. F., Youngren, M. A., & Zeiss, A. M. *Control your depression*. Englewood Cliffs, N.J.: Prentice-Hall, 1978.
Lewinsohn, P. M., Sullivan, J. M., & Grosscup, S. Changing reinforcing events: An approach to the treatment for depression. *Psychotherapy: Theory, Research, and Practice*, 1980, *17*, 322–334.
Lewinsohn, P. M., Breckenridge, J. S., Antonuccio, D. O., & Teri, L. A behavioral group therapy approach to the treatment of depression. In D. Upper & S. Ross (Eds.), *Handbook of behavioral group therapy*. New York: Plenum Press, 1985.
Lewinsohn, P. M., Antonuccio, D. O., Steinmetz, J. L., & Teri, L. *Coping with depression: A psychoeducational approach*. Eugene, Ore.: Castalia, 1984.
Lezak, M. D. Living with the characterologically altered brain injured patient. *Journal of Clinical Psychiatry*, 1978, *39*, 592–598.
Libb, J. W., & Clements, C. B. Token reinforcement in an exercise program for hospitalized geriatric patients. *Perceptual and Motor Skills*, 1969, *28*, 957–958.
MacDonald, M. L., & Butler, A. K. Reversal of helplessness: Producing walking behavior in nursing home wheelchair residents using behavior modification procedures. *Journal of Gerontology*, 1974, *29*, 97–101.
Marks, I. M. Management of sexual disorders. In H. Leitenberg (Ed.), *Handbook of behavior modification and behavior therapy*. Englewood Cliffs, N.J.: Prentice-Hall, 1976.
McLean, P. Therapeutic decision-making in the behavioral treatment of depression. In P. O. David-

son (Ed.), *The behavioral management of anxiety, depression, and pain*. New York: Brunner/Mazel, 1976.
Miller, W. R., & Taylor, C. A. Relative effectiveness of bibliotherapy, individual, and group self-control training in the treatment of problem drinkers. *Addictive Behavior*, 1980, *5*, 13–24.
Mintz, J., Steuer, J., & Jarvik, L. Psychotherapy with depressed elderly patients: Research considerations. *Journal of Consulting and Clinical Psychology*, 1981, *49*, 542–548.
Niederehe, G. Postgraduate training of psychologists for work in aging: Continuing education, retraining, and in-service education. In J. F. Santos & G. R. VandenBos (Eds.), *Psychology and the older adult: Challenges for training in the 1980's*. Washington, D.C.: American Psychological Association, 1980.
Okimoto, J. T., Barnes, R. F., Veith, R. C., Raskind, M. A., Inui, T. S., & Carter, W. B. Screening for depression in geriatric medical patients. *American Journal of Psychiatry*, 1982, *139*, 799–802.
Parkes, C. M. *Bereavement: Studies of grief in adult life*. London: Tavistock, 1972.
Patterson, R. L., & Eberly, D. A. Assessment and training of daily living and social skills in the elderly. In P. M. Lewinsohn & L. Teri (Eds.), *Clinical geropsychology: New directions in assessment and treatment*. New York: Pergamon Press, 1983.
Pfeiffer, E. The psychosocial evaluation of the elderly patient. In E. W. Busse & D. G. Blazer (Eds.), *Handbook of geriatric psychiatry*. New York: Van Nostrand Reinhold, 1980.
Pfeiffer, E., & Busse, E. W. Mental disorders in later life—Affective disorders; paranoid, neurotic, and situational reactions. In E. W. Busse & E. Pfeiffer (Eds.), *Mental illness in later life*. Washington, D.C.: American Psychological Association, 1973.
Pinkston, E., Green, R., & Linsk, N. *Community linkage and behavioral treatment in home based treatment of elderly*. Paper presented at meeting of Gerontological Society of America, Toronto, Canada, November 1981.
Rabins, P. V., Mace, N. L., & Lucas, M. J. The impact of dementia on the family. *Journal of American Medical Association*, 1982, *248*, 333–335.
Redick, R. W., & Taube, C. A. Demography and mental health care of the aged. In J. E. Birren & R. B. Sloane (Eds.), *Handbook of mental health and aging*. Englewood Cliffs, N.J.: Prentice-Hall, 1980.
Rehm, L. P. A self-control therapy program for treatment of depression. In J. F. Clarkin & H. I. Glazer (Eds.), *Depression: Behavioral and directive intervention strategies*. New York: Garland, 1981.
Richards, W. S., & Thorpe, G. L. Behavioral approaches to the problems of later life. In M. Storandt, I. C. Siegler, & M. F. Elias (Eds.), *The clinical psychology of aging*. New York: Plenum Press, 1978.
Roth, M. Epidemiological studies. In R. Katzman, R. D. Terry, & K. L. Bick (Eds.), *Alzheimer's disease: Senile dementia and related disorders*. New York: Raven Press, 1978.
Roth, M. Senile dementia and its borderlands. In J. Cole & E. Barrett (Eds.), *Psychopathology in the aged*. New York: Raven Press, 1980.
Shanas, E., Townsend, P., Wedderburn, D., Friis, H., Milhoj, P., & Stehouwer, J. *Old people in three industrial societies*. New York: Atherton, 1968.
Silver, R. J., Lubin, B., Miller, D. R., & Dobson, N. H. The group psychotherapy literature: 1980. *International Journal of Group Psychotherapy*, 1981, *31*, 469–526.
Silver, R. J., Miller, D. R., Lubin, B., & Dobson, N. H. The group psychotherapy literature: 1981. *International Journal of Group Psychotherapy*, 1982, *32*, 481–554.
Silverman, P. R. The Widow-to-Widow program. *Archives of the Foundation of Thanatology*, 1970, *2*, 133–135.
Smyer, M. The differential usage of services by impaired elderly. *Journal of Gerontology*, 1980, *35*, 249–255.
Spencer, B. Overcoming the age bias of continuing education. In G. Darkenwald & G. Larson (Eds.), *New directions for continuing education: Reaching hard to reach adults*. San Francisco: Jossey-Bass, 1980.
Steinmetz, J. L., Zeiss, A. M., & Thompson, L. W. *The Life Satisfaction Course: An intervention for the elderly*. Paper presented at NIMH State-of-the-Art Workshop on the Prevention of Depression, San Francisco, April 1983.
Steinmetz, J. L., Zeiss, A. M., Hill, J. L., Parke, L. A., & Thompson, L. W. *Leader manual and participant workbook for the Increasing Life Satisfaction Course for the elderly*. Unpublished mimeo, 1983.

Steuer, J. L., Mintz, J., Hammen, C. L., Hill, M. A., Jarvik, L., McCarley, T., Motoike, P., & Rosen, R. *Cognitive-behavioral and psychodynamic group psychotherapy in treatment of geriatric depression.* Unpublished manuscript, University of California, Los Angeles, 1983.

Storandt, M. Clinical psychology of aging. In *A proposal to the APA that a task force on training and aging be formed.* American Psychological Association, Division 20, December 1976.

Stroebe, M. S., & Stroebe, W. Who suffers most? Sex differences in health risks of the widowed. *Psychological Bulletin,* 1983, *93,* 279–301.

Thompson, L. W. *Psychoeducational approaches to reducing depression in the elderly.* Invited address at annual meeting of the American Psychological Association, Los Angeles, August 1981.

Thompson, L., Gallagher, D., Nies, G., Epstein, D., & Machon, R. *Evaluation of an educational model for teaching the elderly skills for coping with depression.* Final progress report submitted to NRTA-AARP Andrus Foundation, Washington, D.C., December 1981.

Thompson, L., Gallagher, D., Nies, G., & Epstein, D. Evaluation of the effectiveness of professionals and nonprofessionals as instructors of "Coping with Depression" classes for elders. *The Gerontologist,* 1983, *23,* 390–396.

VandenBos, G. R., Stapp, J., & Kilberg, R. R. Health service providers in psychology. *American Psychologist,* 1981, *36,* 1395–1418.

Vernon, S. W., & Roberts, R. E. Use of the SADS-RDC in a tri-ethnic community survey. *Archives of General Psychiatry,* 1982, *39,* 47–52.

Zarit, S. *Aging and mental disorders.* New York: The Free Press, 1980.

Zarit, S., & Zarit, J. Families under stress: Interventions for caregivers of senile dementia patients. *Psychotherapy: Theory, Research, and Practice,* 1982, *19,* 461–471.

Zarit, S. E., Reever, K. E., & Bach-Peterson, J. Relatives of the impaired elderly: Correlates of feelings of burden. *The Gerontologist,* 1980, *20,* 649–655.

Zautra, A., Kochanowicz, N., & Goodhart, D. Surveying quality of life in the community. In R. Bell, M. Sundel, J. Aponte, & S. Murrell (Eds.), *Assessing health and human service needs: Concepts, methods, and applications.* New York: Human Sciences Press, 1982.

III

Clinical Applications for Specific Problems

The six chapters in Part III each discuss behavioral group interventions with a specific problem. The problems include depression, addictive behaviors, sexual disorders, anxiety, drunk driving, and chronic pain. Because many of these disorders are commonly encountered by clinicians working in both inpatient and outpatient settings, the material covered in Part III should be of significant relevance and practical utility to those who spend some portion of their time helping clients. Five of the six problem areas constitute formal diagnostic entities, the exception being drunk driving. With the recent advent of tougher drunk driving laws in various states, clinicians are already beginning to see an increase in referrals to mental health settings by the criminal justice system. Thus, although not a diagnostic entity in its own right, it is a significant problem associated with alcoholism and problem drinking and can be expected to occupy an increasing amount of clinicians' time in the near future.

Part III begins with the explication in Chapter 11 of a behavioral group approach to a ubiquitous problem, that of depression. The authors, Lewinsohn, Steinmetz, Antonuccio, and Teri, first present us with an outline of the scope of the problem as well as the importance of, and difficulties in, defining and assessing depression. They discuss four complementary methods for assessing depression and describe instruments and methodologies for each. Next, the literature on cognitive-behavioral approaches to depression is reviewed, as is the evolution of group interventions from individual methods. The remainder of the chapter is devoted to an excellent detailed description of the authors' Coping with Depression (CWD) course, including outcome data and variables found to be associated with successful treatment outcome.

Smoking, obesity, and drug and alcohol abuse have been implicated in a large number of serious medical problems, and, at least for drug and alcohol abuse, psychosocial problems as well. In addition, a large percentage of the population suffers from one or more of these problems. Thus, the practicing clinician can expect to encounter clients who seek assistance for these problems directly and/or for complications of these disorders. Chapter 12, by Barrios, Turner, and Ross, reviews the literature pertaining to behavioral group treatment of each of these problems and comments upon the evidence for the efficacy of the interventions. A strong case is made for further use of group methods, including more experimentation with traditional group notions, for example, cohesiveness and group process. One cannot help but be impressed with the work that still needs to be done in behavioral group treatment of addictive behaviors despite the fact that these problems seem to lend themselves well to a behavioral group approach.

McGovern and Jensen review the treatment of sexual disorders in Chapter 13. Two types of group interventions are described, one for sexual dysfunctions and one for sexual deviations. The bulk of the chapter, however, is devoted to the treatment of deviations, specifically, child molesting, rape, and indecent exposure. Notably, all group participants must first undergo individual aversive counterconditioning of the deviate behavior before entering group treatment. Clients with supportive marital partners are also invited to participate in a marital/sexual enhancement program that is also conducted in a behavioral group format. Thus, the treatment program is composed of several interlocking components, both individual and group, that result in a comprehensive intervention system.

In Chapter 14, Emmelkamp and Kuipers draw upon their substantial clinical experience to provide the reader with a detailed manual for the treatment of anxiety states, agoraphobia, social anxiety, specific phobias, and obsessive-compulsive disorder. Special group procedures are also described, for example, for clients whose anxiety is associated with hyperventilation, and group *in vivo* exposure techniques for agoraphobics. The chapter concludes with several cautions and the identification of specific areas in need of further investigation.

National concern has recently focused on the serious problems of driving while intoxicated, and many states are currently enacting tougher drunk driving laws. Conners, Maisto, Sobell, and Sobell describe a behavioral group intervention strategy in Chapter 15 that deals with this problem. This chapter begins with a discussion of prevention efforts, including distinctions between primary, secondary, and tertiary prevention of drunk driving and the outcome of typical interventions. Next, behavioral approaches are described including skills training, controlled drinking, and self-control training. The chapter ends with an assessment of the current status of the area and needs for further research and clinical intervention.

Chapter 16 also deals with a problem that is commonly encountered in clinical practice—the problem of chronic pain and the serious impact that it has on individuals' lives and the lives of their significant others. Kulich and Gottlieb develop their chapter by first describing the development of chronic pain syndrome and a typical pain patient. Next, they discuss the methodology and importance of a thorough screening and assessment process that is logically related to treatment rationale and goals. Treatment itself is conceptualized in a comprehensive program that includes cognitive-behavioral interventions as well as physical therapy, family involvement, vocational skills training, and interventions designed to maximize compliance and follow-through into aftercare. As with other chapters, this chapter uses behavioral group interventions as one important modality in a complex and sophisticated system of interlocking methods, disciplines, and target problems.

11

A Behavioral Group Therapy Approach to the Treatment of Depression

PETER M. LEWINSOHN, JULIA STEINMETZ BRECKENRIDGE, DAVID O. ANTONUCCIO, AND LINDA TERI

INTRODUCTION

Depression is a significant clinical problem in the United States. The prevalence of clinical depression in this country has typically been estimated at 3 to 4% (Lehman, 1971; Levitt & Lubin, 1975), and the President's Commission on Mental Health has estimated the lifetime incidence of depression at 20% (Task Panel Reports Submitted to the President's Commission on Mental Health, Vol. IV, Appendix, 1978). More recent reports suggest that the point prevalence and lifetime rates are even higher (Amenson & Lewinsohn, 1981; Myers & Weissman, 1980). Depression is twice as likely to occur in women as in men (Amenson & Lewinsohn, 1981; Weissman & Klerman, 1977b), and it is a disorder that exacts a heavy toll in human suffering. It has debilitating effects across all areas of functioning (Weissman & Paykel, 1974), frequently during years of peak responsibility and productivity.

In addition to the sheer numbers of people affected by this disorder, there are a number of other considerations that make availability of prompt and cost-effective treatment for depression important. It is known that an episode of depression is a risk factor for further depression; those who have had an episode are twice as likely to become depressed as those who have not (Amenson & Lewinsohn, 1981). This fact emphasizes the importance of providing prompt help to prevent mild depressions from developing into clinically significant episodes. The development of methods for preventing the occurrence of depression is also important in this regard. The magnitude of the problem makes cost considerations in the administration of such interventions of significant concern.

PETER M. LEWINSOHN • University of Oregon, Eugene, Oregon 97403. JULIA STEINMETZ BRECKENRIDGE • Veterans Administration Medical Center, Palo Alto, California 94304. DAVID O. ANTONUCCIO • Veterans Administration Medical Center, Reno, Nevada 89509. LINDA TERI • University of Washington, Seattle, Washington 98195. This research was supported in part by grant MH33572 from the National Institute of Mental Health.

The development of behavioral, or what are more appropriately called *cognitive-behavioral,* approaches to the treatment of depression is a relatively recent phenomenon, and the development of group behavioral approaches is even more recent.

This chapter briefly reviews issues in the definition and assessment of depression and describes various cognitive-behavioral treatments and related research, with an emphasis on group-administered treatment. Finally, our recent work in developing and evaluating a cost-effective psychoeducational method for treating depression in groups is described, that is, the Coping With Depression course.

Definition and Diagnosis of Depression

The diagnosis of depression is rendered difficult because the term *depression* does not have a single, generally accepted set of referents. Consequently, individuals who are labeled as being *depressed* show quite heterogeneous behaviors. Given this heterogeneity, it is especially important that the criteria used to diagnose patients as depressed are explicitly defined. Fortunately, in the past few years there has been significant progress in the identification of uniform and comparable criteria for the diagnosis of depression. Much confusion can now be avoided by the use of semistructured interviews such as the Schedule for Affective Disorders and Schizophrenia (SADS; Endicott & Spitzer, 1978) and through operational criteria for diagnosis such as those represented by the Research Diagnostic Criteria (RDC; Spitzer, Endicott, & Robins, 1978) and the DSM-III (American Psychiatric Association, 1980).

Clear definition of depression is also important because of the potential confounding between the effects of physical illness and depression. Some depressive symptoms (e.g., irritability, fatigue, lethargy, insomnia, gastrointestinal disturbances, headaches, anorexia) occur in more than 40% of general medical patients (Schwab, Bialow, Clemmons, & Holzer, 1966), and a substantial portion of psychologically depressed individuals have one or more somatic symptoms as their chief complaint (Schwab, Clemmons, Bialow, Duggan, & Davis, 1965). To further complicate the matter, many of the symptoms of depression simulate physical illnesses, and depressive symptoms can be caused by certain medications. All of these diagnostic problems become especially important with elderly depressives, who are much more prone to physical illness and who are much more likely to be taking medications. Ruling out organic involvement is thus an important part of the diagnostic process. Thus, if significant health problems are present, a patient should be asked to consult a physician to rule out purely physical reasons for the distress.

The clinical assessment of depressed patients has the following related goals:

1. *Differential diagnosis.* First, it must be determined whether or not depression is *the,* or at least *a,* problem for the individual. The clinician must use

assessment instruments to evaluate the severity and the duration of the presenting symptoms, to differentiate between different subtypes of depression, and to establish a baseline for evaluating treatment progress and outcome.

2. *Functional diagnosis and identification of targets for intervention.* Assessment should also serve to identify specific events and behavior patterns that are functionally related to the individual's depression. The goal of assessment at this level is to pinpoint areas of person–environment interaction that may contribute to the depression. Such information guides the formulation of a specific treatment plan to change the events and the behavior patterns accounting for the patient's depression and to assist in ongoing treatment decisions.

The presence and severity of the manifestations of depression can be measured through ratings on items presumed to represent symptoms of depression. Such items and their broader dimensions have been identified in descriptive studies of depressed individuals (e.g., Grinker, Miller, Sabshin, Nunn, & Nunnally, 1961). On the basis of such studies, there is considerable agreement as to the constituency of the depression syndrome. The symptoms of depression may be grouped into six general categories: *dysphoria* (i.e., feeling sad, down, or "blue"), *reduced rate of behavior, social-interactional problems, guilt, material burden* (i.e., excessive job or financial responsibilities), and *somatic symptoms*. Depressed patients manifest different combinations of these symptoms.

The assessment of depression can be accomplished with four different but complementary methods: (a) diagnosis; (b) symptom ratings; (c) self-report depression scales; and (d) observations of overt behavior. As mentioned earlier, diagnostic categorization has been simplified and made more reliable since the advent of the SADS interview and the RDC and DSM-III. DSM-III distinguishes among three subtypes of pure (unipolar) depression: chronic (dysthymic), episodic (major), and atypical; and three subtypes of mixed (bipolar) depression: bipolar, cyclothymic, and atypical bipolar. The RDC differentiates four types of unipolar depression (major, minor, intermittent, and labile) and three types of bipolar (with mania, with hypomania, and cyclothymic). The RDC includes numerous nonmutually exclusive subtypes of depression that allow more precise classification for research purposes.

The accurate identification of bipolar depression is particularly important. *Bipolar depression,* that is, a syndrome characterized by a distinct period of elevated, expansive, or irritable mood with other associated manic symptoms alternating with or preceding the dysphoric episode, has been shown to be a distinct disorder requiring quite different treatment. All of the cognitive-behavioral treatments, including the group treatment to be described in this chapter, have been designed primarily for use with unipolar depressives.

The presence and severity of the phenomena of depression may also be assessed by one of several interviewer rating scales. Among the better known scales are the Feelings and Concerns Checklist (Grinker, Miller, Sabshin, Nunn, & Nunnally, 1961), the Hamilton Rating Scale for Depression (Hamilton, 1960,

1967), and the more global Raskin Depression Scales (Raskin, Shulterbrandt, Reatig, Crook, & Odle, 1974). When used by well-trained raters, these scales possess high interrater reliability, differentiate significantly between depressed and nondepressed patients, and differentiate between various intensities of depression.

There are also many self-administered depression scales (Levitt & Lubin, 1975, list 23 such scales). Only the more popular ones are mentioned here, all of which have been shown to correlate significantly with each other (Lubin, 1967; Zung, Richards, & Short, 1965) and to correlate substantially with interview ratings. The best known of the self-report measures for depression is the D-scale of the MMPI. It has been used widely for the measurement of depression for clinical and research purposes. By far the most popular brief self-report depression inventory is the Beck Depression Inventory (Beck, Ward, Mendelson, Mock, & Erbaugh, 1961). This 21-item multiple choice scale is often used as a pre-post measure in depression research. Other widely used self-report instruments are the Zung Self-Rating Depression Scale (Zung, 1965, 1973), the Depression Adjective Checklist (Lubin, 1965, 1967, 1977), and the Center for Epidemiological Studies Depression Scale (Radloff, 1977).

The construct of depression includes a variety of relatively specific overt behaviors, and a number of methods have been used to measure them directly. For instance, many have used a time-sampling procedure to measure the frequency of such behaviors as crying and smiling (Reisinger, 1972), verbal behavior (Lewinsohn, 1974), and social interaction (Fuchs & Rehm, 1977).

A complementary concern to the assessment of presence, severity, and pattern of depressive symptoms is functional assessment: pinpointing the specific person–environment interactions and events related to the depression. This part of the diagnostic process guides the formulation of a treatment plan and provides baseline data for evaluating the progress of therapy. Depression is commonly accompanied by functional problems in regard to social interactions (e.g., Lewinsohn, Biglan, & Zeiss, 1976), depressive cognitions (e.g., Beck, 1967), a low rate of engagement in pleasant activities (e.g., Lewinsohn & Amenson, 1978), and a high rate of occurrence of negative events (e.g., Lewinsohn & Talkington, 1979). On an individual basis, such functional problems may be postulated as being related to the presence of depression if (a) the change in mood is accompanied by a change in the individual's customary level of these behaviors; or (b) the person–environment interaction covaries with daily fluctuations in mood. Measurement of such functional problems is most commonly accomplished by having an individual monitor both the daily occurrence of targeted events and activities and daily mood levels.

Cognitive-Behavioral Approaches to Treatment

During the last 15 years, there have been major advances in the psychosocial treatment of depressed individuals. Over 50 outcome studies have been published, and several major reviews have appeared (Hersen & Bellack, 1982; Hollon & Beck, 1978; Lewinsohn & Hoberman, 1982; Parloff, Wolfe, Hadley, & Waskow, 1978; Rehm & Kornblith, 1979; Weissman, 1983). It is apparent that a variety of cognitive-behavioral treatments are efficacious in ameliorating depression, including those based on cognitive theories of depression (e.g., Rush, Beck, Kovacs, & Hollon, 1977), self-control theories of depression (e.g., Fuchs & Rehm, 1977), reinforcement theories of depression (e.g., Lewinsohn, Youngren, & Grosscup, 1980), other behavioral formulations (e.g., McLean, Ogsdon, & Grauer, 1973; McLean & Hakstian, 1979), social adjustment theories of depression (e.g., Weissman, Prusoff, DiMascio, Neu, Golansky, & Klerman, 1979), and social skills approaches (e.g., Bellack, Hersen, & Himmelhoch, 1981; Sanchez, Lewinsohn, & Larson, 1980). In spite of the fact that each of these treatments employs somewhat different tactics, each has been shown to be more effective than some type of control group.

In particular, four studies (Bellack, Hersen, & Himmelhoch, 1981; Blackburn, Bishop, Glen, Whalley, & Christie, 1981; McLean & Hakstian, 1979; Rush *et. al.*, 1977) have demonstrated the superiority of cognitive and/or behavioral treatments over pharmacotherapy. Traditional expressive or insight-oriented psychotherapies have also not done well in controlled trials (Covi, Lipman, Derogatis, Smith, & Pattison, 1974; Sanchez *et. al.*, 1980; Weinberg, 1978). The evidence is more equivocal on the combined use of psychosocial treatment with pharmacotherapy. Several studies (Roth, Bielski, Jones, Parker, & Osborn, 1982; Weissman, 1979) have reported the combined use to be more efficacious than either treatment alone but these findings were not replicated by Blackburn *et al.* (1981) or by Bellack *et al.* (1981).

Currently available cognitive-behavioral treatments for depression were derived from specific theoretical formulations and posit specific strategies for alleviating depression. In spite of this diversity, commonalities have also been noted (Blaney, 1977; Rehm & Kornblith, 1979). All assume that the depressed patient has *acquired* maladaptive reaction patterns that can be *unlearned.* Symptoms are seen as important in their own right rather than as manifestations of underlying conflicts, and treatments are aimed at modification of relatively specific behaviors and cognitions rather than at a general reorganization of the patient's personality. All cognitive-behavioral treatments are structured and time limited.

The currently most influential theoretical approaches may roughly be divided into those that emphasize *reinforcement* and those that emphasize *cognitions* in the etiology of depression. The first attempt at a behavioral analysis of depression is contained in Skinner's (1953) book *Science and Human Behavior* in which depression is described as a weakening of behavior due to the interruption of established sequences of behavior that have been positively reinforced by the social environment. This conceptualization of depression as an extinction phenomenon and as a reduced frequency of emission of positively reinforced behavior has been central to all behavioral positions. The therapeutic implications of this conceptualization are relatively straightforward. Because the onset of depression is assumed to be preceded by a reduction in positive reinforcement, improvement should follow from an increase in positive reinforcement. Hence the principal goal of treatment should be to restore an adequate schedule of positive reinforcement for the patient by altering the level, the quality, and the range of his or her activities and interpersonal interactions.

A treatment approach ("Decrease Unpleasant Events and Increase Pleasant Activities") that was specifically derived from the *reinforcement* position was developed by Lewinsohn, Sullivan, and Grosscup (1980). The treatment is time limited (12 sessions) and highly structured, and a therapist manual is available. The general goal of the treatment is to teach depressed persons skills they can use to decrease problematic patterns of interaction with the environment, to increase positive patterns, and to maintain these changes after the termination of therapy. To accomplish the goals of treatment, the therapist makes use of a wide range of cognitive-behavioral interventions such as assertion, relaxation training, daily planning, increasing pleasant activities, time-management training, and cognitive procedures intended to allow the person to deal more adaptively with aversive situations. A more detailed description, case illustrations, pre- and posttreatment and follow-up data for three groups of depressed patients treated with this approach are presented elsewhere (Lewinsohn *et al.*, 1980). Most of the participants were substantially improved at the end of treatment, and these improvements were maintained at the 1-month follow-up assessment.

Cognitive theorists such as Beck (1967), Ellis and Harper (1961), Rehm (1977), and Seligman (1974, 1975) have each advanced hypotheses that attribute a causal role to cognitions in the etiology of depression, but they differ in regard to the specific nature of the cognitions that are assumed to lead to depression. Beck (1967, 1976) conceives of depression as a disorder of thinking. The signs and symptoms of depression are assumed to be a *consequence* of the activation of negative cognitive patterns. Several specific cognitive structures are postulated to be central for the development of depression: the cognitive triad, schemata, and cognitive errors (Beck, Rush, Shaw, & Emery, 1979). The cognitive triad consists of three cognitive patterns asserted to dominate ideation: a negative view of oneself, a negative view of the world, and a negative view of the future. Beck also postulates the existence of superordinate schemata or cognitive biases that lead to systematic filtering or distortion of perception and memory. Such distortions are automatic and involuntary, and they include *arbitrary inference* (drawing conclusions without evidence or despite contrary evidence); *selective abstraction* (ignoring the context of an event by fixating on the detailed aspect of the situation while ignoring more salient features); *overgeneralization* (drawing a general conclusion on the basis of limited detail or limited occurrences of an event); *magnification and minimization* (undue exaggerating or limiting of the significance of the information); *personalization* (attaching subjective significance of external events when no basis exists for making such a connection); and *absolutistic thinking* (placing all experiences in one or two opposite categories) (Beck *et al.*, 1979).

Ellis (e.g., Ellis & Harper, 1961) attaches primary importance to *irrational beliefs* for the development of depression. Depression in this view occurs when a particular situation triggers an irrational belief. It is the latter that is hypothesized to cause the person to overreact emotionally to the situation. For example, the person may become depressed after being rejected because he or she believes that "if one is not loved by everyone, one is unloveable."

The most widely used cognitive therapy is described in detail in Beck *et al.* (1979). Cognitive therapy aims to assist the patient in identifying the assumptions and schemata that are supporting recurrent patterns of stereotypical negative thinking and in pointing out specific stylistic errors in thinking. Cognitive therapy is short term and time limited; a maximum of 20 sessions are spread over 10 to 12 weeks. Both behavioral and cognitive techniques are used. Therapy sessions consist of the disucssion of previously assigned homework, a focus on aspects of the patient's thinking, and assignment of homework for the next session.

Rehm (1977) has developed a self-control theory of depression in which negative evaluations and low rates of self-reinforcement and high rates of self-punishment are seen as leading to the low rate of behavior that characterizes depressed individuals. Three processes are postulated to be important in self-control: self-monitoring, self-evaluation, and self-reinforcement. Rehm suggests that depressed persons attend selectively to negative events, that they set too stringent criteria for self-evaluation, and that their self-reinforcement is characterized by low rates of self-reward and high rates of self-punishment.

A treatment based on self-control theory has been described by Fuchs and Rehm (1977). The treatment consists of 6 sessions with 2 sessions devoted to each of the three self-control processes (self-monitoring, self-evaluation, and self-reinforcement). The first session of each phase involves a didactic presentation and discussion of self-control principles relevant to the assumed deficits of depressives plus a behavioral homework assignment. In the second session, patients review the preceding week's assignment. Self-control therapy has been developed as a group approach from the very beginning.

Interpersonal disturbance theories of depression have been advanced by Weissman and Paykel (1974) and by McLean (1976). These formulations consider the depressed person's interactions with his or her social environment to be crucial for the development and for the reversal of depression. Depression is postulated to result when ineffective coping techniques are utilized to remedy problematic life situations. *Interpersonal therapy* attempts to maximize the patient's competence in specific coping skills or life roles. Interpersonal therapy (McLean *et al.*, 1973; McLean & Hakstian, 1979) incorporates behavioral and cognitive techniques. A unique aspect of interpersonal therapy is constituted by an emphasis on therapeutic decision making regarding appropriate intervention components. Interpersonal therapy is also distinguished by its incorporation of procedures for including relevant social network members (e.g., spouse) as integral components of treatment. Thus, a component of interpersonal therapy involves communication training between the patient and his or her spouse, or significant other. Six specific therapeutic tactics are suggested by McLean: communication training, training in skills for behavioral productivity, social interactions, assertiveness, decision making and problem solving, and cognitive self-control.

A fundamental assumption of *interpersonal psychotherapy* (Klerman & Weissman, 1982) is that depressive symptomatology and interpersonal problems are interrelated. Depression can predispose the patient to interpersonal problems, and interpersonal problems can precipitate depression (Rounsaville & Chevron, 1982). In interpersonal psychotherapy (IPT) as developed by Klerman and Weissman (1982), patients are seen weekly for 12 to 16 weeks. This treatment focuses on improving the quality of the depressed patient's interpersonal functioning, with the goal of helping patients develop more productive strategies for dealing with current social and interpersonal problems that are judged to be associated with the onset of depression symptoms. The concept, techniques, and strategies of IPT have been specified in a procedural manual (Klerman, Rounsaville, Chevron, Neu, & Weissman, 1979). Although the goals of IPT are similar, this treatment is less structured than other cognitive-behavioral approaches.

Most studies of cognitive-behavioral treatments have been concerned with the individual treatment of depression. From these studies, it has become very clear that the specific cognitive and social skills deficits of depressed individuals can be pinpointed and that relatively simple methods are available for teaching depressed individuals how to improve these skills. It was, therefore, natural for investigators to try to adapt the available cognitive-behavioral approaches for group application.

The first use of a behaviorally oriented approach to the group treatment of depressed persons was reported by Lewinsohn, Weinstein, and Alper (1970). In this study, the group meetings were used to generate data about specific aspects of the participants' social behavior and its consequences. Feedback was provided to group members in individual therapy sessions that were held between group sessions. The group was structured as a "self-study" group where members would be able to learn about their own behavior and its consequences on others. During the individual therapy sessions, each member was provided with verbal accounts of his or her own behavior in the group (supported by graphs and data) with the aim of defining specific behavioral problems and goals for change.

The most systematic and extensive use of the group approach is represented by the work of Rehm (e.g., Fuchs & Rehm, 1977). Other studies using group cognitive-behavioral approaches with *symptomatic volunteers* (Barrera, 1979; Gioe, 1975; LaPointe & Rimm, 1980; Schmidt & Miller, 1983; Shaw, 1977; Weinberg, 1978), *depressed patients* (Morris, 1975; Roth *et al.*, 1982; Rush & Watkins, 1981; Sanchez *et al.*, 1980; Shaffer, Shapiro, Sank, & Coghlan, 1981; Shaw & Hollon, 1978), and with special populations such as *elderly individuals* (Jarvik, Mintz, Steuer, & Gerner, 1982; Thompson, Gallagher, Nies, & Epstein, 1983), *depressed alcoholics* (Wehl & Turner, 1982), *Puerto Rican women* (Comas-Diaz, 1981), and *chronic depressives* (Antonuccio, Akins, Chatham, Monagen, Tearnan, & Ziegler, 1983) have been reported. Although the kinds of cognitive-behavioral approaches being adapted for group application differ substantially across studies, the results have been very encouraging. It clearly can be done.

An important question needing to be addressed concerns the relative efficacy of group versus individual cognitive-behavior therapy. Brown and

Lewinsohn (1984), Schmidt and Miller (1983), and Teri and Lewinsohn (1981) report no differences. Rush and Watkins (1981), however, found individual cognitive therapy to be somewhat superior to group cognitive therapy, and Wehl and Turner (1982) also found their individual cognitive-behavioral approach superior to the analogous group approach with depressed alcoholic inpatients. In this latter study, 75% of the individual therapy patients were in complete remission following treatment. Individual therapy subjects were also significantly less likely to prematurely terminate therapy. It appears, therefore, that at least with certain patient populations (e.g., those who have suffered some organicity) the individual approach may be more efficacious.

The "Coping with Depression" Course

In the remainder of this chapter, we describe a new approach to the treatment of depression: One that allows outreach, is less stigmatizing, is more affordable, and is easily accessible to a wide variety of depressed persons. A course entitled "Coping with Depression" (CWD) is the vehicle for treatment. The CWD course has been offered through the University of Oregon Depression Research Unit since 1979 to over 300 depressed individuals. The efficacy of the course has been evaluated in a number of treatment outcome studies (Brown & Lewinsohn, 1984; Steinmetz, Lewinsohn, & Antonuccio, 1983; Teri & Lewinsohn, 1981), and additional research is still in progress (Hoberman, Lewinsohn, & Tilson, 1985). It is quite clear that, as a group, individuals who participate in this course show marked improvement both in depression level and diagnosis, and that these changes are maintained to 6 months' posttreatment.

Rationale and Theoretical Foundation

The Coping with Depression course is based on the social learning theory analysis of depression. According to social learning theory (Bandura, 1977), emotional disorders previously considered to be external manifestations of internal (i.e., psychic) conflicts are instead considered to be behaviors that are influenced by the same laws of learning and development that influence normal behavior. Abnormal behaviors are thus considered to be learned phenomena that influence and are influenced by a person's interaction with the environment. In regard to depression, the primary hypothesis (Lewinsohn *et al.*, 1980) is that a low rate of response-contingent positive reinforcement constitutes a critical antecedent for the occurrence of depression. Reinforcement is defined by the quality of the person's interactions with his or her environment. Those person–environment interactions with positive outcomes (i.e., outcomes making the person feel good) constitute positive reinforcement and strengthen the person's behavior. The behavior of depressed persons is assumed not to lead to positive reinforcement to a degree sufficient to maintain their behavior. Hence depressed individuals find it difficult to initiate or to maintain their behavior, and they become increasingly passive. The low rate of reinforcement is also assumed to cause the dysphoric mood that is central to the phenomenology of depression. The experience of little or no rewarding interaction with the environment causes the person to feel sad and blue.

A corollary hypothesis is that a high rate of punishing experience also causes depression. *Punishment* is defined as person–environment interactions with aversive (distressing, upsetting, unpleasant) outcomes. Punishing interactions with the environment may cause depression directly, or indirectly by interfering with the person's engagement in, and enjoyment of, potentially rewarding activities.

There are three reasons why a person may experience low rates of positive reinforcement and/or high rates of punishment: (a) the person's immediate environment may have few available positive reinforcers or have many punishing aspects; (b) the person may lack the skills to obtain available positive reinforcers and/or to cope effectively with negative events; and (c) the positive reinforcement potency of events may be reduced and/or the negative impact of punishing events may be heightened.

Following from these theoretical notions, the goal of treatment (and of the Coping with Depression course) is to increase the quantity and the quality of positively reinforcing interactions between the depressed person and his or her environment and to decrease the quantity and the quality of negative (punishing) interactions.

The CWD course specifically addresses behaviors and cognitions that have been shown to be problematic for depressed individuals. Behavior patterns that have been shown to be functionally related to depression include reduced pleasant activities, social interactional problems, problematic cognitions related to depression, and anxiety. Recognizing the multiplicity and heterogeneity of the types of problems shown by depressed individuals, the CWD course provides a "smorgasbord" of skills training to deal with these problems. Individuals are encouraged to focus on those problems of most direct personal relevance to them.

To train participants in the skills necessary to ameliorate depression, the CWD course utilizes intervention strategies that have been shown to be therapeutically effective singly or in combination, such as cognitive therapy, social skills training, increasing pleasant activities, time-management training, and relaxation. The CWD course also incorporates elements that in a previous publication (Zeiss, Lewinsohn, & Muñoz, 1979) were hypothesized to constitute common and critical components for all of the recent cognitive-behavioral treatments:

1. Therapy should begin with an elaborated, well-planned rationale. This rationale should provide initial structure that guides the patient to the belief that he or she can control his or her own behavior, and thereby his or her depression.
2. Therapy should provide training in skills that the patient can utilize to feel more effective in handling his or her daily life. These skills must be of

some significance to the patient and must fit with the rationale that has been presented.

3. Therapy should emphasize the independent use of these skills by the patient outside of the therapy context and must provide enough structure so that the attainment of independent skills is possible for the patient.
4. Therapy should encourage the patient's attribution that improvement in mood is caused by the patient's increased skillfulness, not by the therapist's skillfulness (Zeiss *et al.*, 1979).

Description of the Coping with Depression Course

Overview

The CWD course is a multimodal, psychoeducational group treatment for unipolar depression. The major vehicle for treatment is an explicit educational experience designed to teach people techniques and strategies for coping with the problems that are assumed to be related to their depression. The CWD course consists of 12 two-hour sessions conducted over 8 weeks. Sessions are held twice a week during the first 4 weeks of treatment, and once a week for the final 4 weeks. One-month and 6-month follow-up sessions, called *class reunions*, are held to encourage maintenance of treatment gains.

The first two sessions of the CWD course are devoted to the definition of course ground rules, the presentation of the social learning view of depression, and instruction in basic self-change skills. The next eight sessions are devoted to the acquisition of skills in four specific areas: learning how to relax, increasing pleasant activities, changing aspects of one's thinking, and improving both the quality and quantity of one's social interactions. Two sessions are devoted to each skill. The final two sessions focus on maintenance and prevention issues.

The course is a highly structured, time limited, skills training program that makes use of a text, *Control Your Depression* (Lewinsohn, Muñoz, Youngren, & Zeiss, 1978), from which reading assignments are made; a *Participant Workbook* (Brown & Lewinsohn, 1984), which was developed to supplement the text; and an *Instructor's Manual* (Steinmetz, Antonuccio, Bond, McKay, Brown, & Lewinsohn, 1979) to insure comparability of treatment across instructors. A more detailed description of the course is provided in Lewinsohn, Antonuccio, Steinmetz, and Teri (1984). The syllabus for the course is shown in Table 1.

The *Participant Workbook* contains goal statements, assignments for each session, and monitoring forms for recording specific behaviors, thoughts, and feelings relevant to the class assignments. Group time is divided between lecture, review of assignments, discussion, role play, and structured tasks. The instructor's main goals are to deliver the course information accurately, promote the effective application of the information, help participants solve problems related to the material, and facilitate a supportive group interaction.

TABLE 1. Coping with Depression—Course Syllabus

Instructor(s):
Text: *Control Your Depression* (Prentice-Hall, 1978)
Hours:
Assignment prior to first session:
- (a) Complete Pleasant Events Schedule and return it.
- (b) Read Chapters 1, 2, and 3 (only after completing Pleasant Events Schedule).
- (c) Begin monitoring daily mood (see Chapter 3, pp. 44–47)

1. Depression and Social Learning
   For next unit: Read Chapter 4
2. Self-Change Methods
   For next unit: Read Chapter 6
3. Relaxation and Depression: Learning to Relax
   For next unit: Review Chapter 6
4. Relaxation in Everyday Situations
   For next unit: Read Chapter 7
5. Pleasant Activities and Depession
   For next unit: Read Chapter 10
6. Formulating a Pleasant Activities Plan
   For next unit: Read Chapter 11
7. Thinking and Depression: Two Approaches to Constructive Thinking
   For next unit: Read Chapter 12
8. Formulating a Plan for Constructive Thinking
   For next unit: Read Chapter 8
9. Social Skills: The Ability to be Assertive
   For next unit: Read Chapter 9
10. Using Your Social Skills
    For next unit: Read Chapter 13
11. Maintaining Your Gains
    For next unit: Read Chapters 14 and 15.
12. Developing a Life Plan
    For next meeting: Review chapters as needed
    1-month Reunion
    For next meeting: Review chapters as needed
    6-month Reunion

Selection Process

Consistent with the educational philosophy of the course, exclusion criteria have been minimal. Individuals are excluded if they show evidence of mental retardation, dyslexia, serious visual or auditory impairment, bipolar disorder, schizophrenia or schizoaffective disorder, or acute substance abuse. Concurrent psychotherapy, counseling, or pharmacotherapy for depression or other problems are not exclusion criteria. Although a current episode of depression is not required for inclusion, approximately 80% of the participants meet criteria for a diagnosis of depression by the RDC (Spitzer *et al.*, 1978) and DSM-III (American Psychiatric Association, 1980) criteria. Typical enrollment is five to eight students, and attrition has been very low.

The typical chain of events is for people to telephone for information about the course. A receptionist provides preliminary information and schedules interested callers for an intake interview. The purposes of this interview are twofold: (a) to determine whether to recommend the course to the particular individual; and (b) to provide the individual with the necessary information to decide whether he or she wants to participate in the course. The general criteria for recommending course participation have been guided by three considerations: (a) whether the individual is going to be able to function well within the treatment format (i.e., can he or she do the readings, carry out the assignments, and function appropriately as a member of a structured group?); (b) whether the individual is likely to benefit from this treatment given the data we have about him or her and about those who tend to benefit from this treatment; and (c) whether the individual seems to be in need of some other treatment. Concurrent psychological or psychiatric treatment and/or psychotropic medication have not been considered to be exclusion criteria, and typically between 30 to 40% of the course participants are also involved in some other form of treatment. People with acute marital conflict are given a choice of first enrolling in the Coping with Depression course with the goal of reducing depression, and following this with working on their marital problems or perhaps with marital therapy. Although the marital relationship may benefit indirectly from the course, it should not be the primary motivation for enrolling.

Following the intake interview, an initial individual meeting with the instructor takes place. We have found this meeting to be important in reducing the dropout rate. It gives each participant an opportunity to "tell his or her story" and to develop rapport with the leader prior to the beginning of the course. It is recommended that each new instructor have basic clinical skills and co-lead the course the first time with an experienced instructor if possible. One training program we have found satisfactory has included having student instructors actually take the CWD course from a trained instructor prior to leading a group themselves.

Session-by-Session Description

Session 1. The first session is particularly important because the ground rules are established. This practice is in sharp contrast to more traditional therapy groups in which process issues are allowed to evolve and are then used for therapeutic interaction. The time-limited and educationally focused nature of the CWD course necessitates that the instructor take a strong role in delineating group norms and ground rules at the outset. Rather than waiting for many problems to evolve and be solved, the most expected issues are predicted, and related ground rules are explicitly described. The ground rules include (a) using the group to learn skills rather than as a sounding board for depression; (b) providing constructive, caring, noncoercive feedback to group members; (c) allowing each group member an equal opportunity to share in the discussions; (d) focusing on practical solutions rather than abstract problems; and (e) keeping shared information confidential.

Session 2. This session is devoted to self-change skills. The instructor thoroughly explains the basic steps in making a self-change plan: pinpointing, baselining, discovering antecedents and consequences, setting goals, contracting, and choosing reinforcers. Hypothetical self-change plans designed by participants as homework are discussed. By the end of this session, it is important that all participants have mastered the basic self-change tools. The mastery of these techniques is a prerequisite for subsequent modules.

Session 3. Because anxiety often accompanies depression, Session 3 begins relaxation training. To supplement the Benson (1975) relaxation technique presented in *Control Your Depression,* the instructor leads the class through the Jacobson (1929) progressive muscle relaxation procedure. The instructor emphasizes the importance of practicing relaxation regularly so that the body may learn to respond with relaxation in problem situations. The instructor also discusses the negative effect that excessive and uncontrolled tension can have on an individual's ability to enjoy activities and social interaction. Participants are asked to monitor their baseline tension level and then to practice relaxation daily. Because relaxation skills are relatively easy to learn, this session provides an early success experience for most participants.

Session 4. The fourth session is devoted to techniques for applying relaxation in problem situations. The instructor discusses covert and "portable" relaxation techniques while working with participants to identify their own "tension situations." The homework consists of monitoring tension in problem situations and the application of relaxation techniques.

Session 5. This session focuses on the demonstrated relationship between level of pleasant activities and mood. During a baseline period, participants are asked to monitor the frequency and enjoyment of their personal list of activities that has been generated from their completed "Pleasant Events Schedule" (MacPhillamy & Lewinsohn, 1982). A graph is provided to visually illustrate the correspondence between level of pleasant activity and mood.

Session 6. In this session, participants use their baseline monitoring to decide on a pleasant activity goal. Participants make a weekly plan of activity, with the idea of attaining a balance each day between activities experienced as negative or neutral and those experienced as positive. They also continue to monitor activities and mood, striving to achieve an improvement in mood level by increasing the rate of pleasant activity.

Session 7. Session 7 deals with the effect negative and nonconstructive thoughts can have on mood. Two different approaches to working on cognitions are presented: (a) methods of increasing positive thoughts and decreasing negative thoughts (e.g., thought interruption, stimulus control techniques for worrying to decrease negative thoughts, and "priming" [i.e., having the person say nice things to him- or herself when he or she does or thinks something positive], and future time projection [i.e., having the person mentally travel forward to a time when he or she is no longer depressed] to increase positive thoughts); and (b) methods for thinking more constructively, involving strategies developed by Beck *et al.* (1979) for identifying and challenging automatic "irrational" thoughts. After being introduced to both methods, participants choose the techniques they prefer and form subgroups to work on whichever strategies they selected. The instructor then works as a consultant, encouraging participants to help each other in the application of the techniques. Although we have no data reflecting on this issue, it is our clinical impression that the former set of strategies is more useful to individuals with obsessive negative or self-critical thoughts, whereas the latter strategies seem to be more effective for people who tend to overreact to situations or become upset easily.

Session 8. Session 8 continues work on cognitive strategies. In addition, participants are exposed to self-instructional strategies developed by Meichenbaum (1975).

Session 9. This session focuses on assertion. The leader discusses typical problems with social interaction that accompany depression. Assertion is presented as a useful skill for interacting with others in a direct, honest, and rewarding way. Participants are encouraged to provide examples of situations in which they tend to be nonassertive and feel more depressed. Modeling and role playing are used to work with the problem situations presented. The homework assignment for this session requires participants to pinpoint problem situations and practice covert rehearsal of assertion.

Session 10. Session 10 presents the notion that low social interaction may result when there is (a) inadequate stimulation (e.g., one gets "into a rut" or one gets out of the habit of being around others); and (b) inadequate reward (e.g., because of tension, nonassertiveness, or some other difficulty social activity is no longer rewarding). Participants discuss activities they may need to increase (e.g., calling friends to suggest getting together), or activities they need to decrease (e.g., watching television) in order to improve their level of pleasant social interaction. Specific plans are then developed for increasing or decreasing problem areas.

Session 11. This session summarizes the course material, and participants begin planning for maintenance of gains. Participants review and set priorities for each problem area covered in the course. They then evaluate the techniques they have learned and, based on their self-monitoring data, determine which strategies have been most effective and which they would like to use on a regular basis.

Session 12. The final session is devoted to the discussion of participants' "life plans." The life plans are written according to guidelines specified in *Control Your Depression.* This task is designed to help participants think about their personal values, goals, and style. Each participant pinpoints problem areas and makes specific plans for continuing to work on his or her difficulties. Many final sessions involve a discussion of treatment gains, and "testimonials" are not uncommon. For participants who have not achieved significant improvement in their depression during the course, this can be a difficult session. The instructor should be sure to emphasize that continued improvement and maintenance of gains is more likely to occur if participants continue to use the coping skills they have learned in the course. Some people will require additional help in mastering these skills, and some may find alternative forms of treatment necessary. It is the instructor's responsibility to discuss plans for the future with members of the group who continue to be depressed. It may be advisable to provide referrals for more intensive forms of treatment for such participants.

Research on the CWD Course

Three treatment outcome studies on the CWD course have been completed (Brown & Lewinsohn, 1984; Steinmetz *et al.*, 1983; Teri & Lewinsohn, 1981), and one is currently in progress (Hoberman, Lewinsohn, & Tilson, 1985). In each of these studies course participants were carefully assessed on a wide range of variables at four points in time: pretreatment, posttreatment, 1 month, and 6 months following treatment. Each of these studies assessed somewhat different variables depending upon the specific hypotheses under investigation. A core assessment battery, however, was constant across studies. Depression was assessed with the Beck Depression Inventory (Beck *et al.*, 1961), a self-report measure of depression symptomatology, and the SADS (Endicott & Spitzer, 1978), a 2-hour semistructured diagnostic interview. The SADS-Change version (SADS-C; Spitzer *et al.*, 1978) was used to measure change from pretreatment to posttreatment and follow-up. Diagnoses of depression and other psychopathological syndromes were obtained by utilizing decision rules specified by the Research Diagnostic Criteria (Spitzer *et al.*, 1978). For each episode of disturbance, the interviewer recorded the diagnosis, age at onset, and duration of the episode. The training of the interviewers and the fact that interrater reliability was high and comparable to that obtained by Spitzer *et al.* (1978) are described in greater detail elsewhere (Amenson & Lewinsohn, 1981).

Four major questions have been posited by these studies: (a) Is the CWD course therapeutically effective? (b) Is the CWD course more (or less) effective in ameliorating depression than other therapeutic approaches? (c) What therapist characteristics contribute to successful CWD courses? and (d) What participant variables are predictive of successful course outcome?

CWD Course Therapeutic Effectiveness

Results of the three completed studies are summarized in Table 2. In each study, depressed individuals participating in CWD course show substantial, and statistically highly significant, improvement at posttreatment and maintain improvement at both 1-month and 6-month follow-up. This was true on self-report and clinical diagnoses (see Tables 2 and 3). Improvement from the CWD course has been comparable in magnitude to that shown by subjects in individual therapy in our own (e.g., Lewinsohn *et al.*, 1980) as well as in other studies of cognitive-behavioral therapy for depression (e.g., Bellack *et al.*, 1981; McLean & Hakstian, 1979; Rush & Beck, 1978; Schmidt & Miller, 1983). Recognizing the usual limitations about generalizing and the need for cross-validation by other centers, it appears that the CWD course as currently constituted is a viable and cost-effective treatment approach for depressed outpatients.

CWD Course Comparative Effectiveness

The CWD course has been evaluated in comparison to other behavioral treatment modalities and in comparison to a wait-list control group. Ethically, it

TABLE 2. Beck Depression Inventory Scores from Three Treatment Outcome Studies Involving the "Coping with Depression" Course[a]

		Pretreat-ment		Posttreat-ment		1 Month follow-up		6 Month follow-up	
Study	Treatment	X	SD	X	SD	X	SD	X	SD
Brown & Lewinsohn, 1984	Class, $N = 31$	19.8	7.7	7.6	7.0	6.6	6.2	6.4	6.9
	Individual, $N = 15$	24.4	8.6	9.5	7.7	11.1	9.4	7.4	7.5
	Phone, $N = 12$	20.1	7.5	10.8	7.2	10.0	9.2	9.5	6.2
	Delayed, $N = 13$	21.5	9.6	13.9	8.7				
Steinmetz, Lewinsohn, & Antonuccio, 1983	Class, $N = 93$	21.1	9.4	6.8	6.1	6.5	6.1	7.9	8.5
Teri & Lewinsohn, 1983	Class, $N = 56$	25.7	14.8	5.9	5.0	5.8	5.3	5.7	4.9
	Individual, $N = 26$	18.7	10.7	6.2	7.1	5.8	5.5	6.5	4.8

[a]Table includes subjects who did not meet criteria for unipolar depression at pretreatment.

is very difficult not to offer treatment to people who are depressed and potentially suicidal. Our solution to this problem was to randomly assign a proportion of the patients in the first study (Brown & Lewinsohn, 1984) to a delayed treatment condition. Their treatment began after an 8 week waiting period during which time they were encouraged to call the course leader if they needed help. During these 8-weeks, these subjects received very little treatment. As can be seen in Table 2, the CWD course was more effective in reducing depression than the delayed treatment condition.

The CWD course was compared to individual tutoring based on the CWD course, a minimal phone contact procedure (Brown & Lewinsohn, 1984), and individual behavior therapy (Teri & Lewinsohn, 1981). The results (shown in Table 3) indicated that differences between all of the active treatment conditions were small and statistically not significant. Thus, the Coping with Depression

TABLE 3. Percentage of Patients Improved As Measured by RDC Criteria for Unipolar Depression (as per RDC) at 1-Month Posttreatment

Study	Percentage no longer meeting RDC criteria for depression[a]
#1 ($N = 50$)	79%
#2 ($N = 75$)	78%
#3 ($N = 66$)	79%

[a]Table includes only subjects who met diagnostic criteria for unipolar depression at pretreatment.

course was as effective as the other treatment conditions. It is also more cost-effective than individual (one-to-one) treatment. From an economic point of view, the class condition was by far the most cost-effective. The instructors also felt most enthusiastic about this condition, finding their classes both challenging and rewarding.

Therapist Variables Related to Outcome

The leaders of the Coping with Depression courses have all been advanced doctoral students in clinical and counseling psychology who, in addition to having had extensive supervised experience in individual psychotherapy as part of their graduate training, have been carefully trained to conduct the course. In two studies (Antonuccio, Lewinsohn, & Steinmetz, 1982; Teri & Lewinsohn, 1981), we were specifically interested in identifying therapist variables that were related to treatment outcome.

We had assumed that there would be systematic differences between therapists in the amount of improvement shown by their clients and that these differences would be related to therapist variables hypothesized to be important on the basis of a literature review (Antonuccio *et al.*, 1982). A repeated measurements design was used. Leaders were evaluated on a large number of variables (pretreatment therapist characteristics, therapist behavior and style during treatment, group behavior, and group process) that were hypothesized to be related to outcome. Each of the eight course leaders conducted two consecutive treatment groups consisting of five to eight subjects per group. The major finding was that, even though the leaders differed significantly on many of the therapist variables (e.g., group cohesiveness, group participation, therapist warmth, therapist enthusiasm, therapist expectations, on-task activities, etc.), the main effect of the ANOVA due to instructor differences did not attain statistical significance. That is, the instructors did not differ in how much improvement their respective students showed at the end of the course.

Teri and Lewinsohn (1981) investigated whether pairing therapists with a co-leader of the same or opposite sex would influence CWD course effectiveness. A repeated measurements design was again used. Four male and four female therapists conducted two consecutive treatment groups consisting of five to eight subjects per group. Therapist pairing was alternated between treatment groups and cohorts so that each therapist led a group with a member of the same sex and a member of the opposite sex. No significant differences were obtained between CWD courses led by same-sex or opposite-sex therapists. That is, therapists paired with members of their own sex were no more or less effective than therapists paired with members of the opposite sex.

Because all of the groups in both studies had shown significant improvement from pre- to posttreatment, we interpret these results to indicate that our criteria for the selection of instructors and our instructor training procedures are quite adequate to insure predictable and high-level success, and to minimize any systematic effects that individual instructor characteristics might have on outcome.

Participant Variables Predictive of Outcome

Although our results show that a majority of depressed individuals are improved at the end of treatment, it is also true that a significant proportion (approximately 20%) are still depressed at the end of treatment. This figure is fairly constant across studies. It would obviously be valuable if one could predict which individuals do not respond to this treatment. In all of our studies, we have included overlapping participant variables with the goal of identifying and cross-validating findings.

Prior to summarizing findings in regard to patient characteristics predictive of improvement, it must be emphasized that our dependent variable so far has been postcourse depression level. Postcourse depression level has been made independent of precourse depression level by using analysis of covariance, computing residual gains scores, or by entering precourse depression level as the first variable into a multiple regression analysis. We have used these methods because our initial interest was in identifying distinguishing characteristics of participants who show the greatest amount of change (improvement) from pre- to posttreatment. What is being summarized, then, are the predictors of improvement as they have emerged in our studies.

As one might expect, the single strongest predictor of postcourse depression level (as measured by the BDI) is pretreatment depression level. Those who are the most depressed at the beginning are still, relatively, the most depressed at the end of treatment. This result supports Garfield's (1978) statement that pretreatment severity should always be taken into account in the prediction of treatment outcome because the correlation between pre- and posttreatment scores is typically positive and substantial.

A number of variables were consistently and positively related to successful treatment outcome (Brown & Lewinsohn, 1984; Steinmetz *et al.*, 1983; Teri & Lewinsohn, 1981):

1. *Expected improvement.* Participants who expected to be the most symptom free at the end of treatment were the most improved, suggesting that self-efficacy expectations (Bandura, 1977) may play an important role in mediating treatment response.
2. *Satisfaction with major life roles.* Participants who had expressed more satisfaction in regard to 18 life areas deemed to be generally important were also most improved.
3. *Lack of concurrent treatment.* Participants who were not concurrently receiving additional psychotherapy and/or antidepressant medications for depression were more improved.
4. *Perceived social support from family members.* Better treatment outcome resulted for those with more perceived social support.
5. *Age.* Younger participants were more likely to improve.

Variables that consistently did *not* predict treatment outcome after correcting for pretreatment depression level were (1) *symptoms:* endogeneity (e.g., early morning awakening, psychomotor retardation, perceiving depression as qualitatively different from ordinary sadness or downcast spirits), number of previous episodes, previous alcohol or drug abuse; (2) *demographics:* sex, income, occupational level, number of children, or marital status; (3) *cognitions:* locus of control, irrational beliefs, or acceptance of course rationale; (4) stressful life events as measured by the Holmes and Rahe (1967) scale; and (5) *other participant characteristics:* "manageability," "treatability," "likeability," motivation, social skills, or emotional reliance on others.

In our studies, the predictor variables accounted for a little more than half the variance in posttreatment BDI scores. Studies are currently underway (Hoberman, Lewinsohn, & Tilson, 1985) to evaluate the contribution of other variables in predicting improvement as well as to cross-validate the findings obtained thus far.

Future Directions

Although it is easy to make enthusiastic statements about the Coping with Depression course (e.g., most participants are improved; these improvements are maintained at 1-month and 6-month follow-up; the dropout rate is quite low), it is equally easy to suggest directions for future research. The issues that seem to us to be the most urgent include (a) evaluating the long-term effects of the course; (b) delineating more carefully the characteristics of those depressives who do and do not respond to the course; and (c) designing and evaluating modifications of the Coping with Depression course for use with populations that are different from those that have been studied so far, and for the prevention of depression.

Even in the absence of long-term follow-up data, it is safe to assume that at least some of the participants who are improved at the end of the course will relapse, that is, develop another episode of depression. At a more general level, there are two issues: (a) In absolute terms, how many of the former participants become depressed again? and (b) Has participation in the course reduced the probability that they will become depressed again in the future?

There have been relatively few studies on the long-term effects of treatment for depression, but the results of a recent study by Keller and Shapiro (1981) suggest that the beneficial effects of treatment may fade with time for many patients. In a 1-year follow-up of persons treated for depression, Keller and Shapiro (1981) showed only 30% to be symptom free during the first year after treatment. Gonzales, Lewinsohn, and Clarke (1983) are currently conducting a long-term follow-up study in which all of the former participants in the CWD courses offered at the University of Oregon will be reassessed for up to 3 years posttreatment. The results of this study will, we hope, not only provide information on the two previously mentioned issues but also will have implications for modifications in the course that might enhance successful long-term outcome. Pending the results of this study, modifications aimed at the generalization and maintenance of treatment gains might include additional therapeutically structured follow-up sessions, such as "booster" sessions or advanced workshops for former participants. Because the CWD course is a "basic" course designed as something of a "smorgasbord" of coping skills, more advanced training in specific areas of difficulties such as cognitions, assertiveness, time management, and relaxation would be a logical next step to encourage maintenance of treatment gains.

Although our research on the Coping with Depression course clearly indicates that most of the participants improve, a significant proportion (approximately 20%) fail to improve. The fact that this figure is consistent with research on other treatments of depression (e.g., Weissman & Klerman, 1977a; Weissman, Klerman, Prusoff, Sholomskas, & Padin, 1981) should not cause one to feel complacent about this very important subgroup of depressives.

The recent literature includes a number of studies that have examined patient characteristics hypothesized to be related to successful and unsuccessful treatment outcome (Bisno, Thompson, Breckenridge, & Gallagher, 1982; Brown & Lewinsohn, 1984; McLean & Hakstian, 1979; Rehm, 1981a,b; Steinmetz, Lewinsohn, & Antonuccio, 1983; Weissman, Prusoff, & Klerman, 1978b), and some promising results have been obtained. However, more efforts are clearly needed to cross-validate these findings and to identify additional distinguishing characteristics that are predictive of outcome.

The fact that attendance and expectancy regarding outcome is predictive of positive treatment response (Steinmetz, Lewinsohn, & Antonuccio, 1983) suggests that the CWD course might be modified to take greater advantage of these variables. The obtained relationships might even be presented to participants as part of pretherapy training and role induction to encourage a positive expectancy and regular attendance.

The combined use of antidepressant medications (and perhaps other psychotherapeutic approaches) with the Coping with Depression course for some participants also deserves further exploration. Our data suggest that the combination is counterproductive. Participants who, concurrently with the course, were taking medication intended to relieve their depression did not respond as well to treatment as did nonmedicated participants. Concurrent use of medication was a negative indicator of both posttreatment depression level and actual improvement; medication use was not significantly correlated with pretreatment depression level. These results are difficult to interpret: it is possible that being on medication somehow interfered with participants' motivation or ability to actively work at learning and using the coping skills presented in the course. However, it is also possible that a third unspecified variable exists that is related both to being on medication and to improving in treatment. Future controlled research is needed to evaluate the efficacy of the course alone and in combination with antidepressant medication to be certain of this finding.

Comparison of the Coping with Depression course with antidepressant medications is an especially important focus for future research. There is strong evidence that pharmacotherapy is also successful in treating unipolar depression (Morris & Beck, 1974; Rush *et al.*, 1977; Weissman *et al.*, 1979), and many depressives are being treated with antidepressant medicines. Because of the wide use and availability of these two very distinct types of treatment, it is of considerable clinical importance to obtain a greater understanding about which persons benefit from which treatment. Future research thus might be directed not only at comparing these two types of treatments but also at identifying factors that predict individual response.

It would also be of interest whether the so-called "chronic" depressives, that is, those individuals who have not responded to other treatments, will respond to the Coping with Depression course. A recent pilot study conducted at the Reno VA Medical Center suggests that many patients with "drug refractory" depression may actually respond favorably to the psychoeducational treatment approach (Antonuccio *et al.*, 1983).

Most of our work to date has been in what has been called *tertiary prevention*, that is, the course has been aimed at people who are already depressed and for whom depression is the major presenting problem. However, the CWD course seems to attract a certain percentage (approximately 20%) of people who do not meet diagnostic criteria for depression but who are taking the course because they would like to avoid becoming depressed again in the future. As of yet, we have no data as to whether or not taking the course actually helps these nondepressed participants to accomplish this goal. However, it may be hypothesized that the course provides a preventive function in that the acquisition of coping skills may help participants reduce both the severity and duration of negative responses to life stress. In other words, the CWD course could be viewed as an effective preventive intervention if it results in people having relatively mild and short-lived future episodes of depression instead of more severe and chronic episodes. An intervention that is capable of doing this would be especially useful in light of the fact that mild episodes have a much better prognosis (Keller, Shapiro, Lavori, & Wolfe, 1982; Steinmetz *et al.*, 1983). People who are mildly depressed are also much less incapacitated (i.e., they continue to be able to function in important life roles).

With these considerations in mind, research aimed at evaluating the preventive function of the CWD course with groups of people known to be at elevated risk for depression appears warranted. On the basis of epidemiological studies by our group (Lewinsohn & Hoberman, 1982) and others (Hirschfeld & Cross, 1982), information is rapidly becoming available with which to select populations at risk. To wit, those who are (a) female, (b) have had previous episodes of depression, (c) are mildly depressed, (d) have weak social support systems, (e) are unemployed and seeking employment, (f) are experiencing marital conflict, and/or (g) have experienced recent life events, especially those involving social exits (e.g., divorce and separation) are at elevated risk for episodes of depression. Another population that is at high risk for depression and for whom the CWD course may serve a preventive role are individuals who are afflicted with medical illnesses (e.g., arthritis) that require major changes in their life-styles. Such individuals might be well-served by being taught coping skills. Other groups of patients for whom the CWD course might serve a preventive function are those who have other psychiatric disorders (e.g., alcoholism) or who are on medications (e.g., antihypertensive medications) that are known to be accompanied by depression symptoms. Of relevance here is a study by Turner, Wehl, Cannon, and Craig (1980) in which techniques similar to those employed in the CWD course were successfully employed to treat depression in alcoholics. A strength of the CWD course is the fact that it can be and has been adapted to different subgroups, for instance elderly people (Breckenridge, Thompson, Breckenridge, & Gallagher, Chapter 10; Thompson *et al.*, 1983) and adolescents (Clarke & Lewinsohn, 1984).

Finally, in regard to primary prevention, the Coping with Depression course could be offered as part of "life skills" or "mental hygiene" courses in high schools and in adult education classes.

The Coping with Depression course holds much potential for adaptation and evaluation with a wide variety of problems and populations. The actualization of this potential awaits future empirical and clinical investigation.

References

Amenson, C. S., & Lewinsohn, P. M. An investigation into the observed sex difference in prevalence of unipolar depression. *Journal of Abnormal Psychology*, 1981, *90*, 1–13.

American Psychiatric Association, Committee on Nomenclature and Statistics. *Diagnostic and statistical manual of mental disorders* (3rd ed.). Washington, D.C.: Author, 1980.

Antonuccio, D. O., Akins, W. T., Chatham, P. M., Monagen, J., Tearnan, B., & Ziegler, B. *An exploratory study: A psychoeducational group treatment of drug refractory unipolar depression.* Unpublished mimeo, VA Medical Center, Reno, Nev., 1983.

Antonuccio, D. O., Lewinsohn, P. M., & Steinmetz, J. Identification of therapist differences in a group treatment for depression. *Journal of Consulting and Clinical Psychology*, 1982, *50*, 433–435.

Bandura, A. *Social learning theory*. Englewood Cliffs, N.J.: Prentice-Hall, 1977.

Barera, M. An evaluation of a brief group therapy for depression. *Journal of Consulting and Clinical Psychology*, 1979, *47*, 413–415.

Beck, A. T. *Depression: Clinical, experimental and theoretical aspects.* New York: Harper & Row, 1967.

Beck, A. T. *Cognitive therapy and the emotional disorders.* New York: International Universities Press, 1976.

Beck, A. T., Ward, C. H., Mendelson, M., Mock, J., & Erbaugh, J. An inventory for measuring depression. *Archives of General Psychiatry*, 1961, *4*, 561–571.

Beck, A. T., Rush, A. J., Shaw, B. F., & Emery G. *Cognitive therapy of depression: A treatment manual.* New York: Guilford Press, 1979.

Bellack, A. S., Hersen, M., & Himmelhoch, J. Social skills training, pharmacotherapy, and psychotherapy for unipolar depression. *American Journal of Psychiatry*, 1981, *138*, 1562–1567.

Benson, H. *The relaxation response.* New York: William Harrow, 1975.

Bisno, B., Thompson, L., Breckenridge, J. N., & Gallagher, D. *Cognitive predictors of outcome for older adults participating in a psychoeducational program for the treatment of depression.* Paper presented at the meetings of the Western Psychological Association, Sacramento, CA, 1982.

Blackburn, I. M., Bishop, S., Glen, A. I. M., Whalley, L. J. & Christie, J. E. The efficacy of cognitive therapy in depression: A treatment trial using cognitive therapy and pharmacotherapy, each alone and in combination. *British Journal of Psychiatry*, 1981, *139*, 181–189.

Blaney, P. H. Contemporary theories of depression: Critique and comparison. *Journal of Abnormal Psychology*, 1977, *86*, 203–223.

Brown, R. & Lewinsohn, P. M. A psychoeducational approach to the treatment of depression: Comparison of group, individual, and minimal contact procedures. *Journal of Consulting and Clinical Psychology*, 1984, *52*, 774–783.

Clarke, G. & Lewinsohn, P. M. *A psychoeducational approach to the group treatment of depressed adolescents*. University of Oregon, 1984.

Comas-Diaz, L. Effects of cognitive and behavioral group treatment on the depressive symptomatology of Puerto Rican women. *Journal of Consulting and Clinical Psychology*, 1981, *49*, 627–632.

Covi, L., Lipman, R. S., Derogatis, L. R., Smith, J. E., & Pattison, J. H. Drugs and group psychotherapy in neurotic depression. *American Journal of Psychiatry*, 1974, *131*, 191–197.

DiMascio, A., Weissman, M., Prusoff, B., Neu, C., Zwilling, M., & Klerman, G. Differential symptom reduction by drugs and psychotherapy in acute depression. *Archives of General Psychiatry*, 1979, *36*, 1450–1456.

Ellis, A., & Harper, R. A. *A guide to rational living*. Hollywood, Calif.: Wilshire, 1961.

Endicott, J., & Spitzer, R. L. A diagnostic interview: The Schedule for Affective Disorders and Schizophrenia. *Archives of General Psychiatry*, 1978, *35*, 837–844.

Fuchs, C. Z., & Rehm, L. P. A self-control behavior therapy program for depression. *Journal of Consulting and Clinical Psychology*, 1977, *45*, 206–215.

Garfield, S. L. Research on client variables in psychotherapy. In S. L. Garfield & A. E. Bergin (Eds.), *Handbook of psychotherapy and behavior change* (2nd ed.). New York: Wiley, 1978.

Gioe, V. J. Cognitive modification and positive group experience as a treatment for depression. *Dissertation Abstracts International*, 1975, *36*, 3039B–3040B.

Gonzales, L., Lewinsohn, P. M., & Clarke, G. Longitudinal follow-up of unipolar depressiveness: An investigation of predictors of relapse. *Journal of Consulting and Clinical Psychology*, in press.

Grinker, R. R., Miller, J., Sabshin, M., Nunn, R., & Nunnally, J. C. *The phenomena of depressions*. New York: Paul B. Hoeber, 1961.

Hamilton, M. A rating scale for depression. *Journal of Neurology, Neurosurgery, and Psychiatry*, 1960, *23*, 56–61.

Hamilton, M. Development of a rating scale for primary depressive illness. *British Journal of Social Clinical Psychology*, 1967, *6*, 278–296.

Hersen, M., & Bellack, A. S. Perspectives in the behavioral treatment of depression. *Behavior Modification*, 1982, *6*, 95–106.

Hirschfeld, R. M. A., & Cross, C. K. Epidemiology of affective disorders: Psychosocial risk factors. *Archives of General Psychiatry*, 1982, *39*, 35–45.

Hoberman, H., Lewinsohn, P. M., & Tilson, M. *Predictors of treatment response in the Coping with Depression course*. Unpublished manuscript, University of Oregon, 1985.

Hollon, S. D., & Beck, A. T. Psychotherapy and drug therapy: Comparisons and combinations. In S. L. Garfield & A. E. Bergin (Eds.), *The handbook of psychotherapy and behavior change: An empirical analysis*. (2d ed.). New York: Wiley, 1978.

Hollon, S. D., & Shaw, B. F. Group cognitive therapy for depressed patients. In A. T. Beck, A. J. Rush, B. F. Shaw, & G. Emery (Eds.), *Cognitive therapy for depression. A treatment manual*. New York: Guilford Press, 1979.

Holmes, T. H., & Rahe, R. H. The social readjustment rating scale. *Psychosomatic Medicine*, 1967, *11*, 213–218.

Jacobson, E. *Progressive relaxation*. Chicago: University of Chicago Press, 1929.

Jarvik, L. F., Mintz, J., Steuer, J., & Gerner, R. Treating geriatric depression: A 26-week interim analysis. *Journal of the American Geriatric Society*, 1982, *30*, 713–717.

Keller, M. B., & Shapiro, R. W. Major depressive disorder: Initial results from a one year prospective naturalistic follow-up study. *Journal of Nervous and Mental Diseases*, 1981, *169*, 761–768.

Keller, M. B., Shapiro, R. W., Lavori, P. W., & Wolfe, N. Recovery in major depressive disorder. *Archives of General Psychiatry*, 1982, *39*, 905–910.

Klerman, G. L., Rounsaville, B., Chevron, E., Neu, C., & Weissman, M. M. *Manual for short-term interpersonal psychotherapy (IPT) for depression*. Unpublished mimeo, 1979.

Klerman, G. L., & Weissman, M. M. Interpersonal psychotherapy: Theory and research. In A. J. Rush (Ed.), *Short term psychotherapies for depression*. New York: Guilford Press, 1982.

LaPointe, K., & Rimm, D. Cognitive, assertive, and insight-oriented group therapies in the treatment of reactive depression in women. *Psychotherapy Theory, Research, and Practice*, 1980, *17*, 312–319.

Lehman, H. E. Epidemiology of depressive disorders. In R. R. Fieve (Ed.), *Depression in the 70's: Modern theory and research.* Princeton, N.J.: Excerpta Medica, 1971.
Levitt, E. G., & Lubin, B. *Depression.* New York: Springer, 1975.
Lewinsohn, P. M. Clinical and theoretical aspects of depression. In K. S. Calhoun, H. E. Adams, & K. M. Mitchell (Eds.), *Innovative methods in psychopathology.* New York: Wiley, 1974.
Lewinsohn, P. M., & Amenson, C. Some relationships between pleasant and unpleasant mood related activities and depression. *Journal of Abnormal Psychology,* 1978, *87,* 644–654.
Lewinsohn, P. M., & Hoberman, H. M. Depression. In A. S. Bellack, M. Hersen, & A. E. Kazdin (Eds.), *International handbook of behavior modification and therapy.* New York: Plenum Press, 1982.
Lewinsohn, P. M., & Talkington, J. Studies on the measurement of unpleasant events and relations with depression. *Applied Psychological Measurement,* 1979, *3,* 83–101.
Lewinsohn, P. M., Weinstein, M., & Alper, T. A behavioral approach to the group treatment of depressed persons: A methodological contribution. *Journal of Clinical Psychology,* 1970, *26,* 525–532.
Lewinsohn, P. M., Biglan, A., & Zeiss, A. Behavioral treatment of depression. In P. O. Davidson (Ed.), *The behavioral management of anger, depression, and pain.* New York: Bruner/Mazel, 1976.
Lewinsohn, P. M., Muñoz, R. F., Youngren, M. A., & Zeiss, A. M. *Control Your Depression.* Englewood Cliffs, N.J.: Prentice-Hall, 1978.
Lewinsohn, P. M., Sullivan, M., & Grosscup, S. J. Changing reinforcing events: An approach to the treatment of depression. *Psychotherapy: Theory, Research and Practice,* 1980, *17,* 322–334.
Lewinsohn, P. M., Youngren, M. A. & Grosscup, S. J. Reinforcement and depression. In R. A. Depue (Ed.), *The psychobiology of the depressive disorders: Implications for the effects of stress.* New York: Academic Press, 1980.
Lewinsohn, P. M., Antonuccio, D. O., Steinmetz, J. L., & Teri, L. *The Coping with Depression course: A psychoeducational intervention for unipolar depression.* Eugene, Oreg.: Castalia, 1984.
Lubin, B. Adjective checklists for measurement of depression. *Archives of General Psychiatry,* 1965, *12,* 57–62.
Lubin, B. *Depression adjective checklists.* San Diego, Calif.: Educational and Industrial Testing Service, 1967.
Lubin, B. *Bibliography for the depression adjective checklists: 1966–1977.* San Diego, Calif.: Educational and Industrial Testing Service, 1977.
MacPhillamy, D., & Lewinsohn, P. M. The Pleasant Events Schedule: Studies on reliability, validity, and scale intercorrelations. *Journal of Consulting and Clinical Psychology,* 1982, *50,* 363–380.
McLean, P. D. Therapeutic decision making in the behavioral treatment of depression. In P. O. Davidson (Ed.), *The behavioral management of anxiety, depression, and pain.* New York: Brunner/Mazel, 1976.
McLean, P. D., & Hakstian, A. R. Clinical depression: Comparative efficacy of outpatient treatments. *Journal of Clinical and Counseling Psychology,* 1979, *47,* 818–836.
McLean, P. D., Ogsdon, K., & Grauer, L. A behavioral approach to the treatment of depression. *Journal of Behavior Therapy and Experimental Psychiatry,* 1973, *4,* 323–330.
Meichenbaum, D. Self-instructional techniques. In F. H. Kanfer & A. P. Goldstein (Eds.), *Helping people change.* New York: Pergamon Press, 1975.
Morris, J. B., & Beck, A. T. The efficacy of anti-depressant drugs: A review of research (1958–1972). *Archives of General Psychiatry,* 1974, *30,* 667–674.
Morris, N. E. A group self-instruction method for the treatment of depressed outpatients. *Dissertation Abstracts International,* 1975, *107,* 4473B–4474B.
Myers, J. K., & Weissman, M. M. Use of a self-report symptom scale to detect depression in a community sample. *American Journal of Psychiatry,* 1980, *137,* 1081–1084.
Parloff, M. B., Wolfe, B., Hadley, S., & Waskow, I. *Assessment of psychosocial treatment of mental disorders: Current status and prospects.* Unpublished mimeo, 1978.
Radloff, L. S. The CES-D scale: A self-report depression scale for research in the general population. *Applied Psychological Measurement,* 1977, *1,* 385–401.
Raskin, A., Schulterbrandt, J. G., Reatig, N., Crook, T. H., & D. Odle. Depression subtypes and response to phenelzine, diazepam, and a placebo. *Archives of General Psychiatry,* 1974, *30,* 66–75.
Rehm, L. P. A self-control model of depression. *Behavior Therapy,* 1977, *8,* 787–804.

Rehm, L. P. Self-management in depression. In P. Karoly & F. H. Kanfer (Eds.), *The psychology of self-management: From theory to practice*. New York: Pergamon Press, 1981. (a)
Rehm, L. P. (Ed.). *Behavior therapy for depression: Present status and future directions*. New York: Academic Press, 1981. (b)
Rehm, L. P., & Kornblith, S. J. Behavior therapy for depression: A review of recent developments. In M. Hersen, R. M. Eisler, & P. M. Miller (Eds.), *Progress in behavior modification* (Vol. 7). New York: Academic Press, 1979.
Reisinger, J. J. The treatment of anxiety-depression via positive reinforcement and response cost. *Journal of Applied Behavior Analysis*, 1972, *5*, 125–130.
Roth, D. M. *Self-control manual for treatment of depression*. Unpublished mimeo, Michigan State University, 1980.
Roth, D., Bielski, R. Jones, M., Parker, W., & Osborn, G. A comparison of self-control therapy and combined self-control therapy and anti-depressant medication in the treatment of depression. *Behavior Therapy*, 1982, *13*, 133–144.
Rounsaville, B. J., & Chevron, E. Interpersonal psychotherapy: Clinical applications. In R. J. Rush (Ed.), *Short term psychotherapies for depression*. New York: Guilford Press, 1982.
Rush, A. J., & Beck, A. T. Behavior therapy in adults with affective disorders. In M. Hersen & A. S. Bellack (Eds.), *Behavior therapy in the psychiatric setting*. Baltimore: Williams & Wilkins, 1978.
Rush, A. J., & Watkins, J. T. Group versus individual cognitive therapy: A pilot study. *Cognitive Therapy & Research*, 1981, *5*, 95–104.
Rush, A. J., Beck, A. T., Kovacs, M., & Hollon, S. Comparative efficacy of cognitive therapy and pharmacotherapy in the treatment of depressed outpatients. *Cognitive Therapy and Research*, 1977, *1*, 17–37.
Sanchez, V. C., Lewinsohn, P. M., & Larson, D. W. Assertion training: Effectiveness in the treatment of depression. *Journal of Clinical Psychology*, 1980, *36*, 526–529.
Schmidt, M. M., & Miller, W. R. Amount of therapist contact and outcome in a multidimensional depression treatment program. *Acta Psychiatrica Scandinavica*, 1983, *67*, 319–332.
Schwab, J. J., Clemmons, R. S., Bialow, M., Duggan, V., & Davis, B. A study of somatic symptomatology of depression in medical inpatients. *Psychosomatics*, 19656, 273–277.
Seligman, M. E. P. Depression and learned helplessness. In R. J. Friedman & M. M. Katz (Eds.), *The psychology of depression: Contemporary theory and research*. New York: Wiley, 1974.
Seligman, M. E. P. *Helplessness: On depression, development, and death*. San Francisco: Freedman, 1975.
Shaffer, C. S., Shapiro, J., Sank, L. I., & Coghlan, D. J. Positive changes in depression, anxiety, and assertion following individual and group cognitive behavior therapy interventions. *Cognitive Therapy and Research*, 1981, *5*, 149–157.
Shaw, B. F. Comparison of cognitive therapy and behavior therapy in the treatment of depression. *Journal of Consulting and Clinical Psychology*, 1977, *45*, 543–551.
Shaw, B. F., & Hollon, S. *Cognitive therapy in a group format with depressed outpatients*. Unpublished mimeo, University of Western Ontario (London), 1978.
Skinner, B. F. *Science and human behavior*. New York: Free Press, 1953.
Spitzer, R. L., Endicott, J., & Robins, E. Research diagnostic criteria: Rationale and reliability. *Archives of General Psychiatry*, 1978, *35*, 773–782.
Steinmetz, J., Antonuccio, D., Bond, M., McKay, G., Brown, R., & Lewinsohn, P. M. *Instructor's manual for "Coping with Depression" course*. Unpublished mimeo, University of Oregon, 1979.
Steinmetz, J. L., Lewinsohn, P. M., & Antonuccio, D. O. Prediction of individual outcome in a group intervention for depression. *Journal of Consulting and Clinical Psychology*, 1983, *51*, 331–337.
Task Panel Reports Submitted to the President's Commission on Mental Health. Vol. IV, Appendix, 1978.
Teri, L., & Lewinsohn, P. M. *A comparison of individual and group treatments for depression*. Unpublished manuscript, University of Oregon, 1981.
Thompson, L. W., Gallagher, D., Nies, G., & Epstein, D. Evaluation of the effectiveness of professionals and nonprofessionals as instructors of Coping with Depression classes for elders. *Gerontologist*, 1983, *23*, 390–396.
Turner, R. W., Ward, M. F., & Turner, D. J. Behavioral treatment for depression: An evaluation of therapeutic components. *Journal of Clinical Psychology*, 1979, *35*, 166–175.

Turner, R. W., Wehl, C. K., Cannon, D. S., & Craig, K. A. *Individual treatment for depression in alcoholics: A comparison of behavioral, cognitive, and nonspecific therapy*. Unpublished mimeo, VA Medical Center, Salt Lake City, 1980.

Wehl, C. K., & Turner, R. W. *Group vs. individual cognitive-behavioral therapy for depressed alcoholics*. Unpublished mimeo, VA Medical Center, Salt Lake City, 1982.

Weinberg, L. Behaviorally and cognitively oriented approaches to the alleviation of depressive symptoms in college students. *Dissertation Abstracts International*, 1978, *38*, 3422B.

Weissman, M. M. The psychological treatment of depression: Evidence for the efficacy of psychotherapy alone, in comparison with and in combination with pharmacotherapy. *Archives of General Psychiatry*, 1979, *36*, 1261–1269.

Weissman, M. M. The psychological treatment of depression: An update of clinical trials. In R. L. Spitzer & J. B. W. Williams (Eds.), *Psychotherapy research: Where we are and where we should be going*. New York: Guilford Press, 1984.

Weissman, M. M., & Klerman, G. Sex differences and the epidemiology of depression. *Archives of General Psychiatry*, 1977, *34*, 98–111.

Weissman, M. M., & Paykel, E. G. *The depressed woman*. Chicago: University of Chicago Press, 1974.

Weissman, M. M., DiMascio, A., Prusoff, B., & Neu, C. *Manual for short term interpersonal psychotherapy for depression*. Unpublished mimeo, Yale/Tufts University, 1977.

Weissman, M. M., Prusoff, B. A., & Klerman, G. L. Application of life table method to naturalistic designs. A comparison of efficacy of tricyclic antidepressants and benzodifazepines in ambulatory depressives. *Comprehensive Psychiatry*, 1978, *19*, 27–36.

Weissman, M. M., Prusoff, B. A., DiMascio, A., Neu, C., Golansky, M., & Klerman, G. L. The efficacy of drugs and psychotherapy in the treatment of acute depressive episodes. *American Journal of Psychiatry*, 1979, *136*, 555–558.

Weissman, M. M., Klerman, G. L., Prusoff, B. A., Sholomskas, D., & Padin, N. Depressed outpatients one year after treatment with drugs and/or interpersonal therapy. *Archives of General Psychiatry*, 1981, *38*, 51–55.

Zeiss, A. M., Lewinsohn, P. M., & Muñoz, R. F. Nonspecific improvement effects in depression using interpersonal, cognitive, and pleasant events focused treatments. *Journal of Consulting and Clinical Psychology*, 1979, *47*, 427–439.

Zung, W. W. K. A self-rating depression scale. *Archives of General Psychiatry*, 1965, *12*, 63–70.

Zung, W. W. K. From art to science: The diagnosis and treatment of depression. *Archives of General Psychiatry*, 1973, *29*, 328–337.

Zung, W. W. K., Richards, C. B., & Short, M. J. Self-rating depression scale in an outpatient clinic. *Archives of General Psychiatry*, 1965, *13*, 508–516.

12

Behavioral Group Treatment for Addictive-Appetitive Disorders

Alcoholism, Smoking, Obesity, and Drug Abuse

BILLY A. BARRIOS, REX W. TURNER, AND STEVEN M. ROSS

Early critics of behavior therapy charged that support for the approach rested largely on studies of the innocuous, transient ailments of college students (e.g., Cooper, Furst, & Bridger, 1969). Naturally, behavior therapists did not take such a slur lying down. Attempts were made by some to logically refute the charge (Levis, 1970; Mahoney, Kazdin, & Lesswing, 1974; McGlynn, 1975) and by others to empirically prove the criticism false. This latter reaction has taken the form of expanding the range of problems and client groups that are amenable to behavioral techniques, among the most aggressively tackled of which have been the addictive and appetitive disorders of alcoholism, smoking, obesity, and drug abuse. As a result, we now have an enormous amount of information on behavior therapy's ability to alter these historically prevalent and intractable patterns. And because the bulk of those treatment outcome studies employed a group format, we also have a wealth of data that is pertinent to the practice of behavioral group therapy *per se*.

The major purpose of the present chapter is to report on the current status of behavioral group treatment for each of the four addictive-appetitive disorders—alcoholism, smoking, obesity, and drug abuse. We do so by first reviewing the relevant research, then by offering a synopsis of their findings. Our survey of the literature is for the most part exhaustive, and in those instances in which it is not, steps have been taken to ensure a healthy representative sample of the studies. The summaries that follow our reviews of the research focus primarily on three issues. One, as you might expect, is the effectiveness of behavioral group procedures. Another is the contribution that the group factor makes to treatment outcome, and the third is the identification of areas that could best profit from further scrutiny. Thus, the present chapter aspires to do

BILLY A. BARRIOS • University of Mississippi, University, Mississippi 38677. REX W. TURNER and STEVEN M. ROSS • Veterans Administration Medical Center, Salt Lake City, Utah 84148.

more than monotonously chronicle the results of one study after another, an exercise that accomplishes little except bore the reader. The present chapter attempts to make manageable and comprehensible what has heretofore been a rich but rather puzzling literature. It is puzzling in terms of what it has to say about behavioral group treatments, their efficacy, and the importance of the group variable. Clarifying those and other related questions is the work of the present chapter, work that if carried out well will also chart for us a course of future research on behavioral group therapy.

Behavioral Group Treatment of Alcoholism

It is impossible to determine the precise number of alcoholics or problem drinkers in need of treatment. Mulford (1982, p. 444) complained that "one can find an alcoholic prevalence rate for all occasions and purposes, and one to fit any of the theories and personal predilections that abound." Estimates of the size of the problem are grossly affected by choosing incidence versus prevalence rates, by the epidemiological methods of study selected, and by whether liberal or conservative assessment criteria are employed. Criteria used to diagnose or count alcoholics range from those loosely defined and tautological to some that are strictly operationalized and empirical. Because there is no empirical referent for *alcoholism,* it is best to explicitly state that the term is used here as an aid to communication.

People who drink too much and suffer severe psychological, medical, and social consequences can be identified and studied, however. Using survey methodology with explicit assessment criteria, Cahalan (1978) concluded that 15% of men and 4% of women (9% of the total representative sample) were in the "high problems" category. Early field trials with the DSM-III indicated that substance use or substance-induced disorders were second only to affective disorder in frequency of diagnosis (Spitzer, Forman, & Nee, 1979). Clearly then, alcoholism or problem drinking is an enormous public health problem, one that virtually every adult clinician will no doubt encounter and have to make decisions concerning its treatment.

Given the extreme demand for alcoholism treatment and insufficient clinical resources, group methods of intervention have obvious appeal. Although economy has been the most frequently cited reason for their employment, the emotional isolation, ineffective social interactions, and excessive dependence associated with alcoholism are perhaps more important reasons for the group approach. The material that follows reviews theoretical issues pertinent to behavioral group therapy with problem drinkers, technical and procedural variations that are available, and empirical results with behavioral group methods. We conclude with practical suggestions for future research on behavioral group therapy with alcoholics.

In his excellent book, Rose (1977) distinguishes between behavior therapy done in groups and behaviorally oriented group therapy. Most of the studies reviewed in this section fell in the first category. That is, they examined the effectiveness of a variety of behavioral techniques and procedures employed with alcoholics in a group format. Despite the popularity of behavioral group interventions among in- and outpatient alcohol treatment facilities, there have been surprisingly few well-controlled investigations of their efficacy. In this section, we review the majority of recently published studies. Where a research team has published a number of reports with highly similar subjects, methods, and results, we review a representative sample of their work.

Behavioral Interventions in the Group Modality

Olson, Ganley, Devine, and Dorsey (1981) studied the long-term effects of behavioral versus insight-oriented therapy with inpatient alcoholics. The experiment involved 150 total patients with 113 completing all components of treatment and up to 4 years of follow-up assessment. The four conditions of the experiment included (a) behavioral group therapy in the form of Cautela's (1967) covert sensitization (2 hours per week) and Bernstein and Borkovec's (1973) progressive relaxation training (2 hours per week); (b) insight-oriented group therapy in the form of Berne's (1961) transactional analysis for 3 hours per week; (c) a combined behavioral and transactional analysis condition (3 hours per week of each); and (d) a milieu control group consisting of multimodal, multidisciplinary interventions such as alcohol education, traditional group therapy, Alcoholics Anonymous meetings, recreation therapy, and the like. The three experimental conditions described in (a) through (c) also received the standard milieu therapy in addition to their specific therapies.

Outcome measures included the MMPI, the Fort Logan Drinking Questionnaire and the Drinking Assessment Battery. The complex outcome measures were administered at pre- and posttreatment intervals as well as at five follow-up periods from 6 months to 1 year in length. The follow-up assessments relied heavily on self-report, supported by a sample-reliability check on collaterals named by the subjects. Agreement between subjects and collaterals was very high at posttest, .94 overall. Follow-up interviews were conducted via telephone by two researchers with 95% agreement on reliability probes. With respect to abstinence figures, there was a clear but nonsignificant trend in favor of the behavioral group followed by the combined behavioral and insight-oriented group. The authors also noted a clear trend for the insight treatment to fare the worst for all evaluation periods. All four groups reduced their absolute quantity of alcohol consumption; again, the combined and behaviorally treated groups fared best. The advantage for the behavioral group treatment endured through $1\frac{1}{2}$ years of follow-up, then washed out. The authors cautioned that several measures of outcome failed to reveal differences between any of the groups and that the amounts of experimental treatments administered were small (3 to 6 hours per week).

Intagliata (1978) evaluated a behavioral group intervention designed to improve interpersonal problem-solving skills and general social competence in alcoholics. Subjects were 64 male inpatients at a Veterans Administration Medical Center. The standard alcoholism treatment program was of 6 months duration. The 64 subjects were assigned to either (a) standard inpatient (control) treatment; or (b) to the standard program with the addition of 10 sessions of interpersonal problem-solving group therapy. Measures of outcome included the Means–Ends Problem-Solving (MEPS) Procedure and assessment of social competence and coping skills in a structured discharge interview. The behavioral problem-solving group showed significantly greater improvement on the MEPS than did controls at the conclusion of treatment. The structured discharge interview also showed that the experimental group improved in general social competence and in the quality of their planning for coping with postdischarge problems. At 1-month follow-up, the majority of these subjects had retained the targeted problem-solving skills and reported successful application of these new coping behaviors outside the hospital environment.

A well-done direct comparison of the efficacy of group versus individual social skills training (SST) was reported by Oei and Jackson (1980). The two SST conditions were compared with group or individual traditional supportive therapy (TST) conditions. The 32 hospitalized "chronic alcoholics" (mean age 33.5 years, 75% male) were matched on age, number of prior admissions for treatment, mean daily alcohol consumption, and scores on an assertiveness/social skills inventory. Measures of outcome in this study included a blind behavioral interview to measure social skills (later rated on 11 dimensions of skill), an alcohol intake inventory to measure consumption, Albert and Emmons's Behavioral Assertion Scale, Watson and Friends's Social Interaction Scale, and nurses' behavioral-observation ratings. Reliability coefficients were acceptable, .80 and .85 for the behavioral interview and nurses' observations, respectively. These measures were taken pre- and posttreatment and at follow-ups of 3, 6, and 12 months. The SST subjects improved significantly more than TST controls on *all* measures at *all* posttreatment intervals. Group SST subjects scored better than individually treated SST subjects on all measures except alcohol consumption. The group SST procedures also required less time to implement. As a whole, the findings support conducting behavioral interventions (at least social skills training) in groups.

Behavioral Self-Control Training

Controlled or reduced consumption of alcohol has been an extremely controversial treatment objective (Marlatt, 1983; Polich, Armor, & Braiker, 1981). The overwhelming majority of providers in substance abuse treatment insist that abstinence is the only viable goal for problem drinkers. Still, more than 100 studies now provide empirical evidence that (a) many alcoholics return to moderate drinking after periods of obvious prior dependence; and (b) many alcoholics have successfully maintained nonproblem drinking for significant periods of time following intensive behavioral training (Heather & Robertson, 1981; Marlatt, 1983; Marlatt & Gordon, 1980; Miller & Hester, 1980). In fact, we even know some of the principal predictors of relapse from controlled to uncontrolled drinking (Polich *et al.*, 1981). Although it is not our purpose to review the literature concerning this controversy nor to presume an answer, there have been a number of studies of behavioral group methods documenting *reduction of consumption* and improvement in the general life functioning of problem drinkers.

Miller and his associates (Miller, Pechacek, & Hamburg, 1981; Miller & Taylor, 1980; Miller, Taylor, & West, 1980) have described a successful Behavioral Self-Control Training (BSCT) program. The BCST treatment has included rate-control training, self-reinforcement training, behavioral assertiveness training, progressive muscle relaxation, and communication skills training in addition to individual consultations.

In one recent representative study (Miller *et al.*, 1981), BSCT was provided to 28 alcoholics (10 were female) in 10 weekly, 90-minute sessions. Over 5 weeks of treatment, mean weekly alcohol intake decreased steadily and remained relatively stable throughout a 3-month follow-up. Zero percentage of the participants were abstinent at termination of treatment and at 3 months follow-up. However, 41 and 48% were rated as considerably improved (defined as at least 50% reduction in drinking) at these respective assessments. An additional 30 and 22% were moderately improved at termination and follow-up. Because alcohol dependence and related problems are inextricably linked with ongoing rate of consumption (Mulford, 1982), the effects of BSCT treatment on consumption with this brief intervention format were encouraging.

In another study, Millet *et al.* (1980) compared BSCT with broad spectrum behavior therapy for problem drinkers. Broad spectrum behavior therapy for alcoholism has been ambitious in purpose, targeting multiple modalities of the drinking response (cf. Lazarus, 1976). BSCT, by contrast, has been described as brief and highly focused on consumption behavior. BSCT administered largely through groups was shown to be equally effective in reducing alcohol intake as the more elaborate broad spectrum approach.

Social Skills/Assertiveness Training Groups

Many researchers have viewed social skills deficits and lack of assertiveness as important links in the etiology and maintenance of problem drinking (Chaney, O'Leary, & Marlatt, 1978; Miller & Mastria, 1977; Miller 1978). Behavioral group therapists have frequently evaluated the effects of correcting these skills deficits on subsequent drinking and psychosocial adjustment.

For example, Ferrell and Galassi (1981) divided 22 chronic alcoholics into 11 pairs matched by age, race, sex, and education. Then, in addition to the standard milieu therapy on the unit, they assigned one member of the matched pair to a behavioral assertiveness training group, the other to a human relations training group. The assertiveness training group ran for 10 consecutive days for 2 hours each day and included modeling, behavioral rehearsal with feedback, practice in "say no" technology, and bibliotherapy. The human relations group focused on verbal and nonverbal exercises designed to improve self-awareness and general communication skills. Posttreatment evaluations occurred 1 day, 6 weeks, and 2 years after the training groups were terminated. Overall abstinence rates at 6 weeks were 73%. The assertiveness training group resulted in greater short-term gains in interpersonal skills. At long-term follow-up, the human relations training group showed a small advantage in interpersonal functioning. This study suffered from small sample size, lack of appropriate control groups, and weak follow-up evaluation procedures.

Oei and Jackson (1982) later compared a social skills package with a cognitive restructuring package administered in group format. The study employed four conditions: (a) social skills training (SST) alone; (b) cognitive restructuring (CR) alone; (c) cognitive restructuring in combination with social skills training (CR-SST); and (d) a traditional supportive therapy (TST) control. The cognitive restructuring group involved didactic presentation of content, use of "rational persuasion," modification of irrational beliefs, and guided practice with Meichenbaum's self-talk procedures. All therapeutic conditions were delivered via 12 two-hour group sessions distributed over 3 weeks of treatment. The SST and CR-SST groups produced significantly greater behavior change than the CR group. As expected, the TST control group showed the least change. At long-term (12-month) follow-up, the trend was reversed with respect to behavioral performance measures (e.g., ability to cope with criticism, nurses' behavior ratings). At 12 months posttreatment, the cognitive restructuring participants also showed the greatest reduction in alcohol consumption. It would appear from these results that social skills training produces the greatest immediate benefit, whereas cognitive restructuring groups may have greater long-term impact. The authors interpreted these findings as support for a multimodal social learning model for the treatment of alcohol dependence.

Relapse Prevention Skills

Another skills acquisition approach to treating problem drinking has been described by Marlatt and associates (Cummings, Gordon, & Marlatt, 1980; Marlatt, 1979, 1983; Marlatt & Gordon, 1980). This relapse prevention model has focused on the identification of life stressors and high-risk situations that threaten abstinence or nonproblem drinking for alcoholics. Relapse risk situations include frustration and anger, social pressure to drink, negative emotional states (e.g., depression), positive emotional states (e.g., celebrations), interpersonal conflict, and others (Marlatt, 1979). The treatment goal of this model is prevention of problem drinking by (a) teaching alcoholics specific cognitive and behavioral skills instrumental in successful coping with high-risk situations and (b) correcting more global "life-style imbalances" (e.g., replacing oppressive *shoulds* with *wants*).

Chaney *et al.* (1978) evaluated a short-term group intervention based on this model. Forty alcoholics were assigned to either (a) a relapse-prevention skills training group; (b) a discussion group; or (c) a no-additional-treatment group. As in other studies in clinical settings, all subjects received standard inpatient treatment while participating in the experimental conditions. The skills training group employed modeling, role playing, and coaching to impart problem-solving skills. Participants learned to identify problems, generate alternatives, and evaluate solutions. They rehearsed desirable coping behaviors in group. Assessment of intervention effects occurred pre- and posttreatment, and at 1, 3, 6, and 12-month follow-ups. Assessment included situational competency tests conducted in follow-up interviews, self-reports of job performance, and records of participation in outpatient (aftercare) treatment. The results indicated that group instruction and rehearsal in relapse prevention skills improved problem-solving behaviors and reduced drinking behavior, as the skills training group showed significant superiority to control groups on these measures. They did not, however, differ on job performance and outpatient participation rates. Thus, the benefits of skills training were specific to problem-solving and drinking behaviors.

Behavioral Group Therapy for Couples/Families

Kaufman and Pattison (1981) have outlined the development of differential treatment modalities for alcoholism with special reference to family and couples therapy. They noted an unfortunate lack of empirical outcome research with these techniques despite the recognition that alcohol abuse has an extremely destructive effect on marital and family relationships. They attribute the paucity of research to (a) negative stereotyped views toward work with alcoholic families; and (b) insufficient awareness and training on the part of mental health professionals regarding marital/family (group) therapy techniques that can be adapted for use with alcoholics. There are virtually no controlled, published studies of behavioral group techniques with alcoholic couples or families. This is quite surprising considering that many broad-spectrum programs have been employing couples therapy groups and family therapy as routine components of treatment programs for over 20 years (Cadogen, 1979: Kaufman & Pattison, 1981).

Steinglass (1979) described an experimental treatment for alcoholic couples combining a number of behavioral and "system" concepts. The program involved conjoint hospitalization, "controlled intoxication," and a multiple-couples group therapy. The study entailed (a) the creation of a simulated environment with direct behavioral observation of the interaction of married alcoholic couples under conditions of intoxication and sobriety; and (b) the creation of an experimental program for evaluating the effectiveness of multiple-couples group therapy. The program involved three treatment phases: (a) 2 weeks outpatient treatment; (b) 10 days of inpatient treatment; and (c) an additional 3-week outpatient phase. All couples participating in the study were provided with a two-room suite and a large common room space with cooking facilities, television, and other comforts of home. The common room space was equipped with videotape cameras and monitors, permitting recording and playback of ongoing interaction and multiple-couples group therapy sessions. Free alcohol intake was limited to the first 7 days of hospitalization with careful monitoring of any behavioral or medical sequelae. Multiple-couples group sessions occurred daily for 90 minutes during hospitalization. Two psychiatrists, one working with a cotherapist, served as therapists for group sessions that included the following procedures: (a) interpretation of patterns of interactional behavior; (b) the use of videotape recording and feedback; (c) role playing; (d) one-way mirror observation with feedback from observers; (e) analysis of speech and communication patterns; and (f) modification of nonverbal behavior.

Steinglass measured changes in individual and marital behavior with an interviewer-administered questionnaire called the Chronological Drinking Record (assessing the type of beverage, amount consumed, times of day, interval since last drink, etc.), the SCL-90, the Structured and Scaled Interview to Assess Maladjustment, the Inventory of Marital Conflicts, and the Subject Is Marriage (a 43-item instrument assessing marital change during therapy across eight behavioral areas). Ten couples completed the therapy program, but only 8 (9 identified alcoholics total) were available at the 6-month follow-up evaluation. Five of the 9 alcoholics were drinking less at the follow-up, 1 had doubled alcohol intake from baseline to follow-up. Changes in nine areas of psychiatric symptomatology measured by the SCL-90 were inconsistent, and interpretation was confounded by therapist-related differences. Changes in interactive behaviors (e.g., conflict negotiation), communication patterns, and marital satisfaction were also inconsistent, lacking in uniform direction.

Variability within and across behavioral and self-report measures and absence of a control/comparison group obscured meaningful interpretation of Steinglass's (1979) results. The author did draw three principal conclusions from the study: (a) the systems or family-level model of alcoholism was supported by the observational and self-report data; (b) interactional behavior is an important target of therapeutic change; and (c) the feasibility and usefulness of directly observing intoxicated behavior in treatment were supported. Steinglass recommended "continued experimentation with the controlled and circumscribed use of alcohol as an adjunct to family-oriented therapy for alcoholism" (p. 180).

Behavioral Group Approaches

Earlier, a reference was made to Rose's (1977) distinction between behavior therapy conducted in group versus behavioral group therapy. We will now focus on progress with behavioral group therapies for alcohol problems.

One method of providing behavioral group therapy in inpatient settings consists of viewing the entire treatment unit, patients and staff, as one group. This conceptualization historically has been referred to as the *therapeutic community* (Jones, 1953). With the rise of behavioral methods in the 1960s, a form of therapeutic community with behavioral emphasis on assessment and data-based interventions became known as the *token economy* (Ayllon & Azrin, 1968). A community-reinforcement system for treating alcoholics was recently described by Hunt and Azrin (1973). Behavioral group therapy on a grand scale or molar level of programming and analysis, this community-reinforcement procedure was based on social learning theory. The intent of the program was (a) to rearrange reinforcers and punishers in the environment to encourage more adaptive, efficient behaviors; (b) to provide sources of reward that would successfully compete with urges to drink alcohol; (c) to encourage community support and generalization of adaptive behavior to the home, job, and community settings; and (d) to prevent or inhibit impulsive drinking through the use of disulfiram (Antabuse[R]).

Hunt and Azrin (1973) used a matched-control design to compare the efficacy of their community-reinforcement program with a more traditional inpatient rehabilitation control group. The community-reinforcement program consisted of behaviorally oriented job-placement methods, marital and family counseling with increases in pleasurable activities, a self-governing social club, disulfiram, and "primed" participation in hobbies and recreational activities. All of these behavioral interventions were designed to compete with drinking behavior. The matched control patients received identical housing and other hospital services. They also participated in alcohol education classes, individual and traditional group psychotherapy, disulfiram, and Alcoholics Anonymous groups. The results of the comparison of programs were impressive. Community-reinforcement subjects spent one-sixth as much time drinking, one-twelfth as much time unemployed, one-half as much time away from home, and one-fifteenth as much time institutionalized compared to traditional treatment controls. According to the authors, these results were evident at a 6-month follow-up as well.

Azrin also (1976) reported on a modification of the earlier program. The improvements consisted of (a) special counseling to increase motivation and compliance with disulfiram prescriptions; (b) development of an early warning system whereby the patient alerts his or her counselor to crises and/or urges to drink; (c) use of a neighborhood advisor to provide practical, life-management assistance as the relationship with the program counselor is faded; and (d) use of the *group* instead of the individual modality for providing counseling. With these improvements over the 1974 model, the modified community reinforcement program further enhanced treatment outcomes by a substantial margin, 2% versus 14% time drinking (55% for controls). Staff time invested in each client dropped from a mean of 50 hours to a mean of 30 hours through the use of group counseling modalities. Azrin claimed that these positive clinical outcomes were stable and maintained over a 2-year follow-up period.

The success rates of these two reports far exceed those typically reported in the alcohol treatment literature (Emrick & Hansen, 1983; Polich *et al.*, 1981). This may reflect the superiority of behavioral community-reinforcement procedures or problems with methodology and interpretation of results. A number of critics (Emrick & Hansen, 1983; Moos & Finney, 1983; Nathan & Lansky, 1978) of the alcohol treatment literature have urged very careful examination of methods and outcome criteria employed by researchers. If community-reinforcement procedures and results described in the studies previously mentioned withstand this cautious scrutiny, they appear to represent an extremely effective behavioral group treatment package for alcohol problems. Because the 1976 study constitutes a *replication* of earlier findings, these methods deserve the attention, perhaps enthusiastic reception, of professionals in the field.

Summary and Recommendations

Although behavioral group treatments such as social skills training have become something of a fixture in most alcohol rehabilitation programs, our review of the literature found very few well-controlled evaluations of their efficacy. Our review also turned up few studies that looked at the group variable *per se* and its contribution to treatment outcome. Those data that are available and that were capsulized in the preceding pages are rather favorable toward the behavioral approach. In general, the evidence points to all variants of behavioral group therapy—group-administered techniques, self-control training, skills training, relapse prevention, couples therapy, community systems—as having promise for reducing alcohol abuse and associated problems. Comparisons with individualized training in social skills, assertiveness, and problem solving add to this promise as they show the group format to be as effective and in some cases superior (Adinolfi, McCourt, & Geoghegan, 1976; Intagliata, 1978; Oei & Jackson, 1980).

Of the interventions reviewed, virtually all can be placed under the umbrella of either the *self-control* or *relapse prevention* model. Behavioral self-control has as its goals reduced consumption and increased personal mastery of and responsibility for drinking (Miller *et al.*, 1981; Miller *et al.*, 1980; Miller & Taylor, 1980). The focus is on arresting current drinking behavior. The relapse prevention model on the other hand emphasizes the adaptive management of future life events (Marlatt, 1979, 1983; Marlatt & Gordon, 1980). It appears then that the relapse prevention approach is concerned more with the correction of so-called "global life-style imbalances." Combining these two minimodels of behavior therapy may have synergistic effects that may lead to more efficacious and enduring treatment of alcohol abuse. Both strategies have been implemented in time- and cost-efficient group modalities; both are data-based interventions; both can accommodate the inclusion of exciting cognitive modification techniques (e.g., McCourt & Glantz, 1980; Turner, Wehl, Cannon, & Craig, 1980; Turner, Wehl, & Moreno, 1983; Wehl, Turner, Cannon & Craig, 1982); and both avoid the paradox inherent in the disease model (e.g., "you are *not responsible* for your disease of alcoholism. Your only hope for cure is to *choose* abstinence). A union of these two models may provide us with a powerful behavioral technology for dealing with alcohol abuse. Given what we know about the disorder, its complexity, and range of impairments, this strikes us as a sensible course of action to pursue. It is also one that warrants critical empirical scrutiny.

Apart from the specific change procedures embodied in behavioral group treatments, there is a tremendous need for further research on their optimum implementation. What effect does incorporating spouses and family members have on treatment outcome? Do booster sessions foster maintenance of therapeutic gains? Does group composition influence attrition rates, which in turn influence the likelihood of positive change? These are but a few of the pressing questions surrounding the mechanics of behavioral group treatment, ones that will probably have complicated answers (e.g., Ahles, Schlundt, Prue, & Rychtarik, 1983). They are, however, questions that if assiduously pursued may lead to marked refinements and advancements in the behavioral group treatment of alcohol abuse.

Behavioral Group Treatment of Smoking

High-rate smoking has been implicated as a major contributor to the development of a host of physical maladies, among which are chronic bronchitis, emphysema, cardiovascular disease, and cancer of the lung and bladder (Surgeon General's Advisory Committee, 1964; United States Public Health Service, 1971, 1973, 1974). In addition to the major health hazards posed, smoking has been found to disrupt social interactions as well as harm the physical well-being of those present in the smoker's immediate environment (Epstein & McCoy, 1975). Previous reviews of behavioral approaches to the treatment of smoking have noted their effectiveness in producing immediate appreciable changes in smoking behavior (e.g., Bernstein, 1969; Bernstein & McAlister, 1976; Hunt & Bespalec, 1974; Hunt & Matarazzo, 1970; Keutzer, Lichtenstein, & Mees, 1968; Lichtenstein & Danaher, 1976). They have also reported disappointing follow-up and maintenance data for these interventions. In the present section, we examine the current status of a subset of these behavioral treatments, specifically those that utilize a group format in their administration. An appraisal of their accomplishments and limitations is offered, along with recommendations for future research. Despite extreme variability in the particulars of the treatments examined, virtually all fell easily into one of the following four categories: self-control, self-monitoring, aversion, and ancillary procedures. The literature on each is reviewed, followed by a critique of behavioral group therapies as a whole. Given the preponderance of professional journals and the salience of smoking as a target behavior, it was necessary to restrict our sample to the outcome investigations appearing in major clinical psychology and psychiatry periodicals through 1982. This somewhat selective search resulted in some studies being excluded from our review. Because, however, the evaluations and conclusions we advance were derived from the general pattern of findings rather than any single study, it is unlikely that our appraisals would be substantially affected by those investigations that were omitted.

Self-Control

Overview of the Findings

The term *self-control* is applied to the various interventions that employ stimulus, cognitive, and affective control techniques to decrease smoking. A uniform self-control program does not exist, but rather a host of interventions differing in the degree to which they draw upon each domain of techniques. They are united, however, in their intent to equip clients with an arsenal of strategies that may minimize the probability of smoking. Thus, any given self-control package may consist of some combination of the following elements:

self-monitoring, stimulus narrowing, response substitution, goal setting, contracting, self-instructions, self-reinforcement, self-punishment, cognitive restructuring, relaxation, systematic desensitization, behavioral rehearsal, covert sensitization, rapid smoking, and sundry other techniques.

A summary of the 22 studies on self-control procedures for the reduction of smoking is presented in Table 1. In general, self-control packages have been found to be superior to no-treatment or wait-list controls across an array of dependent measures (e.g., number of cigarettes per day, percentage of baseline rate, abstinence, attitudes toward smoking), a superiority that has been shown to endure anywhere from 30 days to 6 months. Comparisons with attention-placebo conditions, however, have been less favorable. The four investigations that have pitted a self-control procedure against one controlling for nonspecific factors have yielded mixed findings. In some instances, self-control packages have proven to be more efficacious, in others equivalent. But in no case did the attention placebo surpass the self-control treatment.

A similar picture emerged with respect to the relative effectiveness of self-control procedures and alternative interventions. Although self-control packages have bested negative practice, rapid smoking, self-monitoring, and self-monitoring plus social reinforcement, parity with focused smoking, electrical aversion, transactional analysis, habit reversal, stimulus control, and the American Cancer Society program has been reported. How reliable are the outcomes from these isolated comparative tests is a matter of conjecture, as is the extent to which the findings generalize from one variant of self-control treatment to another.

Ten of the investigations sought to pinpoint variables critical to the short- and long-term effectiveness of self-control programs. Although the simple tacking on of technique onto technique and the inclusion of a maintenance component did not consistently lead to better outcomes, manipulations in the treatment feature of goal setting did. For example, the self-management program of Edinger, Nelson, Davidson, and Wallace (1978) was most successful when the client variable of locus of control was appropriately paired with cient or therapist responsibility for goal setting. Internally controlled subjects achieved greater reductions in smoking when they established their own treatment goals, whereas the externally controlled performed better under the auspices of the therapist's goal setting. The immediacy with which treatment goals were expected to come to pass was also found to be influential, with subjects permitted to delay smoking cessation evidencing greater reductions than those instructed to terminate immediately (Flaxman, 1978). The variable of therapist contact surfaced as another possible moderator of outcome. Although there were exceptions, in general the more intensive the therapist contact the greater the benefits accrued.

Self-Monitoring

Overview of the Findings

Self-monitoring, that is, the process of detecting and recording the occurrence of a specified behavior (Nelson, 1977), is an element of nearly all of the

TABLE 1. Summary of Studies Examining Effectiveness of Behavioral Group Therapy for Smoking: Self-Control Procedures

Author(s)	No., sex, & age of subjects	Group size	Conditions compared	Dependent measures	Results
Bornstein, Carmody, Relinger, Zohn, Devine, & Bugge (1977)	$N = 10$ 8F, 2 M Age range 31–53	$n = 10$	Self-control	% baseline rate	Post: Significant reduction Follow-up (1 yr): Significant reduction
				# cigarettes/day	Post: Significant reduction Follow-up (1 yr): Significant reduction
Brockway, Kleinmann, Edleson, & Gruenwald (1977)	$N = 27$ 13F, 14 M Age range 18–50	$n = 6–7$	Self-control No treatment	# cigarettes/day	Post: Self-control superior to no treatment Follow-up (3 mo): Self-control superior to no treatment Follow-up (6 mo): Self-control superior to no treatment Follow-up (1 yr): No difference
				Blood test for "abstainers"	Follow-up (6 mo): Levels of serum thiocyanate exceeded those of nonsmokers
Delahunt & Curran (1976)	$N = 50$ 50F $\bar{X}$ age 27 News ads	$n = 9–14$	Self-control Negative practice Self-control + negative practice Nonspecific Wait list	% baseline rate	Post: All conditions superior to wait list; no difference between each other Follow-up (6 mo): All conditions superior to wait list; self-control + negative practice superior to self-control, negative practice, and nonspecific
				Abstinence	Post: No differences Follow-up (1 mo): No difference Follow-up (3 mo): No difference

(continued)

Table 1 (*Continued*)

Author(s)	No., sex, & age of subjects	Group size	Conditions compared	Dependent measures	Results
					Follow-up (6 mo): Self-control + negative practice superior to wait list
Edinger, Nelson, Davidson, & Wallace (1978) Exp 1	$N = 14$ 14M $\bar{X}$ age 23	$n = 14$	Self-control	% baseline rate	Post: Significant reduction Follow-up (13 wk): Significant reduction
Edinger, Nelson & Davidson, (1978) Exp 2	$N = 28$ 28M	$n = 14$	Self-control + goal setting by therapist + internal Self-control + goal setting by client + internal Self-control + goal setting by therapist + external Self-control + goal setting by client + external	% baseline rate	Post: Self-control + goal setting by client + internal and self-control + goal setting by therapist + external superior Follow-up (13 wk): Self-control + goal setting by client + internal & self-control + goal setting by therapist + external superior
Elliott & Denney (1978)	$N = 63$ 34F, 29M $\bar{X}$ age 29	$n = 6–9$	Self-control Rapid smoking Nonspecific treatment No treatment	% baseline rate	Post: All conditions superior to no treatment, self-control superior to rapid smoking Follow-up (3 mo): Self-control superior to rapid smoking, nonspecific, & no treatment Follow-up (6 mo): Self-control superior to rapid smoking & no treatment
				Abstinence	Post: Self-control superior to rapid smoking, nonspecific, and no treatment Follow-up (6 mo): Self-control superior to rapid smoking, nonspecific, & no treatment

				Smoking questionnaire	Post: Self-control had more negative attitudes toward smoking than rapid smoking, nonspecific & no treatment Follow-up (3 mo): Self-control had more negative attitudes toward smoking than rapid smoking, nonspecific, & no treatment Follow-up (6 mo): Self-control had more negative attitudes toward smoking than rapid smoking, nonspecific, & no treatment
Flaxman (1978)	$N = 64$ 32F, 32M	$n = 8$	Self-control + gradual reduction + aversion Self-control + partially gradual + aversion Self-control + target date + aversion Self-control + immediate termination + aversion Self-control + gradual reduction + attention Self-control + partially gradual + attention Self-control + target date + attention Self-control + immediate termination + attention	# cigarettes/day	Post: All conditions superior to self-control + immediate termination + aversion & self-control + immediate termination + attention
Hackett & Horan (1979)	$N = 30$ 11F, 19M $\bar{X}$ age 23	$n = 5$	Self-control + focused smoking Self-control Focused smoking	# cigarettes/day	Post: No differences Follow-up (1 mo): No differences Follow-up (3 mo): No differences Follow-up (6 mo): No differences
				Abstinence	Post: No differences

(*continued*)

TABLE 1 (*Continued*)

Author(s)	No., sex, & age of subjects	Group size	Conditions compared	Dependent measures	Results
					Follow-up (1 mo): No differences Follow-up (3 mo): No differences Follow-up (6 mo): No differences
Katz, Heiman, & Gordon (1977)	$N = 29$ 15F, 14M $\bar{X}$ age 40	$n = 9$–10	Cognitive self-control Habit reversal Education + will power	% baseline rate	Post: No differences Follow-up (5–15 wk): No differences
Lando (1978)	$N = 83$ 45F, 38M $\bar{X}$ age 35	$n = 7$–12	Stimulus control Self-monitoring Rapid smoking Weak aversion Contractual maintenance Social support maintenance	% baseline rate Abstinence	Post: Rapid smoking & weak aversion superior to others Follow-up (6 mo): No differences Post: Rapid smoking & weak aversion superior to others Follow-up (6 mo): No differences
Lando & McCullough (1978)	$N = 17$ $\bar{X}$ age 35	$n = 17$	Self-control	Abstinence	Post: Significant effects Follow-up (6 mo): Significant effects
Ober (1968)	$N = 60$ 19F, 41M	$n = ?$	Self-control Electric aversion Transactional analysis	# cigarettes/day	Post: No differences Follow-up (4 wk): No differences
McGrath & Hall (1976)	$N = 29$ 14F, 12M $\bar{X}$ age 24	$n = 5$	Self-control Self-monitoring + social reinforcement No treatment	# cigarettes/day	Post: Self-control & self-monitoring + social reinforcement superior to no treatment Follow-up (80 dy): Self-control superior to self-monitoring + social reinforcement & no treatment

				Smoking questionnaire	Post: No differences Follow-up (80 dy): No differences
Gutmann & Marston (1967)	$N = 76$ 38F, 38M $\bar{X}$ age 31	$n = 10–16$	Self-control Self-monitoring	# cigarettes/day	Post: No difference Follow-up (1 mo): Self-control superior to self-monitoring
Lando (1981), Lando & McGovern (1982)	$N = 100$ 55F, 45M $\bar{X}$ age 37.5	$n = 7–12$	Self-control + intensive therapist contact + abstinence as goal Self-control + minimal therapist contact + abstinence as goal Self-control + intensive therapist contact + reduction as goal Self-control + minimal therapist contact + reduction as goal Abbreviated self-control + intensive therapist contact + abstinence as goal Abbreviated self-control + minimal therapist contact + abstinence as goal Abbreviated self-control + intensive therapist contact + reduction as goal Abbreviated self-control + minimal therapist contact + reduction as goal	% baseline rate	Post: Intensive therapist contact groups superior to minimal contact Follow-up (1 mo): Abbreviated self-control + intensive therapist contact superior to abbreviated self-control + minimal therapist contact Self-control + minimal therapist contact superior to self-control superior to self-control + intensive therapist contact Follow-up (3 mo): Abbreviated self-control + intensive therapist contact superior to abbreviated self-control + minimal therapist contact Self-control + minimal therapist contact superior to self-control + intensive therapist contact Follow-up (6 mo): Abbreviated self-control + intensive therapist contact superior to abbreviated self-control + minimal therapist contact Self-control + minimal therapist contact superior to self-control + intensive therapist contact

(*continued*)

TABLE 1 (*Continued*)

Author(s)	No., sex, & age of subjects	Group size	Conditions compared	Dependent measures	Results
					Follow-up (9 mo): No differences among groups
					Follow-up (1 yr): Abbreviated self-control superior to self-control
					Abbreviated self-control + intensive therapist contact superior to abbreviated self-control + minimal therapist contact
					Self-control + minimal therapist contact superior to self-control + intensive therapist contact
					Follow-up (18 mo): Abbreviated self-control + intensive therapist contact superior to all others
					Follow-up (24 mo): Abbreviated self-control + intensive therapist contact superior to all others
					Follow-up (36 mo): Abbreviated self-control + intensive therapist contact superior to all others
				Abstinence	Post: Intensive therapist contact superior to minimal therapist contact
					Follow-up (1 mo): No differences
					Follow-up (3 mo): No differences
					Follow-up (6 mo): No differences
					Follow-up (9 mo): Abbreviated

					self-control + intensive therapist contact superior to all others Follow-up (12 mo): Abbreviated self-control + intensive therapist contact superior to all others Follow-up (18 mo): Abbreviated self-control + intensive therapist contact superior to all others Follow-up (24 mo): Abbreviated self-control + intensive therapist contact superior to all others Follow-up (36 mo): Abbreviated self-control + intensive therapist contact superior to all others
Colletti & Stern (1980)	Follow-up of 40; Colletti & Kopel (1979); *Ss* plus 32 new *Ss*	n = ?	Self-control + maintenance of self-monitoring Self-control + maintenance of modeling Self-control + maintenance of participant observing	% baseline rate	Follow-up (2 yr): Self-control + maintenance of self-monitoring superior to others
Colletti & Supnick (1980)	N = 29 16F, 13M $\bar{X}$ age 41	n = 5–10	Self-control Self-control + maintenance	% baseline rate	Post: No difference Follow-up (6 mo): Self-control + maintenance superior to self-control Follow-up (1 yr): No difference

(*continued*)

TABLE 1 (*Continued*)

Author(s)	No., sex, & age of subjects	Group size	Conditions compared	Dependent measures	Results
Glasgow, Schafer, & O'Neill (1981)	$N = 88$ 48F, 40M $\bar{X}$ age 37.3	$n = 4–6$	Self-control, Danaher & Lichenstein (1978) manual + self-administered Self-control, Danaher & Lichenstein (1978) manual + therapist administered Self-control, Pomerleau & Pomerleau (1977) manual + self-administered	Abstinence (self-report)	Post: For self-control groups, therapist administered superior to self-administered For minimal treatment, self-administered superior to therapist-administered Follow-up (6 mo): For self-control groups, therapist administered superior to self-administered For minimal treatment, self-administered superior to therapist administered
			Self-control, Pomerleau & Pomerleau (1977) manual + therapist administered Minimal treatment + self-administered Minimal treatment + therapist administered	Abstinence (CO level)	Post: For self-control groups, therapist administered superior to self-administered For minimal treatment, self-administered superior to therapist administered Follow-up (6 mo): Therapist administered superior to self-administered
				# cigarettes smoked (self-report)	Post: No differences Follow-up (6 mo): For self-control groups, therapist administered superior to self-administered For minimal treatment, self-administered superior to therapist administered
				Daily dosage (self-report)	Post: No differences Follow-up (6 mo): No difference
				Daily dosage	Post: No differences

				(CO level)	Follow-up (6 mo): No difference
				Cost & effectiveness	Post: For minimal treatment, self-administered superior to therapist administered Follow-up (6 mo): For minimal treatment, self-administered superior to therapist administered
Paxton (1980)	$N = 60$ 38F, 22M $\bar{X}$ age 40.28	$n = ?$	Self-control Self-control + contract for abstinence	Abstinence	Post: No difference Follow-up (6 mo): No difference
Shipley (1981)	$N = 43$ 22F, 21M $\bar{X}$ age 38	$n = ?$	Self-control Self-control + maintenance letters	Abstinence	Follow-up (3 mo): No difference Follow-up (6 mo): No difference
				% baseline rate	Follow-up (3 mo): No difference Follow-up (6 mo): No difference
Lowe, Green, Kurtz, Ashenberg, & Fisher (1980), Study II	$N = 42$?F, ?M $\bar{X}$ age 40.4	$n = ?$	Self-control Stimulus control Self-control + stimulus control	% baseline rate	Post: No differences Follow-up (3 mo): No difference Follow-up (6 mo): No difference
				Abstinence	Post: No differences Follow-up (3 mo): No difference Follow-up (6 mo): No difference
				% baseline rate + # days abstinent	Follow-up (6 mo): Self-control superior to stimulus control and self-control + stimulus control Stimulus control superior to self-control + stimulus control
Jeffery, Danaher, Killen, Farquhar, & Kinnier (1982)	$N = 40$ 24F, 16M $\bar{X}$ age 46.5	$n = 11$	Self-control Self-control, self-administered Self-control, self-administered + contract Self-control, self-administered + contract + phone contact	% baseline rate	Post: No differences
				Abstinence	Post: No differences
				CO level	Post: No differences

TABLE 2. Summary of Studies Examining Effectiveness of Behavioral Group Therapy for Smoking: Self-Monitoring

Author(s)	No., age, & sex of subjects	Group size	Conditions compared	Dependent measures	Results
Abrams & Wilson (1979)	$N = 40$ Age range 20–55	$n = 5$	Self-monitor cigarettes + health info Self-monitor cigarettes Self-monitor nicotine + health info Self-monitor nicotine	% baseline rate Health questionnaire	Post: Self-monitor nicotine + health info superior to self-monitor cigarettes + health info & self-monitor cigarettes Post: Self-monitor cigarettes + health info and self-monitor nicotine + health info superior to self-monitor cigarettes and self-monitor nicotine
Israel, Raskin, & Peavder (1979)	$N = 18$ Student volunteers	$n = 2$	Self-monitor + feedback Control	# smoking behaviors	Post: Self-monitor + feedback superior to control
Kantorowitz, Walters, & Pezdek (1978)	$N = 27$ $\bar{X}$ age 36	$n = 9$	Self-control + positive self-monitoring Self-control + negative self-monitoring No treatment	# cigarettes/day Abstinence	Post: Self-control + positive self-monitoring and self-control + negative self-monitoring superior to no treatment Follow-up (?): No differences Post: Self-control + positive self-monitoring & self-control + negative self-monitoring superior to no treatment Follow-up (?): Self-control + positive self-monitoring & self-control + negative self-monitoring superior to no treatment
Karoly & Doyle (1975)	$N = 56$	$n = 14$	Self-monitor cigarettes + high expectancy Self-monitor cigarettes + low expectancy Self-monitor urges + high	# cigarettes/day	Post: Self-monitor cigarettes + high expectancy & self-monitor urges + high expectancy superior to self-monitor cigarettes + low expectancy & self-monitor

			expectancy Self-monitor urges + low expectancy		urges + low expectancy Follow-up (2 wk): Self-monitor cigarettes + high expectancy & self-monitor urges + high expectancy superior to self-monitor cigarettes + low expectancy & self-monitor urges + low expectancy
McFall & Hammen (1971)	$N = 36$ 18F, 18M	$n = 9$	Self-monitor cigarettes + cold turkey Self-monitor cigarettes, unresisted urges + cold turkey Self-monitor cigarettes, resisted urges + cold turkey Self-monitor cigarettes, resisted urges + required # resisted urges	# cigarettes/day	Post: No differences Follow-up (3 wk): No differences Follow-up (6 mo): No differences
				Abstinence	Post: Self-monitor cigarettes, unresisted urges + cold turkey & self-monitor cigarettes, resisted urges + required # resisted urges superior to self-monitor cigarettes + cold turkey & self-monitor cigarettes, resisted urges + cold turkey Follow-up (3 wk): Self-monitor cigarettes, unresisted urges + cold turkey & self-monitor cigarettes, resisted urges + required # resisted urges superior to self-monitor cigarettes, resisted urges + cold turkey Follow-up (6 mo): Self-monitor cigarettes, unresisted urges + cold turkey & self-monitor cigarettes, resisted urges + required # resisted urges superior to self-monitor cigarettes + cold turkey & self-monitor cigarettes, resisted urges + cold turkey

interventions reviewed in this section. It has, however, been considered a treatment in its own right and as such has been examined in isolation. A summary of the studies that have tested the utility of self-monitoring is reported in Table 2. Some of these investigations also appear in other tables as their findings were relevant to an appraisal of alternative behavioral change strategies.

Among the studies reviewed not one provided for an unambiguous comparison between self-monitoring and no treatment. In the two studies that did include a no-treatment control (Kantorowitz, Walters, & Pezdek, 1978; McGrath & Hall, 1976), a self-control or self-reinforcement procedure was administered in conjunction with recording, thus precluding an evaluation of the effects of self-monitoring *per se*. This problem of multiple strategies notwithstanding, the findings do not consistently point to superiority over no treatment. The situation is much the same for comparisons with an attention placebo. Although a more pristine form of self-monitoring was tried, the picture remains unclear, for in one case the procedure eclipsed an attention placebo (Israel & Saccone, 1979), but in another the two were indistinguishable (Foxx & Brown, 1979). It is clear, however, that self-monitoring in isolation is not the treatment of choice for smoking. In contests with alternative interventions such as nicotine fading (Foxx & Brown, 1979) and self-management (McGrath & Hall, 1976), self-monitoring has not fared well. Thus across the three types of comparisons—no treatment, attention placebo, alternative intervention—support for self-monitoring is meager if not nonexistent.

The bulk of the research on self-monitoring has been concerned with the impact that type of behavior targeted and instructions delivered have on the procedure's therapeutic effectiveness. Few conclusions, however, can be offered. For although it has been demonstrated that it is irrelevant whether number of cigarettes, urges, resisted urges, or unresisted urges is monitored, it has also been shown that recording of nicotine consumption or number of cigarettes plus urges resisted leads to greater improvement.

Aversive Procedures

Overview of the Findings

Subsumed under the rubric of aversive procedures are five treatments: satiation, rapid smoking, electric aversion, taste aversion, and covert sensitization. A summary of the research on their efficacy is provided in Table 3. An inspection of the table reveals that none of the procedures can claim an advantage over no treatment, an attention placebo, optional therapies, or even one another. In many of these studies differences that were present at posttest disappeared by follow-up. This parity with no treatment and all possible comers is highly discrepant with the literature on individually administered aversive procedures, a discrepancy that may be a red flag for anyone wishing to simply apply these treatments on a group scale.

Much of the research focused on the impact that variations in goal setting, the noxious stimulus, and adjunctive aids have on the effectiveness of aversive

TABLE 3. Summary of Studies Examining Effectiveness of Behavioral Group Therapy for Smoking: Aversive Procedures

Author(s)	No., sex, & age of subjects	Group size	Conditions compared	Dependent measures	Results
Best & Steffy (1975)	$N = 42$ 22F, 20M $\bar{X}$ age 37	$n = 10$	Satiation + cold turkey Satiation + client control Satiation + therapist control Therapist control Client control	% baseline rate	Post: Satiation + client control superior to client control for Ss high on internal locus of control Follow-up (2 wk): No differences Follow-up (4 wk): No differences Follow-up (6 wk): No differences
Lando (1975)	$N = 45$ 27F, 18M $\bar{X}$ age 31	$n = 5–10$	Rapid smoking Satiation Attention placebo	% baseline rate	Post: Rapid smoking & satiation superior to attention placebo Follow-up (1 mo): No differences Follow-up (2 mo): No differences Follow-up (1 yr): No differences
				Abstinence	Post: Rapid smoking & satiation superior to attention placebo Follow-up (1 yr): No differences
Relinger, Bornstein, Bugge, Carmody, & Zohn (1977)	$N = 20$ 12F, 8M	$n = 6–7$	Rapid smoking Rapid smoking + booster Rapid smoking + phone support	# cigarettes/day	Post: No differences Follow-up (3 mo): No differences
				Abstinence	Post: No differences Follow-up (3 mo): No differences
Steffy, Meichenbaum, & Best (1970)	$N = ?$ $\bar{X}$ age 22–35	$n = 6$	Electric shock + overt action verbalization Electric shock + covert action verbalization Electric shock + overt nonaction verbalization Electric shock + insight	# cigarettes/day	Post: Electric shock + covert action verbalization superior to electric shock + overt nonaction & electric shock + insight Follow-up (2 mo): Electric shock + covert action verbalization superior to all others

(continued)

TABLE 3 (*Continued*)

Author(s)	No., sex, & age of subjects	Group size	Conditions compared	Dependent measures	Results
					Follow-up (6 mo): Electric shock + covert action verbalization superior to all others
Whitman (1972)	$N = 158$ 90F, 68M $\bar{X}$ age 41	$n = ?$	Taste aversion, group meetings Taste aversion, individual Wait list	# cigarettes/day	Post: Taste aversion + meetings superior to taste aversion, individual & wait list Follow-up (1 mo): No differences Follow-up (6 mo): No differences
Levenberg & Wagner (1976)	$N = 54$ 26F, 28M $\bar{X}$ age 39	$n = 9$	Rapid smoking Desensitization Relaxation	# cigarettes/day % baseline rate	Post: Rapid smoking superior to desensitization Follow-up (4 mo): No differences
Marsone, Merksamer, & Salzberg (1970)	$N = 32$ 20F, 12M $\bar{X}$ age 36	$n = 11$	Strong satiation Weak satiation No treatment	# cigarettes/day	Post: Strong satiation & weak satiation superior to no treatment Follow-up (4 mo): No differences
				Abstinence	Post: Strong satiation & weak satiation superior to no treatment Follow-up (4 mo): Strong satiation superior to no treatment
Marston & McFall (1971)	$N = 65$ 35F, 30M $\bar{X}$ age 21	$n = 7–10$	Satiation Gradual reduction Pill control Cold turkey	# cigarettes/day	Post: No differences Follow-up (6 mo): No differences
				Smoking questionnaire	Post: No differences Follow-up (6 mo): Satiation reported more positive physical changes
Merbaum, Avimier, & Goldberg (1979)	$N = 52$ 29F, 23M	$n = 8–10$	Strong aversion Strong aversion + self-	% baseline rate	Post: All conditions superior to strong aversion + self-control

	$\bar{X}$ age 34		control Strong aversion + temptation control		Follow-up (2 mo): No differences Follow-up (6 mo): No differences
			Mild aversion	Abstinence	Post: All conditions superior to mild aversion. Strong aversion + self-control superior to strong aversion & strong aversion + temptation control Follow-up (2 mo): All conditions superior to mild aversion. Strong aversion + self-control superior to strong aversion + temptation control. Strong aversion superior to strong aversion + temptation control Follow-up (6 mo): Strong aversion & strong aversion + self-control superior to strong aversion + temptation control & weak aversion
Norton & Barske (1977)	N = 62 40F, 22M $\bar{X}$ age 39	n = 10–12	Strong rapid smoking Weak rapid smoking	% baseline rate	Post: No difference Follow-up (3 mo): Strong rapid smoking superior Follow-up (4 mo): Strong rapid smoking superior Follow-up (5 mo): No difference Follow-up (7 mo): No difference
				Abstinence	Post: No difference Follow-up (3 mo): No difference Follow-up (4 mo): No difference Follow-up (5 mo): No difference Follow-up (6 mo): No difference

(*continued*)

TABLE 3 (*Continued*)

Author(s)	No., sex, & age of subjects	Group size	Conditions compared	Dependent measures	Results
Whitman (1969)	$N = 73$ 39F, 34M $\bar{X}$ age 41	$n = 6$	Electric + taste aversion Incompatible response Info only No treatment	# cigarettes/day	Post: No differences Follow-up (1 wk): All conditions superior to no treatment Follow-up (3 mo): No differences
Wisocki & Rooney (1974)	$N = 28$ 11F, 17M	$n = 3$	Covert sensitization Thought stopping Attention placebo No contact control	# cigarettes/day	Post: Covert sensitization & thought stopping superior to attention placebo and no contact control Follow-up (4 mo): No differences
Lando (1982)	$N = 73$ 33F, 40M $\bar{X}$ age 36.1	$n = 7–13$	Satiation + stimulus control + maintenance Satiation + stimulus control Satiation + maintenance Stimulus control + maintenance Stimulus control Satiation Maintenance	% baseline rate	Post: Stimulus control superior to satiation & maintenance Satiation superior to maintenance Follow-up (1 mo): Stimulus control superior to maintenance & satiation Satiation superior to maintenance All multielement groups superior to single-element groups Follow-up (2 mo): All multielement groups superior to single element groups Follow-up (3 mo): All multielement groups superior to single element groups Follow-up (6 mo): Stimulus control superior to maintenance & satiation

					Maintenance superior to satiation All multielement groups superior to single element groups Follow-up (9 mo): Stimulus control superior to maintenance satiation Maintenance superior to satiation All multielement groups superior to single-element groups Follow-up (1 yr): No difference
				Abstinence	Post: Stimulus control & satiation superior to maintenance Follow-up (1 mo): All multielement groups superior to single-element groups Follow-up (2 mo): All multielement groups superior to single-element groups Follow-up (3 mo): All multielement groups superior to single-element groups Follow-up (6 mo): All multielement groups superior to single-element groups Follow-up (9 mo): Stimulus control superior to satiation & maintenance All multielement groups superior to single-element groups Follow-up (1 yr): No differences
Lowe, Green, Kurtz, Ashenberg, & Fisher (1980), Study I	$N = 33$ 23F, 10M $\bar{X}$ age 40.6	$n = ?$	Self-control + covert sensitization Self-control	% baseline rate	Post: No difference Follow-up (3 mo): No difference Follow-up (6 mo): No difference

(*continued*)

TABLE 3 (*Continued*)

Author(s)	No., sex, & age of subjects	Group size	Conditions compared	Dependent measures	Results
				Abstinence	Post: No difference Follow-up (3 mo): No difference Follow-up (6 mo): No difference
Poole, Sanson-Fisher, & German (1981)	N = 75 40F, 35M $\bar{X}$ age 32.2	n = 3–4	Rapid smoking Rapid smoking + relaxation Rapid smoking + relaxation + contracting Contingent rapid smoking	% baseline rate	Post: No differences Follow-up (1 mo): No differences Follow-up (2 mo): No differences Follow-up (3 mo): No differences Follow-up (6 mo): No differences Follow-up (1 yr): No differences
				Abstinence	Post: No differences Follow-up (1 mo): No differences Follow-up (2 mo): No differences Follow-up (3 mo): No differences Follow-up (6 mo): No differences Follow-up (1 yr): No differences
Raw & Russell (1980)	N = 49 29F, 20M $\bar{X}$ age 39.5	n = 4–5	Rapid smoking Cue exposure Social support	# cigarettes/day	Post: No differences Follow-up (3 mo): No differences Follow-up (6 mo): No differences Follow-up (1 yr): No differences
				% baseline rate	Post: No differences Follow-up (3 mo): No differences Follow-up (6 mo): No differences Follow-up (1 yr): No differences
				Abstinence	Post: No differences Follow-up (3 mo): No differences Follow-up (6 mo): No differences Follow-up (1 yr): No differences
				COHb level	Post: No differences Follow-up (6 mo): No differences

procedures. Here, too, very few substantive remarks can be made. Although degree of client responsibility, severity of noxious stimulation, and the tacking on of other elements such as relaxation, booster sessions, and periodic prompts proved to be inconsequential in some cases (e.g., Best & Steffy, 1975; Lando, 1982; Norton & Barske, 1977; Poole, Sanson-Fisher, & German, 1981; Relinger, Bornstein, Bugge, Carmody, & Zohn, 1977), in others they significantly enhanced the power of the procedures (e.g., Merbaum, Avimier, & Goldberg, 1979). The isolated nature of these comparisons and their sometimes contradictory findings call into question the reliability of the phenomena reported. Until replications are carried out, there is very little we can say about the effect such procedural alterations have on the potency of aversive therapies.

Ancillary Procedures

Overview of the Findings

Those group treatments not falling into any of the previously discussed categories were lumped under the heading of *ancillary procedures*. Among the interventions included in this hodgepodge are systematic desensitization, response cost, breath holding, coverant control, and gradual reduction. A summary of the research on their efficaciousness is presented in Table 4. All of the procedures, with the exception of systematic desensitization, have been contrasted with a no-treatment condition, and all have come out on top in terms of immediate benefits. Over the long run, however, this edge vanished for one of the procedures, that is, gradual reduction, and is suspect for the others given the absence of follow-up assessment. In match ups with an attention placebo, the situation becomes even more disheartening for the four interventions, as not one procedure consistently produced gains beyond those of a control for nonspecific factors.

Tests of the relative effectiveness of distinct treatments have been rare and largely overshadowed by studies concerned with bolstering the therapeutic impact of a given intervention. But those that have been carried out provide us with some insight into their differential outcomes. For example, a program of nicotine fading plus self-monitoring has been shown clearly to outdo nicotine fading alone, self-monitoring, and the smoking cessation tips from the American Cancer Society (Foxx & Brown, 1979; Foxx, Brown, & Katz, 1981), as has systematic desensitization supplemented with group meetings when placed up against self-monitoring (Pyke, Agnew, & Kopperud, 1966). On the other hand, in the sole examination of their relative strength, the treatments of coverant control, breath holding, and negative practice yielded comparable reduction (Keutzer, 1968).

Most noteworthy among the studies of factors that may augment the favorable course of treatment is the emergence of group activity as a contributing variable. Though these examinations of the group factor are few, as are analyses of therapist versus self-administered programs, they shed valuable light on the utility and mechanisms of the group approach. The two studies that looked at

TABLE 4. Summary of Studies Examining Effectiveness of Behavioral Group Therapy for Smoking: Ancillary Procedures

Author(s)	No., sex, & age of subjects	Group size	Conditions compared	Dependent measures	Results
Elliot & Tighe (1968)	$N = 25$ 2F, 23M	$n = 5–11$	Reinforced abstinence + weak response cost Reinforced abstinence + strong response cost	Abstinence	Post: No difference Follow-up (3 mo): No difference
Janis & Hoffman (1971)	$N = 30$ 16F, 14M $\bar{X}$ age 40	$n = 3$	Self-monitoring + hints + high-contact partner Self-monitoring + hints + low-contact partner Self-monitoring + hints	# cigarettes/day	Post: No differences Follow-up (6 wk): Self-monitoring hints + high-contact partner superior to others Follow-up (6 mo): Self-monitoring + hints + high contact partner superior to others Follow-up (1 yr): Self-monitoring + hints + high-contact partner superior to others
				Smoking questionnaire	Post: Self-monitoring + hints + high-contact partner superior to others
Keutzer (1968)	$N = 146$ 118F, 95M Age range 20–69	$n = ?$	Covert control Breath holding	% baseline rate	Post: All conditions superior to no treatment
			Negative practice Drug placebo No treatment	Abstinence	Post: All conditions superior to no treatment
Levinson, Shapiro, Schwartz, & Tursky (1971)	$N = 52$	$n = 4–6$	Gradual reduction + timer + group meetings Gradual reduction + counter + group	Abstinence	Follow-up (3 mo): Gradual reduction + timer + group meetings superior to all conditions. Gradual reduction + timer superior to gradual reduction +

			meetings Gradual reduction + timer Gradual reduction + counter		counter + group meetings & gradual reduction + counter
Pike, Agnew, & Kopperud (1966)	$N = 55$	$n = ?$	Desensitization + group meetings Self-monitoring	# cigarettes/day	Post: Desensitization + group meetings superior to self-monitoring
Upper & Meredith (1970)	$N = 51$	$n = 17$	Gradual reduction + timer Attention placebo No treatment	# cigarettes/day	Post: No differences Follow-up (12 wk): Gradual reduction + timer superior to attention placebo & no treatment Follow-up (1 yr): No differences
				Abstinence	Post: No differences Follow-up (12 wk): No differences Follow-up (1 yr): No differences
Winett (1973)	$N = 45$ 25F, 20M $\bar{X}$ age 37	$n = 7–16$	Response cost contract Attendance contract Response cost + maintenance contract Attendance + maintenance contract	# cigarettes/day	Post: Response cost contract & response cost + maintenance contract superior to attendance contract & attendance + maintenance contract Follow-up (1 wk): Response cost contract & response cost + maintenance contract superior to attendance contract & attendance + maintenance contract Follow-up (2 wk): Response cost contract & response cost + maintenance contract superior to attendance contract & attendance + maintenance contract

(*continued*)

TABLE 4 (*Continued*)

Author(s)	No., sex, & age of subjects	Group size	Conditions compared	Dependent measures	Results
				Abstinence	Follow-up (3 mo): Response cost contract & response cost + maintenance contract superior to attendance contract & attendance + maintenance contract Follow-up (6 mo): Response cost contract & response cost + maintenance contract superior to attendance contract & attendance + maintenance contract
Beaver, Brown, & Lichtenstein (1981)	N = 28 20F, 8M $\bar{X}$ age 30.1	n = ?	Nicotine fading with high anxious *Ss* Nicotine fading with low anxious *Ss* Nicotine fading + anxiety management training with high anxious *Ss* Nicotine fading + anxiety management training with low anxious *Ss*	% baseline rate	Post: No differences Follow-up (1 mo): No differences Follow-up (3 mo): No differences Follow-up (6 mo): All groups superior to nicotine fading + anxiety management training with high anxious *Ss*
				Nicotine intake	Post: No differences Follow-up (1 mo): No differences
				Abstinence	Follow-up (3 mo): Nicotine-fading-only groups superior to nicotine fading + anxiety management training Follow-up (6 mo): Nicotine-fading-only groups superior to nicotine fading + anxiety management training
Foxx & Brown (1979)	N = 44 29F, 15M	n = 11	Nicotine fading Self-monitoring	Abstinence	Post: Nicotine fading + self-monitoring, nicotine fading &

	$\bar{X}$ age 31	Nicotine fading + self-monitoring American Cancer Society program		American Cancer Society program superior to self-monitoring Follow-up (1 mo): Nicotine fading + self-monitoring & American Cancer Society program superior to nicotine fading & self-monitoring Nicotine fading superior to self-monitoring Follow-up (3 mo): Nicotine fading + self-monitoring superior to all conditions American Cancer Society program & nicotine fading superior to self-monitoring Follow-up (6 mo): Nicotine fading + self-monitoring superior to all conditions American Cancer Society program & nicotine fading superior to self-monitoring Follow-up (1 yr): Nicotine fading + self-monitoring superior to all conditions American Cancer Society program & nicotine fading superior to self-monitoring Follow-up (18 mo): Nicotine fading + self-monitoring superior to all conditions American Cancer Society program & nicotine fading superior to self-monitoring
			Tar & nicotine consumption	Post: Nicotine fading + self-monitoring & nicotine fading superior to others

(*continued*)

TABLE 4 (*Continued*)

Author(s)	No., sex, & age of subjects	Group size	Conditions compared	Dependent measures	Results
					Follow-up (1 mo): Nicotine fading + self-monitoring & nicotine fading superior to others
					Follow-up (3 mo): Nicotine fading + self-monitoring superior to all others
					Follow-up (6 mo): Nicotine fading + self-monitoring superior to all others
					Follow-up (1 yr): Nicotine fading + self-monitoring & self-monitoring superior to others
					Follow-up (18 mo): Nicotine fading + self-monitoring & self-monitoring superior to others
				% baseline rate	Post: Nicotine fading + self-monitoring, American Cancer Society program & nicotine fading superior to self-monitoring
					Follow-up (1 mo): Nicotine fading + self-monitoring, American Cancer Society program & nicotine fading superior to self-monitoring
					Follow-up (3 mo): Nicotine fading + self-monitoring, American Cancer Society program & nicotine fading superior to self-monitoring
					Follow-up (6 mo): Nicotine fading + self-monitoring, American Cancer Society program & nicotine fading superior to self-monitoring

					Follow-up (1 yr): Nicotine fading + self-monitoring superior to all Nicotine fading superior to American Cancer Society program & self-monitoring American Cancer Society program superior to self-monitoring Follow-up (18 mo): Nicotine fading + self-monitoring & American Cancer Society program superior to others Nicotine fading superior to self-monitoring
Foxx, Brown, & Katz (1981)	Follow-up on Foxx & Brown (1979)				
	$N = 38$	$n = 8–10$	Nicotine fading Self-monitoring Nicotine fading + self-monitoring American Cancer Society program	Abstinence	Follow-up (30 mo): Nicotine fading + self-monitoring superior to all
				Proportion smoking reduced tar/nicotine	Follow-up (30 mo): No differences
				Proportion smoking baseline or higher tar/nicotine brand	Follow-up (30 mo): All groups superior to nicotine fading
				Proportion smoking reduced tar/nicotine brand & baseline or greater # cigarettes	Follow-up (30 mo): No differences

(continued)

TABLE 4 (Continued)

Author(s)	No., sex, & age of subjects	Group size	Conditions compared	Dependent measures	Results
				Proportion smoking reduced tar/nicotine brand & reduced baseline # cigarettes	Follow-up (30 mo): No differences
				Proportion smoking baseline or higher tar/nicotine brand & baseline or greater # cigarettes	Follow-up (30 mo): No differences
				Proportion smoking baseline or higher tar/nicotine brand & reduced baseline # cigarettes	Follow-up (30 mo): No differences
				% baseline nicotine	Follow-up (30 mo): Nicotine fading + self-monitoring superior to all Nicotine fading superior to self-monitoring & American Cancer Society program Self-monitoring superior to American Cancer Society program

group contact reveal that very simple manipulations can exert considerable influence. Being paired with a fellow client with whom one attended meetings and had daily contact enhanced the effectiveness of an intervention of self-monitoring and cessation tips (Janis & Hoffman, 1971). Similarly, the tacking on of group meetings to a program of gradual reduction brought about greater reductions than a treatment void of the group component (Levinson, Shapiro, Schwartz, & Tursky, 1971).

Summary Evaluation

To date, the bulk of the research on behavioral group treatments for smoking has concentrated on multicomponent self-control packages, mainly teasing out their active ingredients and assessing the properties of sundry maintenance strategies. As such, the mass of what we know about behavioral group approaches is built upon our inquiries into these self-control procedures. As a whole, the behavioral group treatments have not reliably exceeded the effects accrued from wait-list and attention-placebo conditions. A partial exception to this general trend is the self-control strategy, which has repeatedly bested a no-treatment group but has had rather mixed success against procedures equated for nonspecific factors. The only substantive conclusion that arises from the comparative treatment studies is that self-monitoring is the least favored of all the behavioral interventions. This should come as no surprise to rank and file behavior therapists, who nowadays rarely tout and implement self-monitoring as a treatment in and of itself.

The process of collapsing across studies, integrating findings, and venturing forth an assessment of the mettle of behavioral group therapies is an arduous one. The treatments are diverse in their makeup and in their implementation by different researchers. The studies vary in their group size, choice of dependent measures, and follow-up assessment. Among the investigations reviewed, group size ranged from 2 to 17, follow-up intervals from 2 weeks to 36 months. Over a handful of different measures were employed, little of which is known of their psychometric properties and interchangeability. All of this variability in group size, measures, and assessment occasions would be welcomed if the treatments themselves had been carried out in a standardized fashion across studies. If such had been the case we would be in a position to discern whether these factors have much of a hand in the treatments' outcome. But the spotty and unsystematic nature of these investigations makes it impossible to attribute uniform or discrepant findings to fluctuations in the treatment proper, these concomitant procedural variables, or both.

Even more disconcerting than the scattered nature of the research is the inattention paid to the social context in which treatment takes place. This insensitivity is not purely accidental but is largely a function of the prevalent outlook toward the group approach, that being a convenient vehicle for reaching large numbers of clients at a considerable savings in therapists' time and resources. Whether the group format is more cost-efficient remains to be seen, as few investigations have inspected the comparability of group versus individual administration of treatment. Nor have many researchers entertained the group process as a fundamental cog or intensifier of therapeutic outcome. Such disregard on the part of clinicians who place a premium on the controlling properties of the immediate social environment is indeed mystifying. Are we to assume that the group exerts no influence, that the didacticism of the therapist is unaffected by the goings-on in the group, or that client compliance with the therapeutic regimen is unrelated to the interactions among members? We suspect not. We do, however, feel that in our zeal to expand the domain of problems to which our behavioral change principles have been applied, we have overlooked the medium of all this technology. Self-disclosure, interaction, acceptance, cohesiveness, insight, catharsis, guidance, universality, altruism, and vicarious learning are among some of the therapeutic factors posited by theoreticians and practitioners of traditional group psychotherapy, that is, group interactions instigated by the therapist, client, or other members that contribute to the client's betterment (Bloch, Crouch, & Reibstein, 1981). Although many of these notions are an anathema to behavior therapists, they are nevertheless food for thought. They are also reminders that the therapeutic setting is intended to be a learning environment and that a principal task that we as therapists shoulder is arriving at the optimal arrangements for the acquisition of new and adaptive performance patterns.

Behavioral Group Treatment in Obesity

Obesity has been tagged as one of the most prevalent health problems in the United States today, affecting from 15 to 50% of the adult population (Bray, 1976; Van Itallie, 1977). The link between obesity and a host of health complications has been well defined and publicized. Consequently enormous sums of money, energy, and research have been channeled into programs for weight reduction. Previous reviews of the treatment literature have noted both the potential and evident limits of behavioral approaches (e.g., Abramson, 1977; Bellack, 1977; Brownell, 1982; Stunkard & Mahoney, 1977; Wilson & Brownell, 1980). As was the case for smoking, each of the myriad of treatments for obesity conveniently fell into one of the following four categories: self-control, self-monitoring, aversive procedures, and ancillary procedures. The four are critiqued individually then collectively, with innovative efforts to manipulate the group aspect spotlighted.

Self-Control

Overview of the Findings

Self-control programs for the management of obesity come in many forms. They all, however, have as their core the threefold operations of cue elimination, cue suppression, and cue strengthening originally outlined by Stuart and Davis (1972). This tripartite line of attack generally entails self-monitoring caloric intake, narrowing stimulus control, altering the topography of eating, increasing activity level, and programming reinforcement. A potpourri of other techniques from relaxation (Kingsley & Wilson, 1977) to cognitive restructuring (Brownell, Heckerman, & Westlake, 1979) to assertiveness training (Carroll, Yates, & Gray, 1980) has been tacked onto this common framework giving each program some speck of distinctiveness. A summary of the 53 studies on the efficacy of these self-control regimens is presented in Table 5. Against both a no-treatment condition and an attention placebo, self-control strategies consistently came out on top. Though this edge did in some instances diminish if not altogether disappear at follow-up, for the most part it remained throughout the course of assessment. Comparisons with alternative treatments were fewer and less uniform in their support of self-control procedures. Superior to such diverse programs as social pressure (Abrahms & Allen, 1974; Wollersheim, 1970), nutrition plus exercise (Gormally & Rardin, 1981), bibliotherapy (Jeffery & Gerber, 1982), and dynamically oriented treatment (Pearce, LeBow, & Orchard, 1981), self-control procedures failed to transcend a collection of others, for example, pharmacotherapy (Penick, Filion, & Stunkard, 1971; Wilcoxon-Craighead, 1981), psychotherapy (Hall, Hall, DeBoer, & O'Kulitch, 1977), induced affect (Kelly & Curran, 1976). Because of their isolated nature though, these contests offer us only intimations as to the relative merits of self-control strategies and each member in this assortment of competing treatments.

A preponderance of the research has focused on ascertaining either the active ingredients of these elaborate self-control packages or factors that boost their overall effectiveness. Much of this work has touched upon the weight that discrete components, group composition, therapist involvement, and/or size of audience carry in the therapeutic process. With respect to the program's core elements, stimulus narrowing, self-monitoring, and behavioral contracting have all been identified as major determinants of outcome (Beneke, Paulsen, McReynolds, Lutz, & Kohrs, 1978; Carroll & Yates, 1981; Hall, Hall, Borden, & Hanson, 1974; Harris & Bruner, 1971). Whether the reinforcement dispensed is of a social or monetary nature does not appear to be of importance (Abrahms & Allen, 1974); the specific behavior being contracted for, however, does seem to be. Reinforcement contingent upon adaptive eating and prescribed exercise looks to have an advantage over a rewarding of weight loss or eating behavior *per se* (Epstein, Wing, Koeske, Ossip, & Beck, 1982; Harris & Hallbauer, 1973; Mahoney, 1974), an edge though that may be offset or reversed by the influence of other variables such as therapist contact (Coates, Jeffery, Slinkard, Killen, & Danaher, 1982). The sheer adding on of other techniques to the core package does not appreciably alter its outcome. Booster sessions, pharmacotherapy, and restrictive diets all had negligible effect on the magnitude and maintenance of benefits from self-control treatments (Ashby & Wilson, 1977; Brownell & Stunkard, 1981; Kingsley & Wilson, 1977; Wilcoxon-Craighead, Stunkard, & O'Brien, 1981; Wilson & Brownell, 1978; Wing & Epstein, 1981).

A number of investigators looked at the fruits of incorporating significant others into the treatment process. The upshot of this research has been rather disappointing, as the inclusion of family members, be they cooperative or un-

TABLE 5. Summary of Studies Examining Effectiveness of Behavioral Group Therapy for Obesity: Self-Control Procedures

Author(s)	No., sex, & age of subjects	Group size	Conditions compared	Dependent measures	Results
Abrahms & Allen (1974)	$N = 49$ 49F $\bar{X}$ age 34	$n = 6$	Self-control + social reinforcement Self-control + monetary reinforcement Social pressure + reinforcement No treatment	Lb loss	Post: Self-control + social reinforcement & self-control + monetary reinforcement superior to social pressure + reinforcement & no treatment
				Significant loss (> 7½ lb)	Post: Self-control + social reinforcement & self-control + monetary reinforcement superior to social pressure + reinforcement & no treatment Follow-up (8 wk): Self-control + social reinforcement & self-control + monetary reinforcement superior to social pressure + reinforcement & no treatment
Ashby & Wilson (1977)	$N = 75$ 75F $\bar{X}$ age 40	$n = ?$	Self-control + weak booster Self-control + strong booster Self-control + nonspecific weak booster Self-control + nonspecific strong booster Self-control	Reduction quotient	Follow-up (3 mo): No differences Follow-up (6 mo): No differences Follow-up (9 mo): No differences Follow-up (1 yr): No differences
Balch & Ross (1974)	$N = 55$ 53F, 2M $\bar{X}$ age 39	$n = 11–19$	Self-control Partial self-control No treatment	Lb loss	Post: Self-control superior to other conditions
				% body wt loss	Post: Self-control superior to other conditions

Balch & Ross (1975)	$N = 19$ 19F age ?	$n = ?$	Self-control	Lb loss	Post: Significant reductions
Beneke, Paulsen, McReynolds, Lutz, & Kohrs (1978)	$N = 41$	$n = 5–8$	Self-control Stimulus control	Lb loss	Post: Stimulus control superior Follow-up (3 mo): Stimulus control superior Follow-up (6 mo): Stimulus control superior Follow-up (9 mo): Stimulus control superior Follow-up (12 mo): No difference Follow-up (18 mo): No difference
Dilley, Balch, & Balch (1979)	$N = 37$ 34F, 3M $\bar{X}$ age 25	$n = 8–10$	Self-control + group meetings Self-control + individual meetings Bibliotherapy + therapist contact Bibliotherapy No treatment	Wt % overwt Wt loss	Post: All treatments superior to no treatment Follow-up (6 mo): No differences Post: All conditions superior to no treatment Follow-up (6 mo): No differences Post: All conditions superior to no treatment Follow-up (6 mo): No differences
Hall, Hall, Borden, & Hanson (1975)	$N = 62$ 57F, 5M $\bar{X}$ age 40	$n = 6–9$	Self-control Self-control + booster Self-control + self-monitoring No treatment	Reduction index	Post: All conditions superior to no treatment Follow-up (12 wk): Only the 3 treatments included in analyses. Self-control + self-monitoring superior to self-control
Hall, Hall, Hanson, & Borden (1974)	$N = 84$ 64F, 20M	$n = 5–7$	Self-control Self-monitoring	% wt loss	Post: Self-control & self-monitoring superior to attention

(continued)

TABLE 5 (*Continued*)

Author(s)	No., sex, & age of subjects	Group size	Conditions compared	Dependent measures	Results
			Attention placebo No treatment		placebo & no treatment Follow-up (3 mo): Self-control & self-monitoring superior to attention placebo & no treatment Follow-up (6 mo): No differences
Hall, Hall, DeBoer, & O'Kulitch (1977)	$N = 74$ 74F $\bar{X}$ age 43	$n = 5–8$	Self-control External control Self + external control Psychotherapy No treatment	Wt	Post: Self-control, external control, & self + external control superior to psychotherapy & no-treatment Follow-up (3 mo): No differences Follow-up (6 mo): No differences
Hanson, Borden, Hall, & Hall (1976)	$N = 66$ 58F, 8M $\bar{X}$ age 40	$n = 7–13$	Self-control Self-control + manual + high-therapist contact Self-control + manual + low-therapist contact Attention placebo No treatment	% wt loss	Post: Self-control, self-control + manual + high-therapist contact & self-control + manual + low-therapist contact superior to attention placebo & no treatment Follow-up (10 wk): Only four treatments included in analyses. Self-control + manual + low-therapist contact superior to attention placebo Follow-up (1 yr): Only four treatments included in analyses. No differences.
				% lb loss/ideal wt	Post: Self-control, self-control + manual + high-therapist contact & self-control + manual + low-therapist contact superior

					to attention placebo & no treatment Follow-up (10 wk): Only four treatments included in analyses. No differences Follow-up (1 yr): Only four treatments included in analyses. No differences
				Wt loss	Follow-up (10 wk): Only four treatments included in analyses Self-control + manual + low-therapist contact superior to self-control + manual + high-therapist contact & attention placebo Follow-up (1 yr): Only four treatments included in analyses. No differences
Harris & Bruner (1971), Exp 1	*N* = 32 26F, 6M Age range 18–48	*n* = 8–12	Self-control Contract Attention placebo	% wt change	Post: Self-control & contract superior to attention placebo Follow-up (10 mo): Contract superior to self-control & attention placebo
Harris & Bruner (1971), Exp 2	*N* = 18 18F	*n* = 4–6	Self-control Attention control	Lb loss Wt % wt loss	Post: No difference Post: No difference Post: No difference
Harris & Hallbauer (1973)	*N* = 46 35F, 11M Age range 14–50	*n* = 4–11	Self-controlo + contract for eating Self-control + contract for eating & exercise	Lb loss	Post: No differences Follow-up (7 mo): Self-control + contract for eating & self-control + contract for eating & ex-

(*continued*)

TABLE 5 (*Continued*)

Author(s)	No., sex, & age of subjects	Group size	Conditions compared	Dependent measures	Results
			Attention control		ercise superior to attention control Self-control + contract for eating & exercise superior to self-control + contract for eating
Jeffery & Wing (1979)	N = 36 31F, 5M Age range 19–55	n = 11–13	Self-control Self-control + therapist contact Self-control + therapist phone contact	Wt	Post: Self-control + therapist contact & self-control + therapist phone contact superior to self-control
				Caloric intake/day	Post: Self-control + therapist contact & self-control + therapist phone contact superior to self-control
				Caloric expenditure	Post: No differences
Jeffrey & Christensen (1975)	N = 43 35F, 8M $\bar{X}$ age 25	n = 19	Self-control Attention placebo No treatment	Lb loss	Post: Self-control superior to attention placebo & no treatment
Kelly & Curran (1976)	N = 40 40F	n = ?	Self-control Induced affect Info + attention Wait list	Lb loss	Post: Self-control superior to info + attention & wait list Follow-up (26 wk): Self-control superior to info + attention
				Proportion overwt loss	Post: Self-control superior to all other conditions Follow-up (26 wk): No differences
				Eating questionnaire	Post: No differences Follow-up (26 wk): No differences

Kingsley & Shapiro (1977)	$N = 40$ 24F, 16M Age range 10–11	$n = 8$–10	Self-control Self-control + mothers Self-control, mothers only No treatment	Lb loss	Post: All conditions superior to no treatment Follow-up (6 wk): No differences Follow-up (20 wk): No differences
Kingsley & Wilson (1977)	$N = 78$ 78F $\bar{X}$ age 41	$n = ?$	Self-control group Self-control group + booster sessions Self-control individual Self-control individual + booster sessions Social pressure group Social pressure group + booster sessions	Reduction quotient	Post: All conditions superior to social pressure & social pressure group + booster sessions Follow-up (2 mo): No differences Follow-up (4 mo): No differences Follow-up (6 mo): No differences Follow-up (8 mo): No differences Follow-up (10 mo): No differences Follow-up (12 mo): Self-control group & self-control group + booster sessions superior to self-control individual & self-control individual + booster sessions Follow-up (14 mo): No differences
				Lb loss	Post: All conditions superior to social pressure group & social pressure group + booster sessions Follow-up (2 mo): No differences Follow-up (4 mo): No differences Follow-up (6 mo): No differences Follow-up (8 mo): No differences Follow-up (10 mo): No differences Follow-up (12 mo): No differences Follow-up (14 mo): No differences

(*continued*)

TABLE 5 (*Continued*)

Author(s)	No., sex, & age of subjects	Group size	Conditions compared	Dependent measures	Results
Mahoney (1974)	$N = 49$ 48F, 1M Age > 18	$n = 11–14$	Self-control + self-monitoring + self-reward for wt loss Self-control + self-monitoring + self-reward for habit change Self-monitoring Wait list	Reduction quotient	Post: Self-control + self-monitoring + self-reward for habit change superior to all conditions. Self-control + self-monitoring + self-reward for wt loss superior to wait list Follow-up (1 yr): Self-control + self-monitoring + self-reward for habit change superior to all conditions (Wait list not included in analysis)
				Lb loss	Post: Self-control + self-monitoring + self-reward for habit change & self-control + self-monitoring + self-reward for wt loss superior to wait list
				% body wt loss	Post: Self-control + self-monitoring + self-reward for habit change & self-control + self-monitoring + self-reward for wt loss superior to wait list
				Eating questionnaire	Post: Self-control + self-monitoring + self-reward for habit change superior to self-control + self-monitoring + self-reward for wt loss
Murray (1976)	$N = 12$ 12F Age > 21	$n = 6$	Self-control Nonspecific control	Lb loss	Post: No difference Follow-up (3 mo): No difference Follow-up (6 mo): No difference

O'Neil, Currey, Hirsch, Riddle, Taylor, Malcolm, & Sexauer (1979)	$N = 40$ 18F, 22M $\bar{X}$ age 42	$n = 9–11$	Self-control male Self-control male + spouse	Wt	Post: No differences Follow-up (9–14 mo): No differences
			Self-control female Self-control female + spouse	Wt change from pre	Post: No differences Follow-up (9–14 mo): No differences
				% wt change from pre	Post: No differences Follow-up (9–14 mo): No differences
				Reduction index	Post: No differences Follow-up (9–14 mo): No differences
				Eating questionnaire	Post: No differences Follow-up (9–14 mo): No differences
Penick, Filion, Fox, & Stunkard (1971)	$N = 32$ 24F, 8M $\bar{X}$ age 42	$n = 7–10$	Self-control Psychotherapy + info + drug	Lb loss	Post: Self-control superior Follow-up (3 mo): No difference Follow-up (6 mo): No difference
Sonne & Janoff (1979)	$N = 24$ 24F $\bar{X}$ age 45	$n = ?$	Self-control + self-reward + internal attribution External control + external reward + external attribution	Wt	Post: No difference Follow-up (6 wk): Self-control + self-reward + internal attribution superior Follow-up (11 wk): Self-control + self-reward + internal attribution superior
Stuart (1971)	$N = 6$ 6F Age range 27–41	$n = 3$	Self-control Info control	Wt	Post: Self-control superior
Wilson & Brownell (1978)	$N = 32$ 32F	$n = 7–9$	Self-control Self-control + family member	Lb loss	Post: No differences Follow-up (3 mo): No differences Follow-up (6 mo): No differences

(*continued*)

TABLE 5 (*Continued*)

Author(s)	No., sex, & age of subjects	Group size	Conditions compared	Dependent measures	Results
			Self-control + family member + booster sessions Self-control + booster sessions	Reduction quotient	Post: No differences Follow-up (3 mo): No differences Follow-up (6 mo): No differences
Wollersheim (1970)	$N = 79$ 79F Med age 19	$n = 5$	Self-control Nonspecific Social pressure No treatment	Lb loss	Post: Self-control superior to nonspecific & social pressure. All conditions superior to no treatment Follow-up (8 wk): Self-control superior to nonspecific & social pressure. (No treatment not included in analysis.)
				Eating questionnaire	Post: Self-control & nonspecific superior to no treatment. Self-control superior to nonspecific Follow-up (8 wk): Self-control superior to nonspecific & social pressure. (No treatment not included in analysis.)
Zitter & Fremouw (1978)	$N = 56$ 48F, 8M Age range 18–49	$n = 4–8$	Self-control + individual contract Self-control + partner contract Minimal treatment control	Wt	Post: Both conditions superior to minimal treatment control Follow-up (6 wk): Self-control + individual contract superior to minimal treatment control Follow-up (6 mo): Self-control + individual contract superior to all conditions
				% overwt	Post: Both conditions superior to minimal treatment control

					Follow-up (6 wk): Self-control + individual contract superior to minimal treatment control Follow-up (6 mo): Self-control + individual contract superior to all conditions
Brownell, Heckerman, & Westlake (1979)	$N = 147$ 120F, 27M $\bar{X}$ age 44.8	$n = 10–12$	Self-control	Wt loss	Post: $\bar{X}$, 11 lb Follow-up (6 mo): $\bar{X}$, 20 lb
				Change % overwt	Post: $\bar{X}$, 8.5% Follow-up (6 mo): $\bar{X}$, 15.1%
				Wt reduction quotient	Post: $\bar{X}$, 16.1 Follow-up (6 mo): $\bar{X}$, 28.4
Brownell & Stunkard (1981)	$N = 124$ 62F, 62M $\bar{X}$ age 45	$n = 8–24$	Self-control + medication + cooperative spouse + couples training Self-control + medication + cooperative spouse Self-control + medication + uncooperative spouse Self-control + cooperative spouse + couples training Self-control + cooperative spouse Self-control + uncooperative spouse	Wt loss	Post: No differences Follow-up (1 yr): No differences
				Change % above ideal wt	Post: No differences Follow-up (1 yr): No differences
				Wt reduction index	Post: No differences Follow-up (1 yr): No differences
				Change body mass index	Post: No differences Follow-up (1 yr): No differences
				Beck Depression Inventory	Post: No differences Follow-up (1 yr): No differences
				Locke-Wallace Marital Adjustment	Post: No differences Follow-up (1 yr): No differences
Carroll & Yates (1981)	$N = 24$ 24F $\bar{X}$ age 22.4	$n = 12$	Self-control Self-control + stimulus control	Wt loss	Post: No difference Follow-up (8 mo): Self-control + stimulus control superior to self-control

(continued)

TABLE 5 (*Continued*)

Author(s)	No., sex, & age of subjects	Group size	Conditions compared	Dependent measures	Results
				Wt reduction index	Post: No difference Follow-up (8 mo): Self-control + stimulus control superior to self-control
Carroll, Yates, & Gray (1980)	$N = 72$ 72F $\bar{X}$ age 42	$n = 12$	Self-control Social support Wait list	Wt reduction index	Post: Self-control superior to social support & wait list Social support superior to wait list
Castro & Rachlin (1980)	$N = 46$ 43F, 3M Age > 18	$n = ?$	Self-reward Self-monitoring Self-punishment Wait list	Wt reduction quotient	Post: All groups superior to wait list Follow-up (8 wk): No differences; wait list not included in analysis
				% overwt	Post: All groups superior to wait list Follow-up (8 wk): No differences; wait list not included in analysis
				% wt loss	Post: All groups superior to wait list Follow-up (8 wk): No differences; wait list not included in analysis
Coates, Jeffery, Slinkard, Killen, & Danaher (1982)	$N = 38$ 26F, 12M Age range 13–17	$n = ?$	Self-control + contract for wt loss + intensive therapist contact Self-control + contract for wt loss + minimal ther-	% above ideal wt	Post: Self-control + contract for wt loss + intensive therapist contact superior to all others Follow-up (6 mo): Self-control + contract for wt loss + intensive

			apist contact Self-control + contract for calorie change + intensive therapist contact Self-control + contract for calorie change + minimal therapist contact		therapist contact superior to all others
Donke, Lando, & Robinson (1981)	$N = 41$ 39F, 2M $\bar{X}$ age 20.2	$n = ?$	Self-control Self-control, less directive	Wt loss	Post: No difference Follow-up (16 wk): No differences Follow-up (32 wk): Self-control, less directive superior to self-control
Epstein, Wing, Koeske, Andrasik, & Ossip (1981)	Children $N = 56$ 39F, 17M Age range 6–12 Parents $N = 46$ 32F, 14M Age ?	$n = ?$	Self-control, parent & child targets Self-control, child target Self-control, nonspecific target	Wt	Post: For children, no differences For parents no differences Follow-up (8 mo): For children, no differences For parents, self-control, parent & child targets superior to other groups Follow-up (21 mo): For children no differences For parents, no differences
				% overwt	Post: For children, no differences For parents, no differences Follow-up (8 mo): For children, no differences For parents, self-control, parent, & child targets superior to other groups Follow-up (21 mo): For children no differences For parents, no differences

(*continued*)

TABLE 5 (*Continued*)

Author(s)	No., sex, & age of subjects	Group size	Conditions compared	Dependent measures	Results
				Obese/non-obese proportion	Post: For children, self-control, child target superior to self-control, nonspecific target For parents, no differences Follow-up (8 mo): For children, no differences For parents, no differences Follow-up (21 mo): For children, no differences For parents, no differences
Epstein, Wing, Koeske, Ossip, & Beck (1982)	$N = 42$ 34F, 8M $\bar{X}$ age 11	$n = 8–11?$	Self-control + diet + life-style activity Self-control + diet + programmed exercise Self-control + life-style activity	% overwt	Post: Programmed exercise groups superior to life-style activity Follow-up (6 mo): Programmed exercise groups superior to life-style activity Follow-up (17 mo): Programmed exercise groups superior to life-style activity
			Self-control + programmed exercise	Body mass index	Post: Programmed exercise groups superior to life-style activity Follow-up (6 mo): Programmed exercise groups superior to life-style activity Follow-up (17 mo): Programmed exercise groups superior to life-style activity

				HR on fitness test	Post: Programmed exercise groups superior to life-style activity Follow-up (6 mo): No differences Follow-up (17 mo): Life-style activity groups superior to programmed exercise
Foreyt, Mitchell, Garner, Gee, Scott, & Gotto (1982)	N = 648 494F, 154M $\bar{X}$ age 43.3	n = 12–15	Self-control	Wt loss	Post: $\bar{X}$, 10.8 lb Follow-up (1 yr): $\bar{X}$, 12.8 lb
Gormally & Rardin (1981)	N = 100 100F $\bar{X}$ age 39.4	n = ?	Self-control Nutrition + exercise	Wt loss	Post: No difference Follow-up (7 mo): Self-control superior to nutrition + exercise
				Caloric intake	Post: Self-control superior to nutrition + exercise
				% basal level intake	Post: No difference
				Activity level, pedometer	Post: No difference
				Activity level, self-report	Post: Self-control superior to nutrition + exercise
Hartigan, Baker-Strauch, & Morris (1982)	N = 27 19F, 8M $\bar{X}$ age 36.7	n = 9	Self-control + diet Diet Wait list	Wt loss	Post: Self-control + diet superior to diet & wait list Follow-up (4 mo): Self-control + diet superior to diet & wait list
James & Hampton (1982)	N = 80 80F $\bar{X}$ age 37.7	n = 15–20?	Self-control, highly directive Self-control, partially directive	Wt reduction index	Post: Self-control, highly directive superior to all others Self-control, partially directive superior to minimally directive & wait list

(continued)

TABLE 5 (*Continued*)

Author(s)	No., sex, & age of subjects	Group size	Conditions compared	Dependent measures	Results
			Self-control, minimally directive		Follow-up (19 wk): Only highly & partially directive compared, no difference
			Wait list		Follow-up (34 wk): Only highly & partially directive compared; self-control, highly directive superior
				Skinfold	Post: Self-control, highly & partially directive superior to self-control, minimally directive, & wait list
					Follow-up (19 wk): Only highly & partially directive compared, no difference
					Follow-up (34 wk): Only highly & partially directive compared; self-control, highly directive superior
				HR on fitness test	Post: Self-control, highly & partially directive superior to self-control minimally directive & wait list
					Follow-up (19 wk): Only highly & partially directive compared; no difference
					Follow-up (34 wk): Only highly & partially directive compared; self-control, highly directive superior

Jeffery & Gerber (1982)	$N = 175$ 175M age?	$n = 10–20$	Self-control Self-control, correspondence program Minimal treatment	Wt loss	Post: Self-control & compliant self-control, correspondence *Ss* superior to noncompliant self-control, correspondence *Ss*, & minimal treatment Follow-up (6 mo): Self-control & compliant self-control, correspondence *Ss* superior to noncompliant self-control, correspondence *Ss*, & minimal treatment Follow-up (12 mo): Self-control & compliant self-control correspondence *Ss* superior to noncompliant self-control, correspondence *Ss*, & minimal treatment Compliant self-control *Ss* superior to compliant self-control, correspondence
Katahn, Pleas, Thackrey, & Wallston (1982)	$N = 44$ 38F, 6M $\bar{X}$ age, 36.6	$n = 10–14$	Self-control	Wt	Post: Significant reduction Follow-up (12–18 mo): Significant reduction
				Body fat	Post: Significant reduction
				Systolic BP	Post: Significant reduction
				Diastolic BP	Post: Significant reduction
				Resting HR	Post: Significant reduction
				HR on fitness test	Post: Significant reduction
				# situps	Post: Significant increase
				Physical flexibility	Post: Significant improvement

(*continued*)

TABLE 5 (*Continued*)

Author(s)	No., sex, & age of subjects	Group size	Conditions compared	Dependent measures	Results
				Sum of body circumferences	Post: Significant reduction
				Self-esteem Inventory	Post: Significant improvement
				Body Cathexis Scale	Post: Significant improvement
				General well-being schedule	Post: Significant improvement
Murphy, Williamson, Buxton, Moody, Absher, & Warner (1982)	$N = 75$ 50F, 25M $\bar{X}$ age 40.9	$n = 5–7$	Self-control + 1-party contracts Self-control + 2-party contracts Self-control + couples training + 1-party contracts Self-control + couples training + 2-party contracts Supportive group Wait list	Wt loss	Post: All groups superior to wait list Follow-up (5 wk): Only 5 treatments included in analysis, no differences Follow-up (12 wk): Only 5 treatments included in analysis, no differences Follow-up (26 wk): No difference Follow-up (1 yr): Only 5 treatments included in analysis, no differences Follow-up (2 yr): Self-control + couples training + 2-party contracts superior to self-control + 2-party contracts Combined self-control + couples training superior to combined self-control & supportive groups

Change % overwt	Post: All groups superior to wait list Follow-up (5 wk): Only 5 treatments included in analysis, no differences Follow-up (12 wk): Only 5 treatments included in analysis, no differences Follow-up (26 wk): Only 5 treatments included in analysis no differences Follow-up (1 yr): Only 5 treatments included in analysis, combined self-control + couples training groups superior to combined self-control & supportive groups Follow-up (2 yr): Only 5 treatments included in analysis, combined self-control + couples training groups superior to combined self-control & supportive groups
Wt reduction index	Post: All groups superior to wait list Follow-up (5 wk): Only 5 treatments included in analysis, no differences Follow-up (12 wk): Only 5 treatments included in analysis, no differences Follow-up (26 wk): Only 5 treatments included in analysis, no differences

(continued)

TABLE 5 (*Continued*)

Author(s)	No., sex, & age of subjects	Group size	Conditions compared	Dependent measures	Results
					Follow-up (1 yr): Only 5 treatments included in analysis, combined self-control + couples training groups superior to combined self-control & supportive groups
					Follow-up (2 yr): Only 5 treatments included in analysis, combined self-control + couples training superior to combined self-control & supportive groups
				Tricep skinfolds	Post: No differences
					Follow-up (5 wk): Only 5 treatments included in analysis, no differences
					Follow-up (12 wk): Only 5 treatments included in analysis, no differences
					Follow-up (26 wk): Only 5 treatments included in analysis, no differences
					Follow-up (1 yr): Only 5 treatments included in analysis, no differences
					Follow-up (2 yr): Only 5 treatments included in analysis, no differences
Pearce, LeBow, & Orchard (1981)	$N = 68$ 68F Age ?	$n = 6–7$	Self-control Self-control + couples training	Wt loss	Post: No differences
					Follow-up (3 mo): Only 4 treatments included in analysis,

			Self-control + nonparticipating spouse Psychodynamic Wait list		self-control + couples training superior to psychodynamic Follow-up (6 mo): Only 4 treatments included in analysis, self-control + couples training superior to psychodynamic Follow-up (1 yr): Only 4 treatments included in analysis, self-control + couples training superior to psychodynamic Self-control + nonparticipating spouse superior to psychodynamic
				Wt reduction quotient	Post: No differences Follow-up (3 mo): Only 4 treatments included in analysis, self-control + couples training superior to psychodynamic Follow-up (6 mo): Only 4 treatments included in analysis, self-control + couples training superior to psychodynamic Follow-up (1 yr): Only 4 treatments included in analysis, self-control + couples training superior to psychodynamic Self-control + nonparticipating spouse superior to psychodynamic
Pezzot-Pearce, LeBow, & Pearce (1982)	N = 126 ?F, ?M $\bar{X}$ age 39.4	n = ?	Self-control, therapist administered, group format	Wt reduction index	Post: Combined self-control groups superior to combined relaxation + insight groups

(*continued*)

TABLE 5 (*Continued*)

Author(s)	No., sex, & age of subjects	Group size	Conditions compared	Dependent measures	Results
			Self-control, therapist administered, individual Self-control, minimal therapist contact Self-control, self-administered Relaxation + insight, therapist administered, group format Relaxation + insight, therapist administered, individual		Follow-up (3 mo): Combined self-control groups superior to combined relaxation + insight groups Follow-up (6 mo): Combined self-control groups superior to combined relaxation + insight groups Follow-up (16 mo): Combined self-control groups superior to combined relaxation + insight groups Combined group format treatments superior to individual-administered
			Relaxation + insight, minimal therapist contact Relaxation + insight, self-administered Wait list	Body fat	Post: No differences Follow-up (3 mo): No difference Follow-up (6 mo): No difference
				Cost-effectiveness index	Post: Combined self-control groups superior to combined relaxation + insight groups Combined minimal therapist & self-administered groups superior to therapist-administered groups Combined group format superior to individual-administered Follow-up (3 mo): Combined self-control groups superior to combined relaxation + insight groups

					Combined minimal therapist & self-administered groups superior to therapist-administered groups Combined group format treatments superior to individual-administered groups Follow-up (6 mo): Combined self-control groups superior to combined relaxation + insight groups Combined minimal therapist & self-administered groups superior to therapist-administered groups Combined group format treatments superior to individual-administered Follow-up (16 mo): Combined self-control groups superior to combined relaxation + insight groups Combined minimal therapist & self-administered groups superior to therapist-administered groups Combined group format treatments superior to individual-administered
Rodriguez & Sandler (1981)	$N = 15$ 9F, 6M $\bar{X}$ age 25.6	$n = 5$	Self-monitoring + contracting Self-monitoring Attention placebo	Wt loss	Post: Self-monitoring + contracting superior to other groups Follow-up (2 mo): Self-monitoring + contracting superior to other groups

(*continued*)

TABLE 5 (*Continued*)

Author(s)	No., sex, & age of subjects	Group size	Conditions compared	Dependent measures	Results
					Follow-up (6 mo): Self-monitoring + contracting superior to other groups
				% wt loss	Post: No differences Follow-up (2 mo): Self-monitoring + contracting superior to other groups Follow-up (6 mo): Self-monitoring + contracting superior to other groups
				# eating episodes	Post: No differences Follow-up (2 mo): No differences Follow-up (6 mo): No differences
				Min per meal	Post: No differences Follow-up (2 mo): No differences Follow-up (6 mo): No differences
				Type of food eaten	Post: No differences Follow-up (2 mo): No differences Follow-up (6 mo): No differences
Voogt, Riggs, & Kline (1981)	$N = 53$ 53F $\bar{X}$ age 30.3	$n = 11–15$	Self-control, intensive therapist contact Self-control, moderate therapist contact Self-control, minimal therapist contact Wait list	Wt loss	Post: All self-control groups superior to wait list
Wilcoxon-Craighead, Stunkard, & O'Brien (1981)	$N = 134$ 120F, 14M Mdn age $\cong$ 49	$n = 10$	Self-control Pharmacotherapy Self-control +	Wt loss	Post: All treatments superior to wait list Pharmacotherapy & self-control

			Pharmacotherapy Physician control Wait list		+ pharmacotherapy superior to self-control Pharmacotherapy superior to physician control Follow-up (1 yr): Only 3 main treatments included in analysis; self-control superior to pharmacotherapy & self-control + pharmacotherapy
				Eating habits and attitudes about wt loss	Post: Self-control & self-control + pharmacotherapy superior to pharmacotherapy
				Nutrition knowledge	Post: No differences
				Beck Depression Inventory	Post: No differences
Weisz & Bucher (1980)	$N = 30$ 30F Age range 18–50	$n = 7–9$	Self-control Self-control + couples training Wait list	Body wt	Post: Both groups superior to wait list Follow-up (2 mo): Both groups superior to wait list
				% overwt	Post: Both groups superior to wait list Follow-up (2 mo): Both groups superior to wait list
				Eating patterns	Post: Self-control + couples training superior to other groups Self control superior to wait list Follow-up (2 mo): Both groups superior to wait list
				Marital Adjustment Test	Post: Self-control + couples training superior to self-control Follow-up (2 mo): No differences

(*continued*)

TABLE 5 (*Continued*)

Author(s)	No., sex, & age of subjects	Group size	Conditions compared	Dependent measures	Results
				Beck Depression Inventory	Post: Self-control + couples training superior to other groups Self-control superior to wait list Follow-up (2 mo): Self-control + couples training superior to other groups Self-control superior to wait list
Wing & Epstein (1981)	$N = 36$ 28F, 8M	$n = 11–13$	Self-control + small initial intake restriction Self-control + moderate initial intake restriction Self-control + large initial intake restriction	Wt loss	Post: No differences Follow-up (4 mo): No differences
				Caloric intake	Post: Self-control + large initial intake restriction superior to other groups Self-control + moderate initial intake restriction superior to self-control + small initial intake restriction
Wing, Epstein, Marcus, & Shapira (1981)	$N = 38$ 33F, 5M $\bar{X}$ age 38.8	$n = 18–20?$	Self-control + contract for wt loss, then attendance Self-control + contract for attendance, then weight loss	Wt loss	Post: No difference Follow-up (7 mo): No difference Follow-up (13 mo): No difference
Wing, Epstein, & Shapira (1982)	$N = 39$ 36F, 3M $\bar{X}$ age 45.8	$n = ?$	Self-control Scarsdale	Wt loss	Post: No difference Follow-up (6 mo): No difference Follow-up (1 yr): No difference

Jeffery, Danaher, Killen, Farquhar, & Kinnier (1982)	$N = 47$ 38F, 9M $\bar{X}$ age 44.7	$n = 14$	Self-control Self-control, self-administered Self-control, self-administered + contract Self-control, self-administered + contract + phone contact	Wt loss	Post: No differences
Brownell, Heckerman, Westlake, Hayes, & Monti (1978)	$N = 29$ 19F, 10M $\bar{X}$ age 45.3	$n = 9$–18	Self-control + cooperative spouse—couples training Self-control + cooperative spouse—subject alone Self-control + non-cooperative spouse—subject alone	Wt loss	Post: No differences Follow-up (3 mo): Self-control + cooperative spouse—couples training superior to others Follow-up (6 mo): Self-control + cooperative spouse—couples training superior to non-cooperative spouses—subject alone
				Change % over-wt	Post: No differences Follow-up (3 mo): Self-control + cooperative spouse—couples training superior to others Follow-up (6 mo): Self-control + cooperative spouse—couples training superior to others
				Wt reduction quotient	Post: No differences Follow-up (3 mo): No differences Follow-up (6 mo): No differences
				Self-report of habit change	Post: Self-control + cooperative spouse—couples training superior to others
				Knowledge of wt control strategies	Post: No differences

cooperative, has had little discernible impact. For the most part behavior therapists have been unable to bring to pass the promise of spouse involvement and couples training that the Brownell *et al.* (1979) study bred. Nor have they had much luck in extrapolating this strategy to parent–child dyads in their treatment of obese children (Epstein, Wing, Koeske, Andrasick, & Ossip, 1981; Kingsley & Shapiro, 1977). Thus what was initially seen, perhaps a bit too wishfully, as the key to bolstering behavioral treatments of obesity has revealed itself to be no miracle worker.

Self-Monitoring

Overview of the Findings

Summarized in Table 6 is the research on the effectiveness of self-monitoring, the results of which are quite favorable. In comparisons with no-treatment and attention placebo conditions, self-monitoring has invariantly come out on top. Tests with the latter though have been few, in fact, a grand total of only one (i.e., Hall *et al.*, 1974). Investigations of the relative efficacy of self-monitoring and a comprehensive self-control package have been more numerous and, surprisingly, find the two to be quite comparable. These studies, the most recent of which appeared in 1974, are however, quite dated. Since then, self-control programs have become more sophisticated, rendering it doubtful that a treatment composed entirely of self-monitoring would be on an equal footing.

Those studies focusing on parameters of self-monitoring revealed that the recording of the target behavior prior to, as opposed to after, its occurrence was more beneficial (Bellack, Rozensky, & Schwartz, 1974). They also found the monitoring of eating versus weight loss yielded more positive outcome (Israel & Saccone, 1979; Romanczyk, 1974; Saccone & Israel, 1978). The piling of additional techniques such as stimulus narrowing and covert sensitization onto self-monitoring did not, however, noticeably alter its effects (Romanczyk, 1974; Romanczyk, Tracey, Wilson, & Thorpe, 1973).

Therapist contact has also failed to systematically sway the gains accrued from treatment. Intensifying therapist contact has in some instances proven to be profitable (Coates *et al.*, 1982; Jeffery & Gerber, 1982; Jeffery & Wing, 1979), whereas in others it has not (Hanson, Borden, Hall, & Hall, 1976; Jeffery, Danaher, Killen, Farquhar, & Kinnier, 1982; Pezzot-Pearce, Lebow, & Pearce, 1982; Voogt, Riggs, & Kline, 1981). The same holds true for the directiveness of the therapist (Donke, Lando, & Robinson, 1981; James & Hampton, 1982), and the group versus individual administration of treatment (Kingsley & Wilson; Pezzot-Pearce *et al.*, 1982).

Aversive Procedures

Overview of the Findings

Subsumed under the heading of *aversive procedures* are three behavioral treatments—induced anxiety, covert sensitization, and olfactory aversion. A

TABLE 6. Summary of Studies Examining Effectiveness of Behavioral Group Therapy for Obesity: Self-Monitoring Procedures

Author(s)	No., sex, & age of subjects	Group size	Conditions compared	Dependent measures	Results
Bellack, Rozensky, & Schwartz (1974)	$N = 37$ 32F, 5M $\bar{X}$ age 40	$n = 6–10$	Pre self-monitoring + self-control Post self-monitoring + self-control Self-control Wait list	% change in wt	Post: Preself-monitoring + self-control superior to wait list Follow-up (3 mo): Preself-monitoring + self-control & self-control superior to wait list
Israel & Saccone (1979)	$N = 38$ 37F, 1M	$n = 5–7$	Self-monitoring wt Self-monitoring eating behavior Therapist reward for wt loss Therapist reward for eating behavior change Significant other reward for wt loss Significant other reward for eating behavior change	Lb loss	Post: Self-monitoring eating behavior, therapist reward for eating behavior change & significant other reward for eating behavior change superior to other conditions Follow-up (1 yr): Self-monitoring eating behavior, therapist reward for eating behavior change & significant other reward for eating behavior change superior to other conditions
Romanczyk (1974)	$N = 61$ 53F, 8M $\bar{X}$ age 41	$n = 14$	Self-monitor wt Self-monitor calories Self-control Self-control + self-monitor wt & calories No treatment	% overwt loss	Post: Self-monitor calories, self-control & self-control + self-monitor wt & calories superior to other conditions Follow-up (2 wk): No difference (only self-control & self-control + self-monitor wt & calories compared)

(*continued*)

TABLE 6. (*Continued*)

Author(s)	No., sex, & age of subjects	Group size	Conditions compared	Dependent measures	Results
					Follow-up (4 wk): No difference (only self-control & self-control + self-monitor wt & calories compared) Follow-up (13 wk): No difference (only self-control & self-control + self-monitor wt & calories compared)
Romanczyk, Tracey, Wilson, & Thorpe (1973), Exp 1	N = 102 86F, 16M Age range 18–55	n = 5–7	Self-monitor wt Self-monitor calories Self-monitor wt & calories + covert sensitization Self-monitor wt & calories + covert sensitization + relaxation + self-control Self-monitor wt & calories + covert sensitization + relaxation Self-monitor wt & calories + covert sensitization + relaxation + self-control + contract No treatment	% overwt Lb overwt	Post: All conditions superior to self-monitor wt & no treatment Follow-up (2 wk): No differences (only conditions with self-monitor wt & calories + covert sensitization compared) Follow-up (8 wk): No differences (only conditions with self-monitor wt & calories + covert sensitization compared) Post: All conditions superior to self-monitor wt & no treatment Follow-up (2 wk): No differences (only conditions with self-monitor wt & calories + covert sensitization compared) Follow-up (8 wk): No differences (only conditions with self-monitor wt & calories + covert sensitization compared)

Romanczyk *et al.* (1973) Exp 2	$N = 75$ $\bar{X}$ age 42	$n = 15$	Self-monitor + info + relaxation Self-monitor + info + relaxation + self-control + covert sensitization	Lb overwt	Post: Self-monitor + info + relaxation + self-control + covert sensitization superior Follow-up (3 wk): Self-monitor + info + relaxation + self-control + covert sensitization superior Follow-up (12 wk): Self-monitor + info + relaxation + self-control + covert sensitization superior
				% overwt loss	Post: Self-monitor + info + relaxation + self-control + covert sensitization superior Follow-up (3 wk): Self-monitor + info + relaxation + self-control + covert sensitization superior Follow-up (12 wk): Self-monitor + info + relaxation + self-control + covert sensitization superior
Saccone & Israel (1978)	$N = 49$ 48F, 1M $\bar{X}$ age 37	$n = 7$	Self-monitor wt + self-control Self-monitor eating behavior + self-control Self-control + therapist reward for wt loss Self-control + therapist reward for eating behavior change Self-control + significant other reward for wt loss Self-control + significant other reward for eating behavior change No treatment	Lb loss	Post: All conditions superior to no treatment. Self-control + therapist reward for eating behavior change & self-control + significant other reward for eating behavior change superior to all conditions

TABLE 7. Summary of Studies Examining Effectiveness of Behavioral Group Therapy for Obesity: Aversive Procedures

Author(s)	No., sex, & age of subjects	Group size	Conditions compared	Dependent measures	Results
Bornstein & Sipprelle (1973)	N = 40	n = 10	Induced anxiety Relaxation Nonspecific No treatment	Lb loss	Post: Induced anxiety superior to no treatment Follow-up (3 mo): Induced anxiety superior to all conditions Follow-up (6 mo): Induced anxiety superior to all conditions
Elliott & Denney (1975)	N = 75 37F, 8M	n = 2	Covert sensitization Covert sensitization + false physio feedback Attention placebo	% overwt Food questionnaire	Post: No differences Follow-up (4 wk): No differences Post: Covert sensitization superior to attention placebo for target foods Follow-up (4 wk): Covert sensitization superior to attention placebo for target foods
Foreyt & Hagen (1973)	N = 45 45F	n = 6–7	Covert sensitization Placebo	Wt	Post: No differences Follow-up (9 wk): No differences

	Age range 18–24		No treatment	Lb loss	Post: No differences Follow-up (9 wk): No differences
				Food questionnaire	Post: Covert sensitization & placebo superior for target foods
Frohwirth & Foreyt (1978)	$N = 38$ 38F Age range 17–30	$n = 2–5$	Olfactory aversion Attention placebo No treatment	Lb loss	Post: No differences Follow-up (10 wk): No differences
				Food questionnaire	Post: Olfactory aversion & attention placebo superior for target foods
Harris (1969)	$N = ?$	$n = 8$	Covert sensitization Self-control Self-control + covert sensitization No treatment	Lb loss	Post: All conditions superior to no treatment
				% wt loss	Post: All conditions superior to no treatment
Manno & Marston (1972)	$N = 41$ 36F, 5M	$n = 10–11$	Covert sensitization Covert positive reinforcement Attention control	Lb loss	Post: No differences Follow-up (3 mo): No differences
				Food questionnaire	Post: Covert positive reinforcement superior to other conditions

TABLE 8. Summary of Studies Examining Effectiveness of Behavioral Group Therapy for Obesity: Ancillary Procedures

Author(s)	No., sex, & age of subjects	Group size	Conditions compared	Dependent measures	Results
Carter, Rice, & DeJulio (1977)	$N = 48$ 24F, 24M	$n = 8$	Fade therapist + self-punishment Fade therapist + self-reinforcement Therapist + self-punishment Therapist + self-reinforcement Self-punishment Self-reinforcement	Lb loss	Post: Fade therapist + self-punishment & fade therapist + self-reinforcement superior to other conditions Follow-up (6 mo): Fade therapist self-punishment & fade therapist + self-reinforcement superior to other conditions
Epstein, Masek, & Marshall (1978)	$N = 6$ Age range 5–6	$n = 6$	Contingency management	Type of food Caloric intake % overwt	Post: Significant improvement Post: Significant reduction Post: Significant reduction Follow-up (10 mo): Not maintained
Harmatz & Lupac (1968)	$N = 21$ 21M Age range 29–48	$n = ?$	Response cost Caloric diet Caloric diet + social pressure	% baseline rate	Post: Response cost and caloric diet + social pressure superior to caloric diet Follow-up (4 wk): Response cost superior to other conditions
Korman (1973)	$N = 21$	$n = ?$	Contract Info	Wt	Post: No difference Follow-up (8 wk): No difference
Tyler & Straughan (1970)	$N = 57$ 57F $\bar{X}$ age 39	$n = 19$	Covert control Breath holding Relaxation	Lb loss	Post: No difference

summary of the research on their efficacy is presented in Table 7. Relative to self-monitoring, and certainly to self-control programs, these aversive procedures have been largely ignored and therefore remain essentially untested. In induced anxiety and olfactory aversion, for example, each has a body of empirical research composed entirely of a single study (i.e., Bornstein & Sipprelle, 1973; Frohwirth & Foreyt, 1978). Although the situation is not quite as dismal for covert sensitization, a corpus of four investigations does not allow for very many firm conclusions and generalizations. When we put aside the issue of numbers and inspect the studies conducted to date, the picture that emerges is not a flattering one. Though they have been able to hold their own in the few contests with other treatments (Harris, 1969; Manno & Marston, 1972), the aversive procedures as a whole have not performed well against no-treatment and attention placebo conditions. With the exception of induced anxiety, an exception founded upon a single investigation (i.e., Bornstein & Sipprelle, 1973), the aversive procedures have not yet reliably produced effects exceeding those accompanying the mere passage of time and a control for nonspecific factors (Elliott & Denney, 1975; Foreyt & Hagen, 1973; Frohwirth & Foreyt, 1978; Harris, 1969; Manno & Marston, 1972).

Ancillary Procedures

Overview of the Findings

Those techniques that did not conform to any of the categories previously reviewed were lumped under the heading of *ancillary procedures*. Among their ranks are the procedures of covergent control, response cost, self-punishment, and self-reinforcement. Research on their effectiveness is presented in Table 8. Little though can be said about these procedures as not a single investigation contrasted them with a no-treatment condition and a mere one with an attention placebo control. The few comparisons with alternative treatments are also problematic. As solitary investigations, their findings of superiority to dieting (Harmatz & Lupze, 1968) and of the contribution of therapist contact (Carter, Rice, & DeJulio, 1977) await replication before much credence can be assigned to them.

Summary Evaluation

Commentary on the behavioral group treatment of obesity is essentially commentary on self-control procedures, in that they are the most preferred and heavily researched of the four approaches. Today, it is a rarity to come across an intervention program composed exclusively of self-monitoring, aversive techniques, or any of the ancillary procedures. Even more rare is the behavior therapist who purports that such a strategy holds great promise for success. These three modes of treatment have fallen out of favor in part because of the meager support for their efficacy and also because of the growing respect for obesity's multifaceted nature. Self-control procedures, on the other hand, with their multiple techniques and broad-based push, have accumulated impressive evidence attesting to their advantage over both no-treatment and control conditions. And though they have not as of yet been able to outdo alternative active treatments with the same regularity, self-control programs do appear to have had the better of the going.

It is in the area of boosting the effects of these self-control procedures that the picture turns bleak. To date, little has proven to be of much worth in augmenting the benefits accrued from self-control treatments. This sad situation cannot be attributed to neglect and/or simplemindedness on the part of researchers. In fact behavior therapists have been extraordinarily aggressive and imaginative in their efforts to bolster treatment effects. They have experimented with maintenance sessions, tacked on regimens of pharmacotherapy and exercise, prescribed restrictive diets, reduced therapist–client contact, intensified therapist–client contact, rendered treatment less directive, and rendered treatment more directive. Unfortunately, for all their hard work, behavior therapists have ended up empty handed.

A number of researchers have tagged the client's immediate social environment as the key to enhancement and maintenance of treatment effects. Consequently, behavior therapists have gone to considerable lengths to incorporate the client's social nexus into the therapeutic process. This has generally taken the form of including family members, particularly the spouse, into the ongoing stream of therapeutic activities. Despite the mixed findings, this tact of assimilating significant others into the treatment process appears to be the wave of the future. It may not, however, prove to be any more successful than the aforementioned manipulations if the group, be it the therapy or naturalistic one, is attended to in a cursory manner. That is, if it is seen simply as a vehicle for expanding the therapist's didacticism, rather than as a fertile context for the acquisition of adaptive performance patterns. Earlier, we cited factors that may foster productive habit change on the part of group members, factors that have been prominent in traditional group psychotherapy but that have been largely ignored by behavior therapists. It may be that the advancement of behavioral group treatment for obesity, or for that matter all disorders, lies in our ability to mine and utilize such factors as cohesiveness, guidance, and vicarious learning.

Behavioral Group Treatment of Drug Addiction

The number of reports of behavioral group treatment of drug addiction has been extremely limited. Indeed, even the number of reports for all types of group treatment for drug abuse has been miniscule, especially if one looks at the group outcome literature. In their review of the group psychotherapy outcome literature in the period 1966–1975, for example, Parloff and Dies (1977) note only three studies that used drug addicts as subjects. None of these, however, could be classified as a behavioral group intervention. Similarly, in their review of this area, Kaplan and Sadock (1972) cite no behavioral approaches to group treatment of alcoholism or drug abuse. In all, only 10 reports were found despite the fact that addicts are frequently treated in groups (cf. Copemann, 1976) and that behavioral interventions for addictions are becoming both more common and recommended (Ross & Callner, 1982). The reports fell mainly into the self-control category, although three had aversive components and/or used contigency management exclusively. In addition, most group interventions were incorporated into a larger broad-spectrum treatment package or eclectic approach.

Copemann (1976) and Copemann and Shaw (1976) describe a broad-spectrum package that included both individual and group therapy components. During individual sessions, aversive counterconditioning using electric shock was used as the primary technique to reduce overt and covert drug-related responses. Covert sensitization was provided as an alternative for clients not amenable to electric shock. Treatment appears to have been individualized in that relaxation training, shaping, cognitive therapy, or assertiveness training were also provided when deemed necessary. Group therapy was aimed at cognitive restructuring and employed four different group modules. Although the details are sketchy, Copemann and Shaw (1976) state that role playing and role reversal were used to produce cognitive dissonance that, at least theoretically, according to these authors, would result in more efficacious strengthening of prosocial behaviors. The four different group modules specifically addressed were basic social restructuring, rational emotive therapy of cognitive distortions, problem-solving training, and fading of treatment.

In general, the subjects were 50 male and female blacks who were primarily addicted to heroin. As a group, they demonstrated poor educational and employment histories, had criminal records, and came from broken homes. Thus, this report represents one of the few that utilized a representative sample of the drug addict population (Callner & Ross, 1980). Twenty-two remained drug free throughout treatment and continued drug free for 18 to 30 months after treatment. Drug-free status was verified by interview, urinalysis, and checks for fresh needle marks at 6-month intervals. Although these results are encouraging, the authors are quick to remind us that they can only be seen as preliminary because adequate experimental controls were not used.

Cheek (1976) describes a similar broad-spectrum approach for heroin addicts who were being maintained on methadone. Treatment was conducted primarily in eight 1½ hour groups that met twice weekly for four weeks. Individual sessions were conducted at the beginning and end of the program to make cerain participants clearly understood the group material. Lectures, role playing, group discussion, assertion training, structured practice, imagery training, cognitive restructuring, systematic desensitization, relaxation training, and homework assignments were used with the idea of enhancing self-control and social skills. At 6 months clients who underwent this training were compared to clients who did not receive this training but who were also on methadone maintenance. Comparisons were also made on pre- and postprogram measures of anxiety level with respect to inner versus outer control, self-acceptance, and assertiveness. Cheek (1978) reports significant changes in pre- and postprogram data, but specific tests and levels of significance are not reported.

Abrahms (1979) assessed the effectiveness of a cognitive-behavioral (CB) group in teaching methadone maintenance clients skills and attitudes that would compete with drug-abusing behaviors. Fifteen males, 7 black and 8 white, having a mean age of 28 years were randomly assigned to either the CB group or a nondirective discussion group that was used as a comparison to control for nonspecific factors such as therapist attention and maturation. More specifically, the CB group sought to teach management of stress, anxiety, negative self-evaluations, depression, and nonassertiveness. Both groups met weekly for 10 two-hour sessions. Results were analyzed at pre-, post-, and follow-up intervals using a repeated-measures analysis of variance. Significant improvement was obtained for CB group members on self-reported anxiety, depression assertiveness, and group attendance at both posttreatment and at the 16-week follow-up. One of the interesting findings of this study, apart from the effectiveness of the treatment package, is the higher attendance rate of CB group members and the enthusiasm that they had for the helpfulness of the various cognitive-behavioral techniques. In light of the difficulties that many programs have in keeping addicts actively engaged in treatment, this incidental finding has important implications for increasing retention rates.

Although Abrahms (1979) employed a CB group modality to train prosocial skills, Reeder and Kunce (1976) employed a modeling procedure to obtain similar skill-enhancement objectives. Twenty-two black heroin addicts (19 male, 3 female) with a mean age of 29 years were randomly assigned to either a videomodel or videolecture group. Both groups discussed problems related to those that are frequently encountered by addicts upon completing residential treatment, for example, free-time management, job interviewing and employer relations, new life-style adjustment, and the like. The videomaterial was discussed in smaller subgroups with the idea of addicts projecting themselves into the situation and discussing what they would do if faced with the same problems. The models in the videomodeling tapes exhibited a coping attitude but at first appeared pessimistic and ineffective in a particular area. After reflection and discussion with a peer or counselor, the model also displayed more independence in coping and problem-solving behavior. Subjects in the videomodeling group had superior outcomes ($t = 1.75$, $p < .05$, one-tailed) in terms of vocational status 30, 90, and 180 days after treatment than subjects in the videolecture group. Again, it is not clear how much the behavioral group therapy process contributed to the outcome. Specific information on exactly what occurred in the groups is lacking, and it would appear that subjects may have been treated in groups for efficiency as much as for other group therapy advantages.

MacDonough (1976, 1978) reports on the use of an intensive confrontation group session that was used as an addition to both a token economy program and a feedback behavior modification program. Fifty-three active-duty soldiers, 42 polydrug users, and 11 alcoholics served as subjects. Both programs were similar in terms of the phases of treatment (e.g., detox, residential, vocational, and follow-up) and the essential treatment components (structured group, specifying desirable and undesirable behaviors, providing feedback, establishing a social hierarchy, urine surveillance, etc.). The major difference between the token economy program and the feedback behavior modification program appears to have been the way in which positive and negative reinforcers were dispensed or withheld. For example, the token group exchanged tokens for reinforcers, whereas the feedback group was given reinforcers for appropriate behaviors. The actual group therapies themselves, however, were an eclectic mixture of the principles of small group dynamics, confrontation techniques, and behavior therapy techniques. Exactly what behavior therapy techniques were used and how they were intermeshed with the other components is unclear. MacDonough concludes that the intensive confrontation was effective on a short-term basis but that the effect was most pronounced in decreasing inappropriate behavior of drug addicts using the feedback program. For alcohol abusers, the token economy seemed to decrease inappropriate behavior best, whereas programs were equally effective in increasing desirable behaviors.

Polakow and Doctor (1974) describe the results of a general contingency management program with adult drug offenders who were on parole. A group of 26 subjects (15 female and 11 male) with a mean age of 23.5 years was compared to a similar group given traditional probationary counseling. The behavioral program involved three stages—Stage 1 involved awarding points for prompt attendance and appropriate discussion at weekly meetings with the probation officer; Stage 2 involved earning points for participation in group meetings with other probationers; and Stage 3 involved a written contract for achieving prosocial behaviors in exchange for reductions in probation time. The Stage 2 group meetings are of the most relevance to our present discussion. Unfortunately, the exact interventions are not elaborated upon and are described as "experience sharing within a social context, discussions of problems in support for positive self-correction of deviant behavior and behavioral rehearsal" (Polakow & Doctor, 1974, p. 65). Although the behavioral package proved superior to the traditional probationary counseling in terms of probation violations, employment, arrests, and attendance, it is impossible to determine the extent to which behavioral group interventions played a role.

Steinfeld, Rautio, Rice, and Egan (1974) and Steinfeld (1970) anecdotally report the use of group covert sensitization (CS) with incorporated narcotic addicts. As with other group interventions in this section, CS was employed as part of a larger eclectic therapy program that also included seminars, sensitivity workshops, traditional group therapy, and encounter groups. An eight-session CS program was provided to seven volunteers in the later report, all of whom completed treatment. In the earlier report, Steinfeld (1970) does not indicate the number of sessions involved but does indicate that five of seven subjects completed the treatment. Clinical observation and self-report are used to describe the apparent aversions to drug-related stimuli that developed. Steinfeld *et al.* (1974) suggest additional forms of intervention for future research and treatment, for example, "substitute highs" and desensitization of social anxiety.

Ross, Lantinga, Homer, and Malee (1977a, 1977b) describe the use of a skills training curriculum for the combined treatment of alcoholics and drug abusers. The curriculum consisted of group training of relaxation, assertiveness, heterosexual, vocational and general coping skills. Clients were given both didactic and behavior rehearsal experiences supplemented with homework assignments, group modeling, and discussion. As with other reports in this section, the group therapy was also provided in the context of other interventions including individual counseling, contingency contracting, and a point system. Results at 1-, 3-, 6-, 9-, and 12-month follow-up intervals indicated that 65% of all clients had higher incomes after treatment than for comparable pretreatment periods. Similarly, 90% reported fewer legal problems and less actual drug or alcohol use posttreatment. Drug clients tended to return to drug use within the first 3 months after treatment. If they remained drug free for 3 months or more, they appeared to have an increased chance of success at later follow-ups. Alcoholics, however, appeared to have a constant probability of success at each follow-up interval. The net result, however, was approximately equal success rates for both groups. These preliminary results were interpreted as a life-style change hypothesis. That is, addicts who made the change from an addict subculture within the first 3 months increased their chances of success. Alcoholics, on the other hand, may have had a constant chance of success due, in part, to the fact that there is not a drinking subculture from which to separate in our society because drinking is part of the larger culture.

Callner and Ross (1978) describe the use of an assertiveness training group for drug addicts who were concurrently involved in the residential behavioral program described earlier (Ross, Lantinga, Homer, & Malee, 1977a, 1977b). Eight male drug abusers (three heroin, three amphetamine, and two psychedelic abusers) were randomly assigned to either the assertion group or a no-treatment control condition. Four of the eight subjects were court referred. Mean age was 21 years, and mean years of schooling was 12. All subjects were unmarried. All subjects were seen individually for a 30-minute pretest assessment that consisted of an assertion questionnaire designed for drug addicts (Callner & Ross, 1973) and behavioral performance situations. The following sequence was used in the group: discussion of assertion components; specifying verbal, nonverbal, and content objectives; role playing and videotaping situations; receiving feedback from group members; and replaying the scene using modeling and role reversal until the group was satisfied with the performance. Three group sessions averaging 45 minutes in duration were given per week for 3 weeks followed by a posttest assessment that was similar to the pretest. Control subjects were simply administered the pre- and posttests. Groups differed significantly after treatment on each of the three performance measures (duration, fluency, and effect), but not on the questionnaire data. In terms of specific assertion areas, between-group differences in assertiveness following treatment consistently appeared in the areas of drug refusals, positive feedback, and negative feedback.

Finally, Duehn (1978) reports the use of group covert sensitization (CS) in order to eliminate LSD use in seven self-referrred adolescents. Mean LSD use prior to CS was 2.3 times per week during a 14-week period of more traditional group therapy. Subjects were given relaxation training, aversive LSD scenes, and euphoric scenes in eight sessions over a 4-week period. All subjects had terminated LSD use at posttreatment. Six subjects were located at 6- and 18-

months follow-up and reported continued abstinence from LSD, improved academic functioning, and increased self-confidence.

Summary

This latter report was the only one encountered that employed a behavioral group intervention alone to treat drug abusers. All other reports were those in which the group intervention was part of a larger treatment package. In all cases, there was little or no emphasis on the role of the group *per se* in these studies. It appeared that although showing promising results, the reports presented individual techniques applied in a group context. Because peers seem to play such an important role in drug-taking behavior (Albrecht, 1973), one wonders if the role of the group in terms of modeling, shaping, and consequating behaviors of drug abusers could not and should not be more fully explored in a more systematic way with this clinical population. Because the reports were also descriptions of groups within larger treatment packages, one may also ask if the groups added anything to the treatment. It would appear that such component analysis is overdue and warranted.

Conclusion

At the outset of this chapter, we put forth as our main objective that of ascertaining the current status of behavioral group treatment for the addictive-appetitive disorders of alcoholism, smoking, obesity, and drug abuse. Early in our review of the literature, however, it became painfully clear that a monolithic behavioral group treatment does not exist. Instead, what we have is a compilation of diverse interventions that have as their common denominator an educational bent and a group format. This heterogeneity thus prohibits blanket pronouncements concerning the present and future state of behavioral group therapy. Our review of the outcome research reinforces the wisdom of such a ban, as it found not all variants of behavioral group treatment to be of comparable promise in remediating these four maladaptive patterns.

Across the four disorders of alcoholism, smoking, obesity, and drug abuse, our survey points to a broad spectrum, self-control intervention as having the greatest likelihood for success. Given the array of factors that have been implicated in the etiology and perpetuation of these disorders, one might have expected as much. For of all the treatment programs noted in this chapter, only the self-control packages appear to be of sufficient breadth to arrest these destructive patterns. Whether or not they are in fact capable of doing so is a matter for future research to decide.

Research of this nature will undoubtedly find these broad-based programs effective in bringing about rapid, discernible changes in symptomatology. Our review of the literature tells us that this is a relatively safe prediction. Our review also tells us that we can expect these changes to remain quite modest or, worse, completely dissipate with the passage of time. The challenge facing behavioral group researchers is thus one of developing new ways to harness and intensify the power of their technology. And there is perhaps no better place to start than with the group variable itself.

After years of neglect, behavioral researchers are now focusing their attention and energies onto the group factor. Little though is known of the group's contribution to outcome, let alone how we might go about maximizing that input. Efforts to include the spouse, parents, siblings, friends, and the like of the client into the treatment process have so far yielded mixed findings, as has manipulation of other dimensions such as directiveness and cohesion. It is, however, much too early for us to dismiss the potential of this line of research. We have, after all, only just begun to scratch the surface.

In general, the present review hints at an uncertain future for the behavioral group treatment of four addictive-appetitive disorders. Now that most of the initial enthusiasm for the approach has died down, behavioral researchers are settling in on the difficult task at hand, that of empirically demonstrating the effectiveness of their interventions and of coming up with ways to augment those effects. We believe, however, that this will be an exciting period, as conditions appear right for major advancements, if not in the power, then at least in our understanding of behavioral group therapy. Currently, we have sensitive, sound measures of the disorders, a methodology for assessing group process (Flowers, 1979), a growing openness to the work of traditional psychotherapists, and, of course, no shortage of ideas. It is our hope that these forces will coalesce and lead to progress in the practice of behavioral group therapy.

References

Abrahms, J. L. A cognitive-behavioral versus nondirective group treatment program for opioid-addicted persons: An adjunct to methadone maintenance. *The International Journal of the Addictions,* 1979, *14,* 503–511.

Abrahms, J. L., & Allen, G. J. Comparative effectiveness of situational programming, financial payoffs and group pressure in weight reduction. *Behavior Therapy,* 1974, *5,* 391–400.

Abrams, D. B., & Wilson, G. T. Self-monitoring and reactivity in the modification of cigarette smoking. *Journal of Consulting and Clinical Psychology,* 1979, *47,* 243–251.

Abramson, E. E. A review of behavioral approaches to weight control. *Behaviour Research and Therapy,* 1973, *11,* 547–556.

Adinolfi, A. A., McCourt, W. F., & Geoghegan, S. Group assertiveness training for alcoholics. *Journal of Studies on Alcohol,* 1976, *37,* 311–320.

Ahles, T. A., Schlundt, D. G., Prue, D. M., & Rychtarik, R. G. Impact of aftercare arrangements on the maintenance of treatment success in abusive drinkers. *Addictive Behaviors,* 1983, *8,* 53–58.

Albrecht, B. L. The alcoholism process: A social learning viewpoint. In P. Bourne & R. Fox (Eds.), *Alcoholism: Progress in Research and Treatment.* New York: Academic Press, 1973.

Ashby, W. A., & Wilson, G. T. Behavior therapy for obesity: Booster sessions and long-term maintenance of weight loss. *Behaviour Research and Therapy,* 1977, *15,* 451–463.

Ayllon, T., & Azrin, N. H. *The token economy: A motivational system for therapy and rehabilitation.* New York: Appleton-Century-Crofts, 1968.

Azrin, N. H. Improvements in the community reinforcement approach to alcoholism. *Behaviour Research and Therapy,* 1976, *14,* 339–348.

Balch, P., & Ross, A. W. A behaviorally oriented didactic-group treatment of obesity: An exploratory study. *Journal of Behavior Therapy and Experimental Psychiatry*, 1974, *5*, 239–243.
Balch, P., & Ross, A. W. Predicting success in weight reduction as a function of locus of control: A unidimensional and multidimensional approach. *Journal of Consulting and Clinical Psychology*, 1975, *43*, 119.
Beaver, C., Brown, R. A., & Lichtenstein, E. Effects of monitored nicotine fading and anxiety management training on smoking reduction. *Addictive Behaviors*, 1981, *6*, 301–305.
Bellack, A. S. Behavioral treatment for obesity: Appraisal and recommendations. In M. Hersen, R. M. Eisler, & P. M. Miller (Eds.), *Progress in behavior modification* (Vol. 4). New York: Academic Press, 1977.
Bellack, A. S., Rozensky, R., & Schwartz, J. A comparison of two forms of self-monitoring in a behavioral weight reduction program. *Behavior Therapy*, 1974, *5*, 523–530.
Beneke, W. M., Paulsen, B., McReynolds, W. T., Lutz, R. N., & Kohrs, M. B. Long-term results of two behavior modification weight loss programs using nutritionists as therapists. *Behavior Therapy*, 1978, *9*, 501–507.
Berne, E. *Transactional analysis in psychotherapy*. New York: Grove Press, 1961.
Bernstein, D. A. Modification of smoking behavior: An evaluative review. *Psychological Bulletin*, 1969, *71*, 418–440.
Bernstein, D. A., & Borkovec, T. D. *Progressive relaxation training: A manual for the helping professions*. Champaign, Ill.: Research Press, 1973.
Bernstein, D. A., & McAlister, A. The modification of smoking behavior: Progress and problems. *Addictive Behaviors*, 1976, *1*, 89–102.
Best, J. A., & Steffy, R. A. Smoking modification procedures for internal and external locus of control clients. *Canadian Journal of Behavioural Science*, 1975, *2*, 155–165.
Bloch, S., Crouch, E., & Reibstein, J. Therapeutic factors in group psychotherapy: A review. *Archives of General Psychiatry*, 1981, *38*, 591–526.
Bornstein, P. H., Carmody, T. P., Relinger, H., Zohn, C. J., Devine, D. A., & Bugge, I. D. Reduction of smoking behavior: A multivariable treatment package and the programming of response maintenance. *Psychological Record*, 1977, *27*, 733–741.
Bornstein, P. H., & Sipprelle, C. N. Group treatment of obesity by induced anxiety. *Behaviour Research and Therapy*, 1973, *11*, 339–341.
Bray, G. A. *The obese patient*. Philadelphia: Saunders, 1976.
Brockway, B. S., Kleinmann, G., Edleson, J., & Gruenewald, K. Non-aversive procedures and their effect on cigarette smoking. *Addictive Behaviors*, 1977, *2*, 121–128.
Brownell, K. D. Obesity: Understanding and treating a serious, prevalent and refractory disorder. *Journal of Consulting and Clinical Psychology*, 1982, *50*, 820–840.
Brownell, K. D., & Stunkard, A. J. Couples training, pharmacotherapy, and behavior therapy in the treatment of obesity. *Archives of General Psychiatry*, 1981, *38*, 1224–1229.
Brownell, K. D., Heckerman, C. L., Westlake, R. J., Hayes, S. C., & Monti, P. M. The effect of couples training and partner co-operativeness in the behavioral treatment of obesity. *Behaviour Research and Therapy*, 1978, *16*, 323–333.
Brownell, K. D., Heckerman, C. L., & Westlake, R. J. The behavioral control of obesity: A descriptive analysis of a large-scale program. *Journal of Clinical Psychology*, 1979, *35*, 864–869.
Cadogen, D. A. Marital group therapy in alcoholism treatment. In E. Kaufman & P. Kaufman (Eds.), *Family therapy of drug and alcohol abuse*. New York: Halsted Press, 1979.
Cahalan, D. Implications of American drinking practices and attitudes for prevention and treatment of alcoholism. In G. A. Marlatt & P. E. Nathan (Eds.), *Behavioral approaches to alcoholism*. New Brunswick, N.J.: Rutgers Center of Alcohol Studies, 1978.
Callner, D. A., & Ross, S. M. The assessment and training of assertive skills with drug addicts: A preliminary study. *The International Journal of the Addictions*, 1978, *13*, 227–239.
Callner, D. A., & Ross, S. M. Behavioral treatment approaches to drug abuse. In J. M. Ferguson & C. B. Taylor (Eds.), *The comprehensive handbook of behavioral medicine* (Vol. 3). Jamaica, N.Y.: Spectrum, 1980.
Carroll, L. J., & Yates, B. T. Further evidence for the role of stimulus control training in facilitating weight reduction after behavior therapy. *Behavior Therapy*, 1981, *12*, 287–291.

Carroll, L. J., Yates, B. T., & Gray, J. J. Predicting obesity reduction in behavioral and nonbehavioral therapy from client characteristics: The self-evaluation measure. *Behavior Therapy*, 1980, *11*, 189–197.

Carter, E. N., Rice, A. P., & DeJulio, S. Role of the therapist in the self-control of obesity. *Journal of Consulting and Clinical Psychology*, 1977, *45*, 503.

Castro, L., & Rachlin, H. Self-reward, self-monitoring, and self-punishment as feedback in weight control. *Behavior Therapy*, 1980, *11*, 38–48.

Cautela, J. R. Covert sensitization. *Psychological Reports*, 1967, *74*, 459–468.

Chaney, E. F., O'Leary, M. R., & Marlatt, G. A. Skill training with alcoholics. *Journal of Consulting and Clinical Psychology*, 1978, *46*, 1092–1104.

Cheek, F. Behavior modification for addicts on methadone maintenance. *Current Psychiatric Therapies*, 1978, *16*,223–232.

Coates, T. J., Jeffery, R. W., Slinkard, L. A., Killen, J. D., & Danaher, B. G. Frequency of contact and monetary reward in weight loss, lipid change, and blood pressure reduction with adolescents. *Behavior Therapy*, 1982, *13*, 175–185.

Colletti, G., & Stern, L. Two-year follow-up of a nonaversive treatment for cigarette smoking. *Journal of Consulting and Clinical Psychology*, 1980, *48*, 292–293.

Colletti, G., & Supnick, J. A. Continued therapist contact as a maintenance strategy for smoking reduction. *Journal of Consulting and Clinical Psychology*, 1980, *48*, 665–667.

Cooper, A., Furst, J. B., & Bridger, W. H. A brief commentary on the usefulness of studying fears of snakes. *Journal of Abnormal Psychology*, 1969, *24*, 413–414.

Copemann, C. D. Drug addiction: II. An aversive counter-conditioning technique for treatment. *Psychological Reports*, 1976, *38*, 1271–1281.

Copemann, C. D., & Shaw, P. L. A behaviorally-oriented treatment program for drug addiction: A preliminary report. *American Journal of Public Health*, 1976, *66*, 286–287.

Cummings, C., Gordon, J. F., & Marlatt, G. A. Relapse: Prevention and prediction. In W. R. Miller (Ed.), *The addictive behaviors*. Oxford, England: Pergamon Press, 1980.

Delahunt, J., & Curran, J. P. Effectiveness of negative practice and self-control techniques in the reduction of smoking behavior. *Journal of Consulting and Clinical Psychology*, 1976, *44*, 1002–1007.

Dilley, D., Balch, P., & Balch, K. A comparison of strategies for behavioral obesity treatment. *Journal of Behavior Therapy and Experimental Psychiatry*, 1979, *10*, 193–197.

Donke, J. A., Lando, H. A., & Robinson, D. C. A behavioral weight control program for residence hall students. *Journal of Counseling Psychology*, 1981, *28*, 365–368.

Duehn, W. D. Covert sensitization in group treatment of adolescent drug abusers. *The International Journal of the Addictions*, 1978, *13*, 485–491.

Edinger, J. D., Nelson, W. M., Davidson, K. M., & Wallace, J. Modification of smoking behaviors in a correctional institution. *Journal of Clinical Psychology*, 1978, *34*, 991–998.

Elliott, C. H., & Denney, D. R. Weight control through covert sensitization and false feedback. *Journal of Consulting and Clinical Psychology*, 1975, *43*, 842–850.

Elliott, C. H., & Denney, D. R. A multiple-component treatment approach to smoking reduction. *Journal of Consulting and Clinical Psychology*, 1978, *46*, 1330–1339.

Elliott, R., & Tighe, T. Breaking the cigarette habit: Effects of a technique involving threatened loss of money. *Psychological Record*, 1968, *18*, 503–513.

Emrick, C. D., & Hansen, J. Assertions regarding effectiveness of treatment for alcoholism: Fact or fantasy? *American Psychologist*, 1983, *38*, 1078–1088.

Epstein, L. H., & McCoy, J. F. Issues in smoking control. *Addictive Behaviors*, 1975, *1*, 65–72.

Epstein, L. H., Masek, B. J., & Marshall, W. R. A nutritionally based school program for control of eating in obese children. *Behavior Therapy*, 1978, *9*, 766–778.

Epstein, L. H., Wing, R. R., Koeske, R., Andrasik, F., & Ossip, D. J. Child and parent weight loss in family-based behavior modification programs. *Journal of Consulting and Clinical Psychology*, 1981, *49*, 674–685.

Epstein, L. H., Wing, R. R., Koeske, R., Ossip, D., & Beck, S. A comparison of lifestyle change and programmed aerobic exercise on weight and fitness changes in obese children. *Behavior Therapy*, 1982, *13*, 651–665.

Ferrell, W. L., & Galassi, J. P. Assertion training and human relations training in the treatment of alcoholics. *International Journal of the Addictions*, 1981, *16*, 959–968.

Flaxman, J. Quitting smoking now or later: Gradual, abrupt, immediate, and delayed quitting. *Behavior Therapy*, 1978, *9*, 260–270.

Flowers, J. V. Behavioral analysis of group therapy and a model for behavioral group therapy. In D. Upper & S. M. Ross (Eds.), *Behavioral group therapy, 1979: An annual review*. Champaign, Ill.: Research Press, 1979.

Foreyt, J. P., & Hagen, R. L. Covert sensitization: Conditioning or suggestion? *Journal of Abnormal Psychology*, 1973, *82*, 17–23.

Foreyt, J. P., Mitchell, R. E., Garner, D. T., Gee, M., Scott, L. W., & Gotto, A. M. Behavioral treatment of obesity: Results and limitations. *Behavior Therapy*, 1982, *13*, 153–161.

Foxx, R. M., & Brown, R. A. Nicotine fading and self-monitoring for cigarette abstinence or controlled smoking. *Journal of Applied Behavior Analysis*, 1979, *12*, 111–125.

Foxx, R. M., Brown, R. A., & Katz, I. Nicotine fading and self-monitoring for cigarette abstinence or controlled smoking: A two and one-half year follow-up. *The Behavior Therapist*, 1981, *4*, 21–23.

Frohwirth, R. A., & Foreyt, J. P. Aversive conditioning treatment of overweight. *Behavior Therapy*, 1978, *9*, 861–872.

Glasgow, R. E., Schafer, L., & O'Neill, H. K. Self-help books and amount of therapist contact in smoking cessation programs. *Journal of Consulting and Clinical Psychology*, 1981, *49*, 659–667.

Goldman, M. S. Cognitive impairment in chronic alcoholics. *American Psychologist*, 1983, *38*, 1045–1054.

Gormally, J., & Rardin, D. Weight loss and maintenance and changes in diet and exercise for behavioral counseling and nutrition education. *Journal of Counseling Psychology*, 1981, *28*, 295–304.

Gutmann, M., & Marston, A. R. Problems of S's motivation in a behavioral program for reduction of cigarette smoking. *Psychological Reports*, 1967, *20*, 1107–1114.

Hackett, G., & Horan, J. J. Partial component analysis of a comprehensive smoking program. *Addictive Behaviors*, 1979, *4*, 259–262.

Hall, S. M., Hall, R. G., Hanson, R. W., & Borden, D. L. Permanence of two self-managed treatments of overweight in university and community populations. *Journal of Consulting and Clinical Psychology*, 1974, *42*, 731–786.

Hall, S. M., Hall, R. G., Borden, B. L., & Hanson, R. W. Follow-up strategies in the behavioral treatment of overweight. *Behaviour Research and Therapy*, 1975, *13*, 167–172.

Hall, S. M., Hall, R. G., DeBoer, G., & O'Kulitch, P. Self and external management compared with psychotherapy in the control of obesity. *Behaviour Research and Therapy*, 1977, *15*, 89–95.

Hanson, R. W., Borden, B. L., Hall, S. M., & Hall, R. G. Use of programmed instruction in teaching self-management skills to overweight adults. *Behavior Therapy*, 1976, *7*, 366–373.

Harmatz, M. G., & Lapuc, P. Behavior modification of overeating in a psychiatric population. *Journal of Consulting and Clinical Psychology*, 1968, *32*, 583–587.

Harris, M. B. Self-directed program for weight control. *Journal of Abnormal Psychology*, 1969, *74*, 263–270.

Harris, M. B., & Bruner, C. G. A comparison of a self-control and a contract procedure for weight control. *Behaviour Research and Therapy*, 1971, *9*, 347–354.

Harris, M. B., & Hallbauer, E. S. Self-directed weight control through eating and exercise. *Behaviour Research and Therapy*, 1973, *11*, 523–529.

Hartigan, K. J., Baker-Strauch, D., & Morris, G. W. Perceptions of the causes of obesity and responsiveness to treatment. *Journal of Counseling Psychology*, 1982, *29*, 478–485.

Heather, N., & Robertson, I. *Controlled drinking*. London: Metheun, 1981.

Hunt, G. M., & Azrin, N. H. A community-reinforcement approach to alcoholism. *Behaviour Research and Therapy*, 1973, *11*, 91–104.

Hunt, W. A., & Bespalec, D. A. An evaluation of current methods of modifying smoking behavior. *Journal of Clinical Psychology*, 1974, *30*, 431–438.

Hunt, W. A., & Matarazzo, J. D. Habit mechanisms in smoking. In W. A. Hunt (Ed.), *Learning mechanisms in smoking*. Chicago: Aldine, 1970.

Intagliata, J. C. Increasing the interpersonal problem-solving skills of an alcoholic population. *Journal of Consulting and Clinical Psychology*, 1978, *46*, 489–498.
Israel, A. C., & Saccone, A. J. Follow-up of effects of choice of mediator and target of reinforcement on weight loss. *Behavior Therapy*, 1979, *10*, 260–265.
Israel, A. C., Raskin, P. A., & Pravder, M. D. The effects of self-monitoring of smoking and awareness of accuracy feedback upon a concurrent behavior. *Addictive Behaviors*, 1979, *4*, 199–203.
James, J. E., & Hampton, B. A. M. The relative efficacy of directive and nondirective treatment in behavioral weight control. *Behavior Therapy*, 1982, *13*, 463–475.
Janis, I. L., & Hoffman, D. Facilitating effects of daily contact between partners who make a decision to cut down on smoking. *Journal of Personality and Social Psychology*, 1971, *17*, 25–35.
Jeffery, D. B., & Christensen, E. R. Behavior therapy versus "will power" in the management of obesity. *Journal of Psychology*, 1975, *90*, 303–311.
Jeffery, R. W., & Gerber, W. M. Group and correspondence treatments for weight reduction used in multiple risk factor intervention trial. *Behavior Therapy*, 1982, *13*, 24–30.
Jeffery, R. W., & Wing, R. R. Frequency of therapist contact in the treatment of obesity. *Behavior Therapy*, 1979, *10*, 186–192.
Jeffery, R. W. Danaher, B. G., Killen, J., Farquhar, J. W., & Kinnier R. Self-administered programs for health behavior change: Smoking cessation and weight reduction by mail. *Addictive Behaviors*, 1982, *7*, 57–64.
Jones, M. *The therapeutic community*. New York: Basic Books, 1953.
Kanas, N. Alcoholism and group psychotherapy. In E. M. Pattison & E. Kaufman (Eds.), *Encyclopedic handbook of alcoholism*. New York: Gardner Press, 1983.
Kantorowitz, D. A., Walters, J., & Pezdek, K. Positive versus negative self-monitoring in the self-control of smoking. *Journal of Consulting and Clinical Psychology*, 1978, *46*, 1148–1150.
Kaplan, H. I., & Sadock, B. J. *Groups and Drugs*. New York: E. P. Dutton, 1972.
Karoly, P., & Doyle, W. W. Effects of outcome expectancy and timing of self-monitoring on cigarette smoking. *Journal of Clinical Psychology*, 1975, *31*, 351–355.
Katahn, M., Pleas, J., Thackrey, M., & Wallston, K. A. Relationship of eating and activity self-reports to follow-up weight maintenance in the massively obese. *Behavior Therapy*, 1982, *13*, 521–528.
Katz, R. C., Heiman, M., & Gordon, S. Effects of two self-management approaches on cigarette smoking. *Addictive Behaviors*, 1977, *2*, 113–119.
Kaufman, E., & Pattison, E. M. Differential methods of family therapy in the treatment of alcoholism. *Journal of Studies on Alcohol*, 1981, *42*, 951–971.
Kelly, A. H., & Curran, J. P. Comparison of a self-control approach to the treatment of obesity. *Journal of Consulting and Clinical Psychology*, 1976, *44*, 683.
Keutzer, C. S. Behavior modification of smoking: The experimental investigation of diverse techniques. *Behaviour Research and Therapy*, 1968, *6*, 137–157.
Keutzer, C. S., Lichtenstein, E., & Mees, H. L. Modification of smoking behavior: A review. *Psychological Bulletin*, 1968, *70*, 520–533.
Kingsley, R. G., & Shapiro, U. A comparison of three behavioral programs for the control of obesity in children. *Behavior Therapy*, 1977, *8*, 30–36.
Kingsley, R. G., & Wilson, G. T. Behavior therapy for obesity: A comparative investigation of long-term efficacy. *Journal of Consulting and Clinical Psychology*, 1977, *45*, 288–298.
Korman, I. B. The effectiveness of contractual management in weight reduction groups. *Dissertation Abstracts International*, 1973, *33*(9), 4512B.
Lando, H. A. A comparison of excessive and rapid smoking in the modification of chronic smoking behavior. *Journal of Consulting and Clinical Psychology*, 1975, *43*, 350–355.
Lando, H. A. Stimulus control, rapid smoking, and contractual management in the maintenance of nonsmoking. *Behavior Therapy*, 1978, *9*, 962–963.
Lando, H. A. Effects of preparation, experimenter contact, and a maintained reduction alternative on a broad-spectrum program for eliminating smoking. *Addictive Behaviors*, 1981, *6*, 123–133.
Lando, H. A. A factorial analysis of preparation, aversion, and maintenance in the elimination of smoking. *Addictive Behaviors*, 1982, *7*, 143–154.

Lando, H. A., & McCullough, J. A. Clinical application of a broad-spectrum behavioral approach to chronic smokers. *Journal of Consulting and Clinical Psychology*, 1978, *46*, 1583–1585.

Lando, H. A., & McGovern, P. G. Three-year data on a behavioral treatment for smoking: A follow-up note. *Addictive Behaviors*, 1982, *7*, 177–181.

Lazarus, A. A. *Multimodal behavior therapy*. New York: Springer, 1976.

Levenberg, S. B., & Wagner, M. K. Smoking cessation: Long-term irrelevance of mode of treatment. *Journal of Behavior Therapy and Experimental Psychiatry*, 1976, *7*, 93–95.

Levinson, B. L., Shapiro, D., Schwartz, G. E., & Tursky, B. Smoking elimination by gradual reduction. *Behavior Therapy*, 1971, *2*, 477–487.

Levis, D. J. The case for performing research on nonpatient populations with fears of small animals: A reply to Cooper, Furst, and Bridger. *Journal of Abnormal Psychology*, 1970, *76*, 36–38.

Lichtenstein, E., & Danaher, B. G. Modification of smoking behavior: A critical analysis of theory, research, and practice. In M. Hersen, R. M. Eisler, & P. M. Miller (Eds.), *Progress in behavior modification* (Vol. 3). New York: Academic Press, 1976.

Lowe, M. R., Green, L., Kurtz, S. M. S., Ashenberg, Z. S., & Fisher, Jr., E. B. Self-initiated, cue extinction, and covert sensitization procedures in smoking cessation. *Journal of Behavior Medicine*, 1980, *3*, 357–372.

MacDonough, T. S. The relative effectiveness of a medical hospitalization program versus a feedback-behavior modification program in treating alcohol and drug abusers. *The International Journal of the Addictions*, 1976, *11*, 269–282.

MacDonough, T. S. Evaluation of the effectiveness of intensive confrontation in changing the behavior of alcohol and drug abusers. *The International Journal of the Addictions*, 1978, *13*, 529–589.

Mahoney, M. J. Self-reward and self-monitoring techniques for weight control. *Behavior Therapy*, 1974, *5*, 48–57.

Mahoney, M. J., Kazdin, A. E., & Lesswing, N. J. Behavior modification: Delusion or difference? In C. M. Franks & G. T. Wilson (Eds.), *Annual review of behavior therapy, theory, and practice* (Vol. 2). New York: Brunner/Mazel, 1974.

Manno, B., & Marston, A. R. Weight reduction as a function of negative covert reinforcement (sensitization) versus positive covert reinforcement. *Behaviour Research and Therapy*, 1972, *10*, 201–207.

Marlatt, G. A. Alcohol use and problem drinking: A cognitive-behavioral analysis. In P. C. Kendall & S. D. Hollon (Eds.), *Cognitive-behavioral interventions: Theory, research and procedures*. New York: Academic Press, 1979.

Marlatt, G. A. The controlled drinking controversy: A commentary. *American Psychologist*, 1983, *38*, 1097–1110.

Marlatt, G. A., & Gordon, J. R. Determinants of relapse: Implications for the maintenance of behavior change. In P. O. Davidson & S. M. Davidson (Eds.), *Behavioral medicine: Changing health lifestyles*. New York: Brunner/Mazel, 1980.

Marrone, R. L., Merksamer, M. A., & Salzberg, P. M. A short duration group treatment of smoking behavior by stimulus satiation. *Behaviour Research and Therapy*, 1970, *8*, 347–352.

Marston, A. R., & McFall, R. M. Comparison of behavior modification approaches to smoking reduction. *Journal of Consulting and Clinical Psychology*, 1971, *36*, 153–162.

McCourt, W., & Glantz, M. Cognitive-behavior therapy in groups for alcoholics; a preliminary report. *Journal of Studies on Alcohol*, 1980, *41*, 338–346.

McFall, R. M., & Hammen, C. L. Motivation, structure, and self-monitoring: Role of nonspecific factors in smoking reduction. *Journal of Consulting and Clinical Psychology*, 1971, *37*, 80–86.

McGlynn, F. D. *Theory and research in systematic desensitization*. New York: Guilford Press, Behavioral Sciences Tape Library, 1975.

McGrath, M. J., & Hall, S. M. Self-management treatment of smoking behavior. *Addictive Behaviors*, 1976, *1*, 287–292.

Merbaum, M., Avimier, R., & Goldberg, J. The relationship between aversion, group training and vomiting in the reduction of smoking behavior. *Addictive Behaviors*, 1979, *4*, 279–285.

Miller, P. M. Behavior therapy in the treatment of alcoholism. In G. A. Marlatt & P. E. Nathan (Eds.), *Behavioral approaches to alcoholism*. New Brunswick, N.J.: Rutgers Center of Alcohol Studies, 1978.

Miller, W. R., & Hester, R. K. Treating the problem drinker: Modern approaches. In W. R. Miller (Ed.), *The addictive behaviors.* Oxford, England: Pergamon Press, 1980.
Miller, W. R., & Mastria, M. A. *Alternatives to alcohol abuse.* Champaign, Ill.: Research Press, 1977.
Miller, W. R., & Taylor, C. A. Relative effectiveness of bibliotherapy, individual and group self-control training in the treatment of problem drinkers. *Addictive Behaviors,* 1980, *5,* 13–24.
Miller, W. R., Pechacek, T. F., & Hamburg, S. Group behavior therapy for problem drinkers. *International Journal of Addictions,* 1981, *16,* 829–839.
Miller, W. R., Taylor, C. A., & West, J. C. Focused versus broad-spectrum behavior therapy for problem drinkers. *Journal of Consulting and Clinical Psychology,* 1980, *48,* 590–601.
Moos, R. H., & Finney, J. W. The expanding scope of alcoholism treatment evaluation. *American Psychologist,* 1983, *38,* 1036–1044.
Mulford, H. A. The epidemiology of alcoholism and its implications. In E. M. Pattison & E. Kaufman (Eds.), *Encyclopedic handbook of alcoholism.* New York: Gardner Press, 1982.
Murphy, J. K., Williamson, D. A., Buxton, A. E., Moody, S. C., Absher, N., & Warner, M. The long-term effects of spouse involvement upon weight loss and maintenance. *Behavior Therapy,* 1982, *13,* 681–693.
Murray, D. C. Preferred versus nonpreferred treatment, and self-control training versus determination raising as treatments of obesity: A pilot study. *Psychological Reports,* 1976, *38,* 191–198.
Nathan, P. E., & Lansky, D. Common methodology problems in research on the addictions. *Journal of Consulting and Clinical Psychology,* 1978, *46,* 713–726.
Nelson, R. O. Assessment and therapeutic functions of self-monitoring. In M. Hersen, R. M. Eisler, & P. M. Miller (Eds.), *Progress in behavior modification* (Vol. 5). New York: Academic Press, 1977.
Norton, G. R., & Barske, B. The role of aversion in the rapid-smoking treatment procedure. *Addictive Behaviors,* 1977, *2,* 21–25.
Ober, D. C. Modification of smoking behavior. *Journal of Consulting and Clinical Psychology,* 1968, *32,* 543–549.
Oei, T. P. S., & Jackson, P. R. Long-term effects of group and individual social skills training with alcoholics. *Addictive Behaviors,* 1980, *5,* 129–136.
Oei, T. P. S., & Jackson, P. R. Social skills and cognitive behavioral approaches to the treatment of problem drinking. *Journal of Studies on Alcohol,* 1982, *43,* 532–547.
Olson, R. P., Ganley, R., Devine, V. T., & Dorsey, G. D. Long-term effects of behavioral versus insight-oriented therapy with inpatient alcoholics. *Journal of Consulting and Clinical Psychology,* 1981, *49,* 866–877.
O'Neil, P. M., Currey, H. S., Hirsch, A. A., Riddle, F. E., Taylor, C. I., Malcolm, R. J., & Sexauer, J. D. Effects of sex of subject and spouse involvement on weight loss in a behavioral treatment program: A retrospective investigation. *Addictive Behaviors,* 1979, *4,* 167–177.
Parloff, M. B., & Dies, R. R. Group psychotherapy outcome research, 1966–1975. *International Journal of Group Psychotherapy,* 1977, *27,* 281–319.
Paxton, R. The effects of a deposit contract as a component in a behavioural programme for stopping smoking. *Behaviour Research and Therapy,* 1980, *18,* 45–50.
Pearce, J. W., LeBow, M. D., & Orchard, J. Role of spouse involvement in the behavioral treatment of overweight women. *Journal of Consulting and Clinical Psychology,* 1981, *49,* 236–244.
Penick, S. B., Filion, R., Fox, S., & Stunkard, A. J. Behavior modification in the treatment of obesity. *Psychosomatic Medicine,* 1971, *33,* 49–55.
Pezzot-Pearce, T. D., LeBow, M. D., & Pearce, J. W. Increasing cost-effectiveness in obesity treatment through use of self-help behavioral manuals and decreased therapist contact. *Journal of Consulting and Clinical Psychology,* 1982, *50,* 448–449.
Pyke, S., Agnew, N. M., & Kopperud, J. Modification of an overlearned response through a relearning program: A pilot study on smoking. *Behaviour Research and Therapy,* 1966, *4,* 197–203.
Polakow, R. L., & Doctor, R. M. A behavioral modification program for adult drug offenders. *Journal of Research in Crime and Delinquency,* 1974, *11,* 63–69.
Polich, J. M., Armor, D. J., & Braiker, H. B. *The course of alcoholism: Four years after treatment.* New York: Wiley, 1981.
Poole, A. D., Sanson-Fisher, R. W., & German, G. A. The rapid-smoking technique: Therapeutic effectiveness. *Behaviour Research and Therapy,* 1981, *19,* 389–397.

Raw, M., & Russell, M. A. H. Rapid smoking, cue exposure and support in the modification of smoking. *Behaviour Research and Therapy*, 1980, *18*, 363–372.

Reeder, C. W., & Kunce, J. T. Modeling techniques, drug abstinence behavior and heroin addicts: A pilot study. *Journal of Counseling Psychology*, 1976, *23*, 560–562.

Relinger, H., Bornstein, P. H., Bugge, I. D., Carmody, T. P., & Zohn, C. J. Utilization of adverse rapid smoking in groups: Efficacy of treatment and maintenance procedures. *Journal of Consulting and Clinical Psychology*, 1977, *45*, 245–249.

Rodriguez, L., & Sandler, J. The treatment of adult obesity through direct manipulation of specific eating behaviors. *Journal of Behavior Therapy and Experimental Psychiatry*, 1981, *12*, 159–162.

Romanczyk, R. G. Self-monitoring in the treatment of obesity: Parameters of reactivity. *Behavior Therapy*, 1974, *5*, 531–540.

Romanczyk, R. G., Tracey, D. A., Wilson, G. T., & Thorpe, G. L. Behavioral techniques in the treatment of obesity: A comparative analysis. *Behaviour Research and Therapy*, 1973, *11*, 629–641.

Rose, S. D. *Group therapy: A behavioral approach*. Englewood Cliffs, N.J.: Prentice-Hall, 1977.

Ross, S. M., & Callner, D. A. Behavioral treatment of drug addiction. In S. Baker & R. Craig (Eds.), *Drug dependent patient: Treatment and research*. Springfield, Ill.: Charles C Thomas, 1982.

Ross, S. M., Lantinga, L. J., Homer, A. L., & Malee, J. *Behavioral treatment of addictions: I. A curriculum approach for skills training*. Paper presented at the National Drug Abuse Conference, San Francisco, May 1977. (a)

Ross, S. M., Lantinga, L. J., Homer, A. L., & Malee, J. *Behavioral treatment of addictions. II. A progress report of the response of addicts and alcoholics at the Salt Lake City VA Hospital*. Paper presented at the National Drug Abuse Conference, San Francisco, May 1977. (b)

Saccone, A. J., & Israel, A. C. Effects of experimenter versus significant other-controlled reinforcement and choice of target behavior on weight loss. *Behavior Therapy*, 1978, *9*, 271–278.

Shaw, B. F., & Hollon, S. D. *Cognitive therapy in a group format with depressed outpatients*. Unpublished manuscript, University of Western Ontario, London, Ontario, 1978.

Shipley, R. H. Maintenance of smoking cessation: Effect of follow-up letters, smoking motivation, muscle tension, and health locus of control. *Journal of Consulting and Clinical Psychology*, 1981, *49*, 982–984.

Sonne, J. L., & Janoff, D. The effect of treatment attributions on the maintenance of weight reduction: A replication and extension. *Cognitive Therapy and Research*, 1979, *3*, 389–397.

Spitzer, R. L., Forman, J. B. W., & Nee, J. DSM-III field trials: 1. Initial inter-rater diagnostic reliability. *American Journal of Psychiatry*, 1979, *136*, 815–817.

Steffy, R. A., Meichenbaum, D., & Best, J. A. Aversive and cognitive factors in the modification of smoking behaviour. *Behaviour Research and Therapy*, 1970, *8*, 115–126.

Steinfeld, G. J. The use of covert sensitization with institutionalized narcotic addicts. *The International Journal of the Addictions*, 1970, *5*, 225–232.

Steinfeld, G. J., Rautio, E. A., Rice, A. H., & Egan, M. J. Group covert sensitization with narcotic addicts (further comments). *The International Journal of the Addictions*, 1974, *9*, 447–464.

Steinglass, P. An experimental treatment program for alcoholic couples. *Journal of Studies on Alcohol*, 1979, *40*, 159.

Stuart, R. B. A three-dimensional program for the treatment of obesity. *Behaviour Research and Therapy*, 1971, *9*, 177–186.

Stuart, R. B., & Davis, B. *Slim chance in a fat world*. Champaign, Ill.: Research Press, 1972.

Stunkard, A. J., & Mahoney, M. J. Behavioral treatment of eating disorders in H. Leitenberg (Ed.), *Handbook of behavior modification and behavior therapy*. Englewood Cliffs, N.J.: Prentice-Hall, 1976.

Surgeon General's Advisory Committee. *Smoking and Health* (Publ. No. 1103). United States Public Health Service: Washington, D.C., 1964.

Turner, R. W., Wehl, C. K., Cannon, D. S., & Craig, K. A. *Mood-control training for depression in alcoholics: A comparison of behavioral and cognitive therapies*. Paper presented at the National Alcohol and Drug Coalition Conference, Washington, D.C., 1980.

Turner, R. W., Wehl, C. K., & Moreno, J. K. *Long-term outcome for depressed alcoholics in mood-control therapy*. Paper presented at the Annual Convention of the American Psychological Association, Anaheim, California, August 1983.

Tyler, V. O., & Straughan, J. H. Coverant control and breath holding as techniques for the treatment of obesity. *Psychological Record,* 1970, *20,* 473–478.

United States Public Health Service. *Health consequences of smoking.* Washington, D.C.: U.S. Government Printing Office, 1971.

United States Public Health Service. *Health consequences of smoking.* Washington, D.C.: U.S. Government Printing Office, 1973.

United States Public Health Service. *Health consequences of smoking.* Washington, D.C.: U.S. Government Printing Office, 1974.

Upper, D., & Meredith, L. *A timed-interval procedure for modifying cigarette-smoking behavior.* Paper presented at the meeting of the American Psychological Association, September 1970.

Upper, D., & Meredith, L. *A timed-interval procedure for modifying ciagrette-smoking behavior.* Unpublished manuscript, Veterans Administration Medical Center, Brockton, Mass., 1971.

Van Itallie, T. B. *Testimony before Senate Select Committee on Nutrition and Human Needs.* Washington, D.C.: U.S. Government Printing Office, 1977.

Voogt, R. D., Riggs, R. C., & Kline, W. B. Frequency of counselor contact in a behavioral weight control program. *Behavioral Counseling Quarterly,* 1981, *1,* 130–135.

Wehl, C. K., Turner, R. W., Cannon, D. S., & Craig, K. A. *Group vs. individual cognitive-behavioral therapy for depressed alcoholics.* Paper presented at the Annual Convention of the American Psychological Association, Washington, D.C., August 1982.

Weismann, M. M., & Myers, J. K. Clinical depression in alcoholism. *American Journal of Psychiatry,* 1980, *137,* 372–373.

Weisz, G., & Bucher, B. Involving husbands in treatment of obesity—effects on weight loss, depression, and marital satisfaction. *Behavior Therapy,* 1980, *11,* 643–650.

Whitman, T. L. Modification of chronic smoking behavior: A comparison of three approaches. *Behaviour Research and Therapy* 1969, *7,* 257–263.

Whitman, T. L. Aversive control of smoking behavior in a group context. *Behaviour Research and Therapy,* 1972, *10,* 97–104.

Wilcoxon-Craighead, L., Stunkard, A. J., & O'Brien, M. Behavior therapy and pharmacotherapy for obesity. *Archives of General Psychiatry,* 1981, *38,* 763–768.

Wilkinson, D. A., & Sanchez-Craig, M. Relevance of brain dysfunction to treatment objectives: Should alcohol-related cognitive deficits influence the way we think about treatment? *Addictive Behaviors,* 1981, *6,* 253–260.

Wilson, G. T., & Brownell, K. D. Behavior therapy for obesity: Including family members in the treatment process. *Behavior Therapy,* 1978, *9,* 943–945.

Wilson, G. T., & Brownell, K. D. Behavior therapy for obesity: An evaluation of treatment outcome. *Advances in Behaviour Research and Therapy,* 1980, *3,* 49–86.

Winett, R. A. Parameters of deposit contracts in the modification of smoking. *Psychological Record,* 1973, *23,* 49–60.

Wing, R. R., & Epstein, L. H. Prescribed level of caloric restriction in behavioral weight loss programs. *Addictive Behaviors,* 1981, *6,* 139–144.

Wing, R. R., Epstein, L. H., Marcus, M., & Shapira, B. Strong monetary contingencies for weight loss during treatment and maintenance. *Behavioral Therapy,* 1981, *12,* 702–710.

Wing, R. R., Epstein, L. H., & Shapira, B. The effect of increasing initial weight loss with the Scarsdale diet or subsequent weight loss in a behavioral program. *Journal of Consulting and Clinical Psychology,* 1982, *50,* 446–447.

Wisocki, P. A., & Rooney, E. J. A comparison of thought stopping and covert sensitization techniques in the treatment of smoking: A brief report. *Psychological Record,* 1974, *24,* 191–192.

Wollersheim, J. P. The effectiveness of group therapy based upon learning principles in the treatment of overweight women. *Journal of Abnormal Psychology,* 1970, *76,* 462–474.

Zitter, R. E., & Fremouw, W. J. Individual versus partner consequation for weight loss. *Behavior Therapy,* 1978, *9,* 808–813.

13

Behavioral Group Treatment Methods for Sexual Disorders and Dysfunctions

KEVIN B. McGOVERN AND STEVEN H. JENSEN

INTRODUCTION

In the late 1960s, Masters and Johnson's clinical innovations revolutionized treatment approaches for sexual malaise, dissatisfaction, and dysfunction. Although some therapists (Wolpe & Lazarus, 1966) were already utilizing behavioral approaches at that time, traditional insight therapies and psychoanalysis were the primary modes of treatment available for the successful modification of these prolific sexual problems.

Masters and Johnson's exciting treatise awakened the proponents of direct behavioral intervention. At the Reproductive Institute in St. Louis, these dedicated pioneers designed a comprehensive treatment approach for sexually dysfunctional couples. By attending this 2-week program, dissatisfied couples could learn a specific series of behavioral remedies. Through these exciting clinical interventions, the sexually dissatisfied learned how to experience a more rewarding sexual relationship.

As descriptions of these therapeutic approaches were publicized throughout the world (Masters & Johnson, 1970), clinicians decided to design and evaluate other powerful behavioral therapeutic programs. These behavior modification programs were utilized by a significant number of couples and individuals throughout the country who were able to resolve their sexual concerns, dilemmas, and dysfunctions. Although some traditionalists were skeptical, a number of convincing publications discussing the advantages of these treatment approaches were publicized.

As clinicians continued to replicate and modify Masters and Johnson's powerful model, authors began to acclaim that these alternative programs were highly successful. For example, Lobitz and LoPiccolo (1972) developed a self-stimulation program for preorgasmic women. This nine-step behavioral ap-

KEVIN B. McGOVERN and STEVEN H. JENSEN • Private practice, 1225 N. W. Murray Road, Suite 214 and 215, Portland, Oregon 97229.

proach enabled a nonorgasmic woman to achieve orgasim by utilizing a self-stimulation program. Within several years, an array of behavioral programs appeared for the treatment of men and women who were primarily dissatisfied with their sexual functioning. Many of these individuals learned a repertoire of more satisfactory sexual behaviors (LoPiccolo & LoPiccolo, 1978). More recently, the overall ability of these behavioral approaches has been more thoroughly reviewed (Zilbergeld & Kilmann, 1984).

Behavioral Group Therapy Programs for Sexual Dysfunctions

These new therapeutic approaches were gradually incorporated into behavioral group treatment formats. Barbach (1974) designed a behavioral group treatment program for preorgasmic women. While attending these therapy sessions, these women discussed their mutual fears and concerns. During each meeting, they also provided emotional support for each other and discussed their reactions to their weekly behavioral homework assignments. The majority of preorgasmic women attending these and other similar programs (Jankovich & Miller, 1978) were eventually able to experience orgasim during one or more sexual activities and/or interactions.

As these behavioral group treatment programs proved to be effective for preorgasmic women, clinicians began to design and evaluate behavioral group treatment programs for sexually dysfunctional couples (McGovern, Kirkpatrick, & LoPiccolo, 1976). As Barbach had discovered, the sexually dissatisfied could learn how to modify their nonadaptive behaviors while attending group therapy sessions. Although these couples often found the behavioral group therapy meetings to be threatening, initially they were eventually able to discuss their sexual concerns and problematic behaviors.

Through these weekly behavioral group sessions, couples learned that their contemporaries shared similar frustrations about their sexuality. As each additional session progressed, these sexually dysfunctional couples provided each other with support and encouraged the group members to complete their weekly behavioral homework assignments.

As the basic Masters and Johnson program was continuously examined and evaluated, an array of other behavioral group approaches appeared in the literature. These alternate therapeutic modalities were designed for (a) preorgasmic women (Kuriansky & Sharpe, 1982; Schneidman & McGuire, 1976); (b) secondary inorgasmic women (Kilmann, Mills, Bella, Caid, Davidson, Drose, & Wanless, 1983); (c) rapid ejaculating men (Zeiss, Christensen, & Levine, 1978); (d) impotent men (Lobitz & Baker, 1979); and (e) couples impaired by sexual dysfunctions (Powell, Blakeney, Craft, & Pullian, 1974).

Mills and Kilmann (1982) have reviewed and analyzed an array of these group therapy approaches. Of the 37 treatment programs scrutinized, 35 of these therapeutic approaches included some form of direct behavioral intervention, that is, homework assignments, relaxation training, behavioral rehearsal, and/or communication skills. Although there were a number of methodological limitations discussed, these authors indicated the following: "Most of the studies found positive treatment effects on varied aspects of sexual and/or nonsexual functioning" (p. 277). However, they also cautioned that "these studies do not offer an answer to the important question of which treatment methods are most effective in the group format" (p. 277).

Behavioral Group Therapy Programs for Sexual Deviations

Over the last 5 years, there has been a significant escalation in the reported cases of deviant sexual behaviors occurring between adults and minors. Some communities have estimated a 300% increase in the number of reported cases of children who have been sexually abused by a biological parent, a stepparent, a relative, or an individual in a trusted position (i.e., teacher, priest, school counselor, bus driver). Perpetrators of these inappropriate sexual behaviors are often described as sexual psychopaths, pedophiles, incestual parents, or adults impaired by aberrant sexual arousal patterns with characterological deficits. Although the majority of these sexually abusive patterns are perpetrated by men, there are a number of reported cases of women who also engage in aberrant sexual behaviors (Finkelhor, 1979).

As the number of documented cases of deviant sexual behavior increases, clincians are searching for treatment alternatives. At Western State Hospital in Ft. Steilacoom, Washington, the staff has developed a self-help group treatment program for sexual offenders (McDonald & di Furia, 1971). During the last decade, over 500 men have overcome their inappropriate behavioral deficits (Kanfer & Saslow, 1969), such as inappropriate release of anger, deficient social skills, ineffective communication styles, and deviant masturbation habits. In one follow-up study (Saylor, 1979), between December of 1967 and May of 1979, 313 of 402 patients classified as sexual psychopaths were able to successfully complete a comprehensive multiphase treatment program. Of the treatment failures, 13 occurred during a work release phase, 48 during outpatient treatment and 28 after being totally discharged. In 1984, an additional research project (Saylor, 1984) revealed a similar pattern. This study reviewed the recividism rate of 511 men treated in a state hospital program for sexual offenders. Twenty-three percent of these rehabilitated sexual abusers had eventually reoffended. Although this multifaceted treatment approach was highly effective for a large portion of their residents, treatment failures were also noted. These results demonstrate the need for continuous follow-up projects and long-term behavioral maintenance programs (Prithers, Marguis, Gibat, & Marlatt, 1983). Another innovative treatment program designed to correct unhealthy sexual attitudes and behaviors has been adopted by many communities throughout the country. Parents United (Giarretto, 1981), founded in northern California, was established to provide support, assistance, and professional help for sexual offenders who engage in inappropriate sexual behaviors at home. Over the past 5 years, Parents United has endorsed several chapter organizations throughout the USA and in Europe.

In addition, correctional mental health care personnel recognized that many incarcerated sexual offenders do not participate in comprehensive treatment programs. For example, in 1978, the Oregon Departments of Mental Health and Corrections coordinated a study to review the existing state program available for the assessment and treatment of sexual offenders. Following this study, funds were allocated for the creation of a comprehensive treatment program. This inpatient hospital program was designed to clinically assess and treat a population of sexual offenders who were incarcerated in a nearby state penitentiary. The offender's enrolled in this new treatment approach were required to attend a multidimensional therapy program. While participating in this inpatient hospital program, each sexual abuser attends an array of behaviorally oriented group therapy sessions, individual aversive conditioning sessions, and other supplementary rehabilitation programs. Through this multifaceted approach, these men are currently learning how to modify their deviant behavioral patterns. Since this program has just begun, long-term treatment outcome statistics are not yet available. In 1982, the Center for Behavioral Intervention developed an outpatient treatment program for sexual abusers (Jensen, 1983). This treatment program was, in part, designed according to the successful treatment components already developed at Western State Hospital and Oregon State Hospital. The basic treatment premise is that deviant sexual behavior is a product of long-term conditioning, cognitive distortions, and a lack of appropriate social and sexual skills. Each potential treatment candidate's psychological assets and deficits are carefully assessed before the sexual abuser is accepted into this program (McGovern, in press). The habitual and impulsive dangerous sexual offender is referred to other residential care programs such as the Oregon State Hospital Program and the Sexual Psycopathy Program at Western State Hospital.

From this clinical perspective, each sexual abuser is expected to learn adaptive social and sexual behaviors. Many of the sexual abusers attending this program discussed their dissatisfactions with their adult social and sexual relationships. As their past sexual histories, current sexual relationships, and sexual arousal levels were carefully examined, a number of interesting parallels emerged between sexually dysfunctional males and men who had engaged in deviant sexual behaviors.

For example, many of the sexual abusers were also dissatisfied with their adult sexual relationships. Although they initially minimized their dissatisfaction, a thorough examination of their past sexual behaviors revealed that a number of these sexual abusers were dissatisfied with (a) the physical characteristics of their spouse; (b) the frequency of their intimate adult sexual behaviors; and (c) the lack of sexual variety. In addition, a number of the offenders had never acquired a relevant sexual education and felt inadequate as sexual partners.

For example, W. R., a 43-year-old male Caucasian, was referred to the center for engaging in a variety of illegal sexual behaviors with his 15-year-old stepdaughter. During the initial clinical evaluation, a number of serious problems surfaced. W. R. explained that he was aroused and sexually satisfied during the first several years of his marriage. However, during the past 5 years, his wife had gained 50 pounds and developed a number of unattractive physical traits. The sexual relationship deteriorated as he lost interest and both partners became bored and dissatisfied with each other. During this time, W. R. began to notice high levels of sexual attraction toward his stepdaughter, who had begun developing her secondary sex characteristics.

As the sexual components of their relationship continued to deteriorate, W. R. began to develop periodic erectile failure. While engaging in coital behaviors with his overweight, unkept wife, he noticed a decrease in his sexual attraction, arousal, and ability to function. As time went on, this man was unable to obtain and maintain erections. As W. R. became more preoccupied with his sexuality, he experienced erection difficulties on a regular basis. On those occasions when erections were possible, he would ejaculate prematurely. This man's sexuality was now hampered by three forms of sexual dysfunction: (a) premature ejaculation; (b) situational erectile failure; and (c) high levels of sexual dissatisfaction.

As his marital relationship continued to erode, he found himself beginning to fantasize on a more regular basis. While at work, W. R. became sexually aroused by adult female co-workers. Perceiving himself as being shy, retiring, and lacking heterosexual social skills, he was unable to initiate viable social contacts with these women or entice them into sexual encounters. Although he was able to fantasize and masturbate to these erotic sexual fantasies, W. R. was too inhibited to develop sexual relationships with them. In addition, he felt that this would be a direct violation of his marital vows.

As his sexual dysfunction continued to psychologically impair him, W. R. found himself becoming sexually aroused by his stepdaughter. During the middle of the night, he would lie awake and fantasize intimate encounters with her. On some occasions, he would masturbate to these fantasies. As these thoughts became more pronounced, W. R. began to wander into her room under the pretense of checking on his stepdaughter's welfare and safety. During the colder months, he would carefully adjust her bedding and casually rub his hand against her breasts and vagina. As these ritualistic behaviors became more arousing and gratifying, W. R. would spend a greater amount of time touching his stepdaughter inappropriately. On several occasions, this young girl awoke during these fondling incidences. Although pretending to be asleep, she was fully aware of his inappropriate sexual gestures. Afraid to discuss these improprieties with her mother, she eventually discussed them with a girlfriend. These "revelations" were then shared with her friend's mother, who immediately contacted the police.

After a thorough investigation was conducted, W. R. was arrested for engaging in inappropriate sexual behavior with his stepdaughter. He was then referred for a comprehensive clinical assessment that included a physiological evaluation of his sexual arousal patterns (Laws & Osborne, 1983). After his sexual arousal patterns were documented on a chart recorder, a therapist discussed his arousal patterns with him. W. R. was told that he would be taught how to modify his aberrant arousal patterns and enhance his sexual relationship with his wife. This man was then referred to the Center for Behavioral Intervention for treatment. His treatment program included behavioral group therapy sessions with specific homework assignments, physiological monitoring, and individual aversive behavioral therapy sessions. In addition, marital and sexual enhancement group therapy sessions were recommended.

As stated previously, before the sexual abuser is accepted into this multidimensional behavioral treatment program, each treatment candidate must complete a comprehensive assessment (McGovern, in preparation), including a physiological evaluation. During this phase of the assessment, he is placed in a private room and instructed to place a strain gauge on his penis. While listening to an array of audiotapes and viewing a series of erotic materials, his arousal responses are automatically displayed on a chart recorder. After this component of the assessment is completed, he is provided with a summary of his arousal responses, including comparisons between his reactions to normal adult-relevant themes and those arousal responses obtained while viewing or listening to aberrant themes. (Abel, 1976) In addition, comparisons are made between the individual's verbal report of his sexual arousal and the measured changes that occurred during the physiological evaluation.

A physiological arousal assessment (Henson, Rubin, & Henson, 1979; Heiman, 1977) for women sexual abusers has not yet been incorporated into this evaluation approach. However, as the reported cases of female sexual abusers increase (Finkelhor, 1979; Sarrel & Masters, 1982), this clinical procedure may present a viable clinical alternative.

After the physiological assessment has been completed, the sexual abuser is then placed into the first phase of treatment. During these individual behavioral therapy sessions, the sexual abuser learns how to modify his inappropriate sexual patterns through an extensive aversive conditioning approach, which is discussed in detail later in this chapter (Jensen, 1983). When the sexual abuser has learned how to utilize this therapeutic approach, he attends a weekly behavioral group therapy program. During these structured behavioral group meetings, each individual discusses his current psychological problems and thoroughly reviews the weekly homework assignments. Sexual abusers involved in a committed relationship have an opportunity to attend a marital/sexual enhancement program coordinated by a sex therapist. The purpose of this treatment strategy is to teach each individual more effective ways of developing satisfactory adult sexual behaviors with their partners.

Specific components of this behavioral treatment program will now be discussed in greater detail.

Client Selection

Proper client selection is a vital component of this behavioral group treatment approach. Although homogenous groups may be preferred for other types of behavioral group treatment, a homogenous group of deviant offenders tends to accept either passive behavior, such as is seen in incestuous fathers, or highly aggressive behavior, as observed in rapists. More specifically, sexual abusers with various forms of sexual deviations provide the needed mixture of personality types and social experiences to effectively assist other group members in developing new perspectives and social skills. For example, exposers and incestuous fathers can be excessively passive during group therapy and unable to confront each other about their deviant behavior. Rapists, on the other hand, can behave in overtly hostile and confrontive fashions.

These heterogenous groups provide a balance and challenge the members' maladaptive behavioral patterns. Because sexual abusers usually accept these maladaptive coping patterns, they must be continuously confronted and challenged during these behavioral group therapy sessions.

Eligible clients are selected after a comprehensive assessment has been completed. These evaluations consist of psychological testing, physiological evaluations, and a thorough review of the abuser's past social and sexual history. Individuals are rejected when severe psychopathology, mental retardation, brain damage, chronic substance abuse, a long history of multiple incarcerations, and/or when the use of assaultive behavior is observed.

The motivational level of each potential group treatment member is also an extremely important variable to assess. In order to develop a productive behavioral group therapy program, the therapist needs to include motivated clients who will take an active part in therapy, complete homework assignments on time, attend regularly scheduled meetings, and assist other group members in solving their problems. George McDonald, M.D. (1976, personal communication), the founder of the Sexual Psychopathy Program at Western State Hospital in Fort Steilacoom, has stated:

> The key to treating the sexual offender is the individual's acceptance of the existence of his problem and his willingness and ability to work to correct it. This acceptance must be complete, as must the individual's personal commitment to treatment.

This behavioral group treatment approach, like any other form of treatment intervention, will not be effective with unmotivated group members.

During this evaluation, each potential group member is extensively interviewed in order to determine if the abuser is willing to (a) take complete responsibility for his deviant behavior; (b) recognize the need for treatment; (c) spend a significant amount of time modifying his deviant behavioral patterns; (d) accept the guidance and direction of the therapist; (e) resolve his legal problems through the court; and, (f) has been mandated to participate in a treatment program.

When the sexual abuser is initially identified by a legal or social agency, this individual usually experiences an array of negative emotional reactions. During the initial judicial proceedings, the sexual abuser is unable to deny the social unacceptability of his behavior and may exhibit extreme remorse. Unless he experiences actual environmental losses (family, job, fines, and/or incarceration), his discomfort is usually short lived. Most sexual abusers have developed a remarkable denial system that enables them to heal themselves when the judicial scrutiny and external pressures are removed and sufficient time has elapsed. Clinicians have observed that, in these cases, internal motivation by itself is not enough to maintain the sexual abuser in a rigorous treatment program that requires a major modification in his life-style. However, given reasonable external pressures, the abuser will participate in a behavioral group treatment program and/or another therapeutic modality. As his defense mechanisms become less operational and the abuser recognizes significant positive behavioral changes within himself, he often develops internal motivation.

During the early phases of treatment, the sexual abuser should be referred by the courts or other legal agencies, including parole and probation offices and child protective services, in order to provide the necessary levels of initial motivation and commitment. Sexual abusers without external motivation, such as court-mandated therapy, often terminate treatment prematurely. Some of these offenders make the fatal mistake of believing that their problem has been spontaneously resolved through their arrest. During their incarceration, a number of these men also experience religious conversions and/or "see the light." Others profess an immediate cure through jailhouse counseling. These erroneous beliefs often lead to the reenactment of sexually deviant behavioral fantasies and behaviors. Therefore, from this clinical perspective, external controls and mandated therapy often provide the abuser with an opportunity to thoroughly examine the antecedents provoking these disruptive behavioral cycles and ways to control this behavioral disorder.

Compulsive aberrant behaviors cannot be effectively changed without external controls. Without these controls, the transitory guilt may quickly disappear as the abuser recognizes that his participation in this treatment program will disrupt his familiar and comfortable life-style.

One of the earliest steps employed to assess motivation is the development of a contractual agreement among the client, therapist, and court. This contract clearly stipulates that the sexual abuser will participate in a therapy program for a minimum of 1 year. During these 52 weeks, the sexual abuser will attend a minimum of one, 2-hour group behavioral therapy meetings a week. Married offenders with committed spouses will also participate in a weekly sexual enhancement group therapy program with other couples. Specific treatment objectives, methods, and goals are outlined in the contract.

Prior to entering this behavioral group therapy program, each sexual abuser participates in an individual behavioral program. During these weekly meetings, the candidate's level of motivation is further assessed. This program is designed to eradicate compulsive, deviant sexual behaviors that may be reinforced daily through masturbation and fantasy. Because the sexual abuser has engaged in deviant behavior patterns that are both asocial and illegal, this behavioral treatment focuses on the elimination of these deviant arousal patterns and behaviors through an effective treatment vehicle—aversive conditioning. Each client is asked to develop a detailed written description of one of his most erotic incidences that occurred with his victim. He is then fitted with a penile transducer and, as he reads or recites from memory his written description, his arousal is monitered on a penile plethysmograph. The technician notes precisely at what point arousal begins and the specific activity in the description that parallel arousal. The client and technician then review his arousal patterns and identify his earliest arousal point, usually about 5%.

The sexual abuser is then instructed to practice the following procedures two times daily at his home. He first recites the exact description of the sexual behavior that caused his earliest arousal. At that point, he stops and inhales spirits of ammonia. Immediately after his head clears, he repeats this procedure for a minimum of 20 times. The procedure is repeated 2 times a day, separated by at least 4 hours.

The client's progress is monitered weekly on a penile plethysmograph. As the sexual abuser demonstrates complete control over his previous arousal level at each point, he then moves to the next significant point of arousal (5% higher). This procedure is continued until the client can recite his complete sexual scenario without demonstrating any significant arousal (below 2%). If he demonstrates arousal to both sexes or very divergent behavior, several scenarios may be used one after the other in a similar fashion.

After several weeks of demonstrating arousal below 2%, the individual begins the second phase of his individual behavioral treatment program. This maintenance phase is to ensure that the individual maintains continuous control over his arousal. The maintenance procedures are very similar to the above aversion techniques except the ammonia vapor is not used. Instead, aversive fantasy is substituted for the pungent odor. The aversive fantasy is used during the most arousing aspect of the scenario and is described 20 times, as above.

This procedure is practiced every other day and monitored weekly. If arousal remains under control, this assignment is reduced to 20 times a week. The frequency of this procedure is slowly reduced until the sexual abuser is using this approach 2 to 3 times per month and continues to keep the deviant arousal patterns under control. After each homework session, the sexual abuser is asked to record his reaction on a behavioral chart. While evaluating his responses, each individual rates the (a) intensity of arousal to deviant themes; (b) the overall effectiveness of each aversive consequence; and (c) the rate at which he is able to complete each descriptive scenario; and (d) the amount of pleasure associated with the scenario. After the sexual abuser has learned how to control his aberrant arousal patterns by completing his homework assignments on a regular basis, he is then referred to the behavioral group therapy program.

Group Therapist

Each behavioral group therapy session is conducted by a male therapist. One of the more important responsibilities for this therapist is to provide the male abuser with an appropriate role model. The therapist should exemplify both comfort and confidence with his own social skills, gender identity, value systems, and repertoire of adult sexual responses. From our clinical viewpoint, the addition of a female co-therapist may dilute or erode the positive modeling that often occurs between the sexual abusers and the male therapist. In addition, the offenders' acute social sensitivity and lack of adequate social skills may reduce their abilities to actively participate in a behavioral group therapy program coordinated by male and female co-therapists.

Therapists coordinating these behavioral group treatment programs should have already learned, through structured professional training activities and supervised clinical experiences, how to coordinate behavioral group treatment programs. In addition, the group leader should have already acquired specialized training in the areas of sexual deviation and disorders, group therapy techniques, and behavioral treatment approaches.

Unfortunately, the recent increase in clients seeking assistance for their deviant sexual practices has attracted some therapists not fully trained to provide counseling for sexual abusers. Using questionable approaches, they often do not successfully modify their clients' aberrant behaviors. In addition, some group treatment programs are also based on the notion that sexual abusers can learn how to change their sexual habits from other group leaders who have experienced similar disorders.

From our clinical perspective, the therapist should not have a personal history of engaging in deviant illegal sexual behavior. The therapist should be perceived by his group members as a professional with sound ethical standards and an intact value system. The fact that a therapist has experienced legal and psychological problems similar to those of his client may cloud his judgment as a group therapist and leader. In other words, objective decisions may not be made by this therapist. If a group member reoffends, the subjective and biased therapist may decide to conceal the aberrant behaviors from the judiciary system. This questionable policy may lead to a decline in group morale and significantly impede the behavioral group therapy approach.

The "rehabilitated sex offender" group therapist may become a fanatical offender advocate. In this nonproductive role, he may lose his ability to provide a healthy role model. During group therapy meetings, he may not monitor important group guidelines and restrictions.

In addition, if the group leader reoffends, this inappropriate behavior will have a negative effect on the other group members. Some of the sexual abusers may feel that they will never be able to learn adequate behavioral controls. They may begin to believe that if their group therapist cannot learn how to control his behavior, how will they ever learn adaptive behavioral patterns.

In one treatment program, 3 of 6 ex-sex offender counselors eventually reoffended. One of these previously employed counselors was brutally killed by one of his intended victims. If these reoffenses had occurred while these men were conducting behavioral group treatment sessions, this deviant behavior would have had a disasterous effect on the other group members.

Ex-sexual offenders coordinating group treatment programs may develop a false sense of security as therapists; they may begin to believe that they are totally cured. While listening to the autobiographies, and observing the deviant arousal patterns of other group members, they may again experience deviant thoughts, feelings, and sexual arousal patterns.

These stimuli may eventually provoke a relapse. During this phase, the therapist may engage in an array of deviant and harmful sexual behavior including cultivating deviant thoughts, masturbating to these deviant cognitions, exposing, and inappropriately touching and sexually stimulating his victims.

Finally, when the therapist does reoffend, the total treatment program may be publically ostracized by an array of community critics and a group of well-intentioned fanatical citizens. Local referral sources, community agents, and the court may believe that the program director exercised poor judgment by hiring an ex-sec offender to direct and monitor treatment programs for his allies.

Behavioral Group Treatment Setting

The group members meet in a large, well-ventilated room free of obstructions, windows, or distractions. Identical chairs are arranged in a circle in this room. No smoking, eating, or drinking takes place during these structured 2-hour weekly meetings. Most of the group members will attend these meetings for at least 1 year. When a member graduates, new members are introduced into the group. The 2-hour group meetings are divided into two parts: a 1-hour teaching session; and a 1-hour group problem-solving session. An additional weekly meeting is held for offenders with spouses who are involved in a committed relationship, using a similar format.

Behavioral Group Treatment

Several initial problems experienced by group members must be carefully monitored by a therapist such as (a) low self-esteem; (b) depression; (c) minimization; (d) denial; and (e) high levels of anxiety. These defense mechanisms and learned behaviors are major components of the sexual abuser's psychopathology. Some clinicians (Schwartz & Masters, 1983) have implied that offenders participate in self-flagellation due to self-condemnation. From our clinical perspective, the anguish and discomfort is often caused by external factors, including the threat of divorce, incarceration, economical sanctions, community pressures, and other environmental barriers. Although the sexual abuser may initially demonstrate extreme anguish, this response is often superficial. Each member must take full responsibility for his own aberrant behavior and resist blaming authorities for his recent social demise. Therapists must avoid condemning the offender while at the same time identifying his maladaptive behaviors and cognitive distortions.

Throughout the first 2 months of this behavioral group therapy program, each group member is required to write an extensive autobiography and discuss these materials with the other participants. Throughout these discussions, the leader and other group members often confront the writer about the autobiography's accuracy and completeness. This written document serves to help the other group members gain an in-depth understanding of each offender's past sexual history. These written statements serve to help the abuser identify and understand the origin and reinforcing qualities of his deviant behaviors. Each group member must identify the antecedents influencing his pattern of deviant behavior in order to later gain adequate behavioral control.

During another behavioral group activity, each sexual abuser provides a detailed description of his deviant arousal patterns and past deviant behavior. The victim's descriptions in the police reports of the alleged sexual activities are then read aloud to all of the group members. The offender first accepts his deviant sexual behaviors and verbalizes this information to the other group members. This self-disclosure is an important step in learning how to accept responsibility for past deviant patterns. The offender's self-image is often improved when he finds that self-disclosure does not lead to condemnation or social rejection by the other group members.

In addition, the offenders perceive their simularities, dispell the belief that their behavior is unique, and develop a camaraderie with other group members. The sexual abusers begin to internalize the concept of *total responsibility* for their deviant behavior and recognize that there are similar identifiable patterns of deviant sexual behavior. As these insights occur, the group members recognize the need for behavioral change. These behavioral modifications often involve changing specific components of their life-style including (a) jobs; (b) clubs and organizations; (c) recreational activities; (d) friendships; and (e) family practices. The sexual abuser is then instructed to discuss these deviant patterns with other family members and/or close friends. This additional self-disclosure allows each member to demonstrate further acceptance of his deviant behavior. At the same time, each group member discusses his fears of rejection.

In order to understand the factors that reinforced and maintained their deviant sexual behavior, the offenders discuss their deviant behavioral cycles. These cycles are usually identified as each group member discusses his autobiography in group and describes the early components of his sexual deviancy. This self-revelation is then followed by a detailed analysis of the environmental factors and behaviors which preceded the deviant sexual behavior. Because the sexual abuser often experiences great difficulty in identifying his own behavioral patterns, his spouse or close associates are encouraged to assist in identifying these chains of behavior.

The sexual abuser's unrealistic expectations, irrational beliefs, and perceived rejections are assessed and confronted in conjunction with this behavioral cycle. The offender also identifies cognitive distortions that have been used to rationalize coercive, assaultive, and aberrant sexual behavior. The offender often excuses his deviant behavior because he feels "My wife is no longer interested in sex" or "My daughter did not really resist," "I was just teaching my daughter about sex," and "I was just showing my children how much I love them." These forms of distorted thinking are confronted by group members and challenged as to their accuracy, rationality, and alternative ways of interpreting situations. These cognitive distortions are one of the major factors enabling the offender to continue his deviant sexual behavior.

Social Skills Training

The sexual abuser has been previously characterized as a socially immature individual, often displaying deficits in social skills. Because an effective behavioral group therapy program depends on the members' ability to spontaneously and accurately communicate with others, basic communication skills training becomes an important feature of these group meetings. These sexual abusers often cannot initiate and maintain conversations, ask open-ended questions, maintain eye contact, gauge appropriate self-disclosure, actively listen, and give or receive compliments. In addition, some of these men cannot employ a variety of heterosexual dating skills, including asking a woman for a date, enjoying a wide range of recreational activities, and understanding the social reactions of others. They also have limited experience in demonstrating affection, in knowing how to sensitively touch a woman's body, and in understanding the technical aspects of a woman's sexuality. An effective group leader must both identify and teach these individuals these specific behavioral skills (McGovern & Burkhard, 1976). With this training, the offender can more effectively discuss his sexual needs and meet the expectations of his adult sexual partners.

Typical Group Meeting

Meetings are called to order by a specific group member, who is assigned the group leadership responsibility. This leadership role lasts for approximately 2 months and this responsibility is rotated among group members throughout the course of the year. Meetings begin with a brief review of weekly activities, which include a discussion of the behavioral assignments, sexual behaviors, social activities, work responsibilities, and recreational activities. Special problems are identified and placed on the evening agenda for further discussion.

After reviewing individual problems, the second half of the group meeting is devoted to social skills training. Each specific area of training is preceded by an assessment technique and a brief discussion of the importance of acquiring these new skills. This lecture and/or presentation is followed by reading assignments and concurrent behavioral assignments. As each reading assignment is completed, the group members discuss the specific topic, raise questions, and learn new behaviors modeled by the therapist. These skills are then practiced through behavioral rehearsal exercises and discussed by each member in the group. Each individual is encouraged to practice these newly acquired behavioral skills in the community between each behavioral group treatment session. These behavioral homework assignments are discussed during the following therapy meeting. Practice sessions continue until each group member has learned a series of appropriate social skills. Each member continues to rehearse their social skills until a point when the group members perceive that adequate progress has been made.

Each member tracks his behavioral success on specially designed forms for each specific skill area. These forms contain information about the time, date, frequency, setting, and outcome of each specific skill practice. The results are charted weekly on a group bulletin board so that each member can monitor the behavioral successes of other group members, as well as his own. The specific skills areas include, but are not limited to, communication skills, assertiveness training, behavior change strategies, sexual awareness training, dating skills, cognitive restructuring, anger management, and empathy training. Group meetings generally end with homework assignments dealing with the specific behavior and topics under discussion that week.

Homework Assignments

At the end of each group therapy session, the group members are given a set of homework assignments to complete before the next scheduled session. For example, a typical social skills assignment would consist of asking each group member to initiate five different conversations with 5 strangers and to maintain that conversation for at least 1 minute. A behavioral manual with specific communication exercises provides the group members with specialized communication guidelines (McGovern, Arkowitz, & Gilmore, 1975).

After each homework assignment has been completed, the group members are instructed to write out their reactions to these structured exercises on a specific evaluation form. The group members are asked to record the time, place, situation, and reactions of the respondent, as well as the client's perceptions about these social interactions. These completed forms are brought to the next therapy session. These written reports are then reviewed and discussed by group members. By reviewing these materials each week, the group members and therapist will understand what (a) assignments have been completed; (b) problems have occurred; (c) therapeutic gains have been experienced; and (d) skills to be practiced in the future. After these discussions have occurred, the therapist and group members plan their next homework assignment.

Materials

Because group members often lack adequate information about human sexual behavior, the treatment program is complemented by an array of audiovisual materials and books. As the group members begin to discuss their own sexual concerns, feelings, and discomforts, articles, manuals, films, and slides are provided. As the group participants read these materials and discuss their perceptions and attitudes within the group structure, they begin to feel more comfortable about their own sexuality.

By reviewing these resources, they can more effectively examine their attitudes and perceptions. Although the other group members and the therapist can serve as reference points, the group members are often reassured about their belief systems when they have an opportunity to read about their concerns in legitimate books and articles. A specific chapter or article may alleviate more anxiety than any group discussion or statement made by a treating therapist. Some of the books utilized are *Male Sexuality* (Zilbergeld, 1978), which dispels certain sexual myths and reviews a number of sensible components regarding normal sexual functioning, and *Your Perfect Right* (Alberti & Emmons, 1970), which discusses assertiveness training and communication skills. This latter resource is used as a model for those group members who need to develop spontaneous and fluent communication skills. *The New Guide to Rational Living* (Ellis & Harper, 1978) serves to help the group members assess their own irrational thoughts and beliefs. The reader gains a better understanding of how specific cognitive messages can maintain deviant or nonproductive behavior. In addition to these basic texts, each group member reads and discusses a variety of articles, audiovisual materials, and films that are intermittently presented throughout the behavioral group treatment program.

A Farrel Instrument Sexual Plotter (Laws & Osborne, 1983) is used periodically to assess group members' sexual arousal patterns. By utilizing this assessment procedure, the group therapist can consistently assess any changes in each group member's sexual arousal patterns and determine if the homework assignments have been effective. During the course of treatment, each group member learns how to extinguish his deviant patterns and becomes highly aroused by normal and healthy adult sexual materials.

Maintenance Programs

Covert behavioral conditioning is a separate treatment component designed to ensure behavior maintenance. This procedure consists of the periodic practice of covert sensitization and covert modeling techniques that are utilized on a regular basis by each group member once arousal has been reduced to acceptable levels through olfactory aversive conditioning (Jensen, 1983).

To decrease a behavior using covert sensitization, maladaptive behavior (such as sexual contact with children) is paired in the imagination with an aversive event (Cautela, 1966). It is expected that through this pairing the behavior will become aversive and the client will avoid the undesirable behavior. The client is first expected to write down a detailed description of the problematic behavior and the surrounding events. He is then instructed to develop an aversive event that is both meaningful to him and extremely aversive. It is most effective when this aversive event is both a possible consequence to the behavior and is easily maintained in fantasy.

In the case of sexually deviant behavior with children, the client would read his description of the chain of behaviors and thoughts leading up to sexual contact with the child, while attempting to imagine these as clearly as possible. At the point of sexual contact with the child, he then imagines the aversive event, such as being dragged off in handcuffs by the police, having his wife walk in and find him involved sexually with a child, or having the father of the child assault him brutally.

This procedure is practiced 20 times every other day, and arousal is monitored weekly. If arousal remains under control, practice is reduced to 2 times a week. Covert modeling (Hay, Hay & Nelson, 1977) is employed after it has been demonstrated that covert sensitization is maintaining control over undesirable sexual arousal. *Covert modeling* is a technique in which the client imagines himself successfully coping with a previously maladaptive behavior. In the case of a child molestor, a typical example of covert modeling might involve the following fantasy: The client has gone to a playground where he has previously molested children. He is walking through the playground and sees a child isolated from his playmates and very attractive. He begins to approach the child but suddenly increases his stride and walks past the child and continues on out of the area. He feels good that he has controlled his urge to molest and relieved to be away from temptation. This procedure may be alternated with covert sensitization and practiced 20 times once a week.

In addition to this procedure, each offender is instructed to practice avoidance of those particular individuals and/or settings that can evoke or stimulate deviant arousal patterns and behaviors. In a number of cases, the offender may have to limit the degree of physical contact that he has with his own children. He may also have to change his social activities, form of employment, and/or his avocational avenues. The offender cannot place himself in situations where he has access to deviant erotic stimuli, environmental cues, or potential victims.

Each offender is also taught to remove himself from a situation where he begins to become aroused to potential victims. Finally, he should utilize the olfactory aversion conditioning techniques for 3 to 5 days or until such time that the deviant arousal patterns can be corrected.

Because this behavioral group treatment is a long-term program, lasting at least 1 year, this approach ensures the habituation of appropriate recreational, social, and leisure activities as well as constant monitoring of deviant and appropriate sexual behavior. Before each sexual abuser is discharged from his treatment program, he is required to submit a plan which outlines his employment goals, recreational activities, avocational pursuits, his methods to avoid deviant arousal patterns, and guidelines to insure the maintenance of all desirable treatment goals.

In addition to adhering to these maintenance procedures, group participants are encouraged to attend follow-up therapy meetings. Because these behavioral treatment groups are open-ended and ongoing, group sessions are always available to each offender, especially when he feels the need or desire to participate. During these meetings, each participant's accomplishments and particular problems will be discussed and monitored. By attending these follow-up sessions and adhering to these maintenance procedures, group participants can obtain the maximum benefit from their behavioral group therapy program.

Marital-Sexual Enhancement Meetings

In addition to the initial behavioral therapy sessions and the weekly behavioral group therapy programs, the sex offenders with intact marriages, or a committed relationship, attend a second weekly behaviorally orientated group meeting coordinated by a woman sex therapist certified by the American Association of Sex Educators, Counselors and Therapists. These additional group meetings have four primary goals: (a) to better educate the spouse regarding her husband's aberrant behavior; (b) to discuss effective ways to resolve their marital and sexual problems; (c) to help the offender and his spouse identify cycles of problem behavior and effective intervention methods to insure control of problem behavior; and (d) to improve the quality of communication within the family unit. The couples attending these group meetings learn a number of valuable behavioral interventions that enhance their sexual relationship (McGovern, 1979).

The first major problem facing the therapist during these meetings is the spouse's denial and minimization of her husband's deviant behavior. In many cases, the husband has led his wife to believe that the criminal charges are grossly inaccurate and/or overstated. The wife often reinforces her husband's distorted perceptions and unwittingly undermines the treatment program. Consequently, the spouse's distorted perceptions are first reviewed. She is then given a detailed explanation of her husband's deviant arousal patterns, aberrant behaviors, and a summary of his autobiography. The spouse is then informed about his deviant behavioral cycles and how they have been unknowingly reinforced by the spouse.

The couple then learn how to improve their communication and develop higher levels of self-esteem. Each spouse's developmental history is explored in detail, and past sexual patterns are discussed. As these cycles are reviewed, the spouse may become quite angry, shameful, or blatantly distraught about her husband's sexual pathology. As the spouse becomes more communicative, she is able to more directly deal with her anger and frustration. Both husband and wife are encouraged to develop more active social lives together and also a personal support system outside the marital relationship. It is felt that a broad support system offers an opportunity to be more independent and allows each spouse a greater sense of self worth.

During the early phase of this form of intervention, couples often exaggerate their sexual satisfaction with each other. However, after an extensive period of time, the couples more realistically identify and discuss problematic areas. After the couples have carefully assessed their sexual dissatisfactions and concerns, the group is given a series of exercises to complete that will enhance their sexual relationship. These basic behavioral exercises begin with sensate focus exercises, a progressive and gradual form of experiencing tactile pleasure in erogenous and nonerogenous body areas. These sensual activities are discussed during the group meetings and then practiced at home. Each group member learns how to more affectionately touch his partner's body. Through these sensate focus exercises, a previously threatening task may be transformed into an enjoyable sensual experience (Masters & Johnson, 1970). These exercises gradually reduce anxiety and pressure experienced by the sexual abuser.

Although these early touching experiences are often described by the couple as very mechanical, the sexual partners learn how to provide each other with a variety of pleasurable and actually satisfying adult sexual behaviors. As the sexual abuser is able to satisfy his sexual desires with a consenting adult partner and recognizes the harm done to his victim, he is no longer driven to deviant sexual behavior. The sexual abuser begins to realize that aberrant illegal sexual behaviors have acquired too many adverse characteristics including legal sanctions (legal fees and incarceration), adverse social consequences (protective custody agencies), and social ostracization (adverse reactions by employers, relatives, and the local media). The offender recognizes the significant and often lifelong expenses and liabilities related to abusive sexual patterns.

Limitations

The primary limitations of this multidimensional behavioral group therapy program appear to be the extensive amount of time required, the cost, and individual committment on the part of all involved. The offender may spend as many as 5 hours per week involved in treatment and an additional 10 hours completing his homework assignments. His wife will also be involved in at least 2 hours of therapy a week and is expected to complete a series of homework assignments that take her approximately 5 hours per week. This program can also be financially taxing considering the expenses of the individual therapy sessions, the group therapy sessions, the reading materials, and the physiological evaluations. However, the majority of individuals attending this program have acquired, at best, modest incomes.

The other major limitation includes the current size of each treatment group. Each behavioral therapy group for the male offenders normally consists of between 10 and 15 individuals. Some group members complain that the large group interferes with their willingness to discuss their intimate concerns in a timely fashion. However, due to the lengthy involvement with the group therapy sessions, most issues and problems are eventually resolved as each individual learns a multitude of positive skills. Although these programs are time consuming and expensive, they are a sensible alternative to long-term incarceration and to continued sexual abuse of unwilling victims.

Advantages

This multifaceted approach appears to have a number of advantages. Although some clients complain about program restrictions, length of therapy, a multidimensional approach, and financial considerations, this program offers a feasible alternative to long-term residential placement or incarceration. From our clinical perspective, a multidimensional behavioral treatment approach allows the group members to address their numerous problems and concerns. Clients attending these groups will also learn that their past and present sexual thoughts and behaviors are not totally unique. Many are concerned that other individuals with similar backgrounds are not bothered by fears, anxieties, or inadequacies. Although therapists treating sexually deviant individuals in individual therapy normally take a sexual history, these clients do not have an opportunity to contrast their past history with other clients in a group therapy program. With this approach, group participants can compare their sexual histories and their present sexual thoughts and behaviors with other group members. Through self-disclosure, the offenders and therapists realize that most of these abusers have experienced sexual dissatisfaction and have been involved in an array of deviant sexual behaviors.

Another major advantage is that the group serves as an important source of continuous support and reinforcement. As the members identify and change their dysfunctional attitudes, perceptions and/or behaviors, they receive high levels of support and encouragement from other group members. Because group members are working toward similar goals, each of the participants can provide valuable insights, thoughts, and suggestions to enhance the therapeutic process. In many cases, group members provide major contributions that allow significant personal growth and major behavioral changes.

In addition, unwanted sexual arousal patterns are dealt with quickly and effectively. One of the first steps in this treatment program is for each individual to examine and modify his deviant arousal patterns. From the beginning of treatment, the client develops an immediate therapeutic relationship with the therapist. In addition, each group member learns how to effectively and efficiently modify his deviant arousal patterns through aversive conditioning. For most clients, this approach offers each group member his first opportunity to be enrolled in a comprehensive treatment program. Each group member learns a number of important behavioral skills, to enhance his self-concept, modify his distorted perceptions, reverse his deviant arousal patterns, and acquire an array of healthy sexual thoughts, fantasies, attitudes, and behaviors.

Sexual abusers attending this comprehensive program can, in most cases, learn how to control deviant arousal patterns and acquire adaptive sexual attitudes and behaviors. Each member can also acquire more effective marital adult-oriented sexual relationships. Through this behavioral group therapy program, members can overcome their sexual dysfunctions and acquire more positive adult sexual skills.

As the members begin to learn more functional attitudes and/or behaviors, they receive much encouragement from the other group members. They develop close alliances and are, for the first time in their lives, able to fully admit to the extent of their unusual and unacceptable sexual behaviors. As each client moves through the program, he is taught definite behavioral skills. While practicing these positive behaviors on a regular basis, the offender acquires a more comfortable and prosocial life-style, which includes meaningful adult relationships with both men and women. Most importantly, the sexual offender is able to develop a positive self-image, learn a series of appropriate behaviors, and realize that, for the first time in his life, he can control his own destiny.

Finally, the married members with cooperative spouses also learn how to develop more rewarding sexual relationships with their spouses. Their major sexual problems, including orgasmic dysfunctions, arousal disorders, erectile failure, rapid ejaculation, and an array of other sexual concerns, are identified and resolved through a behavioral group treatment program. In addition, the men without cooperating partners are encouraged to develop close intimate relationships with compatible adult partners. Their social and sexual concerns are also identified, discussed, and resolved through the course of their behavioral group treatment program.

Summary

Because the advent of Masters and Johnson's treatment program, clinicians have developed an array of individual and behavioral group treatment programs. Although the initial behavioral group treatment programs were developed for individuals and couples impaired by sexual concerns and dysfunctions, behaviorists are beginning to examine the efficiency of behavioral group treatment approaches for individuals impaired by aberrant sexual arousal patterns and deviant sexual behaviors. Although these innovative approaches are being carefully developed and evaluated, the preliminary results suggest that these approaches provide the clinician with an array of valuable clinical treatment procedures. By utilizing these behavioral treatment modalities, most sexual dysfunctions and disorders can be effectively ameliorated. Individuals experiencing significant sexual dysfunctions, disorders, and/or impairments, can learn healthy and satisfying sexual beliefs, thoughts, attitudes, emotional reactions, and behaviors by acquiring adaptive cognitions and behaviors while attending behavioral group treatment programs.

Acknowledgements

The authors thank Gayla Montgomery, Lannita Coberley, Judy Welch and Cory Jewell for their helpful assistance during the preparation of this manuscript.

References

Abel, G. Assessment of sexual duration in the male. In M. Hersen & A. S. Bellack (Eds.), *Behavioral assessment; A practical handbook.* New York: Pergamon Press, 1976.

Alberti, R. E., & Emmons, M. L. *Your perfect right.* San Luis Obispo, California: Impact, 1970.

Barbach, L. G. Group treatment of preorgasmic women. *Journal of Sex and Marital Therapy,* 1974, *1,* 139–145.

Cautela, J. R. Treatment of compulsive behavior by covert sensitization. *Psychological Record,* 1966, *16,* 33–41.

Ellis, A., & Harper, R. *A new guide to rational living.* Englewood Cliffs, NJ: Prentice-Hall, 1978.

Finkelhor, D. *Sexually victimized children.* New York: Free Press, 1979.

Giarretto, H. A comprehensive child sexual abuse treatment program. In P. B. Mnayck & C. H. Kempe (Eds.), *Sexually abused children and their families.* New York: Pergamon Press, 1981.

Hay, W. M., Hay, L. R., & Nelson, P. O. The adoption of covert modeling procedures to the treatment of chronic alcoholism and obsessive compulsive behavior. *Behavior Therapy,* 1977, *8,* 70–76.

Heiman, J. Use of psycho-physiological exploration of sexual arousal patterns in males and females. *Psychophysiology,* 1977, *14,* 266–274.

Henson, C., Rubin, H. G., & Henson, C. Womens' sexual arousal concurrently assessed by three genital measures. *Archives of Sexual Behavior*, 1979, *8*, 459–469.

Jankovich, R., & Miller, P. R. Response of women with primary orgasmic dysfunction to audiovisual education. *Journal of Sex and Marital Therapy*, 1978, *4*, 16.

Jensen, S. *A behavioral treatment program for residential sexual offenders*. Paper presented at the symposium sponsored by the Northwest Treatment Association, Seattle, WA, September, 1983.

Kanfer, F., & Saslow, G. Behavioral diagnosis. In C. M. Franks (Eds.), *Behavior therapy: Appraisal and status*. New York: McGraw-Hill Book Company, 1969.

Kilmann, P. R., Mills, K. H., Bella, B., Caid, C., Davidson, E., Drose, G., & Wanless, R. *Effectiveness of different treatments on women with secondary orgasmic dysfunction*. Paper presented at the meeting of the American Psychological Association, Anaheim, CA, 1983.

Kuriansky, J. B. & Sharpe, L., Clinical and research implications of the evaluation of women s group therapy for anogasmia: A review. *Journal of Sex and Marital Therapy*, 1981, *7*, 268.

Laws, P. R., & Osborne, C. A. How to build and operate a behavioral laboratory to evaluate and treat sexual deviance. In J. G. Green & I. R., Stuart's *The Sexual aggressor: Current perspectives on treatment*. New York: Von Nostrand Reinhold Company, 1983.

Lobitz, W. C., & Baker, E. L. Group treatment of single males with erectile dysfunction. *Archives of Sexual Behavior*, 1979, *8*, 127.

Lobitz, C., & LoPiccolo, J. L. New methods in the behavioral treatment of sexual dysfunction. *Journal of Behavior Therapy and Experimental Psychiatry*, 1972, *39*, 265.

LoPiccolo, J., & LoPiccolo, L. (Eds.). *Handbook of sex therapy*. New York: Plenum Press, 1978.

MacDonald, G. J., & de Furia, G. (1971). A guided self-help approach to the treatment of the habitual sex offender. *Hospital & Community Psychiatry*, *10*, 34–37.

Masters, W. H., & Johnson, V. E. (1970). *Human sexual inadequacy*. Boston: Little, Brown.

McGovern, K. B. (1979). An analysis of behavioral group treatment programs designed to modify sexual dysfunction. In P. Upper & S. Ross (Eds.), *Behavior group therapy: An annual review*. Champaign, IL: Research Press Company.

McGovern, K. B. The assessment of sexual deviations and disorders. In B. Maletzky (Ed.), *The behavioral treatment of deviant sexual behavior* (in preparation).

McGovern, K. B., Arkowitz, H., & Gilmore, S. The evaluation of social skill training programs for college dating inhibitions. *Journal of Counseling Psychology*, 1975, *22*, 505.

McGovern, K., & Burkhard, J. Initiating social contact with the opposite sex. In J. D. Krumboltz & C. R. Thoresen (Eds.), *Counseling Methods*. New York: Holt, Rinehart & Winston, 1976.

McGovern, K. B., Kirkpatrick, C. C, & LoPiccolo, J. A behavioral group treatment program for sexually dysfunctional couples. *Journal of Marital and Family Counseling*, 1976, *2*, 397.

Mills, K. H., & Kilmann, P. R. Group treatment of sexual dysfunctions: A methodological review of the outcome literature. *Journal of Sex & Marital Therapy*, 1982, *8*, 259.

Powell, L. C., Blakeney, P., Craft, H., & Pullian, G. P. Rapid treatment approach to human sexual inadequacy. *American Journal of Obstetrics & Gynecology*, 1974, *119*, 87.

Prithers, W. D., Marquis, J. K., Gilat, C. C., & Marlatt, A. Relapse prevention with sexual aggressives: A self-control model of treatment and maintenance of change. In J. Green & I. Stuart (Eds.), *The sexual aggressor: Current perspectives on treatment*. New York: Van Nostrand Reinhold Co., Inc., 1983.

Sarrel, P., & Masters, W. Sexual Molestation of men by women. *Archives of Sexual Behavior*, 1982, *11*, 117–132.

Saylor, M. *Guided self-help approach to treatment of the habitual sexual offender*. A paper presented to the *Twelfth Cropwood Conference*, December, 1979.

Saylor, M. Sex offender treatment program: Treatment success and recividism rates between 1967 and 1982. Unpublished manuscript, Western State Hospital, Sexual Psychopathy Program, Ft. Steilacoom, WA, 1984.

Schneidman, B., & McGuire, L. Group therapy for nonorgasmic women: Two age levels. *Archives of Sexual Behavior*, 1976, *5*, 239.

Schwartz, M., & Masters, W. Conceptual factors in the treatment of paraphilias: A preliminary report. *Journal of Sex and Marital Therapy*, 1983, *9*, 1.

Wolpe, J. & Lazarus, A. *Behavior therapy techniques: A guide to the treatment of neurosis.* New York: Pergamon, 1966.

Zeiss, R. A., Christensen, A., & Levine, A. G. Treatment for premature ejaculation through male-only groups. *Journal of Sex and Marital Therapy*, 1978, *4*, 139.

Zilbergeld, B. *Male sexuality*. New York: Bantam Books, 1978.

Zilbergeld, B. & Kilmann, P. R. The scope and effectiveness of sex therapy. *Psychotherapy: Therapy Research & Practice*, 1984, *21*, 319–326.

14

Behavioral Group Therapy for Anxiety Disorders

Paul M. G. Emmelkamp and Antoinette C. M. Kuipers

In this chapter, the group application of behavioral and cognitive procedures in the treatment of anxiety-based disorders will be discussed. Many studies have involved group therapy of mildly disturbed college students, but the emphasis here will be on application in clinical settings. The term *patient* is used throughout this chapter when clinical anxiety or fears are involved; otherwise the term *subject* is used.

We will focus on the group application of treatment procedures, and those readers who are unfamiliar with the treatment of anxiety-based disorders are advised to refer to Emmelkamp (1982) for details of the therapeutic procedures and a review of outcome studies.

The organization of the chapter is as follows. Separate sections are devoted to the group therapy of anxiety states, agoraphobia, social anxiety, specific phobias, and obsessive-compulsive disorder, respectively. In each of these sections studies involving group therapy will be critically evaluated. We will further give some clinical guidelines and discuss issues and problems that are likely to arise in doing group therapy. Finally, general issues and future directions will be discussed, including social cohesion, cost-effectiveness of group therapy versus individual treatment, and indications and contraindications for group therapy.

Anxiety States

According to DSM-III, anxiety states are divided into two categories: generalized anxiety disorder and panic disorder. The essential feature of generalized anxiety disorder is generalized, persistent anxiety. Panic disorders are characterized by recurrent panic attacks for which the person has no explanation himself or herself, and which occur outside typically phobic situations.

PAUL M. G. EMMELKAMP • Academic Hospital, Groningen, Netherlands. ANTOINETTE C. M. KUIPERS • Psychiatric Hospital "Lichten Kracht," Assen, Netherlands.

Generalized Anxiety Disorder

Relatively little attention has been paid to the problem of chronic, general anxiety. Most of the work in this area has focused on relaxation techniques. More recently the group application of cognitive procedures on generalized anxiety has been reported.

Relaxation

Positive results of group treatment by progressive muscle relaxation for general anxiety have been reported by Lehrer, Schoicket, Carrington, and Woolfolk (1980) and Woolfolk, Lehrer, McCann, and Rooney (1982). In both studies relaxation was equally as effective as meditation.

Others have stressed the importance of teaching relaxation as a coping skill. Clients are trained to recognize the physiological cues of tension and to apply relaxation whenever tension is perceived. A fundamental assumption shared by these various relaxation techniques (e.g., applied relaxation, anxiety management, and cue-controlled relaxation) is that patients learn an active coping skill that they can apply in a variety of anxiety-arousing situations in daily life. Applied relaxation, anxiety management, and cue-controlled relaxation conducted in groups all have been found successful in the treatment of generalized anxiety (e.g., Hutchings, Denney, Basgall, & Houston, 1980; Spoth & Meade, 1981). Apart from the subjects in the Lehrer *et al.* (1980) and Woolfolk *et al.* (1982) study, who were recruited through local newspaper advertisements or were referred by mental health professionals, the subjects in the other studies were student volunteers solicited for participation.

Daley, Bloom, Deffenbacher, and Stewart (1983) investigated the relative effectiveness of anxiety management training conducted in large versus small groups with generally anxious students as subjects. Anxiety-management training consisted of seven weekly 60-minute sessions and was either administered in groups of 10 subjects or in a group of 27 subjects. Small-group anxiety management reduced general anxiety, whereas large-group anxiety management evidenced no significant anxiety reduction. Although the studies reviewed here demonstrate the utility of group application of relaxation, there is no information available on the relative efficacy of group versus individual training in relaxation skills.

Clinical Guidelines for Relaxation Groups

In our experience a useful group therapy format is 8 to 10 weekly sessions in groups of six to eight patients, each session lasting about 60 minutes. After group, members introduce themselves, an explanation of the purpose of relaxation training is provided. After this introductory group discussion, patients are trained using a shortened version of the progressive muscle relaxation procedure. In this procedure, the patients learn to relax one muscle group at a time by first tensing the muscles of that group and then releasing tension.

Relaxation is carried out in the group with the patients in comfortable chairs. After 30 minutes of relaxation practice, patients are invited to share their experiences, and at the end of the sessions agreements are made on homework practice. Patients are provided with tapes of relaxation instructions in order to practice the relaxation at home twice daily between sessions for 20 to 30 minutes. In the first sessions, the emphasis is on the learning of the relaxation skills, and the application in stressful situations is not yet recommended.

In the course of the treatment, the time required for patients to become relaxed becomes shorter. The preliminary tensing of muscles can be omitted after a few sessions. It is important not to proceed faster than the level of the patient who makes the least progress in the group. Therefore, we generally use two trainers in order to be able to continuously observe all patients. If a patient makes no progress at all in the group (for example, due to excessive social anxiety), it might be necessary to take this patient out of the group and treat him or her individually; otherwise the progress of the other group members would be unnecessarily delayed.

Patients can be of considerable support to each other. Before actual relaxation practice commences in each session, the group is encouraged to discuss the problems met during practice at home. One of the major problems encountered is the difficulty some patients have in finding the necessary time to do their exercises. Other patients often act as models by showing these patients how they handled this problem in their own family. Further, group members, especially in cohesive groups, motivate each other to do their daily practice. When a patient does not feel attracted to the group and she or he cannot be motivated by the group members to do her or his homework assignments properly, individual treatment may be more appropriate.

After the relaxation exercises have been practiced in the group, the members are asked to share feedback, and the group discussion is centered around experiences and possible problems encountered during these exercises. Group members are asked if they found it more difficult to relax some muscles than others, and if so, they receive special homework assignments to practice relaxing these particular muscle groups.

Once relaxation has been learned, patients are instructed to use it in real-life situations when they feel tense or anxious. In group discussions, patients are taught to identify specific sources of stress related to their anxiety and to apply relaxation as a coping skill.

Anxious patients who are characterized by Type A behavior deserve our special attention. Although relaxation can be particularly suited to reduce their stress and Type A behavior (e.g., Suinn & Bloom, 1978), these patients are often difficult in relaxation groups due to their impatience and sense of time urgency. It is very important that these patients take sufficient time (both in the therapy sessions and at home) to relax and that they do not rush through the exercises in a few minutes.

Cognitive Restructuring

Woodward and Jones (1980) carried out a controlled clinical trial investigating the effectiveness of group cognitive restructuring and a modified systematic desensitization procedure. Subjects were general anxiety patients attending an outpatient clinic. Treatment consisted of eight group sessions (one per week), each session lasting approximately 1¼ hours. Groups were composed of seven patients each. In the cognitive restructuring group, the nature of self-defeating statements and irrational beliefs were discussed, and patients also cognitively rehearsed self-instructional ways of handling anxiety by means of an imagination procedure. Clients were asked to imagine an anxiety-provoking situation as vividly as possible and to replace their negative self-statements with coping self-statements. The desensitization group differed from the cognitive group in the means of coping employed: Relaxation was used instead of coping self-statements. Patients had to visualize themselves in an anxiety-provoking situation and to imagine themselves coping by using relaxation. In a third treatment group, both styles of coping (i.e., relaxation and cognitive self-statements) were trained. The combined procedure improved significantly more than the other two active treatments and the control group. Cognitive restructuring failed to result in any improvement.

Shaffer, Shapiro, Sank, and Coghlan (1981) compared the effectiveness of group cognitive treatment, individual cognitive treatment, and interpersonal group psychotherapy. Subjects were patients who were referred for treatment of anxiety and/or depression. The cognitive group received relaxation, cognitive restructuring, and assertion training. In the individual cognitive treatment condition, the therapist chose only those techniques that were felt to be appropriate. The interpersonal group psychotherapy was nondirective and encouraged group interaction. Although all three treatments resulted in a significant reduction in depression and anxiety, no significant differences between conditions were found. Thus, cognitive therapy conducted in groups was neither superior to individual cognitive therapy nor to interpersonal group psychotherapy. Taken together, the results of these two clinical studies indicate that there is insufficient evidence to assume that a cognitive group is particularly suited to the treatment of general anxiety.

Panic Disorder

Common symptoms of anxiety and panic are dyspnea, palpitations, chest pain, dizziness, sweating, fainting, and fear of dying or going crazy. Many of these symptomes are also common with hyperventilation. Although panic disorders are often associated with hyperventilation, it is unclear whether hyperventilation is a physiological determinant of panic disorder or merely a somatic concomitant of the anxiety experienced. The concept of the vicious circle effect may be helpful to understand the course of the hyperventilation after the first hyperventilation attack. Once initiated, hyperventilation may produce stimuli that lead to reactions that rearouse or intensify the hyperventilation. A hyperventilation attack is usually accompanied by severe anxiety that by itself may provoke hyperventilation in the future.

Clinical Guidelines for Hyperventilation Groups

Recently, we have begun to treat such patients (i.e., those whose anxiety is associated with hyperventilation) in groups. Before starting with such a treatment program, a medical checkup is recommended in order to screen out other organic conditions that may be associated with the symptoms. Further, it might be wise to have patients sign a disclaimer to protect the therapist legally in case a particularly litigious patient were to complain about this form of treatment. Groups of eight patients meet for 10 weeks once a week and are led by two therapists. Each group session lasts 2 hours. The first two sessions are devoted to giving patients a better understanding of the relationship between hyperventilation and anxiety. A videotape of the treatment of hyperventilation is shown, and patients receive a booklet with information on the hyperventilation syndrome. Most patients believe that they have a serious medical disease (e.g., heart attack, tumor). For a number of patients, just being informed about the nature of the symptoms is sufficient to let them relabel the somatic symptoms as *hyperventilation,* which can result in reduced anxiety (cognitive restructuring).

During the group discussions, each patient is given time to express himself or herself. Patients who monopolize the discussion by complaining about their somatic symptoms have to be cut short. A useful strategy is to ask another patient what she or he thought about what the other person was saying. Group members are often better able than therapists to convince another group member that the problem is psychological rather than medical because most of them have previously had similar thoughts themselves. Starting with the first session, patients are requested to keep a structured diary of the hyperventilation attacks, anxiety level, and the condition under which the hyperventilation occurs. It is important for the patient to fill out his or her diary regularly so that he or she does not need to recall events. Inspection of the diary may reveal significant associations between hyperventilation and particular stressful events.

In the third session, the marital partner or another trusted person is invited to join in the group session. Most significant others are willing to participate. The nature of the hyperventilation syndrome is theoretically explained. The relationship between breathing and the symptoms is shown by provoking a hyperventilation attack with each patient individually in the presence of her or his partner. Partners are instructed how they can assist in stopping the hyperventilation by having the patient breathe for a few minutes into a small plastic bag.

In the following sessions, the provocation of hyperventilation is repeated, first with each patient individually, later with all the group members together. The provocation is quite useful to directly show the patients the relationship between hyperventilation and their symptoms, and thus this may lead to relabeling of the symptoms and hence to a reduction of the anxiety associated with them. The symptoms usually appear within a few minutes of provoked hyperventilation, although often to a lesser degree than when the patients are at home. Starting with the fourth session, patients are trained in self-control techniques to deal with the hyperventilation; these include relaxation and breathing exercises. Patients are trained to breathe out passively and to insert a short rest period after each respiratory cycle. Further, in discussing the diaries of each patient, group members help each other to trace connections between stressful conditions and hyperventilation.

Although a formal evaluation has not yet been conducted, most patients appear to benefit from these groups. Generally, at the end of treatment the frequency of the hyperventilation attacks and the anxiety accompanying them are reduced. However, not all patients are suited for group treatment. For example, patients who continuously complain about their somatic symptoms or who really faint may have a negative influence on the group and can be better treated individually. Other patients who may benefit more from individual treatment are patients who are excessively socially anxious in groups.

Agoraphobia

Agoraphobia refers to a syndrome in which the most characteristic feature is attacks of anxiety or panic in a variety of public places such as streets, crowds, stores, buses, and the like that cause "fear of fear" and lead to an avoidance of these situations.

Group treatment of agoraphobia has become quite popular in the last few years. Group therapy has involved exposure *in vivo,* cognitive restructuring, and assertive training.

Exposure *in Vivo*

The first pilot study investigating behavioral group therapy for agoraphobics was reported by Watson, Mullett, and Pillay (1973). Three groups of patients (5–7 per group) received three weekly sessions, each of which included 3 hours of active treatment consisting of exposure to imaginal phobic stimulation (flooding) and exposure to real phobic situations. Although this group program was quite effective, analyses revealed that the imaginal part was superfluous.

Hand, Lamontagne, and Marks (1974) investigated whether social cohesion could facilitate improvement in exposure *in vivo* groups. Twenty-five agoraphobics were randomly assigned to two differing group exposure *in vivo* conditions. In the *cohesive* groups, the patients met as a group with the therapist. Task-oriented group discussion was stimulated before, during, and after exposure sessions. Therapist–patient interaction was kept to a minimum. Exposure *in vivo* consisted of exposing patients in groups to situations that are anxiety arousing for agoraphobics (e.g., walking in busy streets, buses, shopping, etc.). In the cohesive groups, patients supported each other during exposure *in vivo*. In the *unstructured* groups, attempts were made to prevent group cohesion from developing. Patients met each other only before they were taken out into the phobic situation. During exposure *in vivo,* patients were separated as much as possible and were asked not to talk together about their phobias or other problems. Before, during and after exposure sessions the patients discussed therapeutic problems individually with their therapist.

The two forms of group exposure *in vivo* led to differential social cohesion. Group cohesion as measured by questionnaires during treatment sessions was significantly greater in cohesive groups than in structured groups. Patients rated the group as more helpful than the therapist, and patients in the cohesive groups reported fewer urges to escape than did those in the unstructured groups. However, contrary to prediction, unstructured groups did as well as cohesive groups at posttest. At 3 and 6 months follow-up, patients from the cohesive groups continued to improve, whereas some patients from the unstructured groups relapsed. Follow-up data from one of the three cohesive groups were not gathered. If this group of patients contained more severe patients than the other two groups, the apparent continuing improvement at follow-up could be due to artifactual reasons, as suggested by Teasdale, Walsh, Lancashire, and Mathews (1977).

Teasdale *et al.* (1977) attempted to replicate the finding of Hand *et al.* (1974) that cohesive groups resulted in continuing improvement at follow-up. Three groups, each containing 5 to 8 patients, were treated along the lines of Hand *et al.*'s cohesive groups. Results of social cohesion ratings were intermediate between Hand *et al.*'s cohesive and unstructured groups. Results at the posttest were similar to those of Hand *et al.* However, the continuing improvement

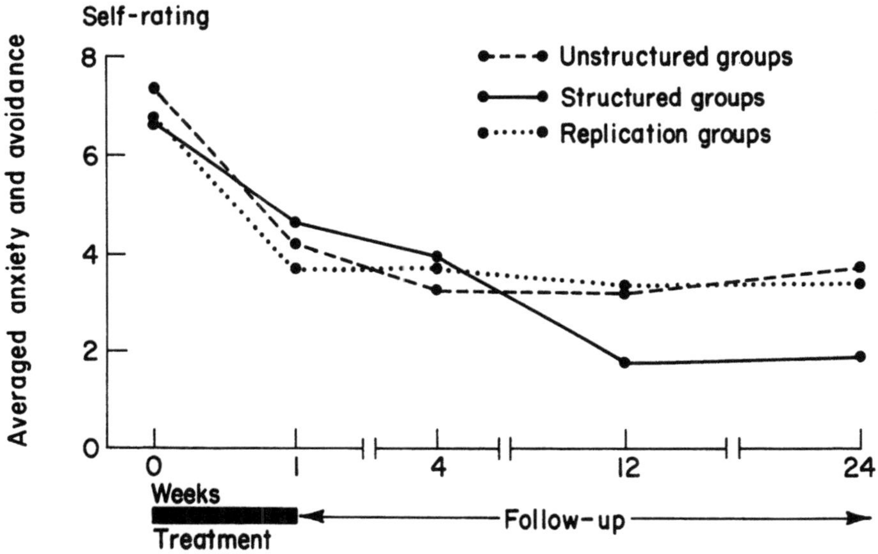

FIGURE 1. Averaged self-ratings of anxiety and avoidance in unstructured and structured (cohesive) groups of Hand *et al.* (1974) and replication (cohesive) groups of Teasdale *et al.* (1977). The continuing improvement in the cohesive groups of Hand *et al.* was not replicated. From "Group exposure for agoraphobics: A replication study" by J. D. Teasdale, P. A. Walsh, M. Lancashire, & A. M. Mathews, 1977, *British Journal of Psychiatry*, *130*, p. 188. Copyright by The British Psychological Society. Reprinted by permission.

shown by Hand *et al.*'s cohesive groups was not replicated. Figure 1 shows the results of Hand *et al.*'s cohesive groups (structured) and unstructured groups and the replication groups of Teasdale *et al.* before and immediately after treatment and at 4, 12, and 24 weeks follow-up. To account for their failure to replicate the findings of Hand *et al.*, Teasdale *et al.* suggested that possibly a certain minimum level of social cohesion is necessary to produce further improvement during follow-up and that the groups in their replication study were still below this minimum.

Emmelkamp and Emmelkamp-Benner (1975) compared individual and group treatment directly. The exposure *in vivo* procedure ("self-observation") involved a systematic graduated approach by the patient to the actual phobic situation; the patient was allowed to turn back on experiencing undue anxiety. The patient had to record the duration of each trial and to write this down in a notebook. This procedure was repeated until the 90-minute session was over. This procedure had proven to be effective with agoraphobics treated individually (Emmelkamp, 1974; Emmelkamp & Ultee, 1974). At the beginning of each treatment session, homework was discussed (either individually or in the group). Next, the 90-minute self-observation procedure was carried out individually, and this was then discussed for half an hour (either individually or in group). Group treatment was about equally effective as individual treatment. Social cohesion was not measured, but this was probably lower than in the cohesive groups of Hand *et al.* due to the fact that *during* actual exposure *in vivo*, group interactions were minimal because each patient did his or her exercises on his or her own.

A second study comparing individual and group treatment was reported by Hafner and Marks (1976). They compared the effectiveness of moderately cohesive groups with individual treatment. Treatment consisted of exposure *in vivo*. Although group treatment was not rated at less anxiety provoking than individual treatment, there was a consistent trend for individually treated patients to improve slightly less than group-treated patients. Further, individually treated patients requested more additional treatment sessions after the experimental part of the study.

Taken together, the results of the studies discussed here indicate that there is now considerable evidence that exposure *in vivo* conducted in groups is at least equally effective as individual treatment. Thus, in terms of cost-effectiveness, group treatment is to be preferred. Usually, group sessions are conducted by two therapists in tandem, but this is not strictly necessary. Another advantage of group treatments is that it may prevent dropout. For example, Hafner and Marks (1977) reported that all dropouts during treatment were from individual sessions. Further, exposure *in vivo* sessions are often easier to conduct in groups than with individual patients because it usually takes longer to persuade individual patients to enter phobic situations than patients treated in a group. The more easy application of exposure in groups may be due to social pressure from other group members or modeling.

The self-observation procedure (Emmelkamp & Emmelkamp-Benner, 1975) was difficult to carry out in groups because group interaction is limited during actual exposure. Prolonged exposure *in vivo* is much more suited for group treatment, and this approach has been applied successfully in a number of other studies (e.g. Emmelkamp, Kuipers, & Eggeraat, 1978; Emmelkamp & Mersch, 1982; Emmelkamp, van de Hout, & de Vries, 1983; Sinnott, Jones, Scott-Fordham, & Woodward, 1981).

Sinnott *et al.* (1981) selected agoraphobic patients for treatment by group exposure according to their residential neighborhood. Because most agoraphobics have lost social contacts due to their long-standing avoidance, it was hypothesized that patients selected according to proximity of residence would benefit more from treatment than patients who were randomly selected: the neighborhood group would have realistic targets (i.e., the homes of other group members) that could serve as the basis for the practice of short journeys from home and could lead to social contact that reinforces the likelihood of successful completion of homework assignments. In their study neighborhood-based treatment, clinic-based treatment, and no-treatment control were compared. All exposure patients received homework assignments, but the patients in the neighborhood groups were encouraged to use each other's residences as "target destinations." The authors had the impression that the neighborhood groups were more cohesive than the randomly selected groups, but cohesiveness was not measured. Further, the neighborhood groups were found to have more social contacts at the end of treatment as compared to the other conditions. Neighborhood groups resulted in more improvement in phobic measures than the other conditions.

The frequency and spacing of exposure sessions varied from study to study. Patients in the Hand *et al.* (1974) and Teasdale *et al.* (1977) studies received three 5-hour treatment sessions on separate days of a single week, whereas patients in the Sinnott *et al.* (1981) study were given 11 sessions once a week. It is conceivable that group cohesion can be fostered more easily when treatment is conducted within a short interval than when the treatment sessions are spread over a prolonged period.

Foa, Jameson, Turner, and Payne (1980) compared 10 sessions of massed and spaced practice. Treatment consisted of exposure *in vivo* conducted in a group setting. In the massed practice condition, treatment was conducted on 10 consecutive days, whereas in the spaced condition, 10 sessions were held once a week only. Results indicated that massed practice was more effective than spaced practice. Foa *et al.* (1980) suggested that the superiority of the massed condition may be due to the fact that massed practice provides less opportunity for accidental exposure between treatment sessions and for the reinforcement of avoidance or escape behavior. An alternative explanation to account for the differential effectiveness of massed and spaced exposure could be different levels of cohesiveness in the two conditions; the massed exposure condition probably is the most cohesive. However, cohesiveness was not measured in this study, thus making the latter interpretation of the results difficult to evaluate.

Several authors reported adverse treatment effects after group exposure *in vivo*. Hand and Lamontagne (1976) found that in some cases improvement of phobia was followed by a marital crisis. Hafner (1977) found that some spouses were adversely affected by their wives' improvement but improved when their partner relapsed. Barlow, Mavissakalian, and Hay (1981) described a pilot study in which agoraphobic women and their partners participated in a group therapy program consisting of exposure *in vivo* and cognitive restructuring. The husband acted as co-therapist. Results were positive. However, because no control groups were employed, it is unclear whether the results of this program are superior to group treatment of agoraphobics without spouse involvement.

Clinical Guidelines

The following section provides some practical guidelines for carrying out an exposure *in vivo* program in groups. In our exposure groups, treatment usually consists of 8 to 10 treatment sessions, 3 sessions a week, each session lasting about 3 hours. The first half hour and the last half-hour of each session are devoted to task-oriented group discussion, in which patients exchange information about their exercises. Although the emphasis throughout the treatment program is on "walking the walk rather than talking the talk," the group discussions are felt to be very important, especially in fostering group cohesiveness.

The first treatment day starts with group discussion that centers around the onset and development of agoraphobia. Patients are usually very talkative. The task of the therapist is to have the patients tell their stories to the other group members rather than to the therapist and to keep the discussion task oriented. Patients who speak very circumstantially have to be interrupted and focused in order to leave enough room for other patients to relate their experiences, This introductory discussion often results in feelings of surprised awareness in the patients, who often did not know that many patients have problems similar to their own. After this group discussion, the therapist presents the following rationale for the exposure treatment (Emmelkamp, 1982, pp. 285–286):

> You have all come here with similar problems. You all become anxious when walking, shopping, etc. You are afraid of panic attacks or of fainting spells. Most of you start to tremble or get palpitations when you find yourself in such situations and some of you even may fear going crazy.
>
> Anxiety is in principle a useful mechanism. Anxiety leads to physical sensations like palpitations, shortness of breath, tightness of the chest, dizziness, trembling, etc. These sensations are quite terrible and make you want to get out of such dangerous situations. Anxiety as a reaction to real danger (e.g., a loose tiger) can be extremely useful and a very functional warning signal. This can be compared with toothache. The pain can be terrible, but useful because it is an indication that you have a cavity. Unfortunately, you become anxious in situations in which this warning signal is of no use.
>
> In fact, your anxiety arises from experiences in the past. Most of you reported on the first anxiety attack. After that traumatic experience you started to avoid the situations in which it had occurred and subsequently you avoided other situations as well in which it possibly could happen also. Because of this sort of experience you now become anxious in situations like walking alone, shopping in busy stores, waiting, travelling by bus, etc., which in fact are not dangerous at all. It is this anxiety that causes your physical sensations like dizziness, palpitations, and shortness of breath. These sensations themselves are likely to make you even more anxious: "Oh, I am

going to faint, . . . have a heart-attack, . . . going to die." So, even though you are all healthy, you think you have to be careful because something might happen to you.

In this group we will not go into the development of your anxiety. Rather we will deal with the situation which currently maintains your anxiety. In certain situations you become anxious because you are convinced that something terrible is going to happen. You continuously avoid or try to escape from such situations. In this way you will never notice that nothing terrible happens when you remain in these situations long enough. You will continue to be convinced that terrible things are going to happen if you go on avoiding these situations. The more you avoid these situations, the more convinced you become. The very reason your anxiety does not diminish is because you have never tried to see whether the terrible things which you expect really occur.

This treatment is focused on helping you to get through these anxiety arousing situations so that you may see that your anxiety is unfounded. You might have some pretty bad times and it will cost you a lot of effort to stay in the phobic situations. A lot of patients before you have gone through this as well with quite good results.

What we are going to do is put ourselves in these difficult situations and stay there till the anxiety has subsided. Thus, you are no longer allowed to escape from these situations, since doing so will maintain or perhaps even increase your anxiety. Take, for example, the case of a housewife who decides to enter a supermarket after some hesitation and becomes anxious. If she immediately runs out, it will cost her more effort to enter the supermarket a next time. She may even send her son or daughter to avoid going to the supermarket. The next time when she is forced to go shopping it will be very difficult if not impossible for her to do so. Thus, when you become anxious in certain situations it is very important for you to stay there and not try to escape. Of course, as a result of your anxiety you may experience palpitations, start to perspire, become dizzy, etc. However, the anxiety and the accompanying sensations will gradually diminish when you stay in the anxiety-arousing situations long enough.

It is explained to the patients that they can be of much support to each other and that no one will be put in a situation against his or her will. Then, group and therapist leave the hospital for a short walk to the center of the town. Patients are encouraged to walk without holding each other or the therapist for support. In town, patients are requested to walk a few minutes behind each other through the main street, thus often walking alone for the first time in many years. In all groups treated so far, very few patients insisted that this was impossible. The few patients who could not be persuaded to walk alone eventually joined a fellow patient. After having walked with the group for about 20 minutes, patients start short walks on their own in the city until the exposure session is over (2 hours). Patients then return as a group to the hospital. Here, an often lively group discussion starts, most patients being astonished about their achievements. The patients then receive detailed homework instructions for a walk from their own homes of similar difficulty as the exercises executed in the group session.

The following sessions typically start with a group discussion centered around the homework assignments and the program for that day. During the exposure part, patients have to enter situations that are difficult, at first in groups of two or three, but as treatment progresses more and more on their own. Difficult situations for the patients are, for example, walking in crowded areas, shopping in department stores and supermarkets, and riding in buses. Deliberate anxiety provocation is not necessary. Prolonged exposure can best be accomplished along a hierarchy from less to more distressing situations. The therapist is less and less frequently present during the exposure *in vivo* periods; he consciously fades from the group and after the third session is usually only present at the discussions preceding and following the exposure periods. In the group discussion following the exposure parts, patients receive homework assignments to be completed before the next session. As a general rule it makes sense not to go beyond what has been practiced during the therapy sessions.

The speed at which exposure *in vivo* can be carried out varies from patient to patient. It is important for every patient to practice at his or her own pace and not to hurry so that anxiety reduction can be clearly felt. Some patients are jealous of the progress of other patients. Therefore, it is important for the therapist to keep explaining that the patients' problems cannot be compared.

Cognitive Restructuring

Group cognitive restructuring programs for agoraphobia have usually employed one or more of the following two cognitive strategies: (a) self-instructional training, and (b) rational emotive therapy.

With *self-instructional* training, patients are instructed to substitute positive coping self-statements for the anxiety-engendering self-statements. Generally, four stages are differentiated: preparing for a stressor, confronting or handling a stressor, possibly being overwhelmed by a stressor, and, finally, reinforcing oneself for having coped (Meichenbaum, 1975). During treatment sessions, patients cognitively rehearse self-instructional ways of handling anxiety by means of an imagination procedure in the group.

Ellis (1962) uses an ABC framework of *rational emotive therapy*. *A* refers to an *A*ctivating event or experience, *B* to the person's *B*elief about the activating (A) event, and *C* to the emotional or behavioral *C*onsequence, assumed to result from the *B*eliefs (B). The critical elements of treatment involve determining the (irrational) thoughts that mediate the anxiety and confront and modify them so that undue anxiety is no longer experienced. According to Ellis (1962), there are certain irrational beliefs that are quite common. To give two examples: the idea that if something seems dangerous or fearsome, you must become terribly occupied with and upset about it"; and "the idea that your past remains all-important and that, because something once strongly influenced your life, it has to keep determining your feelings and behavior today."

In rational emotive therapy the therapist challenges the underlying irrational beliefs in a Socraticlike fashion. In group therapy patients can assist in confronting other patients' irrational beliefs.

So far, four studies have evaluated the efficacy of group cognitive restructuring programs with agoraphobics. In our first study (Emmelkamp *et al.*, 1978), cognitive restructuring was compared with prolonged exposure *in vivo* in a crossover design. Half of the groups received cognitive restructuring as the first treatment and exposure *in vivo* as the second. The order of treatment in the other groups was reversed. Both prolonged exposure and cognitive restructuring were conducted in groups. Cognitive restructuring consisted of self-instructional training and group discussion of eight "irrational beliefs" of Ellis (1962). Exposure *in vivo* was found to be far more effective than cognitive restructuring both on the behavioral measure and phobic anxiety and avoidance scales. However, treatment was conducted in a relatively short time period (five sessions in one week) that might be too short to result in significant cognitive changes. Moreover, the use of a crossover design precluded conclusions about the long-term effectiveness of the cognitive package. Thus, the study might not have been a fair test for cognitive restructuring because it might be possible that cognitive restructuring becomes effective only after the passage of some time.

In our following study (Emmelkamp & Mersch, 1982), we compared cognitive restructuring and exposure *in vivo* in a between-group design. About 30 chronic agoraphobics were randomly assigned to three types of groups: (a) exposure *in vivo;* (b) cognitive restructuring; and (c) self-instructions and exposure *in vivo.* The latter group package was included to investigate whether cognitive modification (i.e., self-instructional training) would enhance the effectiveness of exposure *in vivo.* Treatment consisted of eight 2-hour sessions and was conducted in small groups. A follow-up took place 1 month after the posttest. No treatment was provided during this period.

The cognitive group treatment consisted of two components: (a) insight into irrational beliefs; and (b) self-instructional training. In contrast with our earlier study, more emphasis was placed on insight into unproductive thinking, and patients had to analyze their own feelings in terms of Ellis's ABC model. The second phase of cognitive restructuring was designed to train the patients to emit more productive self-statements. Examples of productive self-statements are "I can handle the situation"; "Anxiety will dissipate with time"; "Don't think about fear: just think about what you have to do"; "Don't try to eliminate fear totally; just keep it manageable." In the groups, the patients cognitively rehearsed self-instructional ways of handling anxiety by means of an imagination procedure. Situations that were cognitively rehearsed were, for example, walking in the street, traveling by bus or train, and being in a crowded restaurant or supermarket.

With the combined procedure involving self-instructional training and exposure *in vivo,* the first three sessions consisted of self-instructional training. Starting with the fourth session, the first half-hour of each session was devoted to self-instructional training, with the rest of the session devoted to prolonged exposure *in vivo.* The exposure treatment was conducted along the same lines as the exposure-alone condition with the important addition being that the groups were instructed to use their productive self-statements during practice *in vivo.* At the posttest, prolonged exposure *in vivo* and the combined procedure (self-instructional training plus exposure *in vivo*) were clearly superior to cognitive restructuring. At 1-month follow-up, however, the differences between the treatments partly disappeared, due to a continuing improvement in the cognitive restructuring condition and a slight relapse in the exposure *in vivo* condition (see Figure 2). Thus, although the short-term effects were similar to the results of the earlier study, in the long run cognitive modification groups were about equally effective.

Finally, self-instructional training did not enhance the effects of exposure *in*

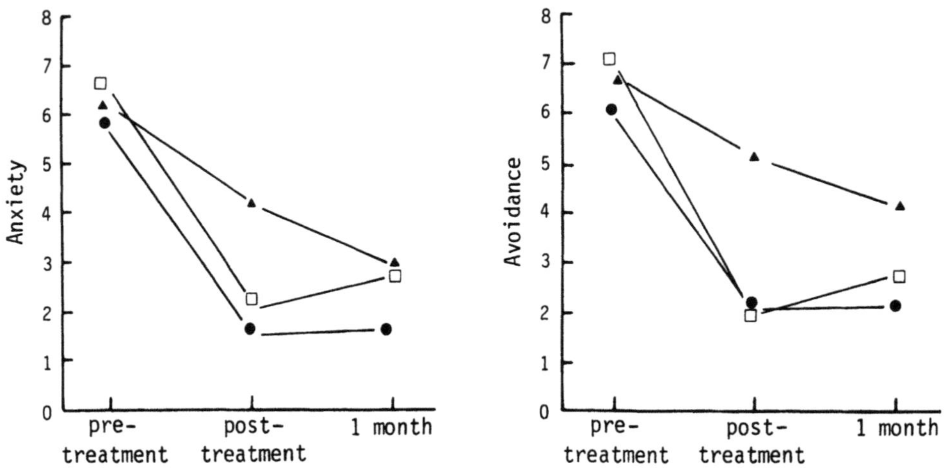

FIGURE 2. The effects of various group treatments on the phobic anxiety and avoidance scales: □ = exposure groups; ▲ = cognitive groups; ● = combined therapeutic package groups. From "Cognition and exposure in vivo in the treatment of agoraphobia: Short-term and delayed effects" by P. M. G. Emmelkamp & P. P. Mersch, 1982, *Cognitive Research and Therapy, 6,* p. 85. Copyright by Plenum Publishing Corporation. Reprinted by permission.

vivo. On no variable were the combined groups found to be more effective than the exposure *in vivo* groups.

In our following study (Emmelkamp, Brilman, Kuipers, & Mersch, 1985), 41 patients were randomly assigned across the following three groups: (a) prolonged exposure *in vivo;* (b) rational emotive therapy; and (c) self-instructional training. After six treatment sessions, a 4-week period followed in which no treatment was given. Then, all groups received prolonged exposure *in vivo.* After the first block of treatment, prolonged exposure *in vivo* groups were superior to either self-instructional training or rational emotive therapy groups on a behavioral measure and on phobic anxiety and avoidance. During the month without treatment, results remained stable. Continuing treatment by exposure *in vivo* for all groups resulted in further improvement.

Mavissakalian, Michelson, Greenwald, Kornblith, and Greenwald (1983) investigated the impact of self-instructional training and paradoxical intention on exposure *in vivo.* With paradoxical intention, patients were instructed to welcome the fear and to attempt to exaggerate it and to become as panicky as possible. Patients practiced these procedures twice during each group therapy session and were encouraged to practice their newly learned cognitive coping strategies regularly and to apply them in actual anxiety-provoking situations. Treatment consisted of 12 weekly 90-minute group sessions. At the end of the treatment period, paradoxical intention resulted in greater gains than self-instructional training. However, groups that were treated with self-instructional training continued to improve after the posttest, which resulted in equivalent long-term effectiveness of the two treatments. Because an exposure-only group was not included, it is unclear whether the cognitive strategies enhanced the effects of exposure.

Assertiveness Training

In many instances, it is insufficient to focus exclusively on the modification of phobic anxiety and avoidance. Because, in a number of patients, agoraphobia is associated with other problems, the latter may become therapeutic goals on their own. For example, Andrews (1966) considers phobic patients as generally shy, anxious, and dependent in many other situations than the typically phobic situations. Fodor (1974) holds that most agoraphobics are unassertive. In her view, feeling of being dominated with no outlet for assertion leads to the development of agoraphobia. Chambless and Goldstein (1980) note that agoraphobics are generally unassertive people with marked social anxieties.

These views on agoraphobia suggest that a behavioral approach that focuses only on the phobic anxiety and avoidance—as in the case of exposure *in vivo*—may be less appropriate for agoraphobics whose phobic complaints are related to unassertiveness. Such patients may profit more from behavioral approaches that focus on broader therapeutic targets as, for example, assertive training.

To study the effectiveness of assertiveness training in groups, we (Emmelkamp, van der Hout, & De Vries, 1983) recently compared the effectiveness of (a) assertiveness training; (b) prolonged exposure *in vivo*; and (c) a combination of assertiveness training and prolonged exposure *in vivo*. Treatment was conducted in small groups. Patients were 21 unassertive agoraphobics. The median score on the Adult-Self-Expression Scale (ASES; Gay, Hollandsworth, & Galassi, 1975) was used as criterion for participation. Each session lasted 3 hours, and each condition received 10 sessions.

With assertiveness training, patients had to report on social situations in which they were unassertive or felt uneasy. During treatment sessions, these situations were discussed, and a more adequate handling of these situations was trained through modeling by the therapist or by one of the other patients and through behavior rehearsal. About half of the time was devoted to structured exercises such as making eye contact, giving a small speech, refusing requests, and the like. In the combined treatment, half of the time was devoted to assertiveness training, whereas the other half consisted of exposure *in vivo*. During the exposure *in vivo* phase of the combined treatment, patients had to practice the newly-learned assertive skills.

As for the main measures (behavioral measurement and ratings for phobic anxiety and avoidance), exposure *in vivo* was found to be superior. On the other hand, assertiveness training was found to be more effective on assertive measures (e.g., ASES). The combined procedure was not more effective than each of the individual treatments on its own.

In summary, expsoure *in vivo* groups are recommended for the treatment of the anxiety and avoidance behavior of agoraphobics. Cognitive groups generally result in less clinical improvement. If unassertiveness is the target of treatment, as assertiveness group is the best option.

Social Anxiety

Clinical social anxiety or *social phobia* consists of disabling fears in social situations that cause patients to avoid such situations. Clinical social anxiety is distinguished from the shyness and social anxiety many individuals experience by the intensity of the fears and the abnormal avoidance of situations involved. A large number of studies have evaluated group application of various cognitive-behavioral interventions in the treatment of social evaluative anxiety (including speech anxiety, communication apprehension, interpersonal anxiety, dating anxiety, and unassertiveness) in academic settings with mildly disturbed college students. Here, the focus will be on the application of group therapy in clinical settings.

Generally, three models are distinguished to explain the functioning of social anxiety, each emphasizing different aspects of the disorder. The *skills deficit model* asserts that social anxiety results from a lack of social skills within the patients' behavioral repertoire. This model suggests that the appropriate goal of treatment should be to assist patients to acquire the skills that they currently lack. Assuming that such lack of social skills provokes anxiety, then anxiety may be overcome through social skills training. If patients have adequate social skills but are inhibited in social situations by anxiety that has become conditioned to interpersonal settings and avoidance of social situations, the principal goal of treatment should be the direct reduction of social anxiety and avoidance (*conditioned anxiety model*). Others have stressed that faulty evaluation of one's performance in social situations or "irrational beliefs" mediate social anxiety. Thus, the *cognitive inhibition model* suggests that maladaptive cognitions rather than conditioned anxiety or skills deficits are responsible for the impairments in social situations. The emphasis on various aspects of social anxiety has led to a number of different treatment strategies of which only those that have been applied in groups will be discussed.

Social Skills Training Approaches

Most studies on group therapy with socially anxious patients have involved social skills training. Ullrich de Muynck and Ullrich (1975) developed a standardized assertive training program for use with groups. Subjects were 20 inpatients. Training was administered in groups of 5 to 7 patients. Patients who considered a particular social situation relatively easy began the role playing. Other patients followed the example of these patients later on. Social skills training in groups was found to result in greater anxiety reduction than a control group of 20 patients who received individual therapy.

Falloon, Lindley, McDonald, and Marks (1977) investigated whether the addition of modeling and role playing (social skills training) enhanced the effects of a cohesive goal-directed small-group discussion. Their patients were patients with social interaction difficulties, including social phobics. Social skills training proved to be superior to group discussion alone. Falloon (1981) reported on attraction for group and leaders rated at the end of each session in the Falloon *et al.* (1977) study. The mean attraction to the group was significantly higher in the social skills training groups than in the discussion groups (see Figure 3.). Thus, social skills training appeared to increase group cohesiveness. In both groups there was a trend toward progressively greater attraction for the group in the course of the 10 sessions. Attraction for the leader and attraction for the group both were significantly related to improved self-image after treatment. Attraction for the leader but not attraction for the group was related to reduction of target anxiety. This study had a substantial dropout rate (21%). It was found that the dropouts showed less attraction for the group and leaders than those completing the 10 sessions (see Figure 3).

Rose (1981) had subjects (recruited from a normal population by means of advertisements) rate satisfaction after each assertive training group session and found that satisfaction had *no* significant relationship with outcome. However, participation in behavior rehearsal and carrying out of homework assignments was related to outcome. The importance of homework assignments was also demonstrated by Falloon *et al.* (1977). Social skills groups that received daily social homework resulted in better outcome than social skills groups without such homework assignments.

Because social skills training had also been applied successfully as individual treatment (see Emmelkamp, 1982), the question is whether skills training is more useful as individual or as group treatment. Only one study (van Son, 1978) addressed this issue. There was a consistent trend for the group therapy patients to improve more than individually treated patients, but the difference between the two conditions did not reach statistical significance.

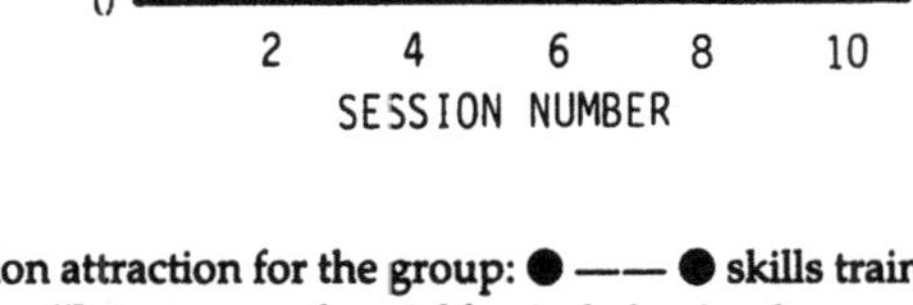

FIGURE 3. Mean postsession attraction for the group: ● —— ● skills training, ● - - - ● discussion, ● • • • • ● dropouts. From "Interpersonal variables in behavioral group therapy" by I. R. H. Falloon, 1981, *British Journal of Medical Psychology, 54,* p. 138. Copyright by The British Psychological Society. Reprinted by permission.

Enhancing Effects of Cognitive Restructuring

Several therapists have developed therapeutic packages that focus both on the dysfunctional cognitions and behavioral skills deficits, but few studies investigated such a therapeutic package in groups with socially anxious patients. Wolfe and Fodor (1977) compared (a) social skills training; (b) social skills training plus cognitive therapy; (c) consciousness raising; and (d) a wait-list control group using unassertive women in an outpatient clinical setting. Both skills training and the combined procedure were superior to the consciousness-raising group and control group on the behavioral measure. Only patients who had received the combined treatment showed anxiety reduction. However, treatment involved two sessions only, which limits the conclusions to be drawn.

A second study investigating this issue was reported by Frisch, Elliott, Atsaides, Salva, & Denney (1982). Thirty-four male outpatients who evidenced marked interpersonal impairments or social avoidance were randomly assigned to (a) social skills training; (b) social skills training plus "stress management"; and (c) a minimal treatment control condition. Stress management included applied relaxation training and cognitive restructuring. Both active treatment groups resulted in improved social skills at the end of treatment. However, on the anxiety measures, no significant improvements were found. The combined approach was about equally effective as social skills training alone.

Exposure *in Vivo*

It should be noted that exposure *in vivo* may account for part of the effects achieved with social skills training. The role played by modeling in social skills training is unclear: it is quite possible that modeling is superfluous with most social phobics and that the essential therapeutic ingredients are repeated behavior rehearsal *in vivo* in the group and the structured homework practice involving real-life rehearsal of feared situations. Falloon, Lloyd, and Harpin (1981) reported a pilot study with 16 socially anxious outpatients who received a treatment program that attempted to maximize rehearsal in real-life settings. Treatment was conducted in small groups. Each patient was grouped with one other patient and a nonprofessional therapist. After behavior rehearsal of problem situations in the clinic, the small group left the clinic and repeatedly rehearsed the same behavior in a real-life setting. Results of this 4-week program were similar to those achieved with social skills training conducted over a 10-week period (Falloon *et al.*, 1977).

Emmelkamp, Mersch, Vissia, and van der Helm (1985) compared the effects of (a) exposure *in vivo*; (b) rational emotive therapy; and (c) self-instructional training. Subjects were 34 socially anxious outpatients. Treatment was conducted in small groups (n = 4–7) for six sessions of 3 hours duration each. In the exposure *in vivo* sessions, patients had to confront their feared situations in the group. For example, patients who were afraid of blushing had to sit in front of others with an open-necked blouse until anxiety dissipated. Others who feared that their hands would tremble had to write on the blackboard and to serve tea to the group. All patients had to give speeches in front of the group. An important part of treatment consisted of actual exposure *in vivo* in real social situations in the town center. Patients had to perform a number of difficult assignments such as making inquiries in shops and offices, speaking to strangers, visiting bars, and the like. Role playing was not applied. Generally, exposure was equally effective as the cognitive treatments. Only on the physiological measure (pulse rate) during an actual social interaction, exposure resulted in more improvement than both cognitive treatments. Thus, contrary to our findings with agoraphobics, in our socially anxious patients, cognitive therapy proved to be as effective as exposure *in vivo*. Presumably, cognitive processes play a more important part in mediating social anxiety than in the case of agoraphobia.

It should be noted that group therapy of socially anxious patients is by definition exposure *in vivo*, irrespective of the actual content of the group therapy program. Thus, in social skills training groups and cognitive restructuring groups, exposure to social interaction with peer patients forms an integral part of the treatment, and it is difficult to discriminate the effects due to specific therapeutic strategies applied and the common factor of exposure *in vivo*. For most patients the first group sessions are very distressing, but the anxiety usually dissipates with time.

The selection of patients for groups is very important. Excessive social anxiety often inhibits the proper application of therapeutic exercises in the groups. For example, a number of social phobics find it very distressing to close their eyes in the group as is typically done during self-instructional training. In rational emotive therapy groups, patients have to bring in their homework into the group. This usually consists of written self-analyses of their own emotional problems, which are discussed and corrected, if necessary, by other group members and the therapist. Patients with an excessive fear of failure find this very difficult and are inclined to avoid possible criticism in the group by not making their homework analyses at all. In such cases, it is better to start treatment individually and proceed later to group therapy when the patient can more adequately cope with these anxieties.

Specific Phobias

The essential feature of specific or simple phobia is a persistent, irrational fear of and compellig desire to avoid specific objects and situations other than those involved in agoraphobia and social anxiety.Examples of simple phobias are claustrophobia, acrophobia, animal phobias, sexual phobias, test anxiety, death anxiety, fear of flying, and the like. Group therapy has involved systematic desensitization, flooding, cognitive restructuring and modeling, and exposure *in vivo*. However, it should be noted that most specific phobias are seen relatively infrequently in clinical settings to make treatment in groups that are homogeneous with respect to type of phobia worthwhile. Most of the studies reported here were of an analog nature: mildly distressed subjects were solicited for participation in experimental studies.

Systematic Desensitization

Several studies report on the application of systematic desensitization in groups consisting of individuals with heterogeneous phobias (Burnett & Ryan, 1964; Deffenbacher, 1974; Lazarus, 1961). Before formal group desensitization starts, anxiety hierarchies were constructed in individual or group sessions and printed on separate cards. When all clients were relaxed, they were instructed to visualize their first item. A client moved to his or her next item only after he or she had imagined the previous scene several times without experiencing anxiety.

A few studies have been conducted that studied group systematic desensitization with subjects having homogeneous phobias. For example, Denholz and Mann (1974) reported group systematic desensitization for fear of flying, using a sound film of flight scenes and accompanying instructional tape. Two studies were conducted to investigate the effectiveness of group systematic desensitization in reducing death anxiety in nonterminal populations. Peal, Handal and Gilner (1981) found systematic desensitization superior to both a relaxation and no-treatment group in reducting death anxiety. Desensitization was conducted in small groups using a standardized hierarchy. Working through the hierarchy was geared to the slowest person in each group. In contrast, Testa (1981) reported negative results of group desensitization of death anxiety of nurses. Desensitization did not have any effect.

The conflicting results between the Peal *et al.* and Testa studies can perhaps best be explained by the fact that the nurses in the Testa study were not selected on the basis of showing high death anxiety, whereas Peal *et al.* used only highly death-anxious subjects.

Elsewhere (Emmelkamp, 1982), we have expressed our view that sexual dysfunctions often can be conceptualized as phobic reactions. Most behavioral treatment procedures for the treatment of sexual dysfunctions involve elements that aim at anxiety reduction. For example, the Masters and Johnson program can be viewed as a gradual exposure *in vivo* program that aims at reduction of performance anxiety related to the sexual situation. Systematic desensitization also focuses explicitly on anxiety.

Group systematic desensitization (often including gradual *in vivo* exercises) has been found to be effective in improving the performance of sexually dysfunctional couples, although the effects on anxiety are less clear (Adelson & Peress, 1979; Andersen, 1981; Auerbach & Kilmann, 1977; Lazarus, 1961, 1968; Lobitz & Baker, 1979; O'Gorman, 1978). To date, only one study (Andersen, 1981) compared the relative efficacy of directed masturbation, involving a series of extratherapy sensuality and masturbatory activities, and systematic desensitization. Both treatments were conducted in small groups (five members per group). Subjects were females with primary orgasmic dysfunction. Although both treatments were equally effective in increasing sexual pleasure, changes in anxiety were negligible. Another controlled study that investigated the efficacy of a masturbation program in groups composed of preorgasmic women was reported by Ersner-Hershfield and Kopel (1979). Masturbation training was found to be significantly more effective than no treatment. Unfortunately, sexual anxiety was not assessed. Thus, it is unclear whether the treatment program affected anxiety. Other behavioral group treatments for sexual dysfunctions are discussed by Mills and Kilmann (1982) and McGovern (chapter 13, this volume) and will not be reiterated here.

Many more studies have applied systematic desensitization in groups, but, as was noted by Upper and Ross (1977) and Grawe (1978), most studies dealt with parametric issues, and groups were used here primarily for the sake of efficiency in generating sufficient numbers of subjects to compare various treatment strategies. Typically, subjects were volunteer students who did not really have a serious problem. Two examples of specific fear reactions being treated by group systematic desensitization in analog studies involved test anxiety (e.g., Deffenbacher and Michaels, 1981; Leal, Baxter, Martin, & Marx, 1981; Russell & Lent, 1982) and snake anxiety (e.g., Odom, Nelson, & Wein, 1978).

Few studies have addressed issues that are particularly relevant to group treatment. Cohen (1969) studied whether group discussion would enhance systematic desensitization in a group context with test-anxious subjects. The discussion was oriented toward test anxiety and included discussion of the process of relaxation and of the subjects' performance during actual tests outside experimental sessions, thus providing group members alternative means of handling these problems. Students in groups given an opportunity to interact with each other reported greater anxiety reduction than those who were not allowed to interact. Further, group-interaction subjects rated their group as more desirable than the noninteraction subjects, although this difference was not statistically significant. Similarly, Katahn, Strenger, and Cherry (1966) and Paul and Shannon (1966) suggested that group interaction could contribute to systematic desensitization in the treatment of test anxiety and social-evaluative anxiety, respectively, but they did not investigate this particular issue.

Two studies, both with test-anxious students, made a direct comparison between group and individual systematic desensitization (Ihli & Garlington, 1969; Scissons & Njaa, 1973). Both approaches were found to be about equally effective.

In summary, group desensitization in imagination is about equally effective as individually administered desensitization. Generally, more sessions are required for groups because the group procedure is slower than individual treatment. However, because imaginal systematic desensitization is less effective than other behavioral procedures (e. g., exposure *in vivo*), group administered systematic desensitization is probably more of historical interest than of interest because it will be often applied in the future.

Flooding

Flooding in imagination—a technique in which the patient has to imagine situations and experiences that she or he finds frightening for a prolonged period of time until anxiety declines—has also been applied in a group context. For example, Dawley and Wenrich (1973) and Graff, MacLean, and Loving

(1971) treated test anxiety, Testa tested (1981) death anxiety, and Stone (1971) tested snake phobia by imaginal flooding in groups. Results were meagre, which is not surprising given the fact that an important basic condition of flooding can not be met when this treatment is conducted in groups. The duration of exposure to the stimulus variable within a session is crucial (Emmelkamp, 1982). Too early termination of flooding sessions may lead to an exacerbation instead of a reduction of fear. In fact, the subject is then allowed to escape the fearful situation that may lead to an immediate anxiety reduction (negative reinforcement) and prevent habituation from occurring. Group presentation of flooding scenes can not take into account the individual variability of exposure time necessary for habituation to occur. Therefore, group application of flooding in imagination is discouraged.

Cognitive Methods

Several studies report on the use of cognitive coping methods in groups with specific phobias. For example, Girodo and Roehl (1978) studied the effectiveness of stress-inoculation training in subjects with fear of flying. During treatment, subjects shared in small groups events in which they experienced anxiety and recalled negative thoughts that accompanied these situations. Then, subjects had to imagine stressful situations and to replace their negative thoughts with more constructive ones. The total training took 2½ hours. Anxiety ratings obtained during a normal flight indicated that self-instructional training was no more effective than prior information giving. However, anxiety ratings during an unexpected event (a missed landing) showed that the subjects who had received stress-inoculation training coped better than did the information and control subjects.

Graziano and Mooney (1980) investigated the application of group cognitive and coping skills training with children who suffered from excessive nighttime fear. Children, ranging in age from 6 to 12 years were in small age-matched groups instructed in the following coping skills to deal with their fear at nighttime: (a) relaxation; (b) pleasant imagery; and (c) positive self-statements (e.g., "I am brave; I can take care of myself when I am in the dark"). The children had to practice these exercises every night with their parents and whenever they started to become afraid. After 3 weeks of training, the treated group had significantly less nighttime fear that did a no-treatment control group. Other fears that have been treated successfully with cognitive group therapy include test anxiety (e.g., Bistline, Jaremko, & Sobleman, 1980; Cooly & Spiegler, 1980; D'Alelio & Murray, 1981; Deffenbacher & Hahnloser, 1981; Goldfried, Linehan, & Smith, 1978; Leal *et al.*, 1981; Wise & Haynes, 1983), snake fear (Odom *et al.*, 1978), and musical performance anxiety (Acevedo & Horan, 1982).

Modeling and Exposure *in Vivo*

Lineham, Rosenthal, Kelley, and Theobald (1977) investigated the effectiveness of modeling in groups. Three types of subjects were included: (a) spider phobics; (b) height phobics; and (c) subjects with public-speaking fear. Subjects from each fear type were randomly assigned to homogeneously or heterogeneously composed groups. Homogeneous groups watched videotapes of models performing coping behavior in fear-relevant situations. The heterogeneous group instead observed tapes of models performing coping behavior in each of the three feared situations, two of which were irrelevant for their particular fear. After two group sessions, subjects received homework to practice feared events (exposure *in vivo*). Both therapeutic strategies were equally effective, but subjects with public-speaking anxiety worsened in the course of treatment. Although the results suggest that watching fear-irrelevant coping models in heterogeneous groups might be equally effective as observing coping in fear-relevant situations only, it should be noted that both groups received exposure *in vivo* instructions as homework assignments. Thus, it is quite possible that modeling did not contribute very much to the treatment outcome but that exposure *in vivo* did (Emmelkamp, 1982).

A clinically more relevant study (Matson, 1981) concerns participant modeling (*in vivo* exposure plus modeling). Mildly mentally retarded adults received group treatment for fear associated with going to stores in the community. Treatment was conducted in small groups ($n = 5$) and was provided in a sheltered workshop and a shopping area in the community. In the first phase of treatment, adequate shopping skills were modeled by the therapist and had to be rehearsed by each patient in the group. *In vivo* training consisted of taking the patients to the shopping area to engage them in various shopping behaviors in a graduated hierarchy. This group exposure *in vivo* program proved to be significantly more effective than no treatment.

Prolonged exposure *in vivo* is the most effective treatment for phobic disorders (Emmelkamp, 1982), but almost no study has been conducted to investigate *group* exposure *in vivo* with specific phobias. Roosen (1975) described an exposure *in vivo* treatment of "specific phobic" patients in heterogeneous groups. Treatment was successful in most cases, but this study was uncontrolled.

In summary, few studies have been reported that investigated the effectiveness of behavioral group therapy on *patients* with homogeneous or heterogeneous phobias. In light of the small prevalence and the idiosyncratic nature of most specific phobias in clinical settings, group therapy seems not to be particularly suited for this category of patients.

Obsessive-Compulsive Behavior

No controlled studies have been published on group treatment with obsessive-compulsives. Marks, Hodgson, and Rachman (1975) reported beneficial effects of booster sessions conducted in groups with patients who had been treated individually with exposure *in vivo* and response prevention, but no data were provided. Hand and Tichatzky (1979) treated 17 obsessive-compulsives in three groups. The group treatment dealt with obsessive-compulsive problems as well as with additional problems. Treatment started with 12 weeks of group sessions in the hospital twice weekly. In addition, patients received five *in vivo* training sessions at home, with members of the family, at least one peer patient, and the therapist present. Apart from the patient group, the therapist met the spouses as a group. In the second phase, the therapist attempted to fade out by having patients take over responsibility for treatment (6 weeks); finally, the patients continued to meet together as a group for another 12 weeks without a therapist present (self-help group). Throughout the therapy, group cohesion was fostered. However, ratings of group cohesion made by the patients were generally low, much lower than in the cohesive exposure *in vivo* groups with agoraphobics of Hand *et al.* (1974). Actually, ratings of cohesion were similar to or even less than ratings of the *un*cohesive groups of agoraphobics. Because the study was uncontrolled, no conclusions can be drawn with respect to the value of group treatment. However, it should be noted that outcome of this intensive treatment program in terms of reduction of obsessive-compulsive complaints was meager when compared to that achieved in individual exposure *in vivo* programs with obsessive-compulsives (Emmelkamp, 1982).

Because relatively few obsessive-compulsives apply for treatment (1 or 2% of outpatients), group treatment will be difficult to organize for most treatment agencies. Therefore, studies investigating the value of group therapy for obsessive-compulsives are difficult to organize. Further, even if such a study should demonstrate that group treatment enhances treatment effectiveness, such a finding would probably be of little clinical utility because of the small availability of suitable patients.

Concluding Remarks and Future Directions

The findings reviewed in this chapter suggest that group therapy might be a useful program for patients with anxiety-based disorders. However, the data presented here are meager, and continued research is necessary. Basic questions that still need to be addressed are whether group therapy is any more effective than individual treatment, and if so, which patients are particularly suited for group therapy and which not.

There is a clear need for research into patient characteristics that are related to refusal to attend and failure of behavioral group therapy. Emmelkamp and van der Hout (1983) noted that a number of agoraphobics refused the group therapy offered to them because they found the group not suited for their particular problems. Further, most patients who dropped out of therapy reported that group therapy had made them anxious. Clearly, not every patient is suited for group treatment. Some patients are better off with an individualized treatment program from the start. For example, there is now some evidence that such an individualized approach may be necessary for patients with marital complications (Emmelkamp and van der Hout 1983). Other examples have been offered throughout this chapter.

Group therapy appears to be an economical way to treat patients. It is generally assumed that group therapy is more efficient than individual therapy, but this proposition requires further empirical support. Often group therapy sessions last longer than individual sessions and are conducted by two rather than one therapist. Future research should use cost-benefit analyses of therapist time requirements in individual and group therapy programs.

Group cohesion is held to be an important factor in contributing to the outcome of group therapy by group therapists of various theoretical orientations, including behavior therapists (e.g., Flowers & Booraem, 1980; Liberman, 1970). However, few studies have addressed the issue in group therapy of anxiety-based disorders (e.g., Falloon, 1981; Hand *et al.*, 1974; Hand & Tichatzky, 1979; Rose, 1981; Teasdale *et al.*, 1977). Results of these studies are inconclusive. Although Hand *et al.* (1974) and Falloon (1981) found a relationship between group cohesion and anxiety reduction, this finding does not necessarily mean that group cohesion was causal in effecting the favorable outcome. The relationship can also be the other way around, with the patients' ratings of cohesion being reflections of their overall satisfaction with treatment. Further, these studies have tended to measure group cohesion by a single measure (attraction to the group or satisfaction), but group cohesion can better be studied as a construct consisting of a network of variables that covary over group sessions, as has been suggested by Flowers and Booraem (1980). Nevertheless, the preliminary results are intriguing and indicate that group cohesion and group processes deserve more attention in future studies.

Clinically, it is important to note that group cohesion does not necessarily have to lead to positive outcome. For example, in one of our most cohesive exposure *in vivo* groups of agoraphobics, patients decided to spend their time drinking coffee rather than doing their anxiety-provoking *in vivo* tasks. This suggests that the effect of group cohesion on therapeutic outcome is related to the norm of a particular group. Furthermore, the norm does not necessarily have to be similar to that of the therapist. Further, a few (especially socially anxious) patients experience high levels of group cohesion as threatening. Such patients may feel forced by group pressure to do activities against their will, which may lead to dropout from the group. Further studies are needed to investigate under which conditions group cohesion is therapeutic and under which conditions it is not.

Another issue that needs to be studied is whether homogeneous groups are more effective than heterogeneous groups or vice versa. Homogeneity may refer to the target problem, but also to age, sex, socioeconomic class, and so forth. Most of the treatments reviewed in this chapter have been conducted with groups that were homogeneous as far as target problem is concerned, but heterogeneous with respect to age, sex, and socioeconomic class. Johnson (1975) has suggested that heterogeneity of the latter variables is required to maximize group resources. What is needed is an empirical investigation of the effects that various group compositions have upon treatment outcome. The optimal group constellation may differ across various intervention strategies. For example, with rational emotive therapy it might be wise to select patients who are matched with respect to intelligence, whereas this variable may be of less importance with exposure *in vivo* groups.

The numbers of patients that participate in a group varies from study to study and is partially dependent on the availability of suitable patients. Generally, six to eight patients seem to be a workable number, enabling each individual to participate actively in the group activities. With smaller numbers, dropouts may cause serious problems. As to duration of the group therapy, time-limited groups are preferred to "open" groups. Prolonging the therapy after a certain number of sessions does not seem to add substantially to treatment outcome. Time limitation provides a motivating condition that may enhance treatment effectiveness. A second advantage of time-limited groups is that patients are better prepared to function independently from the therapist and the group. Finally, time-limited groups are organized like an adult education program. Such an educational approach, emphasizing the role of homework assignments, requires a much more active participation from the individual group members than in more traditional group therapies.

In summary, behavioral group therapy may offer several advantages over individual treatment of anxiety disorders, but research in this area is in an embryonic stage. Further studies are needed to investigate the value of the clinical hunches and recommendations made throughout this chapter. Research into guidelines concerning the selection of group members should have the highest priority.

References

Acevedo, G., & Horan, J. Separate and combined effects of cue-controlled relaxation and cognitive restructuring in the treatment of musical performance anxiety. *Journal of Counseling Psychology*, 1982, *29*, 486–497.

Adelson, G., & Peress, E. Single-couple and group sex therapy: A comparison. *Social Case Work: Journal of Contemporary Social Work*, 1979, *60*, 471–478.

Andersen, B. L. A comparison of systematic desensitization and directed masturbation in the treatment of primary orgasmic dysfunction in females. *Journal of Consulting and Clinical Psychology*, 1981, *49*, 568–570.

Andrews, J. D. W. Psychotherapy of phobias. *Psychological Bulletin*, 1966, *66*, 455–480.

Auerbach, R., & Kilmann, P. R. The effects of group systematic desensitization on secondary erectile failure. *Behavior Therapy*, 1977, *8*, 330–339.

Barlow, D. H., Mavissakalian, M., & Hay, L. R. Couples treatment of agoraphobia: Changes in marital satisfaction. *Behaviour Research and Therapy*, 1981, *19*, 245–255.

Bistline, J. L., Jaremko, M. E., & Sobleman, S. The relative contribution of covert reinforcement and cognitive restructuring to test anxiety reduction. *Journal of Clinical Psychology*, 1980, *36*, 723–728.

Burnett, A., & Ryan, E. Conditioning techniques in psychotherapy. *Canadian Psychiatric Association Journal*, 1964, *9*, 140–146.

Chambless, D. L., & Goldstein, A. The treatment of agoraphobia. In A. Goldstein & E. B. Foa (Eds.), *Handbook of behavioral interventions*. New York: Wiley, 1980.

Cohen, R. The effects of group interaction and progressive hierarchy presentation on desensitization of test anxiety. *Behaviour Research and Therapy*, 1969, *7*, 15–26.

Cooley, E. J., & Spiegler, M. D. Cognitive versus emotional coping responses as alternatives to test anxiety. *Cognitive Therapy and Research*, 1980, *4*, 159–166.

D'Alelio, W. A., & Murray, E. J. Cognitive therapy for test anxiety. *Cognitive Therapy and Research*, 1981, *5*, 299–307.

Daley, P. C., Bloom, L. J., Deffenbacher, J. L., & Stewart, R. Treatment effectiveness of anxiety management training in small and large group formats. *Journal of Counseling Psychology*, 1983, *30*, 104–107.

Dawley, H., & Wenrich, W. W. Implosive group therapy in the treatment of test anxiety. *Behavior Therapy*, 1973, *4*, 261–263.

Deffenbacher, J. L., & Hahnloser, R. M. Cognitive and relaxation coping skills in stress inoculation. *Cognitive Therapy and Research*, 1981, *5*, 211–215.

Deffenbacher, J. L., & Michaels, A. C. Anxiety management training and self-control desensitization—15 months later. *Journal of Counseling Psychology*, 1981, *28*, 459–462.

Denholtz, M. S., & Mann, E. T. An audiovisual program for group desensitization. *Journal of Behavior Therapy and Experimental Psychiatry*, 1974, *5*, 27–29.

Ellis, A., *Reason and emotion in psychotherapy*. New York: Lyle-Stuart, 1962.

Emmelkamp, P. M. G. Self-observation versus flooding in the treatment of agoraphobia. *Behaviour Research and Therapy*, 1974, *12*, 229–237.

Emmelkamp, P. M. G. *Phobic and obsessive-compulsive disorders: Theory, research and practice*, Plenum Press: New York, 1982.

Emmelkamp, P. M. G. & Emmelkamp-Benner, A. Effects of historically portrayed modeling and group treatment on self-observation: A comparison with agoraphobics. *Behaviour Research and Therapy*, 1975, *13*, 135–139.

Emmelkamp, P. M. G., & Mersch, P. P. Cognition and exposure in vivo in the treatment of agoraphobia: Short-term and delayed effects. *Cognitive Research and Therapy*, 1982, *6*, 77–90.

Emmelkamp, P. M. G., & Ultee, K. A. A comparison of successive approximation and self-observation in the treatment of agoraphobia, *Behavior Therapy*, 1974, *5*, 605–613.

Emmelkamp, P. M. G., & van der Hout, A. Failure in treating agoraphobia. In E. B. Foa & P. M. G. Emmelkamp (Eds.), *Failures in behavior therapy*. New York: Wiley, 1983.

Emmelkamp, P. M. G., Kuipers, A., & Eggeraat, J. Cognitive modification versus prolonged exposure in vivo: A comparison with agoraphobics. *Behaviour Research and Therapy*, 1978, *16*, 33–41.

Emmelkamp, P. M. G., van der Hout, A., & De Vries, K. Assertive training for agoraphobics, *Behaviour Research and Therapy*, 1983, *21*, 63–68.

Emmelkamp, P. M. G., Brilman, E., Kuipers, H. & Mersch, P. P. A comparison of self-instructional training, rational-emotive therapy, and exposure *in vivo* in the treatment of agoraphobia. *Behavior Modification*, in press.

Emmelkamp, P. M. G., Mersch, P. P., Vissia, E., & van der Helm, M. Social phobia: A comparative evaluation of cognitive and behavioral interventions. *Behaviour Research and Therapy*, 1985, *23*, 365–369.

Ersner-Hershfield, R., & Kopel, S. Group treatment of preorgasmic women: Evaluation of partner involvement and spacing of sessions. *Journal of Consulting and Clinical Psychology*, 1979, *47*, 750–759.

Falloon, I. R. H. Interpersonal variables in behavioral group therapy. *British Journal of Medical Psychology*, 1981, *54*, 133–141.

Falloon, I. R. H., Lindley, P., McDonald, R., & Marks, I. M. Social skills training of out-patient groups: A controlled study of rehearsal and homework. *British Journal of Psychiatry*, 1977, *131*, 599–609.

Falloon, I. R. H., Lloyd, G. G., & Harpin, R. E. The treatment of social phobia: Real-life rehearsal with nonprofessional therapists. *Journal of Nervous and Mental Disease*, 1981, *169*, 180–184.

Flowers, J. V., & Booraem, C. D. Three studies towards a fuller understanding of behavioral group therapy: Cohesion, client flexibility, and outcome generalization. In D. Upper & S. M. Ross (Eds.), *Behavioral group therapy, 1980: An annual review*. Champaign, Ill.: Research Press, 1980.

Foa, E. B., Jameson, J. S., Turner, R. M., & Payne, L. L. Massed vs. spaced exposure sessions in the treatment of agoraphobia. *Behaviour Research and Therapy*, 1980, *18*, 333–338.

Fodor, I. G. The phobic syndrome in women. In V. Franks & V. Burtle (Eds.), *Women in therapy*. New York: Brunner/Mazel, 1974.

Frisch, M. B., Elliott, C. H., Atsaides, J. P., Salva, D. M., & Denney, D. R. Social skills and stress management training to enhance patients' interpersonal competencies. *Psychotherapy: Theory, Research and Practice*, 1982, *19*, 349–358.

Gay, M. L., Hollandsworth, J. G., & Galassi, J. P. An assertiveness inventory. *Journal of Counseling Psychology*, 1975, *22*, 340–344.

Frisch, M. B., Elliott, C. H., Atsaides, J. P,, Salva, D. M., & Denney, D. R. Social skills and stress management training to enhance patients' interpersonal competencies. *Psychotherapy: Theory, Research and Practice*, 1982, *19*, 349–358.

Girodo, M., & Roehl, J. Cognitive preparation and coping self-talk: Anxiety management during the stress of flying. *Journal of Consulting and Clinical Psychology*, 1978, *46*, 978–989.

Goldfried, M. R., Linehan, M. M., & Smith, J. L. The reduction of test anxiety through rational restructuring. *Journal of Consulting and Clinical Psychology*, 1978, *37*, 228–234.

Grawe, K., Verhaltenstherapeutische Gruppentherapie. In H. Thomas (Ed.), *Handbuch der Psychologie* (Vol. 8). Verlag für Psychologie. Dr. C. J. Hogrefe, Göttingen, 1978.

Graziano, A. M., & Mooney, K. C. Family self-control instruction for children's nighttime fear reduction. *Journal of Consulting and Clinical Psychology*, 1980, *48*, 206–213.

Hafner, R. J. The husbands of agoraphobic women and their influence on treatment outcome. *British Journal of Psychiatry*, 1977, *131*, 289–294.

Hafner, R. J., & Marks, I. M. Exposure in vivo of agoraphobics: Contributions of diazepam, group exposure, and anxiety evocation. *Psychological Medicine*, 1976, *6*, 71–88.

Hand, I., & Lamontagne, Y. The exacerbation of interpersonal problems after rapid phobia-removal. *Psychotherapy: Theory, Research and Practice*, 1976, *13*, 405–411.

Hand, I., & Tichatzky, M. Behavioral group therapy for obsessions and compulsions: First results of a pilot study. In P. O. Sjöden, S. Bates, & W. S. Dockens (Eds.), *Trends in behavior therapy*. New York: Academic Press, 1979.

Hand, I., Lamontagne, Y., & Marks, I. M. Group exposure (flooding) in vivo for agoraphobics. *British Journal of Psychiatry*, 1974, *124*, 588–602.

Hutchings, D. F., Denney, D. R., Basgall, J., & Houston, B. K. Anxiety management and applied relaxation in reducing general anxiety. *Behaviour Research and Therapy*, 1980, *18*, 181–190.

Ihli, K. L., & Garlington, W. R. A comparison of group vs. individual desensitization of test anxiety. *Behaviour Research and Therapy*, 1969, *7*, 207–209.

Johnson, W. G. *Group therapy:* A behavioral perspective. *Behavior Therapy*, 1975, *6*, 30–38.

Katahn, M., Strenger, S., & Cherry, N. Group counseling and behaviour therapy with test anxious college students. *Journal of Consulting Psychology*, 1966, *30*, 544–549.

Lazarus, A. A. Group therapy of phobic disorders by systematic desensitization. *Journal of Abnormal and Social Psychology*, 1961, *63*, 505–510.

Lazarus, A. A. Behavior therapy in groups. In G. M. Gazda (Ed.), *Basic approaches to group psychotherapy and group counseling*. Springfield, Ill.: Charles C. Thomas, 1968.

Leal, L. L., Baxter, E. G., Martin, J., & Marx, R. W. Cognitive modification and systematic desensitization with test anxious high school students. *Journal of Counseling Psychology*, 1981, *28*, 525–528.

Lehrer, P. M., Schoicket, S., Carrington, P., & Woolfolk, R. L. Psychophysiological and cognitive responses to stressful stimuli in subjects practicing progressive relaxation and clinically standardized meditation. *Behaviour Research and Therapy*, 1980, *18*, 293–304.

Liberman, R. P. A. A behavioral approach to group dynamics: I. Reinforcement and prompting of cohesiveness in group therapy. *Behavior Therapy*, 1970, *1*, 141–175.

Lineham, K. S., Rosenthal, T. L., Kelley, J. E., & Theobald, D. E. E. Homogeneity and heterogeneity of problem class in modeling treatment of fears. *Behaviour Research and Therapy*, 1977, *15*, 211–215.

Lobitz, W. C., & Baker, E. L. Group treatment of single males with erectile failure. *Archives of Sexual Behavior*, 1979, *8*, 127–138.

Marks, I. M., Hodgson, R., & Rachman, S. Treatment of chronic obsessive-compulsive neurosis by in vivo exposure. *British Journal of Psychiatry*, 1975, *127*, 349–364.

Matson, J. L. A controlled outcome study of phobias in mentally retarded adults. *Behaviour Research and Therapy*, 1981, *19*, 101–108.

Mavissakalian, M., Michelson, L., Greenwald, D., Kornblith, S., & Greenwald, M. Cognitive-behavioral treatment of agoraphobia: Paradoxical intention vs. self-statement training. *Behaviour Research and Therapy*, 1983, *21*, 75–86.

Mills, K. H., & Kilmann, P. R. Group treatment of sexual dysfunctions: A methodological review of the outcome literature. *Journal of Sex and Marital Therapy*, 1982, *8*, 259–296.

Odom, J. V., Nelson, R. O., & Wein, K. S. The differential effectiveness of five treatment procedures on three response systems in a snake phobia analog study. *Behavior Therapy*, 1978, *9*, 936–942.

O'Gorman, E. C. The treatment of frigidity: A comparative study of group and individual desensitization. *British Journal of Psychiatry*, 1978, *132*, 580–584.

Paul, G. L. & Shannon, D. F. Treatment of anxiety through systematic desensitization in therapy groups. *Journal of Abnormal Psychology*, 1966, *71*, 124–135.

Peal, R. L., Handal, P. J., & Gilner, F. H. A group desensitization procedure for the reduction of death anxiety. *Omega*, 1981, *12*, 61–70.

Roosen, C. J. A. Gedragstherapeutische behandeling in een groep. *Tijdschrift voor de Psychiatrie*, 1975, *17*, 205–212.

Rose, S. D. How group attributes relate to outcome in behavior group therapy. *Social Work Research and Abstracts*, 1981, *16*, 25–29.

Russell, R. K., & Lent, R. W. Cue-controlled relaxation and systematic desensitization versus nonspecific factors in treating test anxiety. *Journal of Counseling Psychology*, 1982, *29*, 100–103.

Scissons, E. H., & Njaa, L. J. Systematic desensitization of test anxiety: A comparison of group and individual treatment. *Journal of Consulting and Clinical Psychology*, 1973, *41*, 470.

Shaffer, C. S., Shapiro, J., Sank, L. I., & Coghlan, D. J. Positive changes in depression, anxiety and assertion following individual and group cognitive behavior therapy intervention. *Cognitive Therapy and Research*, 1981, *5*, 149–157.

Sinnott, A., Jones, R. B., Scott-Fordham, A., & Woodward, R. Augmentation of in vivo exposure treatment for agoraphobia by the formation of neighbourhood self-help groups. *Behaviour Research and Therapy*, 1981, *19*, 539–347.

Spoth, R., & Meade, C. Differential application of cue-controlled relaxation in the reduction of general anxiety. *Journal of Behavior Therapy and Experimental Psychiatry*, 1981, *12*, 57–61.

Stone, W. R. *Individual and group implosive therapy*. Unpublished doctoral dissertation, University of South Dakota, 1971.

Suinn, R. M., & Bloom, L. J. Anxiety management training for pattern A behavior. *Journal of Behavioral Medicine*, 1978, *1*, 25–35.

Teasdale, J. D., Walsh, P. A., Lancashire, M., & Mathews, A. M. Group exposure for agoraphobics: A replication study. *British Journal of Psychiatry*, 1977, *130*, 186–193.

Testa, J. A. Group systematic desensitization and implosive therapy for death anxiety. *Psychological Reports*, 1981, *48*, 376–378.

Ullrich de Muynck, R., & Ullrich, R. The efficiency of a standardized assertive training program. In J. Brengelman (Ed.), *Progress in behavior modification*. Munich: Urban &Schwarzenberg, 1975.

Upper, D., & Ross, S. M. Behavioral group therapy: I. Emotional, avoidance, and social skills problems of adults. In M. Hersen, R. M. Eisler, and P. M. Miller (Eds.), *Progress in behavior modification* (Vol. 5). New York: Academic Press, 1977.

van Son, M. J. M. *Sociale vaardigheidstherapie*. Amsterdam: Swets und Zeitlinger, 1978.

Watson, J. P., Mullett, G. E., & Pillay, H. The effects of prolonged exposure to phobic situations upon agoraphobic patients treated in groups. *Behaviour Research and Therapy*, 1973, *11*, 531–546.

Wise, E. H., & Haynes, S. N. Cognitive treatment of test anxiety: Rational restructuring versus attentional training. *Cognitive Therapy and Research*, 1983, *7*, 69–78.

Wolfe, J. L., & Fodor, I. G. Modifying assertive behavior in women: A comparison of three approaches. *Behavior Therapy*, 1977, *8*, 567–574. Woodward, R., & Jones, R. B. Cognitive restructuring treatment: A controlled trial with anxious patients. *Behaviour Research and Therapy*, 1980, *18*, 401–408.

Woolfolk, R. L., Lehrer, P. M., McCann, B. S., & Rooney, A. J. Effects of progressive relaxation and meditation on cognitive and somatic manifestations of daily stress. *Behaviour Research and Therapy*, 1982, *20*, 461–468.

15

Behavioral Group Therapy with Drunk-Driving Offenders

GERARD J. CONNORS, STEPHEN A. MAISTO, LINDA C. SOBELL, AND MARK B. SOBELL

INTRODUCTION

Motor vehicle accidents have become the major cause of accidental mortality and morbidity in industrial nations (Havard, 1975), and alcohol consumption has been cited as the most significant contributor to such accidents (Seppala, Linnoila, & Mattila, 1979). Of the approximately 50,000 traffic accident mortalities that occur yearly in the United States, it has been estimated that as many as 78% of these victims are drivers with some level of alcohol in their blood (Reed, 1982). Of course, a measurable blood alcohol level does not necessarily mean that a driver is "drunk" nor that there is a causal relationship between alcohol consumption and accident involvement. In fact, Zylman (1975) has suggested that perhaps only 30% of traffic deaths can be linked to alcohol consumption in some causal manner. Nevertheless, when all is taken into account, the impact of drinking drivers assuredly remains immense.

Neither the drinking driver problem nor efforts to remedy it are new. In fact, the problem was recognized shortly after the introduction of the automobile (Heise, 1934; Holcomb, 1938; Monroe, 1947; "Motor Wagons," 1904). The most common approach to counteract drinking drivers has been secondary prevention projects. In this regard, there has been, in recent years, a marked increase in the use of educational programs or educationally-oriented treatment programs for persons arrested for driving while intoxicated (DWI) (Israelstam & Lambert, 1975; Zelhart & Schurr, 1977). Much less attention has been given to the use of other treatment approaches, although recent data suggest that behaviorally oriented techniques hold promise in working with drinking drivers.

GERARD J. CONNORS • University of Texas Medical School at Houston, Houston, Texas 77025. STEPHEN A. MAISTO • Veterans Administration Medical Center, Providence, Rhode Island 02908. LINDA C. SOBELL and MARK B. SOBELL • Addiction Research Foundation, Toronto, Ontario, Canada M5S2S1.

The present chapter is divided into three sections. First, treatment approaches used to date with drinking drivers are briefly summarized, and data regarding the efficacy of these approaches are reviewed. Second, the use of behavioral group therapies with DWI offenders is discussed. The benefits of behavioral group approaches are outlined, and treatment strategies are delineated. The closing section presents a summary and suggestions for future research.

Before discussing treatment approaches used with DWI offenders, some discussion of prevention efforts is in order. Prevention programs are typically classified into three categories based upon their intended objectives. The first is *primary prevention,* which refers to the prevention of any occurrence of a health problem. *Secondary prevention* refers to the treatment of a health problem shortly following its initial development. Finally, the term *tertiary prevention* is used to describe treatment of a health problem that has already become well established (i.e., chronic). Strategies used to prevent drunk driving are typically classified as primary or as secondary efforts, depending on their aims and target populations. According to Klajner, Sobell, and Sobell (1984), primary prevention efforts are designed to prevent an initial DWI arrest, whereas secondary prevention efforts are intended to prevent subsequent DWI offenses among those once convicted. This chapter focuses on secondary prevention efforts; primary prevention efforts are described in more detail elsewhere (e.g., Klajner *et al.*, 1984; Waller, 1982).

Secondary Prevention

The most common nonpunitive approach to the problem of drinking and driving has been secondary prevention projects. Within the past decade, there has been a rapid increase in the use of educational or educationally oriented treatment programs for persons arrested for DWI. Unfortunately, there has been little concomitant empirical support for the efficacy of such programs (Nichols, Weinstein, Ellingstad, & Struckman-Johnson, 1978; Whitehead, 1975; Zador, 1976). The best examples of secondary prevention programs have been the Alcohol Safety Action Projects (ASAP) established and operated throughout the United States in the early and mid-1970s. Over 200,000 DWI offenders were referred to ASAP education and rehabilitation programs (Nichols *et al.*, 1978). The ASAPs were intended to coordinate through a "systems approach" a variety of DWI countermeasures (e.g., law enforcement, public education, judicial efforts, legislative mandates, rehabilitative strategies). In addition, the efforts of various community agencies were coordinated by a "special management office," and special efforts were directed toward identifying and referring problem drinkers for specific clinical services (Levy, Voas, Johnson, & Klein, 1978). If the offender followed through with the referral, the courts generally reduced the DWI charge and/or related penalties.

The San Antonio (Texas) Alcohol Safety Action Project was representative of the ASAPs using the "systems approach" to reduce the prevalence of drinking and driving. As described by Nathan and Turnbull (1974), the San Antonio ASAP included five principal components: (a) dissemination of information on drinking and driving (e.g., flyers, newspaper articles, presentations); (b) more stringent enforcement of the existing statutes regarding driving under the influence of alcohol; (c) coordination of various judicial system divisions (e.g., judges, prosecuting attorneys, probation officers); (d) a 10-hour alcohol education program; and (e) development of a "presentence psychosocial evaluation" of DWI offenders referred by the judicial system. This evaluation was used to identify offenders in need of treatment and to make recommendations to the judiciary regarding such cases.

The alcohol education course described by Nathan and Turnbull (1974) as one component of the San Antonio ASAP is a near-universal feature of ASAP programs. The prototypic alcohol education course has been the DWI Phoenix program. As discussed by Malfetti (1975), the DWI Phoenix course has been the model upon which hundreds of other DWI programs in the United States and Canada have been based. The course was developed "to provide information on the consequences of drinking and driving, and to consider why people drink and what countermeasures they can take" (Malfetti, 1975, p. 256). The DWI Phoenix course included four 2½-hour sessions. The first focused on data demonstrating "the seriousness of the [DWI] problem" (p. 256). The effects of varying amounts of alcohol on driving behaviors are addressed in the second session, whereas the third focused on the general issue of problem drinking. The final session emphasized the development of individualized countermeasure strategies for avoiding future DWI arrests. As with other ASAP programs, additional treatment services were recommended for persons having more serious alcohol problems.

There have been many evaluations of the ASAP programs, but they have varied considerably in their designs and data analyses, follow-up periods, and types of outcome data collected. This research on the ASAPs, as well as on the few programs that preceded them and the many others that followed, has yielded mixed results at best. For example, although Levy *et al.* (1978) found that ASAP programs decreased the number of nighttime fatal crashes in several settings, there was no evidence that efforts to rehabilitate problem drinkers contributed in any meaningful way to the decrease. Nichols, Ellingstad, and Struckman-Johnson (1979) studied 11 ASAP programs that randomly assigned "moderate-problem-drinker" DWI offenders to either a treatment group or to a no-treatment control group. Program effectiveness was evaluated using a variety of traffic safety (e.g., tickets, recidivism, accidents) and nontraffic safety (e.g., drinking data, life activities) criteria. The results were not encouraging, leading Nichols *et al.* (1979) to conclude that "laws that require the attendance of the convicted DWIs at education and/or rehabilitation programs in lieu of losing their licenses cannot be objectively supported on the basis that they result in a safer driving environment" (p. 176). In yet another assessment of ASAP programs, Nichols *et al.* (1978) studied treatment effectiveness according to the type of drinker targeted. They found that social drinkers derived a small positive effect, but that problem drinkers generally derived no benefit. Finally, Ellingstad and Springer (1976) summarized the findings of a variety of ASAP programs. They reported that increases in knowledge and alterations in attitudes have been demonstrated, but there is no evidence for reductions in DWI arrests or alcohol-related motor vehicle accidents.

There are several possible reasons for the general ineffectiveness of DWI educational/treatment programs. One likely factor is that these programs serve a heterogeneous population (Donovan & Marlatt, 1982; Scoles & Fine, 1977; Yoder & Moore, 1973), suggesting that a diversity of approaches may be warranted. A second factor that may contribute to the ineffectiveness of secondary prevention efforts is that persons arrested for DWI frequently are problem drinkers (Bell, Warheit, Bell, & Sanders, 1978; Fine & Scoles, 1976; Fine, Scoles, & Mulligan, 1975; Selzer & Barton, 1977; Waller, 1967), although clearly not all of these drinkers would concur with such an assessment (e.g., Sandler, Palmer, Holmen, & Wynkoop, 1975). One of the reasons for this supposed "denial" would be that the extent of their use of alcohol and related problems is often less serious than that exhibited by alcoholics (Bell *et al.*, 1978; Calsyn, Reynolds, O'Leary, & Walker, 1982). However, that DWI offenders may be problem drinkers in general is an important point, because these drinkers appear to be the least likely to benefit from educational programs (Hayslip, Kapusinski, Darbes, & Zeh, 1976; Scoles & Fine, 1977). Taken together, these data strongly suggest a need for the differential assessment of DWI offenders and the development of treatment approaches to address the needs of different DWI subgroups. One further reason that DWI educational programs may not have been particularly effective is that these programs seem to have been developed in the absence of a theoretical conceptualization of the variables that cause and maintain DWI behaviors.

In summary, secondary prevention activities designed to reduce DWI recidivism have generally not been effective. Additional evaluative research is needed to investigate alternative treatment methods that may be more effective with DWI offenders in general and perhaps with particular subgroups of offenders. Given the efficacy of behavioral approaches to problem drinking in general (Marlatt & Nathan, 1978; Miller, 1976; Nathan & Briddell, 1977; Sobell, Sobell, Ersner-Hershfield, & Nirenberg, 1982), it has been argued (e.g., Brown, 1980) that behaviorally oriented treatments are a logical alternative to educational DWI programs. In the next section, specific examples of behavioral group approaches are described and discussed.

Behavioral Group Treatments

Although there is an extensive literature regarding the behavioral group treatment of addictive behaviors in general (see Barrios, Turner, & Ross, Chapter 12, this volume), behavioral treatments presented within a group format have not been frequently used with DWI offenders. However, such an approach may be a viable and effective treatment approach for persons arrested for drunk driving.

There are multiple advantages to using group versus individual behavioral treatments for DWI offenders. The most obvious advantages are time efficiency and cost-effectiveness. However, of greater potential value are several more clinically relevant attributes. To begin with, clients are given an opportunity to recognize that they are not uniquely different, and that others share parallel experiences. Larazus (1968) has noted that groups can reduce a client's feelings of isolation and may provide some relief from the alienation sometimes experienced when treated individually. A second advantage to group treatment of DWI offenders is that groups typically represent a range of experiences, values, inputs, and opinions. Such diverse experiences and viewpoints can importantly influence an individual's assessment of his or her drinking behavior and subsequent development of strategies for avoiding future DWI arrests. Group input, and especially group consensus, may also allow more natural or spontaneous sociobehavioral changes to occur. Finally, group formats provide multiple opportunities for modeling, role playing, and behavioral rehearsal (Rose, 1977). Group input to individualized problem-solving exercises (D'Zurilla & Goldfried, 1971) and drink refusal training (Foy, Miller, Eisler, & O'Toole, 1976) can be central to the acquisition of new drinking-related behaviors.

Although a well-developed body of literature does not exist regarding the behavioral treatment of DWI offenders, this area is receiving increasing attention. In this section, three behavioral group treatment approaches for DWI offenders will be described. The first protocol, developed by Donovan and his colleagues (Salzberg, Queisser, & Donovan, 1980), currently is being used with first DWI offenders, whereas the second two programs (Brown, 1980; Connors, Maisto, & Ersner-Hershfield, 1983) have been tested with populations of DWI recidivists (i.e., those with more than one DWI arrest).

A Skills Training Program

The Skills Training Program developed by Donovan and his colleagues (Salzberg *et al.*, 1980; see also Donovan, Marlatt, & Salzberg, 1983) was designed to address personality factors, drinking behavior, and high-risk driving. The program is currently being evaluated in the state of Washington as a potential means of reducing subsequent accidents and DWI recidivism among DWI first offenders. In this regard, the specific objective of the intervention is "to teach effective problem solving skills and alternative adaptive responses to problematic situations which are likely to lead to drinking and high-risk driving" (Salzberg *et al.*, 1980). The participants are first offenders who have completed a standard 2-hour alcohol education course sponsored by the state of Washington Department of Licensing and who are classified as nonalcoholic drinkers (or who refuse alcoholism treatment). Potential participants are randomly assigned either to the Skill Training Program, to a group receiving only the 2-hour alcohol education program, or to a no-contact group.

Part of the rationale behind the Skill Training Program is that there exists a group of heavy alcohol consumers who have deficient capabilities for coping with anger and stress and/or who have an aggressive disposition. It is hypothesized that when stressors are not adequately confronted and dealt with, increased frustration and decreased self-efficacy result (see Bandura, 1977). These perceptions, in turn, are hypothesized to lead to drinking and/or driving as a means of reducing frustration and tension and of increasing one's feelings of control. It is the interaction of these maladaptive coping strategies that places the individual at risk for drinking and driving and subsequent arrest. Donovan and his colleagues postulate that if these individuals can acquire and use appropriate coping skills to deal effectively with stressful situations, they will then be less likely to drink and/or drive in order to increase perceived self-efficacy. Consequently, in the Skill Training Program, a particular focus is placed on problem-solving strategies (see D'Zurilla & Goldfried, 1971; Goldfried & Davison, 1976) and on the development of techniques for dealing with stressful situations.

The Skill Training Program itself is divided into four 2-hour segments, each of which includes six to eight participants. The first session includes presentation of the components of effective problem solving (e.g., developing an orientation, defining the problem, generating and evaluating alternatives, decision making, and verification and reevaluation as necessary). In addition, a creative "road-map concept" is used to break down life events into a series of interrelated components, each of which involves discrete decision-making requirements. This process is used to identify the best times for interventions to alter maladaptive patterns or chains of behavior. Finally, participants are given instruction in monitoring their drinking behavior. Self-monitoring is a procedure that is commonly used for collecting baseline data and making clients more aware of their behavior, its antecedents, and its consequences. Self-monitoring additionally serves to place problem-solving activities in the present, permits focusing on critical events, and engages clients quickly in the process of behavior change (Kanfer, 1980).

The second session of the Skill Training Program begins with discussion on the self-monitoring homework and with training in calculating blood alcohol concentrations. Further, participants are asked to identify their drinking limits for occasions on which driving is likely. Strategies for drinking within these limits (including abstinence) are developed to assure that the established drinking limits are achievable. The final topic covered in this second session is learning to resist social pressures to drink. Role playing with group feedback is used to aid in the integration of these new behavioral options.

The third and fourth sessions of the Skill Training Program (Salzberg *et al.*, 1980) focus on dealing with negative emotional states. The third session includes a presentation of the previously described model regarding drinking, interpersonal conflict, and traffic accidents. This session also focuses on the use of assertive behavior and anger management as techniques that can be used in situations involving interpersonal conflict. The final session is similar in structure to the third session, in that strategies for mediating such states as anxiety and depression are discussed. For example, relaxation techniques are described as self-control strategies effective in reducing tension. What is important also is that each participant also develops a detailed plan of action for avoiding future drinking and driving.

The Skill Training Program proposed by Donovan and his colleagues comprises a variety of strengths. To begin with, the program is based on sound theoretical conceptions drawn from a comprehensive review of the research on the interrelationship among personality characteristics, high-risk driving behavior, and drinking behavior (see also Donovan & Marlatt, 1982, and Donovan *et al.*, 1983). Based on that conceptualization, it is hypothesized that individuals who maladaptively drink and/or drive in order to cope with various life stressors are at significant risk for DWI arrests and that alternative coping strategies can be beneficial. The value of the Skill Training Program remains to be established, however, and treatment outcome data are currently being collected to assess the program's effects. A final strength of the Skill Training Program is that in addition to empirically assessing the efficacy of the program relative to the alcohol education course or no treatment, it may also be possible to assess which individuals are more likely to benefit from the experimental treatment (Donovan & Marlatt, 1982). Thus, the findings of this innovative and theoretically sophisticated endeavor are eagerly awaited.

Controlled Drinking Education

Another innovative behavioral program used with DWI offenders in New Zealand has been described by Brown (1980). He reasoned that controlled drinking training might be an effective treatment option for DWI offenders, given that they frequently exhibit problem drinking in general (Fine & Scoles, 1976; Selzer & Barton, 1977). There is a large body of literature demonstrating the efficacy of moderate drinking treatment approaches with problem drinkers (for a review see Miller & Hester, 1980).

Subjects participating in the Brown (1980) study were males convicted of DWI. Most of these offenders apparently were recidivists, as the subjects averaged about three previous convictions for DWI (no range was provided). They were randomly assigned to one of three conditions: an educational course on controlled drinking, a conventional driver education course, or a no-education control condition. Subjects in the conventional driver education course participated in five weekly 3-hour sessions. These sessions included invited speakers, films, and discussion about alcohol-related topics. The fifth session included review and the development of individualized strategies for avoiding DWIs. The no-treatment control subjects received no educational instruction.

The participants assigned to the educational drinking condition received specific training in controlled drinking. Their five weekly 3-hour sessions were conducted in an experimental bar setting. Subjects' drinking behaviors initially were recorded and assessed during ad lib access to alcohol in the experimental bar facility. They later were given feedback on their drinking behavior, and received instruction on its moderation. In this regard, they received instruction on reducing drink strength and sip rate and increasing the amount of time between drinks to reduce alcohol intake. The subjects also received training in blood alcohol level discrimination and self-monitoring of daily drinking behavior.

Brown's 1-year posttreatment follow-up revealed three major findings. First, the subjects in the controlled drinking educational groups showed significant changes in their drinking behavior. Only the subjects in this group significantly reduced their frequency of uncontrolled drinking days over the follow-up period, with uncontrolled drinking operationally defined as consumption of greater than 80 g of absolute alcohol per day. Further, this change in drinking was evident during the first 90-day posttreatment and was maintained through the 12-month follow-up contact. The second finding was that the frequency of drinking and driving decreased from base-line to follow-up for subjects in all three groups. However, the controlled drinking subjects showed the greatest reduction in the frequency of this behavior. The third major finding was that subjects in the two treatment groups showed improved "psychosocial adjustment" (based on an assessment of participants' "domestic, vocational, interpersonal, and health status and contact with community agencies" during months 10 through 12 of the follow-up period), whereas no changes were noted for the no-treatment control subjects.

Brown's (1980) results indicate that the DWI offenders (many of whom were recidivists) in his study were responsive to educational interventions designed to change drinking behavior and to decrease the likelihood of recidivism. Only the controlled drinking training subjects showed a marked decrease in uncontrolled drinking days and improved psychosocial adjustment. However, it would be premature to assess the impact of this training program on DWI recidivism. Arrests for DWI are relatively infrequent events (e.g., Beitel, Sharp, & Glauz, 1975), and only 2 of the 60 subjects in Brown's (1980) project were convicted on another DWI charge during follow-up. It is for this reason that Maisto, Sobell, Zelhart, Connors, and Cooper (1979) have recommended the use of a 36-month follow-up period when assessing DWI recidivism.

Behavioral Self-Control Treatment

A third behavioral group treatment study was conducted by Connors *et al.* (1983). This study was designed to evaluate the effects of a behavioral group treatment on knowledge and attitude change and on rearrest for drunk driving among court-referred DWI recidivists (i.e., only those referrals with multiple past arrests for DWI were included). The final sample included 62 males and 5 females; most had either two or three prior DWI arrests.

The participants in this study were randomly assigned to a program focusing on behavioral self-control principles or to a general educational program. A refund deposit manipulation was also included (see Ersner-Hershfield, Connors, & Maisto, 1981) but was found to have no consistent effect in the treatment outcome evaluation. Participants attended eight weekly treatment groups (8–10 individuals per group), and then attended two "booster" sessions held 8 and 16 weeks after completion of the eighth weekly group session. The total treatment spanned 24 weeks.

Each of the two treatment conditions was designed to provide the participants with the knowledge and techniques to change problem behavior, specifically drinking and driving under the influence of alcohol. However, the behavioral program was based on principles of self-control (Mahoney & Thoresen, 1974; Thoresen & Mahoney, 1974) and behavioral assessment, and it included an individualized functional analysis (Sobell & Sobell, 1981) of situations that posed high risk for a subsequent DWI arrest. It was hypothesized that behavioral self-control and self-management strategies could be used by DWI offenders to prevent recidivism, just as these strategies have been used with other populations to modify a variety of other target behaviors (see Kanfer & Goldstein, 1980). In contrast, the general educational treatment program components were alcohol education, relaxation training, and a general evaluation of situations typically associated with DWI arrests. Unlike the behavioral groups, the educational groups did not cover principles of self-control and the regulation of behavior, and were not individually tailored to the specific high-risk situations for drinking and driving faced by each group member.

Several dependent variables reflecting knowledge and attitude changes were assessed over the course of the 24-week treatment period. In addition, Connors *et al.* (1983) collected 3-year follow-up DWI recidivism (i.e., rearrest) data on their subjects. The data generally revealed positive effects of the treatment programs. The short-term data showed that subjects in both treatment conditions perceived an increased likelihood of their being rearrested if they drove while drinking. The subjects also reported more frequent use of portable breath-testing devices (Sobell, VanderSpek, & Saltman, 1980), which were made available to all participants at modest cost. These significant increases occurred from pre- to posttreatment assessments (over the eight weekly sessions) and were maintained at least through the 24th week of treatment (the second booster assessment). There also was a trend ($p < .10$) for subjects to increase their use of alternative forms of transportation (instead of drinking and driving) from pre- to posttreatment, and to maintain such behavior through the second booster session. Taken together, these data suggest that DWI recidivists in both groups experienced important changes in treatment, according to both cognitive and behavioral variables. However, the Connors *et al.* study did not include a no-treatment control group because the judicial system where this study was conducted would not sanction a no-treatment control condition. Thus, it is not possible to determine whether the observed changes were a direct result of participating in the treatment programs.

Connors *et al.* (1983) did, however, provide some data suggesting that there were differential effects of treatment. Specifically, it was found that subjects in the behavioral group thought about avoiding DWIs to a greater extent than did subjects in the educational group. It was hypothesized that this may have reflected the highly individualized nature of the behavioral groups in developing strategies for avoiding DWIs. For example, subjects in the behavioral self-control group received specific training in generating and evaluating alternatives to drinking and driving on an individual, situation-specific basis. On the other hand, subjects in the educational group were exposed only to a general evaluation of situations typically associated with DWI arrests. The focus on principles of self-control and the regulation of behavior, in conjunction with the tailoring of problem-solving strategies to individual needs, may have accounted for behavioral subjects spending more time thinking about avoiding drinking and driving.

The long-term effects of the treatments are perhaps the more critical issue. In this regard, the arrest recidivism data showed that rearrest for subjects in both treatment conditions was a relatively infrequent event in any given year during the 36-month posttreatment follow-up. No more than four individuals from either treatment group were rearrested in any given year. Nevertheless, 34% of the educational treatment subjects and 32% of the behavioral treatment subjects were rearrested over the 36-month follow-up. Only three subjects had more than one rearrest over the follow-up period.

Connors *et al.* (1983) offered several considerations in interpreting their recidivism data. First, the outcome rates were based on arrest data rather than convictions that appear on driver license records. In contrast, previous studies assessing recidivism typically have used state driver license records. Arrest records, however, are probably a more sensitive measure of drinking–driving behavior than driving license records because driver licence records often do not reflect reduced charges, cases purged from records, and clerical errors or ommissions in the posting of violations onto the records. A second issue dealt with the length of time between successive DWI arrests. Maisto *et al.* (1979) previously reported findings based on driver license records that included DWI convictions. Those data were collected in the same state in which the Connors *et al.* study was later conducted. Maisto *et al.* (1979) found that the average periods of time between second and third, third and fourth, and fourth and fifth DWI convictions were 16.8, 10.7, and 8.0 months, respectively. Thus, assuming consistent enforcement, it would be expected on the basis of the Maisto *et al.* (1979) actuarial data that the subjects in the Connors *et al.* study would typically have had their third, fourth, and fifth DWI convictions after time intervals similar to the previous study. However, the recidivists in the Connors *et al.* sample were rearrested, on the average, after 18 months (range = 1–33 months), and only 3 of the 21 recidivists had more than one rearrest over the 36-month follow-up period. If subjects' convictions (and not arrests) in the Connors *et al.* (1983) study were compared to Maisto *et al.*'s (1979) actuarial data, these intervals would probably have averaged even longer than 18 months. It is possible, therefore, that the interventions in the Connors *et al.* study may have served to extend the length of time before recidivists were rearrested. But such an effect can only be speculated about in the absence of a no-treatment control group.

Taken together, the Connors *et al.* (1983) data suggest that DWI recidivists are responsive to treatment interventions, and that the inclusion of behavioral self-control principles as a group treatment component may have engendered additional positive benefits in short-term results. The results of this study, as suggested by the investigators, call for additional research to identify techniques for maintaining treatment gains over extended periods of time.

Conclusions

Researchers and clinicians have been slow to use behavioral group treatment interventions with DWI offenders. Nevertheless, encouraging results of such methods have begun to appear, and considering the lack of effective DWI treatment programs and the vast resources that have been invested in ineffective programs, further development and evaluation of behavioral group treatments for DWI offenders is warranted. In this chapter, the programs reported by Donovan and his colleagues (e.g., Donovan *et al.*, 1983; Salzberg *et al.*, 1980), Brown (1980), and Connors *et al.* (1983) were described in some detail. What is important is that these programs have been developed within theoretical frameworks. However, additional research is required to demonstrate the effectiveness of behavioral group treatments with DWI offenders and to refine treatment procedures. It is hoped that the programs described herein are but harbingers of more extensive research efforts.

There are at least four areas warranting systematic attention in research on behavioral group treatments for DWI offenders. The first is the determination of whether such treatment packages are effective and the evaluation of alternative behavioral treatment strategies. Researchers subsequently may wish to conduct analyses within particular approaches to assess the contribution of different treatment components to the overall process of behavior change. It also may be useful to study, as a strategy for effecting behavior change, the involvement of significant others in the treatment process (e.g., spouse, family, employers, friends). O'Farrell and Cutter (1984), for example, have used conjoint behavior group therapy with alcoholics and their spouses. However, significant others typically are not involved in the treatment of alcohol abusers (Regan, Connors, O'Farrell, & Jones, 1983), and such approaches have not been applied to DWI offenders.

A second, related domain deserving of attention is the differential assessment of DWI offenders in an effort to match DWI offenders to treatments. For example, differences between first and multiple DWI offenders have been noted (e.g., Steer & Fine, 1978; Yoder & Moore, 1973), but these distinctions have not played any systematic role in the differential provision of treatment services. Only a handful of more sophisticated efforts have been conducted to more precisely differentiate among subgroups of DWI offenders (e.g., Donovan & Marlatt, 1982; Steer, Fine, & Scoles, 1979; Sutker, Brantley, & Allain, 1980). Such research will be needed if a patient-to-treatment matching process is to be effected.

A third area warranting attention is the use of multiple measures of outcome (Maisto & McCollam, 1980). For example, studies that simply report pre-post treatment changes in knowledge and attitudes are not likely to contribute in any major way to the long-term goal of reducing recidivism rates. It also is worth noting that recidivism, although important, is not the most sensitive of treatment outcome measures. Nonrecidivism rates for DWI first offenders are quite high, and a very powerful treatment would be required to impact significantly on this baseline level. Moreover, arrest rates will vary with the intensity of police efforts to enforce drunk-driving laws. Thus, alternative measures and measures that are less sensitive to enforcement differences over time need to be developed and assessed. The investigation reported by Brown (1980), for example, is noteworthy in that data on drinking behavior and not just recidivism were collected as part of the long-term follow-up efforts.

The fourth area needing further study is the maintenance of changes resulting from treatment. In this regard, one strategy, as noted earlier, would be the evaluation of alternative treatment methods. A second approach would be to assess the effect of various aftercare strategies. For example, only limited attention has been given to length of treatment and the progressive spacing of treatment contacts (see, for example, Noel, Sobell, Celluci, Nirenberg, & Sobell, 1982). It may be that participation at booster sessions will reinforce the continued use of strategies developed during the formal phase of treatment and allow patients to discuss any risks or problem situations related to avoiding drinking and driving. It appears that aftercare strategies can enhance the endurance of positive behavioral changes (e.g., Ahles, Schlundt, Prue, & Rychtarik, 1983; Davidson, 1976; Pittman & Tate, 1969; Pokorny, Miller, Kanas, & Valles, 1973; Ritson, 1969), but their use with DWI offenders has not been assessed.

In summary, promising steps have been taken in the behavioral group treatment of DWI offenders. Continued research is needed to specify the parameters of these behavior change principles and to enhance the long-term maintenance of behavior change to reduce the incidence of DWI recidivism.

References

Ahles, T. A., Schlundt, D. G., Prue, D. M., & Rychtarik, R. R. Impact of aftercare arrangements on the maintenance of treatment success in abusive drinkers. *Addictive Behaviors*, 1983, *8*, 53–58.

Bandura, A. Self-efficacy: Toward a unifying theory of behavioral change. *Psychological Review*, 1977, *84*, 191–215.

Beitel, G. A., Sharp, M. C., & Glauz, W. D. Probability of arrest while driving under the influence of alcohol. *Journal of Studies on Alcohol*, 1975, *36*, 109–116.

Bell, R. A., Warheit, G. J., Bell, R. A., & Sanders, G. An analytic comparison of persons arrested for driving while intoxicated and alcohol detoxification patients. *Alcoholism: Clinical and Experimental Research*, 1978, *2*, 241–248.

Brown, R. A. Conventional education and controlled drinking education courses with convicted drunken drivers. *Behavior Therapy*, 1980, *11*, 632–642.

Calsyn, D. A., Reynolds, R. D., O'Leary, M. D., & Walker, R. D. Differential drinking patterns, personality characteristics, and field articulation of court-referred and non-court-referred male alcoholics in treatment. *International Journal of the Addictions*, 1982, *17*, 249–257.

Connors, G. J., Maisto, S. A., & Ersner-Hershfield, S. M. *Treating drunk-driving recidivists: Short and long-term effects of a behavioral treatment*. Paper presented at the annual meeting of the Association for Advancement of Behavior Therapy, Washington, D.C., December 1983.

Davidson, A. F. An evaluation of the treatment and aftercare of a hundred alcoholics. *British Journal of Addictions*, 1976, *71*, 217–224.

Donovan, D. M., & Marlatt, G. A. Personality subtypes among driving-while-intoxicated offenders: Relationship to drinking behavior and driving risk. *Journal of Consulting and Clinical Psychology*, 1982, *50*, 241–249.

Donovan, D. M., Marlatt, G. A., & Salzberg, P. M. Drinking behavior, personality factors and high-risk driving: A review and theoretical formulation. *Journal of Studies on Alcohol*, 1983, *44*, 395–428.

D'Zurilla, T. J., & Goldfried, M. R. Problem-solving and behavior modification. *Journal of Abnormal Psychology*, 1971, *78*, 107–126.

Ellingstad, V. A., & Springer, T. J. *Program level evaluation of ASAP diagnosis, referral and rehabilitation efforts: Volume III—Analysis of rehabilitation countermeasure effectiveness*. Prepared for Department of Transportation, National Highway Traffic Safety Administration. (Report No. DOT-HS-802-044). Springfield, Va.: National Technical Information Service, 1976.

Ersner-Hershfield, S. M., Connors, G. J., & Maisto, S. A. Clinical and experimental utility of refundable deposits. *Behaviour Research and Therapy*, 1981, *19*, 455–457.

Fine, E. W., & Scoles, P. Secondary prevention of alcoholism using a population of offenders arrested for driving while intoxicated. *Annuals of the New York Academy of Science*, 1976, *273*, 637–645.

Fine, E. W., Scoles, P., & Mulligan, M. Under the influence. *Public Health Reports*, 1975, *90*, 424–429.

Foy, D. W., Miller, P. M., Eisler, R. M., & O'Toole, D. H. Social skills training to teach alcoholics to refuse drinks effectively. *Journal of Studies on Alcohol*, 1976, *37*, 1340–1346.

Goldfried, M. R., & Davison, G. C. *Clinical behavior therapy*. New York: Holt, Reinhart & Winston, 1976.

Havard, J. D. The drinking driver and the law: Legal countermeasures in the prevention of alcohol-related road traffic accidents. In R. J. Gibbins, Y. Israel, H. Kalant, R. E. Popham, W. Schmidt, & R. G. Smart (Eds.), *Research advances in alcohol and drug problems* (Vol. 2). New York: Wiley, 1975.

Hayslip, B., Kapusinski, D., Darbes, A., & Zeh, R. Evaluation of driving-while-intoxicated programs: Some methodological considerations. *Journal of Studies on Alcohol*, 1976, *37*, 1742–1746.

Heise, H. A. Alcohol and automobile accidents. *Journal of the American Medical Association*, 1934, *103*, 739–741.

Holcomb, R. L. Alcohol in relation to traffic accidents. *Journal of the American Medical Association*, 1938, *111*, 1076–1085.

Israelstam, S., & Lambert, S. (Eds.). *Alcohol, drugs and traffic safety: Proceedings of the 6th International Conference on Alcohol, Drugs, and Traffic Safety, Toronto, September 1974*. Toronto: Addiction Research Foundation, 1975.

Kanfer, F. H. Self-management methods. In F. H. Kanfer & A. P. Goldstein (Eds.), *Helping people change* (2d ed.). New York: Pergamon Press, 1980.

Kanfer, F. H., & Goldstein, A. P. *Helping people change* (2d ed.). New York: Pergamon Press, 1980.

Klajner, F., Sobell, L. C., & Sobell, M. B. Secondary prevention of drunk-driving: Pitfalls, pratfalls, and prescriptions. In P. M. Miller and T. D. Nirenberg (Eds.), *Prevention of alcohol abuse*. New York: Plenum Press, 1984.

Lazarus, A. A. Behavior therapy in groups. In G. M. Gazda (Ed.), *Basic approaches to group psychotherapy and group counseling*. Springfield, Ill.: Charles C Thomas, 1968.

Levy, P., Voas, R., Johnson, P., & Klein, T. M. An evaluation of the Department of Transportation's Alcohol Safety Action Projects. *Journal of Safety Research*, 1978, *10*, 162–176.

Mahoney, M. J., & Thoresen, C. E. *Self-control: Power to the person*. Monterey, Calif.: Brooks/Cole, 1974.

Maisto, S. A., & McCollam, J. B. The use of multiple measures of life health to assess alcohol treatment outcome: A review and critique. In L. C. Sobell, M. B. Sobell, & E. Ward (Eds.), *Evaluating alcohol and drug abuse treatment effectiveness: Recent advances*. New York: Pergamon Press, 1980.

Maisto, S. A., Sobell, L. C., Zelhart, P. F., Connors, G. J., & Cooper, T. Driving records of persons convicted of driving under the influence of alcohol. *Journal of Studies on Alcohol*, 1979, *40*, 70–77.

Malfetti, J. L. Reeducation and rehabilitation of the drunken driver. *Journal of Drug Issues*, 1975, *5*, 255–269.

Marlatt, G. A., & Nathan, P. E. *Behavioral approaches to alcoholism*. New Brunswick, N.J.: Rutgers Center of Alcohol Studies, 1978.

Miller, P. M. *Behavioral treatment of alcoholism*. New York: Pergamon Press, 1976.

Miller, W. R., & Hester, R. K. Treating the problem drinker: Modern approaches. In W. R. Miller (Ed.), *The addictive behaviors: Treatment of alcoholism, drug abuse, smoking, and obesity*. New York: Pergamon Press, 1980.

Monroe, D. G. The drinking driver: Problems of enforcement. *Quarterly Journal of Studies on Alcohol*, 1947, *8*, 385–405.

"Motor wagons." *Quarterly Journal of Inebriety*, 1904, *26*, 308–309.

Nathan, H., & Turnbull, J. The psychiatrist's role in combating drunken driving. *Canadian Psychiatry Association Journal*, 1974, *19*, 381–385.

Nathan, P. E., & Briddell, D. W. Behavioral assessment and treatment of alcoholism. In B. Kissin &

H. Begleiter (Eds.), *The biology of alcoholism: Treatment and rehabilitation of the chronic alcoholic.* (Vol. 5). New York: Plenum Press, 1977.

Nichols, J. L., Weinstein, E. B., Ellingstad, V. S., & Struckman-Johnson, D. L. The specific deterrent effect of ASAP education and rehabilitation programs. *Journal of Safety Research,* 1978, *10,* 177–187.

Nichols, J. L., Ellingstad, V. S., & Struckman-Johnson, D. L. An experimental evaluation of the effectiveness of short-term education and rehabilitation programs for convicted drinking drivers. In M. Galanter (Ed.), *Currents in alcoholism: Treatment and rehabilitation and epidemiology* (Vol. 6). New York: Grune & Stratton, 1979.

Noel, N. E., Sobell, L. C., Celluci, T., Nirenberg, T., & Sobell, M. B. Behavioral treatment of outpatient program drinkers: Five clinical case studies. In W. M. Hays & P. E. Nathan (Eds.), *Clinical case studies in the behavioral treatment of alcoholism.* New York: Plenum Press, 1982.

O'Farrell, T. J., & Cutter, H. S. G. Behavioral marital therapy for male alcoholics: Clinical procedures from a treatment outcome study in progress. *American Journal of Family Therapy,* 1984, *12,* 33–46.

Pittman, D. J., & Tate, R. L. A comparison of two treatment programs for alcoholics. *Quarterly Journal of Studies on Alcohol,* 1969, *30,* 888–899.

Pokorny, A. D., Miller, B. A., Kanas, T., & Valles, J. Effectiveness of extended aftercare in the treatment of alcoholism. *Quarterly Journal of Studies on Alcohol,* 1973, *34,* 435–443.

Reed, D. S. Drinking and driving programs. In *Prevention, intervention, and treatment: Concerns and models* (Alcohol and Health Monograph No. 3). Rockville, Md.: National Institute on Alcohol Abuse and Alcoholism, 1982.

Regan, J. M., Connors, G. J., O'Farrell, T. J., & Jones, W. C. Services to the families of alcoholics: A survey of treatment agencies in Massachusetts. *Journal of Studies on Alcohol,* 1983, *44,* 1072–1082.

Ritson, B. Involvement in treatment and its relation to outcome amongst alcoholics. *British Journal of Addictions,* 1969, *64,* 23–29.

Rose, S. D. *Group therapy: A behavioral approach.* Englewood Cliffs, N.J.: Prentice-Hall, 1977.

Salzberg, P. M., Queisser, H. R., & Donovan, D. M. *Skill training: An intervention program for DWI offenders.* Paper presented at the annual conference of the National Council on Alcoholism, Seattle, May 1980.

Sandler, I., Palmer, S., Holmen, M., & Wynkoop, R. Drinking characteristics of DWIs screened as problem drinkers. *Alcohol Health and Research World,* Fall 1975.

Scoles, P., & Fine, E. W. Short-term effects of an educational program for drinking drivers. *Journal of Studies on Alcohol,* 1977, *38,* 633–637.

Selzer, M. L., & Barton, E. The drunken driver: A psychosocial study. *Drug and Alcohol Dependence,* 1977, *2,* 239–253.

Seppala, T., Linnoila, M., & Mattila, M. J. Drugs, alcohol and driving. *Drugs,* 1979, *17,* 389–408.

Sobell, L. C., VanderSpek, R., & Saltman, P. Utility of portable breath alcohol testers for drinking driver offenders. *Journal of Studies on Alcohol,* 1980, *41,* 930–934.

Sobell, M. B., Sobell, L. C., Ersner-Hershfield, S., & Nirenberg, T. Alcohol and drug problems. In A. S. Bellack, M. Hersen, & A. E. Kazdin (Eds.), *International handbook of behavior therapy.* New York: Plenum Press, 1982.

Sobell, M. B., & Sobell, L. C. Functional analysis of alcohol problems. In C. K. Prokop & L. A. Bradley (Eds.), *Medical psychology: Contributions to behavioral medicine.* New York: Academic Press, 1981.

Steer, R. A., & Fine, E. W. Mood differences of men arrested once and men arrested twice for driving while intoxicated. *Journal of Studies on Alcohol,* 1978, *39,* 922–925.

Steer, R. A., Fine, E. W., & Scoles, P. E. Classification of men arrested for driving while intoxicated, and treatment implications. *Journal of Studies on Alcohol,* 1979, *40,* 222–229.

Sutker, P. B., Brantley, P. J., & Allain, A. N. MMPI response patterns and alcohol consumption in DWI offenders. *Journal of Consulting and Clinical Psychology,* 1980, *48,* 350–355.

Thoresen, C. E., & Mahoney, M. J. *Behavioral self-control.* New York: Holt, Reinhart & Winston, 1974.

Yoder, R. D., & Moore, R. A. Characteristics of convicted drunken drivers. *Quarterly Journal of Studies on Alcohol,* 1973, *34,* 927–936.

Waller, J. A. Identification of problem drinking among drunken drivers. *Journal of the American Medical Association,* 1967, *200,* 114–120.

Waller, P. F. Alcohol and highway safety. In E. M. Pattison & E. Kaufman (Eds.), *Encyclopedic handbook of alcoholism*. New York: Gardner Press, 1982.

Whitehead, P. C. DWI programs: Doing what's in or dodging what's indicated? *Journal of Safety Research*, 1975, *7*, 127–134.

Yoder, R. D. & Moore, R. A. Characteristics of convicted drunken drivers. *Quarterly Journal of Studies on Alcohol*, 1973, *34*, 927–936.

Zador, P. Statistical evaluation of the effectiveness of "Alcohol Safety Action Programs." *Accident Analysis and Prevention*, 1976, *8*, 51–66.

Zelhart, P. F., & Schurr, B. C. People who drive while impaired: A review of research on the drinking-driver problem. In N. Estes & E. Heinemann (Eds.), *Alcoholism: Physiological and psychological bases*. St. Louis: Mosby, 1977.

Zylman, R. Drinking-driving and fatal crashes: A new perspective. *Journal of Alcohol and Drug Education*, 1975, *21*, 1–10.

16

The Management of Chronic Pain

A Cognitive-Functioning Approach

RONALD J. KULICH AND BRUCE S. GOTTLIEB

INTRODUCTION

Despite a vast array of treatment efforts from medical, psychological, and rehabilitation sources, chronic pain problems continue to plague society. In the United States, the management of chronic pain, including hospital and health-care services, loss of work productivity, insurance compensation, medication, and litigation costs an estimated $40 to $50 billion annually (U.S. Department of Health, Education and Welfare, 1979). It has been estimated that 700 million work days are lost per year due to chronic pain (Brena, Chapman, Stegall, & Chyatte, 1979). In addition to these financial costs, there is a significant level of emotional distress suffered by the patients and their families.

Traditional medical and surgical approaches that have attempted to eliminate the individual's pain have met with only limited success. It has become clear that traditional approaches have employed too narrow a perspective, overlooking the complexity of the chronic pain problem (see review by Turner & Chapman, 1982). However, increasingly effective treatment has been developed by integrating principles of behavioral science in comprehensive pain management programs that can provide treatment for the multiple difficulties that comprise the chronic pain problem. This approach, explicated in the present chapter (a) describes the chronic pain patient and the particular needs of this population; (b) reviews a cognitive-functioning formulation of chronic pain (Gottlieb, 1984) based on Beck's applications to depression and anxiety (Beck & Emery, 1979; Beck, Rush, Shaw, & Emery, 1979); (c) outlines a program that integrates this cognitive approach with approaches to deal with the various aspects of the chronic pain patient's problem; and (d) discusses the advantages involved in the group treatment of these patients.

RONALD J. KULICH • Lahey Clinic Medical Center, Burlington, Massachusetts 01805. BRUCE S. GOTTLIEB • Pain Management and Behavioral Medical Center, Farmington, Connecticut 06032.

Development of the Chronic Pain Syndrome

The chronic pain syndrome discussed in this chapter typically begins following an injury, but can also be a result of arthritis, fibrositis, pancreatitis, headaches, or other disorders. As noted in Figure 1, the chronic pain syndrome begins when the patient's injury has occurred, and the pain phase persists, despite multiple treatments.

Most patients with back injuries do show significant improvement with conservative management techniques, and patients eventually return to work and to avocational activities. However, in certain situations, an increase in the activity level may result in more severe pain. The patient then returns to a state of inactivity in an attempt to reduce the pain. This pattern may occur a number of times, and the individual may begin to believe he or she can accurately predict the pain he or she will experience following activity.

Once the patient begins to anticipate that certain events will exacerbate his or her condition, he or she may tend to avoid those events, thus promoting his or her disability. Whenever pain occurs, he or she will attempt to terminate it by discontinuing the activity and will often apply some treatment. A negative reinforcement paradigm is thereby established wherein the patient successfully terminates the pain by inactivity. Eventually, this inactivity will only terminate the pain intermittently, and a chronic pain problem will develop.

The situation is further complicated by the attention and concern provided by family members who inadvertently reinforce the person's pain problem and by health-care providers who instruct the patient to engage in activities to "tolerance". This tends to exacerbate the individual's disability as the patient learns that an increasingly wide range of behaviors falls above the anticipated tolerance level.

Figure 2 represents the phase in which the chronic pain patient has dramatically reduced most activity in order to avoid any possible painful stimuli. However, pain persists, and self-applied treatments eventually become habitual avoidance responses regardless of their lack of effectiveness.

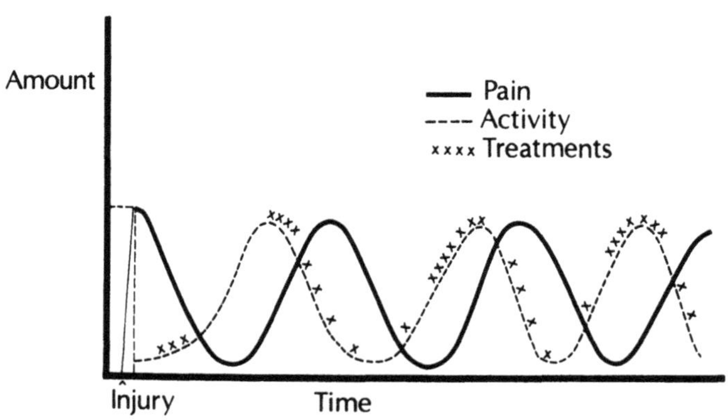

FIGURE 1. Pain-related activity levels.

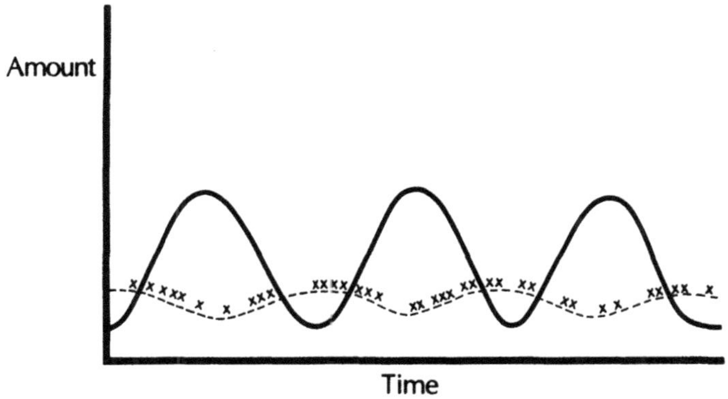

FIGURE 2. Chronic avoidance of activity and seeking multiple treatments.

Weakness, muscle spasms, and various psychosocial difficulties then ensue. Any efforts to return to activity often may be conducted in nonpaced spurts, interrupted by pain, leading the individual to conclude that he or she should not engage in those activities at all.

The individual's motivation to avoid pain is exponentially increased by the belief that the pain represents physical danger. When the injury is first incurred, the pain sensation indicates that the individual has sustained an insult, and guarding as well as inactivity of the damaged body part is desired in order for it to heal. As the individual's pain persists, the resting and guarding response also persists because the individual cannot discriminate between pain that signals danger and benign chronic pain. Indeed, the individual may conclude that because his or her pain has continued so long, the problem is even more serious than was initially believed.

The belief that *any* pain is dangerous is reinforced by family and physicians, who tell patients to stop an activity and to rest when they experience pain. Extensive attempts to reduce pain or continued referrals to other physicians, even when negative results are expected, reinforce the idea that there has to be some procedure that will eliminate the pain. Finally, because there are so many people trying to do so much to eliminate the pain, the individual may conclude that his or her pain *really* is as terrible a problem as he or she initially believed.

Additional cognitive distortions are often present, depending on the person's proclivities. Unrealistic expectations of health-care providers and family members, exaggerated fears of what the pain means, tendencies to view the problems in all-or-nothing terms (e.g., completely disabled or completely well), and other dysfunctional cognitive phenomena that may contribute to the individual's disability and distress are commonly observed in chronic pain patients.

A "TYPICAL" CHRONIC PAIN PATIENT

Research and clinical experience have shown chronic pain to be a particularly complex problem. Although the characteristics of chronic pain patients may vary markedly, the following illustrates a typical profile of individuals who are selected for treatment in a comprehensive pain management program.

1. Most patients have sustained an injury, usually in a work-related setting, and subsequently complain of low back pain. The location of the pain may become more diffuse as chronicity progresses, and it is not uncommon for some individuals to complain of virtual total-body pain.

2. The individual's pain has resisted multiple traditional forms of treatment for a period of 6 months or more. Typical treatments that may have been attempted include bed rest, chiropractic manipulation, various braces, traction, heat, ice, massage, transcutaneous neural stimulation, various nerve blocks, hypnosis, exercise, psychotherapy, and often, multiple surgeries. Furthermore, Brena (1983) reported that 73% of chronic pain patients also suffer from iatrogenic complications related to unnecessary surgery or other treatments.

3. Some degree of disability is present with all work activities usually terminated due to pain. Many patients' lives consist of little more than seeking treatment, spending large amounts of time in bed, and engaging in multiple overt pain behaviors, such as complaining, grimacing, and limping. Often, family members assume the pain patient's former responsibilities or admonish the individual not to engage in activities that they fear may result in further injury. This type of response inadvertently promotes the individual's disability and makes rehabilitation more difficult. In order to avoid pain or try to reduce it, the chronic pain patient no longer engages in sports, recreational hobbies, or social activities. Medically, such long-term muscle disuse may exacerbate fibrositis and degenerative changes (Cailliet, 1983).

4. Difficulty with dependence on medication is often reported, and it is estimated that 90% of chronic pain patients misuse prescription medications (see Brena, 1983). These difficulties are compounded when the individual sees several physicians, each of whom will try to manage his or her patient's complaints with various medications. This can be further complicated in cases where the individuals attempt to medicate themselves.

5. Psychological disturbances are often associated with chronic pain states. The presence of depression or anxiety is often evident in this population, and many patients report sleep disturbances, tearfulness, helplessness, lethargy, or concentration difficulties (see Fordyce, 1976; Sternbach, 1974). In addition, family relationships may be strained by the necessity for others to assume the pain patient's former responsibilities and the tendency for family communications to center around strategies for seeking pain relief (see Block, Kremer, & Gaylor, 1980; Shanfield, Heiman, Cope, & Jones, 1979; Swanson & Maruta, 1980).

6. Multiple health-care providers may present conflicting opinions and treatment recommendations regarding the possible outcome of surgeries, how the patient should cope with his or her problem on a day-to-day basis (e.g., whether or not to wear his or her corset), and other issues. This adds to the frustration of the health-care professionals dealing with the patient and to the distress of the patients and their families.

7. Financial and legal difficulties may complicate the chronic pain problem, particularly when attorneys reinforce decreases in functioning in order to obtain

as great a settlement as possible. The patient may perceive that the treatment gains will jeopardize chances to resolve a suit, or the patient may fear the possible termination of desperately needed compensation payments if his or her condition should improve.

8. The typical chronic pain patient subscribes to a number of beliefs that serve to promote physical disfunction (Gottlieb, 1984). These dysfunctional beliefs include misinterpretations of data (e.g., "It feels as though something is ripping apart my back"); overgeneralizations, (e.g., "I will be completely disabled tomorrow if I clean the house today"); negative predictions ("If I have more pain I will cripple myself"); and arbitrary statements (e.g., "I should stop my activity as soon as my pain increases"). In addition to promoting the individual's disability, such cognitions tend to engender psychological distress (Beck *et al.*, 1979).

The preceding description illustrates a complex picture of suffering experienced by the chronic pain patient and his or her family, a situation that is unlikely to be ameliorated by any narrowly focused treatment intervention offered by a single discipline. Comprehensive treatment must be offered to address the multiple problem areas.

Screening Issues

There are a number of chronic pain patients who are not appropriate for a comprehensive intervention program that targets the previously mentioned areas. Although exclusion criteria tend to remain somewhat subjective (see Keefe, Block, Williams, & Surwit, 1981), there are several factors that should be evaluated when considering a patient for a comprehensive chronic pain treatment program.

1. Often, chronic pain patients indicate that they want only to eliminate the pain, despite being told by numerous physicians that it is not possible to do so. Individuals can usually be disabused of this idea by reviewing their medical history and noting the results of past treatments. When individuals note that all pain-relieving attempts have provided only temporary relief at best, they are usually unable to conclude that further treatment will likely result in failure. Individuals who insist that they want to continue to search for someone to get rid of their pain would not be appropriate candidates.

2. Occasionally, there is minimal or no distress associated with the individual's disability. If the individual is not highly motivated to change his or her lifestyle, it is unlikely that he or she will be able to put forth the effort needed to succeed in treatment. In some cases, obvious satisfaction with disability may be present. Patients may enter an initial evaluation smiling and making statements such as "although my pain is terrible, it seems to have brought my wife and me together," or "I've never done much in the way of activity anyway." In such cases, intervention can be directed toward helping the primary care physician to minimize health-care utilization, medication abuse, and so forth.

3. Patients who display erratic vocational histories and do not believe that they can return to work may be very ambivalent about a treatment program designed to return them to work. Many individuals believe that because of their limitations, they cannot earn a living. Such individuals may conclude that they would be better off to try to maintain their disability payments and defer their efforts at trying to overcome their disability.

4. An adequate social support system or significant other may not be present. Presence of a supportive family member has been shown to be important to providing reinforcement for treatment gains *outside* of the treatment setting, as well as maintenance of treatment gains after the completion of the program.

5. The patient may possess a history of significant psychiatric difficulties that preclude or severely inhibit the learning of appropriate, cognitive coping responses, for example, a major affective disorder or thought disorder.

6. The patient may possess covert or overt treatment agendas that conflict with the goals of the treatment program. For example, the patient may make statements such as "The program sounds good, but the medication works . . . and I'll have to just keep taking it unless my pain stops."

7. Although not precluding a patient's appropriateness in every case, many patients present with major issues of compensation or legal complications. Patients are told that gradual gains within the program are documented on a daily and weekly basis, and it is not a question of "seeing if I am all better in the end." In this regard, they are made aware that participation may impair the outcome of lawsuits or compensation cases.

8. Some patients present with additional medical issues that have not achieved satisfactory resolution (e.g., sufficient testing to rule out a ruptured disc). In such cases, increases in activity are contraindicated as pain may not be benign in nature. Thus, a complete medical evaluation is critical prior to the onset of any active treatment program. In these cases, the patient would not be appropriate for treatment until these problems are resolved.

Assessment Protocol

The chronic pain literature has been replete with a variety of instruments for addressing screening factors, identifying treatment targets, and assessing treatment outcome (Johnson, 1983). We will briefly state the assessment strategies that are employed in a pre-post format as well as those that are employed throughout the treatment process. From a treatment planning point of view, the primary focus is usually on the need to conduct an adequate functional analysis, identifying the antecedents and consequences of the patient's pain behavior. The first stage of assessment involves an initial interview that addresses each of the screening issues, identifies treatment goals, and maximizes commitment to the treatment process. It is important to note that a "significant other" is required to attend this interview because information from this additional source is often very valuable.

In addition to an assessment interview, patients are administered a series of self-monitoring activity diaries in which to record daily physical activity, pain behaviors, medication usage, social interaction, and cognitive appraisals of performance. Patients are also given a series of activity graphs that they maintain as visual indicators of their step-by-step progress. Each health-care provider can review the graphs and provide feedback on the patient's progress within the program. In addition to the preceding measures, patients complete a series of questionnaires pre- and posttreatment. These include the Sickness Impact Profile, a measure of physical, emotional, and social functioning (Gibson, Gilson, Bergner, Bobbitt, Kreisel, Pollar, & Vesselaso, 1975), measures of marital functioning, and a videotaping sequence of specific functional activities (see Kulich, Follick, Miller, & Conger, 1983).

Prior to initiating a treatment regimen, the physical and occupational therapists evaluate the patient's range of motion, muscle strength, and elasticity. Multiple muscle spasms and disuse atrophy may be present, and comprehensive assessment is needed to determine the contributory nature of these factors (for evaluation format, see Grabois, 1979; Roesch & Ulrich, 1980).

Treatment Goals

The rehabilitation of chronic pain patients entails helping them to live as normal a life-style as possible despite pain. Consequently, we need to help these individuals accept the fact of the pain persisting and to help them see that there are ways of reducing the impact of their pain on their lives. The following represents the goals that we can help the patient achieve. All goals are generated with as much input from the patient as possible.

1. *Reconceptualize the various aspects of the pain problem as problems that the individual can solve.* Many patients believe that their life-style will always be determined by the level of their pain. They conclude their situation is hopeless unless their pain is eliminated. Thus, patients search for pain relief even when it is not possible. The problem is reconceptualized so that the goal becomes how the person can change *what he or she does* instead of changing *how he or she feels.*

2. *Improve physical functioning and body mechanics.* As the majority of chronic pain patients have spent considerable time in sedentary pursuits, muscle atrophy and joint stiffness is common. Patients complete a comprehensive physical reconditioning program designed to increase their strength, endurance, and range of motion. Patients are also taught proper posture, lifting and bending techniques, and body mechanics needed to compensate for physical limitations.

3. *Develop a more "normal" activity level.* Activities that constitute a normal life-style for the individual (e.g., household chores, shipping, socializing, etc.) are gradually introduced. These "well behaviors" are usually those activities that the individual discontinued or has not pursued because of pain.

4. *Return to gainful employment.* Vocational functioning is promoted with the help of a vocational counselor. This may entail returning to a former job, modification of that job, or vocational retraining.

5. *Reducing reliance on pain behaviors.* All verbal and nonverbal pain behaviors are gradually eliminated. These include complaining of pain, using medication, limping, grimacing, lying down, and others.

6. *Psychological problems resulting from the pain problem are treated.* Psychological responses to chronic pain, such as anxiety or depression, are targeted in order to reduce the distress associated with the problem. This may include improving sleep habits or concentration, or reducing muscle tension.

7. *Reducing family and marital discord.* Block *et al.* (1982) have argued the importance of addressing spouse and family distress in this population. Significant others may enhance treatment efficacy by providing patients with encouragement and reinforcement for engaging in newly learned behaviors in the home environment.

8. *Reducing unnecessary health-care utilization.* Many patients believe that someone ought to be able to eliminate the pain and thus persist in seeking further medical care. As they are disabused of this idea and alternatively learn that there are effective ways of improving their life-style, they are usually willing to discontinue their search for a cure. Appropriate uses of the health-care system are discussed.

9. *Decatastrophizing the pain problem.* Many pain patients regard their pain and associated disability as "terrible," "catastrophic," or "overwhelming." This tendency makes the individual's pain problem appear unsolvable and results in increased anxiety and depression. Individuals are taught to conceptualize the pain problem more objectively and attend to changes that they can effect rather than ruminating about the pain problem.

All of the preceding goals are designed to help the individual develop a sense of control over the pain problem. Generating lists of goals with the patient, in terms of what the individual can do differently in order to improve his or her life-style, helps to make the pain problem less overwhelming. The patient is encouraged to develop a problem-solving set whereby he or she learns to generate alternative ways to deal with problems and to set specific goals that will help him or her to resolve those problems.

Given the complexity of the chronic pain problem, the successful treatment of the patient requires a coordination of multiple sources of expertise. This often includes the involvement of physicians, psychologists, physical therapists, vocational counselors, occupational therapists, and others.

Treatment Rationale

Nearly all chronic pain patients have had an extensive history of medical treatments designed to reduce their pain. The expectation that there must be some way of eliminating the pain is promoted by family, friends, and physicians, until the primary care provider indicates that the pain will probably continue despite further treatment. For the person to relinquish his or her search for pain relief and adopt an approach designed to modify his or her life-style despite pain, it is imperative to present a rationale that the person can understand and accept.

Both Fordyce (1976) and Genest and Turk (1979) present rationales that suggest that the individual's pain is controlled by environmental events. But, whereas Fordyce suggests that changing the behavior's consequence will alter the individual's pain experience, Genest and Turk suggest that the person can reduce his or her pain by developing various coping skills.

An alternative rationale is offered at the authors' programs consistent with the cognitive-functioning formulation presented in this chapter. Using a Socratic approach, the rationale is first presented in the initial interview between therapist and client:

T: [*Following a review of the individual's medical history*] So, after all of these procedures, you still say that you have had most of your pain for years. How much has all of this treatment helped you?
C: I guess not much. Usually I feel a bit better for only a few hours if I do something like take a pill.
T: So, at this point, do you really think any treatment will be able to eliminate your pain?
C: I guess not—at least that's what my doctors tell me.
T: You've had this pain for a while, and it seems like it will probably continue. But what about all of the things you stopped doing? Do you really want to do those again?
C: Sure, I'd love to, but I really can't; not with all of this pain!
T: It sounds like you really believe that you can't change your functioning much as long as you have pain; and that you have concluded that as long as you have pain, you will have to be disabled.
C: Well, that's the way it's been for years, and it's not getting any better—in fact, it seems worse all of the time.
T: Well, let's look at specifics, taking one step at a time. You say that you can't go running like you used to, but what about walking? If you were able to get used to walking further distances—say, a mile or so—do you think you'd be ready to try a little running?
C: Well, it's probably worth a try.

Note that the therapist is educating the patient, disabusing him or her of the idea that the pain can be eliminated by examining the patient's own past experiences. The alternative is then generated—learning to resume activities despite pain and a plausible method of doing so is introduced—a gradual, stepwise approach. The interview is conducted with the individuals' drawing the conclusions themselves as much as possible, rather than the therapist's imposing his or her own constructions on the patient. This engenders a cooperative approach with the therapist in the role of facilitator rather than an individual who can "cure" the patient. This also helps the individual to realize that treatment gains will ultimately be a function of his or her own efforts. This is particularly important as most patients expect the same kind of treatment they received in the past, where they essentially took their bodies to a physician's office and expected him or her to eliminate their pain.

In fact, many patients respond favorably to a treatment approach that indicates that they can exert control over the course of treatment and ultimately over their disability. To be sure, many patients are distressed at the prospect of having to assume more responsibility for their pain problem. These patients need to be assured that treatment progresses as gradually as needed for them to accomplish their treatment goals and that the staff will provide ample direction and support.

Review of the treatment rationale is conducted at the first group meeting. Group members are asked to relate their expectations of treatment, and fellow group members are invited to comment. It appears to be very encouraging for these individuals to hear that other pain patients are willing to test the hypothesis that they can improve their life-style despite the fact that their pain will probably continue.

Cognitive Techniques

Cognitive-behavioral approaches have been employed in group settings with chronic pain patients designed to help the individual to influence the level of his or her pain (Genest & Turk, 1979; Meichendaum & Turk, 1976; Tan, 1982; Turner & Chapman, 1982). Patients are taught attention diversion techniques, relaxation procedures, techniques to reconceptualize pain experience (e.g., thinking of the painful areas as being numb), and coping self-statements (e.g., "I won't think about the pain. I will focus my attention on remembering details of the movie I saw last night" [Genest & Turk, 1979, p. 266]) The focus of this approach is to provide the individual with some sense of control over his or her pain.

One of us has developed an alternative approach that focuses on the individual's *activities* and teaches the patient to recognize and evaluate cognitions that interfere with activities of daily living (Gottlieb, 1984). In contrast, Genest and Turk (1979) have the individual respond to his or her *pain* by generating self-statements designed to reduce the pain sensations. As noted earlier in the treatment rationale, the patient is disabused of the idea that it is possible to eliminate the pain. It is suggested that although it is not possible to eliminate this pain, patients can learn to improve their functioning. Rather than concluding that they should not do some activity at all because they have been unsuccessful in the past, they should conclude that they should do it differently because they are not attaining success with their current methods, The present model was developed following repeated observations of patients verbalizing reasons why they were so limited, and noting that many statements represented cognitive distortions of one type or another. Often, patients would report past experiences (e.g., trying to mow the lawn and then being bedridden for days) and the conclusions they drew (e,g,, "I should never try that again. I wouldn't be able to take the pain") that would promote their disability.

Given the perception of their problem that chronic pain patients have, it is easy to see why chronic pain syndromes have been so resistant to treatment.

When success is observed in behavioral pain management programs, it may take place as a function of the changes of cognitions resulting from experiences of a gradual shaping process where the individual finally realizes that "I can really do that activity after all." However, the current model suggests that treatment will be less anxiety provoking if the individual realizes that beliefs that promote the use of pain behaviors or overuse of the health-care system and ideas that support their disability may be inaccurate (e. g., "Maybe I won't hurt myself if I start by mowing only part of the lawn").

Cognitions that relate to the patient's functioning are assessed and discussed in a group setting so that patients see that others share their concerns, and to provide the opportunity for patients to model appropriate responses. The following five-step cognitive treatment approach is used.

1. The first objective of treatment is to disabuse patients of the idea that their pain can be eliminated and instead, have him or her consider the idea that it is feasible to improve one's life-style, despite pain. These notions are presented in the treatment rationale and throughout the program. The individual is encouraged to stop dwelling on the pain and limitations and to generate specific goals toward which to work.

2. Daily planning is initiated that is designed to increase normative activities (e.g., household cleaning) and reduce reliance on pain-related behaviors (e.g., taking medication, lying down).

3. Whenever the individual does not accomplish his or her daily goals, he or she identifies any cognitions that inhibited performance. For example, the person may believe that he or she will further damage his or her body if he or she tries to engage in certain activities or that he or she necessarily has to lie down when in pain.

4. The individual determines the accuracy of his or her beliefs usually asking, "How do I know that?" or "Is it really as likely to happen as it seems?" and then adopts a more objective viewpoint, for example "Just because I couldn't do it last time doesn't mean that I'll never be able to do it."

5. The consequences of the belief are then determined (e.g., "As long as I believe that, I will always be limited"), and the individual generates a more useful idea to apply to that situation (e.g., "I have nothing to lose by trying; perhaps I will be able to get it done"). This serves to further reinforce the idea that the disability is largely a result of a dysfunctional thought pattern rather than completely veridical perceptions.

The idea that the individual can control his or her life-style is stressed throughout the program. An experimental approach is encouraged wherein hypotheses regarding the ability to modify the individual's life-style are tested. This is done primarily by gradually reducing pain behaviors, improving activity level, and learning that having a pain problem does not have to be so distressing.

Reducing Pain Behaviors

When an individual develops a pain problem, he or she is likely to engage in any number of pain behaviors in order to reduce the pain. These may include taking medication, lying down to rest, taking hot baths or showers, using a heating pad or transcutaneous neural stimulator. The patient may complain of pain, moan, groan, grimace, or sigh. Nearly all pain behaviors have deleterious consequences: the addiction to medication; increased muscle atrophy with prolonged rest; hot baths, showers, and other devices being incompatible with activities of daily functioning; and complaints that alienate family and friends. In addition, many pain behaviors preclude most types of employment.

Unfortunately, patients seem to attend to only the short-term consequences (i.e., feeling a bit better for a while) that maintain these behaviors. Rather than insisting that patients eliminate these behaviors as they "may reinforce their pain problem," patients in the treatment group are asked to examine all of the facts about pain behaviors and decide what course of action to take. Patients do this be generating lists of advantages and disadvantages of continuing their pain behaviors, as in the following example:

Advantages	*Disadvantages*
• Some temporary reduction of pain • Tension reduction	• Possibility of addition to medication • Muscle atrophy • Costliness • Ruins social relationships; people don't ask you to get involved in activities • Can't plan activities ahead (as may have to engage in pain behaviors) • Can't get a job • Gets you to focus more on pain • Gets you more depressed

Group members are then encouraged to discuss these results and indicate which list is more important to them. Nearly all patients decide the disadvantages outweigh the advantages and learn to gradually reduce their reliance on pain behaviors (e.g., using a heating pad on a lower heat setting for a shorter period of time). In addition to eliminating the deleterious consequences of the pain behavior, patients find out that they can gain greater control over their pain problem than they had previously believed they could. Contrary to their initial beliefs, many patients discover than they can manage to improve functioning without these pain behaviors.

Improving Activity Levels

As noted earlier, many people believe they should not be engaging in activities that increase their pain—that they will only make themselves worse. These individuals believe this very strongly as they have attempted to resume some activities only to fail, while exacerbating their pain. Some individuals are able to readily list activities that they cannot do (e.g., vacuum floors). They are encouraged to view these situations as problems to be solved by generating lists of initial steps that would help them accomplish their long-range goals (e.g., vacuum one-half of a room). Thus, the individual develops a list of things that he or she *can* do, that will help him or her accomplish the things he or she cannot do, *now*.

Such a list may include

1. Playing ball with his or her children
2. Eating at a restaurant once a week
3. Returning to bowling
4. Sitting through a movie
5. Doing volunteer work

Weekly goals are established, and a gradually shaping procedure is employed to resume these activities. It is not important *how much* is accomplished, but that the individual begins to develop a sense of greater control over his or her daily activities and realizes that he or she need not be as limited as he or she had been.

Occasionally patients may indicate that although they can do some of the activity, they will never be able to do it as they would like. This would be responded to by noting that there is no such certainty; that they may be able to do that activity over time and that if they cannot, they can learn to be satisfied with what they have accomplished. It is helpful for many patients to adopt the attitude, "What do I have to lose by trying?"

Decatastrophizing the Pain Problem

The greater majority of patients experience some distress associated with their pain problem. The experience of having an interminable aversive sensation and some continued activity limitation often serves to engender frustration, depression, and anxiety. As these reactions apparently make the pain experience more stressful, patients are taught to minimize their distress.

Patients are asked how they feel about their pain-related experiences (e.g., being limited physically) and are then asked *why* they feel that way, what makes it so upsetting for them. First, it is established that it is not their pain or limitations *per se* but rather their perceptions that engender their distress. Second, patients are instructed to determine if their perceptions are accurate and to correct them if they are not. For example, patients may feel depressed thinking that as long as they have pain they will never be happy. They can then determine that this is an exaggeration as most patients are able to recall experiences that they have had that contradict this belief.

Lastly, if the disadvantages outweigh the advantages of maintaining that belief, they are instructed to generate equally plausible ideas that are more useful. Thus, the individual who believes that "I can't stand the pain anymore" may learn to respond to that idea with the idea that "I really don't like this pain and it's too bad it doesn't go away, but in fact, I can stand it and can even try to improve my life in spite of it. At least I'll feel that I'm doing all that I can." The format that patients use is illustrated next:

Situation	*Emotional response*	*Upsetting thoughts*	*Useful responses*
Noticing sharp pains	Depressed	I'm getting worse.	This probably isn't true; I've had these a lot and my doctor says it's part of the problem. It doesn't mean that I'm doing more damage to myself.
		I'll never get better.	I don't know that. Certainly, thinking this way doesn't help; let me see what I can get done this week and see if I can do something productive.
		I can't stand this.	Of course I can stand it even if I don't like it. Although it may be hard, I can even keep working at improving things to see if things can get better for me.

Additional Treatment Groups

In addition to group sessions on learning how to modify their life-styles and coping more effectively with distress, multiple group sessions are devoted to developing a number of specific skills to address deficits common in chronic pain patients. In addition to the relaxation and vocational skills training groups described later, patients receive training in assertiveness, social skills, and Type A stress management, among other skills. Chronic pain patients may attend such skills training groups with nonpain patients to be exposed to models who may be functioning more effectively.

Relaxation Group

Chronic pain patients often complain of sleeplessness, muscle tightness and spasms, and lack of flexibility. These difficulties are treated with progressive muscle relaxation (Chapman, 1983). Although the relative contribution of relaxation training for the modification of chronic pain remains unclear, investigators generally have agreed that it is an efficacious treatment component (Sanders, 1983).

Often specialized relaxation exercises are developed for a patient to facilitate progress on a certain goal. For example, patients may employ relaxation techniques during gradual increases in sitting tolerance or during walking or cycling programs. The focus is placed on maximizing the patient's control over anxiety rather than reducing pain. Electromyographic biofeedback training may also be offered as an adjunct for improving control of muscular tension. However, it may be easier to promote generalization using progressive muscle relaxation as additional equipment is not needed.

Particular emphasis is also placed on the transfer of the relaxation response from the group to the patient's natural setting. Patients are encouraged to employ differential relaxation (Goldfried & Davison, 1976), whereby they relax only the muscles they find to be particularly tense. They would use this initially in situations with few other demands (e.g., watching a TV commercial) and would gradually employ it in more stressful situations (e.g., socializing during an exacerbation in their pain).

Vocational Skills Training

Early in treatment, patients undergo an evaluation by a vocational counselor who can assist in designing a treatment program including tasks that are required in the eventual work site (see Catchlove & Cohen, 1982). The physical demands of the job are assessed along with job stressors that can be addressed in the treatment program (e.g., communication or assertion problems with coworkers or supervisors).

Vocational groups are usually held in the last third of the pain management program, helping the individual develop skills to help him or her return to work or pursue other employment options. Specific techniques including modeling, behavioral rehearsal via taped feedback, and various homework assignments are provided. Typical topic areas include handling difficult questions, communication with the boss, and asking for help. Cognitions that would interfere with job search (e.g., "No one is going to hire someone with a back problem") are assessed, distortions are identified, and more functional cognitions are generated.

Physical Therapy

Physical and occupational therapy programs consist of exercises designed to improve the patient's activity tolerance rather than reduce or cure the pain (see Fordyce, 1976, for a review of a typical exercise regimen). Based on the initial evaluation, usually consisting of two or three sessions with the physical and occupational therapists, an individualized exercise regimen is established.

Each exercise is recorded on a graph with the starting point at minimum number of repetitions. For example, the patient may initiate a walking program at 2 minutes with an eventual goal for 45 minutes at the termination of the program. A generalization component is built into the exercise program often with the requirement that patients establish a membership in an organization such as a health club or YMCA/YWCA prior to the conclusion of the full treatment program.

The exercise regimen is gradually integrated into activities of daily living to promote generalization. For example, patients can rearrange materials in a closet, park further from the front of the building when they arrive for their appointments, and climb stairs rather than taking an elevator.

In addition to reconditioning the patient, the exercise program serves to disabuse the individual of the belief that his or her pain has to be eliminated in order for him or her to do more physically. Their daily charts and feedback from the physical and occupational therapist shows them that it is possible for them to effect significant changes in their physical capabilities once they are motivated to do so. Furthermore, the individual's fear of further injury gradually diminishes once he or she has an authority figure instructing him or her to gradually do more. As most patients were told by their physicians to do *less* whenever they have pain, they often need to be assured that it is not dangerous to now do more, if done in a gradual, structured fashion. In a short time, their own experience bears this out, and patients feel more relaxed completing their exercises.

Family and Spouse Involvement

A spouse or significant family member may sabotage any treatment regimen by continued reinforcement of disability behavior or conversely provide an ideal source of reinforcement for continued gains after the termination of the treatment program. Furthermore, family members may be worried about a loss of financial compensation or about changes in life-style if the patient does get better. Thus, investigators are paying greater attention to other family members when developing treatment programs (see Block *et al.*, 1980; Shanfield, *et al.*, 1979; Swanson & Maruta, 1980).

In order to address these and other issues, family involvement is required, and family members are encouraged to attend physical therapy sessions and group educative sessions. Joint marital therapy sessions also occur on a weekly basis with approximately 70% of the patients, and the focus is placed on improved communication strategies and planning of pleasant events.

Group members and their families discuss how they interact with the patients when they have pain as well as the advantages and disadvantages of their approach. Often, both the patients and their families feel quite frustrated by the problem and want to change the way that they cope with it. However, they both may think that if family members do not express concern about the patient's pain, it means that they do not care about the patient. They need to be disabused of this idea and determine what are more normative ways of expressing caring.

Maximizing Compliance

An emphasis is placed on maximizing the patient's commitment to the treatment process and adherence to the treatment regimen. This is addressed at the inception of the pain management program as well as throughout the treatment process. The patient is told that the treatment program requires more than "just bringing your body to your doctor's office for him to take care of it," but rather requires a consistent effort in order for patients to benefit.

Patients may be challenged regarding their motivation to resume various activities in order to determine whether or not these activities are important enough for them to expend the effort needed to achieve their goals. For example, a patient may be asked why he or she wants to return to work if his or her current workman compensation payments covers his or her expenses. The individual's commitment is formalized in a treatment contract (Fordyce, 1976) wherein the specific target behaviors and treatment goals for the patient and family are outlined. As noted earlier, the majority of these patients have received multiple treatments and conflicting messages regarding appropriate ways to deal with their pain problem. The clarity of a written treatment agreement assists in maximizing adherence to the treatment regimen.

Commitment is further enhanced by encouraging the patient to test out hypotheses rather than simply accepting the therapist's perspective. The patient develops an experimental approach in which he or she tries out different approaches to see which will best help him or her to develop more control over his or her pain problem. Moreover, patients are taught that treatment gains are ultimately a function of their own efforts.

Aftercare Groups

Posttreatment structured groups are employed to assist with the maintenance of treatment gains. We have attempted to address the important issue of aftercare by encouraging patients to continue with ongoing monthly group sessions that review previously outlined treatment gains and principles. Many patients have developed a commitment to assisting new candidates to the program while participating in problem-solving sessions about new difficulties that may have arisen for them. Family members are encouraged to attend when relevant topics are covered. One or more components of the program also may be reinstituted as a brief treatment booster (e.g., a 10-day relaxation or vocational group sequence).

Concluding Remarks

The present chapter has presented a model for a cognitive-functioning approach to the treatment of chronic pain patients in group settings. The current approach is different from others that attempt to teach patients to modify their pain. In the current model, the goal is strictly a modification of the person's functioning; patients are explicitly told that nothing will be done to directly reduce their pain. Rather, treatment is designed to modify behaviors and cognitions in such a fashion that the individual develops as satisfying a life-style as possible despite pain. The assessment of cognitions is designed to determine why the person responds as he or she does to his or her pain, and why he or she fails to adopt a more satisfying existence (e.g., "I'll hurt myself more if I try"). The individual is trained to articulate those cognitions that promote disability and those cognitions that interfere with rehabilitation. This represents an alternative to treatments where cognitions that precipitate or exacerbate the pain are assessed in order to develop a program to reduce the individual's pain.

The current model represents an extrapolation from Beck's (Beck *et al.*, 1979) work with depression and anxiety disorders. Our clinical observations have repeatedly indicated that our patients subscribe to a number of dysfunctional beliefs that exacerbate their disability and engender psychological distress. These observations led us to try assisting patients in examining cognitions regarding their pain problem and develop an alternative view that would facilitate their functioning. We believe that the particular appeal of this model is that the method of questioning beliefs, determining the nature of the cognitive distortions, and testing out more adaptive beliefs are skills that are particularly well suited for reducing the emotional distress often associated with chronic pain states.

Chronic pain is a problem that appears to be particularly amenable to group treatment. The modeling effect that occurs as other group members work through their rehabilitation and the social reinforcement provided for treatment gains are powerful intervention methods that would be missing in individual treatment. Moreover, the groups provide settings in which dysfunctional beliefs can be challenged and more adaptive ones generated. For example, many patients had believed that having a pain problem meant that something was wrong with them personally—that no one could understand how they feel (never having met someone else with a chronic pain problem)—or that one cannot be happy, sociable, or productive with a pain problem. Having these beliefs corrected by other pain patients and having the opportunity to observe effective models appear to be highly powerful ways to effect change in the patients' level of functioning.

References

Beck, A. T. & Emery, G. *Cognitive therapy of anxiety and phobic disorders*. Philadelphia: Center for Cognitive Therapy, 1979.

Beck, A. T., Rush, A. J., Shaw, B. F., & Emery, G. *Cognitive therapy of depression*. New York: The Guilford Press, 1979.

Block, A. R. An investigation of the response of the spouse to chronic pain behavior. *Psychosomatic Medicine*, 1981, *43*, 415–422.

Block, A. R., Kremer, E. F., & Gaylor, M. Behavioral treatment of chronic pain: The spouse as a discriminative cue for pain behavior. *Pain*, 1982, *9*, 243–252.

Brena, S. F. Pain control facilities: Roots, organization, and function. In S. F. Brena & S. L. Chapman (Eds.), *Management of patients with chronic pain*. New York: Spectrum, 1983.

Index

Brena, S. F., Chapman, S. L., Stegall, P. G., & Chyatte, S. B. Chronic pain states: Their relationship to impairment and disability. *Archives of Physical Medicine and Rehabilitation*, 1979, *60*, 387–389.

Cailliet, R. Disuse syndrome: Fibrositic and degenerative changes. In S. F. Brena & S. L. Chapman (Eds.), *Management of patients with chronic pain*. New York: Spectrum, 1983.

Catchlove, R., & Cohen, K. Effects of directive return to work approach in the treatment of workman's compensation patients with chronic pain. *Pain*, 1982, *14*, 181–191.

Chapman, S. L. Behavior modification. In S. F. Brena & S. L. Chapman (Eds.), *Management of patients with chronic pain*. New York: Spectrum, 1983.

Fordyce, W. E. *Behavioral methods for chronic pain and illness*. St. Louis: C. V. Mosby, 1976.

Genest, M., & Turk, D. C. A proposed model for behavioral group therapy with pain patients. In D. Upper & S. M. Ross (Eds.), *Behavioral group therapy: An annual review*. Champaign, Ill.: Research Press, 1979.

Gibson, B., Gilson, J., Bergner, M., Bobbitt, R., Kreisel, S., Pollar, W., & Vesselaso, M. The sickness impact profile. Development of an outcome measure of health care. *American Journal of Public Health*, 1975, *65*, 1304–1310.

Goldfried, M. R., & Davidson, G. C. *Clinical behavioral therapy*. New York: Holt, Rinehart & Winston, 1976.

Gottlieb, B. S. *Cognitive therapy approach to chronic pain*. Manuscript submitted for publication, 1984.

Grabois, M. Treatment of pain syndrome through exercise. In D. T. Lowenthal, K. Bharadwaja, & W. W. Oaks (Eds.), *Therapeutics through exercise*. New York: Grune & Stratton, 1979.

Johnson, J. J. Psychological assessment of chronic pain. In S. F. Brena & S. L. Chapman (Eds.), *Management of patients with chronic pain*. New York: Spectrum, 1983.

Keefe, F. J., Block, A. R., Williams, R. B., & Surwit, R. S. Behavioral treatment of chronic low back pain: Clinical outcome and individual differences in pain relief. *Pain*, 1981, *11*, 221–231.

Kulich, R. J., Follick, M. J., Miller, A., & Conger, A. J. *Development of a pain behavior classification system: Importance of multiple data sources*. Paper presented at the annual meeting of the American Pain Society, Chicago, 1983.

Meichenbaum, D. H., & Turk, D. The cognitive-behavioral management of anxiety, anger, and pain. In P. O. Davidson (Ed.), *The behavioral management of anxiety, depression and pain*. New York: Brunner/Mazel, 1976.

Roesch, R., & Ulrich, D. E. Physical therapy management in the treatment of chronic pain. *Physical Therapy*, 1980, *60*, 53–57.

Sanders, S. H. Component analysis of a behavioral treatment program for chronic low back pain. *Behavior Therapy*, 1983, *14*, 697–705.

Shanfield, S. B., Heiman, E. M., Cope, D. N., & Jones, J. R. Pain and the marital relationship: Psychiatric distress. *Pain*, 1979, *7*, 343–351.

Sternbach, R. A. *Pain patients: Traits and treatments*. New York: Academic Press, 1974.

Swanson, D. W., & Maruta, T. The family's viewpoint of chronic pain. *Pain*, 1980, *8*, 163–166.

Tan, S. Y. Cognitive and cognitive-behavioral methods for pain control: A selective review. *Pain*, 1982, *12*, 201–228.

Turner, J. A., & Chapman, C. R. Psychological interventions for chronic pain: A critical review. I. Relaxation training and biofeedback. *Pain*, 1982, *12*, 1–21.

Turner, J. A., & Chapman, C. R. Psychological interventions for chronic pain: A critical review. II. Operant conditioning, hypnosis, and cognitive-behavioral therapy. *Pain*, 1982, *12*, 23–46.

U.S. Department of Health, Education and Welfare. *National Research strategy for neurological and communicative disorders*. Washington, D.C.: National Institute of Neurological and Communicative Disorders and Stroke, 1979.

GPSR Compliance
The European Union's (EU) General Product Safety Regulation (GPSR) is a set of rules that requires consumer products to be safe and our obligations to ensure this.

If you have any concerns about our products, you can contact us on

ProductSafety@springernature.com

In case Publisher is established outside the EU, the EU authorized representative is:

Springer Nature Customer Service Center GmbH
Europaplatz 3
69115 Heidelberg, Germany

www.ingramcontent.com/pod-product-compliance
Ingram Content Group UK Ltd.
Pitfield, Milton Keynes, MK11 3LW, UK
UKHW051451290926
15471UKWH00008B/1134

* 9 7 8 1 4 6 8 4 4 9 5 9 4 *